UPDATE ON MECHANISMS OF HORMONE ACTION – FOCUS ON METABOLISM, GROWTH AND REPRODUCTIONS

Edited by **Gianluca Aimaretti**
Co-Editors: **Paolo Marzullo** and **Flavia Prodam**

Update on Mechanisms of Hormone Action – Focus on Metabolism, Growth and Reproductions
Edited by Gianluca Aimaretti with Paolo Marzullo and Flavia Prodam

Published by InTech

Janeza Trdine 9, 51000 Rijeka, Croatia

Publishing Process Manager Petra Nenadic

Technical Editor Teodora Smiljanic

Cover Designer InTech Design Team

Additional hard copies can be obtained from orders@intechopen.com

Update on Mechanisms of Hormone Action – Focus on Metabolism, Growth and Reproductions, Edited by Gianluca Aimaretti with Paolo Marzullo and Flavia Prodam
p. cm.
ISBN 978-953-307-341-5

For EU product safety concerns:
IN TECH d.o.o., Prolaz Marije Krucifikse Kozulić 3, 51000 Rijeka, Croatia,
info@intechopen.com or visit our website at intechopen.com.

Meet the editors

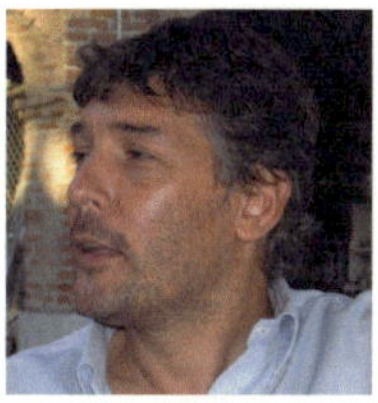

Gianluca Aimaretti has been professor of Endocrinology at the University of Piemonte Orientale, Novara, Italy, since 2006. He was graduated in Medicine from the University of Turin in 1992 and gained his post-graduate qualification in Endocrinology and Metabolism from the University of Turin in 1998. In 2004, he was awarded as PhD in Endocrinology and Metabolism from the University of Milan.His research interests are the control of growth hormone secretion throughout the human life span, the diagnosis of growth hormone deficiency in children and adults, endocrine alterations in central nervous system diseases, growth hormone-releasing peptides (GHRPs) and thyroid tumors. He has written more than 120 original articles that have been published in international journals and 38 book chapters or letters to the editor. He has been an invited speaker at more than 120 national and international meetings.

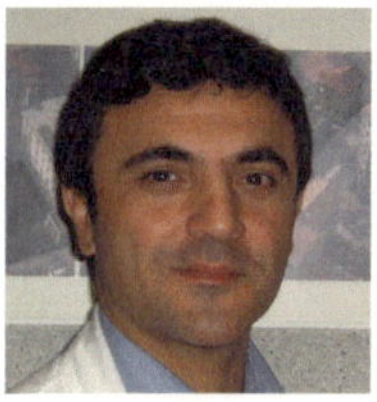

Dr. Paolo Marzullo graduated in 1993 from the School of Medicine of the University of Naples "Federico II", became Specialist in Endocrinology in 1999 and achieved his Ph.D. in 2004. At the time, he partook in clinical research activity on pituitary diseases, mainly GH disorders. In 1999-2001, he attended as postdoc Dr. Rosenfeld's lab at the OHSU in Portland, Oregon. Since 2001, Dr. Marzullo is Consultant in the Division of General Medicine of Istituto Auxologico Italiano, Piancavallo. From 2008, he is Lecturer of Endocrinology at the University of Eastern Piedmont "A. Avogadro", Novara, Italy. His research is mostly focused on endocrine aspects of extreme obesity.

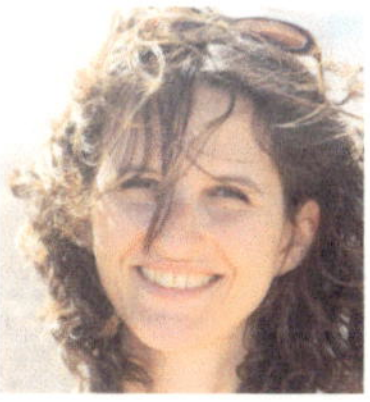

Dr. Flavia Prodam has been Assistant Professor of Pediatrics at the University of Piemonte Orientale, Italy, since 2011. She was graduated in Medicine from the University of Turin in 2001 and gained her post-graduate qualification in Endocrinology and Metabolism in 2006. In 2010, he was awarded as PhD from the University of Piemonte Orientale.Her research interests are: ghrelin, obesity, GH, genetics in hypopituitarism and short stature. She has written more than 47 original articles and 46 book chapters or reviews. She acts as referee for several international journals, and is an associate faculty member of F1000.

Contents

Preface

The purpose of the present volume is to focus on more recent aspects of the complex regulation of hormonal action, in particular in 3 different hot fields: metabolism, growth and reproduction.

Modern approaches to the physiology and pathology of endocrine glands are based on cellular and molecular investigation of genes, peptide, hormones, protein cascade at different levels. In all of the chapters in the book all, or at least some, of these aspects are described in order to increase the endocrine knowledge.

In the first section, the chapters are focused on gastrointestinal hormones and their interactions with food intake and energy expenditure, adipose tissue function and metabolism, regulation of glucose metabolism and their clinical alterations in human and animal models.

The second section on growth and reproduction show new advances in these field with specific focus on pediatric endocrinology, with contributions on reproduction and pubertal development.

The third section is on gynecological endocrinology, related in particular on common clinical problem.

We are grateful to all contributors to this volume for sharing their in-depth insight and wisdom. These will undoubtedly make it as a successful reference for all the readers interested in endocrinology: physiology, patho-physiology, comparative and clinical aspects.

We hope that the reader of this book will be inspired by the scientific contributions from the forefront of research to further their own scientific and clinical achievements for the ultimate purpose of benefiting in their scientific work, inducing new creative ideas that will stem from reading it.

Novara, 2011

Editor: **Gianluca Aimaretti**
Co-Editors: **Paolo Marzullo** and **Flavia Prodam**
University "A. Avogadro" of the Eastern Piedmont, Novara, Italy

Part 1

Metabolism

1

The Gut Peptide Hormone Family, Motilin and Ghrelin

Ichiro Sakata and Takafumi Sakai
Saitama University
Japan

1. Introduction

Endocrine hormones are a system of glands, each of which secretes a type of hormone into the bloodstream to regulate multiple physiology of the body. In the past several decades, many hormones from the gastrointestinal tract has been identified and cloned, and their physiological functions have been studied. Although the pituitary gland was considered to be the main endocrine organ of the body in early studies, there are other organs that produce endocrine hormones such as adipose tissue, reproductive organ, adrenal gland, and gastrointestinal tract. Among those, the gastrointestinal tract is the largest endocrine organ of the body in volume, and hormones produced in the gastrointestinal tract are physiologically important for their roles in development, growth, cardiovascular, gastric motility, behavior and maintenance of energy homeostasis. Many hormones have been identified in each different parts of the gastrointestinal tract. For instance, in the stomach, gastrin, histamine (Dornonville de la Cour, et al. 2001), somatostatin (Bolkent, et al. 2001), neuropeptide Y (Wang, et al. 1987), ghrelin (Sakata, et al. 2002) and leptin (Bado, et al. 1998) are produced in the mucosal layer and/or myentric plexus, and cholecystokinin (CCK) (Miyamoto and Miyamoto 2004), glucagon-like peptide-1 (Theodorakis, et al. 2006), motilin (Sakai, et al. 1994a) (Satoh, et al. 1995), serotonin (Ku, et al. 2004) and $PYY_{3\text{-}36}$ (Rozengurt, et al. 2006) are produced in the upper and lower intestine. Motilin and ghrelin are considered to comprise a peptide family based on similarity of their structures and also their similarity in each specific G protein coupled receptor, growth hormone secretagogue receptor (GHS-R) and motilin receptor (MTL-R, also known as GPR38). In this chapter, we review recent research and knowledge of the peptides, motilin and ghrelin regarding their structures, distribution of motilin- and ghrelin-producing cells, distribution of their receptors, plasma profies and secretion of motilin and ghrelin, and the role of motilin and ghrelin in gastric motility. However, there is a lack of basic information for motilin study such as information on the detailed distribution of motilin and motilin receptor in the body and changes in motilin release under some physiological states. One of the reasons for the difficulty in motilin study is that rodents such as rats and mice cannot be used for motilin study because the motilin gene is inactivated in the common ancestor of mice and rats (He, et al. 2010). For this reason, motilin has been studied using relatively large- sized animals, such as dogs and rabbits, which has made it difficult to investigate in detail the mechanisms underlying the actions of motilin. Recently, we characterized the *house musk shrew* (Suncus murinus, order: Insectivora, suncus named as laboratory strain) as a motilin- and ghrelin-producing small animal model for studies on gastric motility, and we therefore also provide some information on suncus motilin and ghrelin.

2. Structures of motilin and ghrelin

Motilin was initially isolated from a side fraction produced during the purification of secretin by Brown et al. in 1971 (Brown, et al. 1971), and the complete amino acid sequence of motilin was determined in 1973 (Brown, et al. 1973). Mature motilin is a 22-amino-acid polypeptide with a molecular weight of 2698, and motilin has been isolated from humans (Strausberg, et al. 2002), pigs (Khan, et al. 1990) (Bond, et al. 1988), dogs (Ohshiro, et al. 2008), cats (Xu, et al. 2003), guinea pigs (Xu, et al. 2001), rabbits (Banfield, et al. 1992), and chickens (De Clercq, et al. 1996). We recently identified and cloned suncus motilin as a useful small animal model, and the mature region of suncus motilin is highly conserved between these species (Tsutsui, et al. 2009). The precursor of motilin consists of 133 amino acids and includes a 25-amino-acid signal peptide followed by a 22-amino-acid motilin sequence and a motilin-associated peptide (MAP) (Banfield et al. 1992). The amino acid sequence of MAP is also conserved between species, but the functional and physiological roles of MAP have not been elucidated.

Ghrelin was identified from rat and human stomach extracts by Kojima et al. in 1999 using a "reverse pharmacology" strategy (Kojima, et al. 1999). In mice, rats and humans, ghrelin is a 28-amino-acids polypeptide and, interestingly, ghrelin has an acyl modification at the third serine by *n*-octanoate, one of the medium chain fatty acids (Kojima et al. 1999). Ghrelin exists as two different molecular forms, acyl ghrelin (modified form) and des-acyl ghrelin (unmodified form), in both gastric ghrelin-producing cells and circulation (Ariyasu, et al. 2001; Fujimiya, et al.). Ghrelin has been identified in many species, including mammlas, avians (Kaiya, et al. 2002; Wada, et al. 2003), amphibians (Kaiya, et al. 2001; Kaiya, et al. 2006), reptilian (Kaiya, et al. 2004), and fish (Kaiya, et al. 2009; Kaiya, et al. 2003; Miura, et al. 2009), and the sequence of first seven amino acids of the N-terminal region of ghrelin are highly conserved between species (Kojima, et al. 2008). In addition, it has been reported that the first four or five amino acids are sufficient for calcium mobilization *in vitro* (Bednarek, et al. 2000).

3. Distributions of motilin- and ghrelin-producing cells

The distribution of motilin-producing cells in the gastrointestinal tract has been studied by using immunohistochemistry and *in situ* hybridization techniques. Since motilin is genetically knockdown in rats and mice, the distribution and morphology of motilin-producing cells were investigated using rabbits (Satoh et al. 1995), monkeys, and humans (Helmstaedter, et al. 1979). In rabbits, motilin-immunopositive cells were found in the epithelia of the crypts and villi throughout the gastrointestinal tract from the gastric antrum to the distal colon, but no immunostaining was observed in the gastric body (Satoh et al. 1995), and motilin-producing cells were localized abundantly in the upper small intestine. Cell densities (cells/mm^2, mean ± SE) were 0.41 ± 0.16 in the gastric antrum, 8.2 ± 0.8 in the duodenum, 1.9 ±0.5 in the jejunum, 0.62 ± 0.14 in the ileum, 0.19 ± 0.05 in the cecum, 0.13 ± 0.03 in the proximal colon, and 0.39 ± 0.18 in the distal colon (Satoh et al. 1995). Immunoelectron microscopic observations revealed that the motilin-producing cell is characterized by relatively small (180 nm in man; 200 nm in the dog) solid granules with a homogeneous core and closely applied membrane, round in man and round to irregularly-shaped in the dog. Recently, we succeeded in identification of suncus motilin cDNA and amino acid sequence (Tsutsui et al. 2009), and immunohistochemical analysis was performed in all regions of the gastrointestinal tract and also *in situ* hybridization analysis was performed to detect motilin mRNA-expressing cells. Motilin-immunopositive and expressing cells in suncus were observed in the mucosal layer but not in the myenteric plexus and were abundantly distributed in the upper intestine. However, the density of motilin mRNA-expressing cells was slightly higher than that of motilin-immunopositive cells, suggesting low accumulation of motilin in the cytoplasm. In addition, motilin-producing cells in suncus were closed- and opened-type cells as previously reported in other mammals.

Gastric ghrelin cells had been classified as X/A-like cells by their round, compact, electron-dense secretory granules that distinguish them electron-microscopically from other previously characterized gastric endocrine cell types before the discovery of ghrelin (Dornonville de la Cour et al. 2001) (Date, et al. 2000). The distribution of ghrelin-producing cells in the gastrointestinal tract has been studied in many species. Ghrelin-producing cells were most dense in the gastric body and were found in the mucosal layer but not in the myenteric plexus in all of the examined regions of rats (Sakata et al. 2002). In the stomach, most of the ghrelin cells were observed in the glandular base to body of the fundic gland, and a few ghrelin cells were observed in the glandular neck. In rodents, in addition to the stomach, ghrelin-producing cells were observed in all regions of the gastrointestinal tract, including the duodenum, ileum, cecum and colon (Sakata et al. 2002). In the duodenum, ileum, cecum and colon, ghrelin cells were scattered in the epithelia of crypts and villi, and the densities of ghrelin cells were dramatically decreased toward the lower gastrointestinal tract. In the stomach, ghrelin-producing cells were observed as small and round-shaped cells (called closed-type cells). On the other hand, in the duodenum, ileum, cecum and colon, ghrelin cells were found as two different types of endocrine cells, closed-type cells with triangular or elongated shapes and opened-type cells with their apical cytoplasmic process in contact with the lumen. In suncus, ghrelin-producing cells were abundant in the stomach and most of the ghrelin cells were closed-type cells with relatively rich cytoplasm and scattered in the glandular body and base of the gastric mucosa (Ishida, et al. 2009). Using electron microscopic observation, immunogold labeling for ghrelin has been shown to be localized on round and electron-dense granules in gastric mucosal cells. The diameters of granules containing ghrelin in mice (277.7 ± 11.1 nm) and rats (268.8 ± 13.0 nm) were similar; however, those in hamsters (200.8 ± 8.8 nm) were significantly smaller than those in mice or rats. Rindi et al. demonstrated that mouse and canine ghrelin-immunoreactive cells closely resembled those of the human stomach, though it has been shown that dog ghrelin cells have obviously larger granules (273 ± 49 nm) than those of rats (183 ± 37 nm) and humans (147 ± 30 nm).

Co-localization of motilin and ghrelin was examined in the human biopsy and tissues from pig by immunohistochemistry and *in situ* hybridization in a study by Wierup et al. (Wierup, et al. 2007). They showed that ghrelin and motilin are coproduced in the same cells in the duodenum and jejunum of humans and pigs and that ghrelin and motilin are stored in all secretory granules of such cells in humans, suggesting that motilin and ghrelin are co-secreted by the same stimulus (Wierup et al. 2007). As mentioned above, suncus is a small laboratory animal that produces both motilin and ghrelin, and further studies are therefore needed to examine the co-localization of motilin and ghrelin in the duodenum and lower intestine of suncus.

4. Distributions of motilin and ghrelin receptors

The receptor for motilin was identified from the human gastrointestinal tract by Feighner et al. in 1999 (Feighner, et al. 1999) and it is now called GPR38 or motilin receptor. Growth hormone secretagogue receptor (GHS-R) was initially identified from the pituitary gland and brain in 1996 (Howard, et al. 1996), and GHS-R had been known as the orphan receptor until ghrelin was discovered. In the process of exploring the natural ligand for the GHS-R using reverse pharmacology, ghrelin was discovered as an endogenous ligand for GHS-R. Both motilin and ghrelin receptors belong to the seven transmembrane G protein-coupled receptor family (McKee, et al. 1997), and these receptors showed high sequence homology of 52 % to each other in humans (Takeshita, et al. 2006). The tissue distribution of motilin and ghrelin receptors has been mainly examined using binding assays or mRNA analysis with RT-PCR. Motilin binding sites were found on smooth muscle layers of the gastric antrum, duodenum and colon, but no positive binding reaction was detected in the smooth muscle layer of the cecum (Sakai, et al. 1994b). Specific binding sites were particularly abundant in the circular muscle layers, with low concentrations in longitudinal muscle layers of the gastric antrum, duodenum and colon, and no motilin binding sites were found in the mucosa of the gastrointestinal tract and pancreas (Sakai et al. 1994b). mRNA analysis showed that motilin receptor was expressed in the gastrointestinal tract in humans (Takeshita et al. 2006; Ter Beek, et al. 2008), dogs (Ohshiro et al. 2008), guinea pigs (Xu, et al. 2005) and chickens (Yamamoto, et al. 2008). It has also been shown that motilin receptor immunoreactivity was present in muscle cells and the myenteric plexus, but not in mucosal or submucosal cells in humans (Takeshita et al. 2006). In dogs, motilin receptor immunoreactivity was observed among muscle fibers on both the longitudinal and circular muscle layers (Ohshiro et al. 2008). In the guinea pig stomach, motilin receptor immunoreactivity was also found in the myenteric plexus, consistent with findings in humans and dogs (Xu et al. 2005). In addition to gastrointestinal tract, Depoortere et al. reported that specific binding sites for the motilin receptor were observed in the hippocampus, thalamus, hypothalamus and amygdaloid body in the central nervous system (Depoortere, et al. 1997).

On the other hand, distribution of the ghrelin receptor (GHS-R) has been studied in detail in several species, and it has been shown that the ghrelin receptor is expressed widely in the body from the central nervous system to peripheral organs. In rodents, expression of ghrelin receptor mRNA was observed in the various of regions of the brain, with high expression levels in Arcuate nucleus (Arc), Ventromedial nucleus, Ventral tegmental area (VTA), hippocampus and the nucleus of solitary tract (NTS) (Zigman, et al. 2006) (Mondal, et al. 2005) (Guan, et al. 1997). In addition, high expression levels of GHS-R were found in the pituitary gland (Kamegai, et al. 2001) (Gnanapavan, et al. 2002) and pancreas (Kageyama, et al. 2005) (Volante, et al. 2002). In the gastrointestinal tract, ghrelin receptor mRNA expression was also found throughout the stomach and intestines, and expression of the ghrelin receptor was detected in the muscle layer but not in the mucosal layer in the stomach (Date et al. 2000). Moreover, it has been reported that ghrelin receptor immunoreactivity was found within neuronal cell bodies and fibers in rats (Dass, et al. 2003) and that ghrelin receptor mRNA transcripts were found in longitudinal muscle/myenteric plexus preparations and in cultured myenteric neurons of the guinea pig (Xu et al. 2005)

5. Roles of motilin and ghrelin in gastric motility

According to the origin of its name, the main function of motilin is to stimulate gastric motility. Migrating motor complex (MMC) is characterized by the appearance of gastrointestinal motility in the interdigestive state. It has been reported that these coordinated contractions consist of three phases, phase I (period of motor quiescence), phase II (period of preceding irregular contractions) and phase III (period of clustered potent contractions). It has been shown that plasma concentration of motilin changed in a cyclic fashion and that it has rhythmus occurring every 90-100 min. In fact, administration of motilin has been shown to induce phase III-like contraction via the cholinergic pathway, and endogenous motilin is thought to be physiologically important for phase III contraction (Vantrappen, et al. 1979) (Itoh, et al. 1978).

Since the ghrelin receptor is expressed in the gastrointestinal tract, the effect of ghrelin on gastric motility has also been examined. In rats, ghrelin exerts stimulatory effects on motility of the antrum and duodenum in both fed and fasted states (Fujimiya, et al. 2008), and Taniguchi et al. reported that ghrelin infusion significantly increased motility index of phase III-like contractions at the antrum and jejunum in a dose dependent manner (Taniguchi, et al. 2008). As well as the rat stomach, phase III-like contractions in mice were observed in the interdigestive state, and no spontaneous phase III-like contractions were found in vagotomized mice, suggesting that ghrelin-induced gastric phase III-like contractions are mediated via vagal cholinergic pathways in mice (Zheng, et al. 2009). In humans, administration of ghrelin induced a premature gastric phase III of the MMC, which was not mediated through release of motilin (Tack, et al. 2006).

As a new model to study gastric motility, we established an *in vitro* and *in vivo* functional assay system using suncus. Administration of suncus motilin showed almost the same contractile effect as that of human motilin *in vitro* (Tsutsui et al. 2009). During the fasted state, the suncus stomach and duodenum showed clear migrating phase III contractions (intervals of 80-150 min) as found in humans and dogs, and motilin injection also increased the gastric motility index in a dose-dependent manner (Sakahara, et al. 2010). Moreover, pretreatment with atropine completely abolished the motilin-induced gastric phase III contractions (Sakahara et al. 2010). Since suncus has almost the same GI motility and motilin response as those found in humans and dogs, suncus would be a suitable model to analyze the interaction of motilin and ghrelin in gastric motility.

6. Plasma profiles and secretion of motilin and ghrelin in the gastrointestinal tract

Motilin is mainly produced in the duodenum and secreted into the blood stream. During the interdigestive state, it was found that plasma motilin concentration increased in complete accordance with the cyclical interdigestive contractions of the stomach in dogs (Itoh et al. 1978). Furthermore, plasma motilin concentration was lowered by ingestion of food, and it remained low as long as the gastric motor activity was in the digestive pattern (Itoh et al. 1978). It has been demonstrated that plasma motilin is released at about 100-min intervals in the interdigestive state in humans (Vantrappen et al. 1979) and dogs (Itoh et al. 1978). Zietlow et al. also reported that the peak of plasma motilin levels was always observed in the period of gastric phase III contractions (Zietlow, et al. 2010).

Inverse correlations were found between plasma motilin concentration and glucose and between motilin concentration and insulin, suggesting that glucose and/or insulin are important in suppressing motilin secretion during feeding (Funakoshi, et al. 1985). Dopamine infusion caused a significant decline of plasma motilin levels, and dopamine antagonism with domperidone caused a significant elevation of motilin (Funakoshi, et al.

1983). Atropine suppressed the basal levels of motilin but did not alter the increment of motilin levels after domperidone administration, suggesting that dopaminergic mechanisms exert a tonic inhibitory effect on motilin secretion in normal subjects (Funakoshi et al. 1983). Using an enzymatic method, dispersed cells from the canine duodenojejunal mucosa were separated by centrifugal counterflow elutriation to enrich motilin content, and carbachol dose-dependently stimulated the release of motilin from its enriched cells (Poitras, et al. 1993). Moreover, bombesin, morphine, and erythromycin stimulated motilin release *in vivo*, but did not influence the secretion of motilin *in vitro* (Poitras et al. 1993). Serotonin, GIP, CCK, pentagastrin, cisapride, neosynephrine, isoproterenol, and muscimol also had no effect on motilin release in an *in vitro* model (Poitras et al. 1993). The response to carbachol was abolished by atropine but was not affected by somatostatin, serotonin, secretin, CCK, or GIP (Poitras et al. 1993). These results suggest that muscarinic receptors are present on the motilin cell membrane and that acetylcholine is a major regulator of motilin release.

It is well known that the stomach is a major source of circulation plasma ghrelin, and the levels were elevated in a fasting state and returned to basal levels after re-feeding (Cummings, et al. 2001; Cummings, et al. 2002). In contrast, peptide content of ghrelin in the stomach decreased after fasting, indicating that cytoplasmic ghrelin released from gastric ghrelin cells caused an increase in plasma ghrelin levels (Toshinai, et al. 2001). The effects of nutrients on ghrelin release have been studied in detail. Oral and intravenous glucose administration sharply reduced plasma ghrelin concentration in rodents, and this effect of glucose on ghrelin inhibition was similar to that found in humans (Broglio, et al. 2004; Soriano-Guillen, et al. 2004). In addition to glucose, it has been reported that duodenal and jejunal infusions of lipids reduced ghrelin levels in rats and that infusion of amino acids also induced ghrelin suppression in rats (Overduin, et al. 2005). Although further studies are needed to elucidate the molecular mechanisms of ghrelin secretion from the stomach by nutrients, nutrients may be directly involved in the rapid decline of plasma ghrelin concentration after feeding.

Ghrelin secretion is regulated by peptide and steroid hormones. For example, ghrelin cells are located close to somatostatin-producing D cells, and somatostatin inhibits ghrelin secretion in rats and humans (Broglio, et al. 2002; Shimada, et al. 2003). Ghrelin secretion from the perfused stomach was also stimulated by glucagon treatment in a dose-dependent manner (Kamegai, et al. 2004), and this effect was shown to be mediated by glucagon receptors on ghrelin cells (Katayama, et al. 2007). de la Cour et al. found that epinephrine, norepinephrine, endothelin and secretin stimulated ghrelin release (de la Cour, et al. 2007). In addition, steroid hormone is involved in ghrelin regulation. In humans, estrogen regulates plasma ghrelin concentration (Paulo, et al. 2008) (Kellokoski, et al. 2005). In female rats, the levels of gastric ghrelin mRNA and plasma ghrelin and the number of ghrelin cells were found to be transiently increased by ovariectomy (Matsubara, et al. 2004), and treatment of gastric mucosal cells with estrogen showed that estrogen stimulated ghrelin expression and ghrelin secretion (Sakata, et al. 2006) (Zhao, et al. 2008). Recently, ghrelin-producing cell lines have been generated by different two groups. Iwakura et al. generated ghrelin cell lines from the stomach and showed that insulin decreased ghrelin secretion into culture medium (Iwakura, et al. 2010). Zhao et al. also established different ghrelin cell lines from the stomach and pancreas, and they showed that adrenaline and noradrenaline stimulated ghrelin secretion and that ghrelin-secreting cells express high levels of mRNA encoding beta(1)-adrenergic receptors (Zhao, et al. 2010). Moreover, they reported that fasting-induced increase in plasma ghrelin was blocked by treatment with reserpine to deplete adrenergic neurotransmitters from sympathetic neurons and that inhibition was also seen following administration of atenolol, a selective beta1-adrenergic antagonist, suggesting that sympathetic neurons are involved in ghrelin secretion by directly acting on beta1 receptors (Zhao et al. 2010).

7. Conclusion and future perspectives

Although ghrelin was discovered more than twenty years after motilin was identified, the biological and physiological functions of ghrelin have been studied in more detail than those of motilin. The major reason for this is due to the lack of a motilin gene in experimental rodents like mice and rats, which are used for biological and physiological analysis. So far, dogs and/or rabbits have been used for motilin studies, but these animals are too large to perform detailed analysis. Research has also been limited by the ban on use of genetically engineered mice. To resolve this problem and expand studies on motilin and its relationship with ghrelin, we established suncus as a novel motilin- and ghrelin-producing laboratory animal for motilin study. It has been shown that suncus motilin exerted phase III contraction in MMC using *in vivo* and *in vitro* experiments. This new suncus model will enable the detailed molecular and physiological analysis that were difficult using dogs and rabbits, and suncus will therefore be a powerful tool to understand the detailed mechanisms of motilin- and/or ghrelin-induced gastrointestinal motility.

8. References

Ariyasu H, Takaya K, Tagami T, Ogawa Y, Hosoda K, Akamizu T, Suda M, Koh T, Natsui K, Toyooka S, et al. 2001 Stomach is a major source of circulating ghrelin, and feeding state determines plasma ghrelin-like immunoreactivity levels in humans. *J Clin Endocrinol Metab* 86 4753-4758.

Bado A, Levasseur S, Attoub S, Kermorgant S, Laigneau JP, Bortoluzzi MN, Moizo L, Lehy T, Guerre-Millo M, Le Marchand-Brustel Y, et al. 1998 The stomach is a source of leptin. *Nature* 394 790-793.

Banfield DK, MacGillivray RT, Brown JC & McIntosh CH 1992 The isolation and characterization of rabbit motilin precursor cDNA. *Biochim Biophys Acta* 1131 341-344.

Bednarek MA, Feighner SD, Pong SS, McKee KK, Hreniuk DL, Silva MV, Warren VA, Howard AD, Van Der Ploeg LH & Heck JV 2000 Structure-function studies on the new growth hormone-releasing peptide, ghrelin: minimal sequence of ghrelin necessary for activation of growth hormone secretagogue receptor 1a. *J Med Chem* 43 4370-4376.

Bolkent S, Yilmazer S, Kaya F & Ozturk M 2001 Effects of acid inhibition on somatostatin-producing cells in the rat gastric fundus. *Acta Histochem* 103 413-422.

Bond CT, Nilaver G, Godfrey B, Zimmerman EA & Adelman JP 1988 Characterization of complementary deoxyribonucleic acid for precursor of porcine motilin. *Mol Endocrinol* 2 175-180.

Broglio F, Gottero C, Prodam F, Destefanis S, Gauna C, Me E, Riganti F, Vivenza D, Rapa A, Martina V, et al. 2004 Ghrelin secretion is inhibited by glucose load and insulin-induced hypoglycaemia but unaffected by glucagon and arginine in humans. *Clin Endocrinol (Oxf)* 61 503-509.

Broglio F, Koetsveld Pv P, Benso A, Gottero C, Prodam F, Papotti M, Muccioli G, Gauna C, Hofland L, Deghenghi R, et al. 2002 Ghrelin secretion is inhibited by either somatostatin or cortistatin in humans. *J Clin Endocrinol Metab* 87 4829-4832.

Brown JC, Cook MA & Dryburgh JR 1973 Motilin, a gastric motor activity stimulating polypeptide: the complete amino acid sequence. *Can J Biochem* 51 533-537.

Brown JC, Mutt V & Dryburgh JR 1971 The further purification of motilin, a gastric motor activity stimulating polypeptide from the mucosa of the small intestine of hogs. *Can J Physiol Pharmacol* 49 399-405.

Cummings DE, Purnell JQ, Frayo RS, Schmidova K, Wisse BE & Weigle DS 2001 A preprandial rise in plasma ghrelin levels suggests a role in meal initiation in humans. *Diabetes* 50 1714-1719.

Cummings DE, Weigle DS, Frayo RS, Breen PA, Ma MK, Dellinger EP & Purnell JQ 2002 Plasma ghrelin levels after diet-induced weight loss or gastric bypass surgery. *N Engl J Med* 346 1623-1630.

Dass NB, Munonyara M, Bassil AK, Hervieu GJ, Osbourne S, Corcoran S, Morgan M & Sanger GJ 2003 Growth hormone secretagogue receptors in rat and human gastrointestinal tract and the effects of ghrelin. *Neuroscience* 120 443-453.

Date Y, Kojima M, Hosoda H, Sawaguchi A, Mondal MS, Suganuma T, Matsukura S, Kangawa K & Nakazato M 2000 Ghrelin, a novel growth hormone-releasing acylated peptide, is synthesized in a distinct endocrine cell type in the gastrointestinal tracts of rats and humans. *Endocrinology* 141 4255-4261.

De Clercq P, Depoortere I, Macielag M, Vandermeers A, Vandermeers-Piret MC & Peeters TL 1996 Isolation, sequence, and bioactivity of chicken motilin. *Peptides* 17 203-208.

de la Cour CD, Norlen P & Hakanson R 2007 Secretion of ghrelin from rat stomach ghrelin cells in response to local microinfusion of candidate messenger compounds: a microdialysis study. *Regul Pept* 143 118-126.

Depoortere I, Van Assche G & Peeters TL 1997 Distribution and subcellular localization of motilin binding sites in the rabbit brain. *Brain Res* 777 103-109.

Dornonville de la Cour C, Bjorkqvist M, Sandvik AK, Bakke I, Zhao CM, Chen D & Hakanson R 2001 A-like cells in the rat stomach contain ghrelin and do not operate under gastrin control. *Regul Pept* 99 141-150.

Feighner SD, Tan CP, McKee KK, Palyha OC, Hreniuk DL, Pong SS, Austin CP, Figueroa D, MacNeil D, Cascieri MA, et al. 1999 Receptor for motilin identified in the human gastrointestinal system. *Science* 284 2184-2188.

Fujimiya M, Asakawa A, Ataka K, Chen CY, Kato I & Inui A Ghrelin, des-acyl ghrelin, and obestatin: regulatory roles on the gastrointestinal motility. *Int J Pept* 2010.

Fujimiya M, Asakawa A, Ataka K, Kato I & Inui A 2008 Different effects of ghrelin, des-acyl ghrelin and obestatin on gastroduodenal motility in conscious rats. *World J Gastroenterol* 14 6318-6326.

Funakoshi A, Ho LL, Jen KL, Knopf R & Vinik AI 1985 Diurnal profile of plasma motilin concentrations during fasting and feeding in man. *Gastroenterol Jpn* 20 446-456.

Funakoshi A, Matsumoto M, Sekiya K, Nakano I, Shinozaki H & Ibayashi H 1983 Cholinergic independent dopaminergic regulation of motilin release in man. *Gastroenterol Jpn* 18 525-529.

Gnanapavan S, Kola B, Bustin SA, Morris DG, McGee P, Fairclough P, Bhattacharya S, Carpenter R, Grossman AB & Korbonits M 2002 The tissue distribution of the mRNA of ghrelin and subtypes of its receptor, GHS-R, in humans. *J Clin Endocrinol Metab* 87 2988.

Guan XM, Yu H, Palyha OC, McKee KK, Feighner SD, Sirinathsinghji DJ, Smith RG, Van der Ploeg LH & Howard AD 1997 Distribution of mRNA encoding the growth hormone secretagogue receptor in brain and peripheral tissues. *Brain Res Mol Brain Res* 48 23-29.

He J, Irwin DM, Chen R & Zhang YP 2010 Stepwise loss of motilin and its specific receptor genes in rodents. *J Mol Endocrinol* 44 37-44.

Helmstaedter V, Kreppein W, Domschke W, Mitznegg P, Yanaihara N, Wunsch E & Forssmann WG 1979 Immunohistochemical localization of motilin in endocrine non-enterochromaffin cells of the small intestine of humans and monkey. *Gastroenterology* 76 897-902.

Howard AD, Feighner SD, Cully DF, Arena JP, Liberator PA, Rosenblum CI, Hamelin M, Hreniuk DL, Palyha OC, Anderson J, et al. 1996 A receptor in pituitary and hypothalamus that functions in growth hormone release. *Science* 273 974-977.

Ishida Y, Sakahara S, Tsutsui C, Kaiya H, Sakata I, Oda S & Sakai T 2009 Identification of ghrelin in the house musk shrew (Suncus murinus): cDNA cloning, peptide purification and tissue distribution. *Peptides* 30 982-990.

Itoh Z, Takeuchi S, Aizawa I, Mori K, Taminato T, Seino Y, Imura H & Yanaihara N 1978 Changes in plasma motilin concentration and gastrointestinal contractile activity in conscious dogs. *Am J Dig Dis* 23 929-935.

Iwakura H, Li Y, Ariyasu H, Hosoda H, Kanamoto N, Bando M, Yamada G, Hosoda K, Nakao K, Kangawa K, et al. 2010 Establishment of a novel ghrelin-producing cell line. *Endocrinology* 151 2940-2945.

Kageyama H, Funahashi H, Hirayama M, Takenoya F, Kita T, Kato S, Sakurai J, Lee EY, Inoue S, Date Y, et al. 2005 Morphological analysis of ghrelin and its receptor distribution in the rat pancreas. *Regul Pept* 126 67-71.

Kaiya H, Kodama S, Ishiguro K, Matsuda K, Uchiyama M, Miyazato M & Kangawa K 2009 Ghrelin-like peptide with fatty acid modification and O-glycosylation in the red stingray, Dasyatis akajei. *BMC Biochem* 10 30.

Kaiya H, Kojima M, Hosoda H, Koda A, Yamamoto K, Kitajima Y, Matsumoto M, Minamitake Y, Kikuyama S & Kangawa K 2001 Bullfrog ghrelin is modified by n-octanoic acid at its third threonine residue. *J Biol Chem* 276 40441-40448.

Kaiya H, Kojima M, Hosoda H, Moriyama S, Takahashi A, Kawauchi H & Kangawa K 2003 Peptide purification, complementary deoxyribonucleic acid (DNA) and genomic DNA cloning, and functional characterization of ghrelin in rainbow trout. *Endocrinology* 144 5215-5226.

Kaiya H, Sakata I, Kojima M, Hosoda H, Sakai T & Kangawa K 2004 Structural determination and histochemical localization of ghrelin in the red-eared slider turtle, Trachemys scripta elegans. *Gen Comp Endocrinol* 138 50-57.

Kaiya H, Sakata I, Yamamoto K, Koda A, Sakai T, Kangawa K & Kikuyama S 2006 Identification of immunoreactive plasma and stomach ghrelin, and expression of stomach ghrelin mRNA in the bullfrog, Rana catesbeiana. *Gen Comp Endocrinol* 148 236-244.

Kaiya H, Van Der Geyten S, Kojima M, Hosoda H, Kitajima Y, Matsumoto M, Geelissen S, Darras VM & Kangawa K 2002 Chicken ghrelin: purification, cDNA cloning, and biological activity. *Endocrinology* 143 3454-3463.

Kamegai J, Tamura H, Shimizu T, Ishii S, Sugihara H & Oikawa S 2001 Regulation of the ghrelin gene: growth hormone-releasing hormone upregulates ghrelin mRNA in the pituitary. *Endocrinology* 142 4154-4157.

Kamegai J, Tamura H, Shimizu T, Ishii S, Sugihara H & Oikawa S 2004 Effects of insulin, leptin, and glucagon on ghrelin secretion from isolated perfused rat stomach. *Regul Pept* 119 77-81.

Katayama T, Shimamoto S, Oda H, Nakahara K, Kangawa K & Murakami N 2007 Glucagon receptor expression and glucagon stimulation of ghrelin secretion in rat stomach. *Biochem Biophys Res Commun* 357 865-870.

Kellokoski E, Poykko SM, Karjalainen AH, Ukkola O, Heikkinen J, Kesaniemi YA & Horkko S 2005 Estrogen replacement therapy increases plasma ghrelin levels. *J Clin Endocrinol Metab* 90 2954-2963.

Khan N, Graslund A, Ehrenberg A & Shriver J 1990 Sequence-specific 1H NMR assignments and secondary structure of porcine motilin. *Biochemistry* 29 5743-5751.

Kojima M, Hosoda H, Date Y, Nakazato M, Matsuo H & Kangawa K 1999 Ghrelin is a growth-hormone-releasing acylated peptide from stomach. *Nature* 402 656-660.

Kojima M, Ida T & Sato T 2008 Structure of mammalian and nonmammalian ghrelins. *Vitam Horm* 77 31-46.

Ku SK, Lee HS & Lee JH 2004 An immunohistochemical study of gastrointestinal endocrine cells in the BALB/c mouse. *Anat Histol Embryol* 33 42-48.

Matsubara M, Sakata I, Wada R, Yamazaki M, Inoue K & Sakai T 2004 Estrogen modulates ghrelin expression in the female rat stomach. *Peptides* 25 289-297.

McKee KK, Tan CP, Palyha OC, Liu J, Feighner SD, Hreniuk DL, Smith RG, Howard AD & Van der Ploeg LH 1997 Cloning and characterization of two human G protein-coupled receptor genes (GPR38 and GPR39) related to the growth hormone secretagogue and neurotensin receptors. *Genomics* 46 426-434.

Miura T, Maruyama K, Kaiya H, Miyazato M, Kangawa K, Uchiyama M, Shioda S & Matsuda K 2009 Purification and properties of ghrelin from the intestine of the goldfish, Carassius auratus. *Peptides* 30 758-765.

Miyamoto Y & Miyamoto M 2004 Immunohistochemical localizations of secretin, cholecystokinin, and somatostatin in the rat small intestine after acute cisplatin treatment. *Exp Mol Pathol* 77 238-245.

Mondal MS, Date Y, Yamaguchi H, Toshinai K, Tsuruta T, Kangawa K & Nakazato M 2005 Identification of ghrelin and its receptor in neurons of the rat arcuate nucleus. *Regul Pept* 126 55-59.

Ohshiro H, Nonaka M & Ichikawa K 2008 Molecular identification and characterization of the dog motilin receptor. *Regul Pept* 146 80-87.

Overduin J, Frayo RS, Grill HJ, Kaplan JM & Cummings DE 2005 Role of the duodenum and macronutrient type in ghrelin regulation. *Endocrinology* 146 845-850.

Paulo RC, Brundage R, Cosma M, Mielke KL, Bowers CY & Veldhuis JD 2008 Estrogen elevates the peak overnight production rate of acylated ghrelin. *J Clin Endocrinol Metab* 93 4440-4447.

Poitras P, Dumont A, Cuber JC & Trudel L 1993 Cholinergic regulation of motilin release from isolated canine intestinal cells. *Peptides* 14 207-213.

Rozengurt N, Wu SV, Chen MC, Huang C, Sternini C & Rozengurt E 2006 Colocalization of the alpha-subunit of gustducin with PYY and GLP-1 in L cells of human colon. *Am J Physiol Gastrointest Liver Physiol* 291 G792-802.

Sakahara S, Xie Z, Koike K, Hoshino S, Sakata I, Oda S, Takahashi T & Sakai T 2010 Physiological characteristics of gastric contractions and circadian gastric motility in the free-moving conscious house musk shrew (Suncus murinus). *Am J Physiol Regul Integr Comp Physiol* 299 R1106-1113.

Sakai T, Satoh M, Koyama H, Iesaki K, Umahara M, Fujikura K & Itoh Z 1994a Localization of motilin-immunopositive cells in the rat intestine by light microscopic immunocytochemistry. *Peptides* 15 987-991.

Sakai T, Satoh M, Sonobe K, Nakajima M, Shiba Y & Itoh Z 1994b Autoradiographic study of motilin binding sites in the rabbit gastrointestinal tract. *Regul Pept* 53 249-257.

Sakata I, Nakamura K, Yamazaki M, Matsubara M, Hayashi Y, Kangawa K & Sakai T 2002 Ghrelin-producing cells exist as two types of cells, closed- and opened-type cells, in the rat gastrointestinal tract. *Peptides* 23 531-536.

Sakata I, Tanaka T, Yamazaki M, Tanizaki T, Zheng Z & Sakai T 2006 Gastric estrogen directly induces ghrelin expression and production in the rat stomach. *J Endocrinol* 190 749-757.

Satoh M, Sakai T, Koyama H, Shiba Y & Itoh Z 1995 Immunocytochemical localization of motilin-containing cells in the rabbit gastrointestinal tract. *Peptides* 16 883-887.

Shimada M, Date Y, Mondal MS, Toshinai K, Shimbara T, Fukunaga K, Murakami N, Miyazato M, Kangawa K, Yoshimatsu H, et al. 2003 Somatostatin suppresses ghrelin secretion from the rat stomach. *Biochem Biophys Res Commun* 302 520-525.

Soriano-Guillen L, Barrios V, Martos G, Chowen JA, Campos-Barros A & Argente J 2004 Effect of oral glucose administration on ghrelin levels in obese children. *Eur J Endocrinol* 151 119-121.

Strausberg RL, Feingold EA, Grouse LH, Derge JG, Klausner RD, Collins FS, Wagner L, Shenmen CM, Schuler GD, Altschul SF, et al. 2002 Generation and initial analysis of more than 15,000 full-length human and mouse cDNA sequences. *Proc Natl Acad Sci U S A* 99 16899-16903.

Tack J, Depoortere I, Bisschops R, Delporte C, Coulie B, Meulemans A, Janssens J & Peeters T 2006 Influence of ghrelin on interdigestive gastrointestinal motility in humans. *Gut* 55 327-333.

Takeshita E, Matsuura B, Dong M, Miller LJ, Matsui H & Onji M 2006 Molecular characterization and distribution of motilin family receptors in the human gastrointestinal tract. *J Gastroenterol* 41 223-230.

Taniguchi H, Ariga H, Zheng J, Ludwig K & Takahashi T 2008 Effects of ghrelin on interdigestive contractions of the rat gastrointestinal tract. *World J Gastroenterol* 14 6299-6302.

Ter Beek WP, Muller ES, van den Berg M, Meijer MJ, Biemond I & Lamers CB 2008 Motilin receptor expression in smooth muscle, myenteric plexus, and mucosa of human inflamed and noninflamed intestine. *Inflamm Bowel Dis* 14 612-619.

Theodorakis MJ, Carlson O, Michopoulos S, Doyle ME, Juhaszova M, Petraki K & Egan JM 2006 Human duodenal enteroendocrine cells: source of both incretin peptides, GLP-1 and GIP. *Am J Physiol Endocrinol Metab* 290 E550-559.

Toshinai K, Mondal MS, Nakazato M, Date Y, Murakami N, Kojima M, Kangawa K & Matsukura S 2001 Upregulation of Ghrelin expression in the stomach upon fasting, insulin-induced hypoglycemia, and leptin administration. *Biochem Biophys Res Commun* 281 1220-1225.

Tsutsui C, Kajihara K, Yanaka T, Sakata I, Itoh Z, Oda S & Sakai T 2009 House musk shrew (Suncus murinus, order: Insectivora) as a new model animal for motilin study. *Peptides* 30 318-329.

Vantrappen G, Janssens J, Peeters TL, Bloom SR, Christofides ND & Hellemans J 1979 Motilin and the interdigestive migrating motor complex in man. *Dig Dis Sci* 24 497-500.

Volante M, Allia E, Gugliotta P, Funaro A, Broglio F, Deghenghi R, Muccioli G, Ghigo E & Papotti M 2002 Expression of ghrelin and of the GH secretagogue receptor by pancreatic islet cells and related endocrine tumors. *J Clin Endocrinol Metab* 87 1300-1308.

Wada R, Sakata I, Kaiya H, Nakamura K, Hayashi Y, Kangawa K & Sakai T 2003 Existence of ghrelin-immunopositive and -expressing cells in the proventriculus of the hatching and adult chicken. *Regul Pept* 111 123-128.

Wang YN, McDonald JK & Wyatt RJ 1987 Immunocytochemical localization of neuropeptide Y-like immunoreactivity in adrenergic and non-adrenergic neurons of the rat gastrointestinal tract. *Peptides* 8 145-151.

Wierup N, Bjorkqvist M, Westrom B, Pierzynowski S, Sundler F & Sjolund K 2007 Ghrelin and motilin are cosecreted from a prominent endocrine cell population in the small intestine. *J Clin Endocrinol Metab* 92 3573-3581.

Xu L, Depoortere I, Tang M & Peeters TL 2001 Identification and expression of the motilin precursor in the guinea pig. *FEBS Lett* 490 7-10.

Xu L, Depoortere I, Thielemans L, Huang Z, Tang M & Peeters TL 2003 Sequence, distribution and quantification of the motilin precursor in the cat. *Peptides* 24 1387-1395.

Xu L, Depoortere I, Tomasetto C, Zandecki M, Tang M, Timmermans JP & Peeters TL 2005 Evidence for the presence of motilin, ghrelin, and the motilin and ghrelin receptor in neurons of the myenteric plexus. *Regul Pept* 124 119-125.

Yamamoto I, Kaiya H, Tsutsui C, Sakai T, Tsukada A, Miyazato M & Tanaka M 2008 Primary structure, tissue distribution, and biological activity of chicken motilin receptor. *Gen Comp Endocrinol* 156 509-514.

Zhao TJ, Sakata I, Li RL, Liang G, Richardson JA, Brown MS, Goldstein JL & Zigman JM 2010 Ghrelin secretion stimulated by {beta}1-adrenergic receptors in cultured ghrelinoma cells and in fasted mice. *Proc Natl Acad Sci U S A* 107 15868-15873.

Zhao Z, Sakata I, Okubo Y, Koike K, Kangawa K & Sakai T 2008 Gastric leptin, but not estrogen and somatostatin, contributes to the elevation of ghrelin mRNA expression level in fasted rats. *J Endocrinol* 196 529-538.

Zheng J, Ariga H, Taniguchi H, Ludwig K & Takahashi T 2009 Ghrelin regulates gastric phase III-like contractions in freely moving conscious mice. *Neurogastroenterol Motil* 21 78-84.

Zietlow A, Nakajima H, Taniguchi H, Ludwig K & Takahashi T 2010 Association between plasma ghrelin and motilin levels during MMC cycle in conscious dogs. *Regul Pept* 164 78-82.

Zigman JM, Jones JE, Lee CE, Saper CB & Elmquist JK 2006 Expression of ghrelin receptor mRNA in the rat and the mouse brain. *J Comp Neurol* 494 528-548.

2

Functions of Adipose Tissue and Adipokines in Health and Disease

Francisca Lago[1], Rodolfo Gómez[2], Javier Conde[2], Morena Scotece[2], Carlos Dieguez[3] and Oreste Gualillo[2]
[1]SERGAS Santiago University Clinical Hospital, Research Laboratory 7 (Molecular and Cellular Cardiology), Santiago de Compostela,
[2]SERGAS Santiago University Clinical Hospital, Research Laboratory 9 (NEIRID LAB, Laboratory of Neuro Endocrine Interactions in Rheumatology and Inflammatory Diseases), Santiago de Compostela,
[3]University of Santiago de Compostela, Department of Physiology, Santiago de Compostela,
Spain

1. Introduction

The notion of white adipose tissue (WAT) as an active contributor to whole-body homeostasis, rather than as a mere fat depot, began to take identity with the discovery of leptin in 1994 [1]. This 16 kDa protein secreted by adipocytes was found to be the product of the gene obese (ob), which is mutated in a murine form of hereditary obesity. From this point on, WAT has been found to produce more than 50 cytokines and other molecules. These "adipokines" participate, through endocrine, paracrine, autocrine or juxtacrine mechanisms of action, in a wide variety of physiological or physiopathological processes, including food intake, insulin sensitivity, vascular sclerotic processes, immunity and inflammation [2,3,4]. They are currently considered to play a crucial role in crosstalk among the adrenal, immune and central and peripheral nervous systems, among others.

Obesity, the condition originally motivating the spate of research on WAT, is now regarded as a pro-inflammatory state, several markers of inflammation having been found to be elevated in obese subjects [5]. It is thought that excess WAT can contribute to the maintenance of this state in three ways: through inflammation-inducing lipotoxicity; by secreting factors that stimulate the synthesis of inflammatory agents in other organs; and by secreting inflammatory agents itself. Adipokines include a variety of pro-inflammatory peptides (including TNFα, secretion of which by adipocytes was observed even before the discovery of leptin [6]). These pro-inflammatory adipokines appear to contribute significantly to the "low-grade inflammatory state" of obese subjects with metabolic syndrome [7], a cluster of metabolic abnormalities including insulin resistance, dyslipidaemia and alteration of coagulation that is associated with increased risk of cancer, type II diabetes, cardiovascular complications and autoimmune inflammatory diseases.

WAT also produces, possibly as an adaptive response, anti-inflammatory factors such as IL1 receptor antagonist (which binds competitively to the interleukin 1 receptor without triggering activity within the cell) and IL10 (circulating levels of which are also elevated in obese individuals).

2. Cellular and molecular alterations of white adipose tissue in obesity

One of the consequences of the production and local release of cytokines and adipokines by adipocytes is the recruitment of large numbers of immune cells, including monocytes and T-lymphocytes, into adipose tissue. In particular, pro-inflammatory cytokine levels and macrophage density in visceral fat depots are much higher than in subcutaneous adipose tissue. While the mechanisms underlying the recruitment and activation of macrophages in adipose tissue remain poorly understood, there is emerging evidence that adipose tissue-secreted chemokines are largely responsible for the recruitment, retention and activation of macrophage precursors (monocytes) in fat. Monocyte chemoattractant protein-1 (MCP-1) has been implicated as one of the major mediators of the monocyte recruitment that occurs in adipose tissue, while macrophage colony stimulating factor (M-CSF) is believed to mediate the conversion of monocytes to macrophages in adipose tissue. Other candidate adipocyte-derived molecules that have also been implicated in macrophage recruitment/activation in adipose tissue include free fatty acids and lipoprotein lipase.

The primary function of resident macrophages of adipose tissue remains still unclear. It has been proposed that macrophages clear dead (apoptotic and necrotic) cells. Actually, adipocytes undergoing necrosis secondary to hypertrophy may lead to macrophage activation (with the accompanying release of inflammatory mediators) and their subsequent elimination from adipose tissue Another potentially important role of adipose tissue macrophages is modulation of adipocyte function. Cross-talk between adipocytes and macrophages is evidenced by the ability of each cell type to enhance the production of protein mediators by the other. For instance, adipocyte conditioned media can elicit large increases in the production/release of TNFa, IL-6 and NO by macrophages, while TNF-a released from macrophages inhibits the production of adiponectin by adipocytes. Likely consequences of this cross-talk between macrophages and adipocytes include amplification and perpetuation of the inflammatory phenotype that is induced by the expanding mass of body fat.

In humans, macrophage infiltration is correlated with both adipocyte size and BMI and is reduced after surgery-induced weight loss in morbidly obese subjects. There is also a preferential infiltration of macrophages into omental *vs.* subcutaneous fat, a phenomenon exaggerated by central. The majority of macrophages in obese adipose tissue aggregates in "crown-like structures" completely surrounding dead (necrotic-like) adipocytes and scavenging adipocyte debris.

3. Leptin

Leptin is a 16 kDa non-glycosylated peptide hormone encoded by the gene obese (ob), the murine homologue of the human gene LEP [1]. Structurally, it belongs to the class I cytokine superfamily, consisting of a bundle of four α-helices. It is mainly produced by adipocytes, and circulating leptin levels are directly correlated with WAT mass. It decreases food intake and increases energy consumption by acting on hypothalamic cell populations [8,9], inducing anorexigenic factors (CART, POMC) and inhibiting orexigenic neuropeptides

(NPY, AGRP and orexin), and leptin levels are negatively correlated with glucocorticoids [10] and positively with insulin [11]. Its own synthesis is mainly regulated by food intake and eating-related hormones, but also depends on energy status, sex hormones (being inhibited by testosterone and increased by ovarian sex steroids) and a wide range of inflammation mediators [12, 13] (being increased or suppressed by pro-inflammatory cytokines depending on whether their action is acute or chronic). Through the mediation of these latter agents, leptin synthesis is increased by acute infection and sepsis. As a result of the effects of sex hormones, leptin levels are higher in women than in men even when adjusted for BMI, which may be relevant to the influence of sex on the development or frequency of certain diseases [14], such as osteoarthritis [56]. Thus leptin appears to act not only as an adipostatin, the function in relation to which it was discovered, but also as a general signal of energy reserves [2] that is involved in a wide variety of other functions, including glucose metabolism, the synthesis of glucocorticoids, the proliferation of CD4+ T lymphocytes, cytokine secretion, phagocytosis, regulation of the hypothalamic-pituitary-adrenal axis, reproduction, and angiogenesis [15]. It can accordingly be described as a cytokine-like hormone with pleiotropic actions.

Leptin exerts its biological actions by binding to its receptors. These are encoded by the gene diabetes (db) and belong to the class I cytokine receptor superfamily, which includes receptors for IL6, LIF, CNTF, OSM, G-CSF and gp130. Alternative splicings of db give rise to six receptor isoforms: the soluble form Ob-Re, which lacks a cytoplasmic domain; four forms with short cytoplasmic domains (Ob-Ra, Ob-Rc, Ob-Rd and Ob-Rf); and the long form Ob-Rb, which is found in almost all tissues and appears to be the only form capable of transducing the leptin signal.

As in the case of other class I cytokine receptors, the main routes by which Ob-Rb appears to transmit the extracellular signal it receives are JAK-STAT pathways [16], which involve JAK2 phosphorylating tyrosines in the cytoplasmic domain of the receptor. In particular, mutation of the intracellular tyrosine Y1138 of murine Ob-Rb prevents STAT3 activation and results in hyperphagia, obesity and impaired thermoregulation, and replacing Y1138 with a serine residue likewise causes pronounced obesity in knock-in mice. However, since Y1138S knock-in mice do not exhibit other defects of db/db mice, such as infertility, the role of leptin in the processes that are disrupted in these latter conditions must be independent of STAT3 [17]. Indeed, the other two cytoplasmic tyrosines of murine Ob-Rb, Y985 and Y1077, have been shown to bind other intracellular signalling molecules [16, 18]. The early studies of leptin focused on its anorexigenic action. Both in humans and rodents, leptin levels are closely correlated with body mass index, and defects of the genes encoding for leptin and its receptors give rise to severe obesity and diabetes. Treating leptin-deficient mice with leptin induces a reduction in food intake accompanied by an increase in metabolic rate and weight loss. Mutations of these genes in humans appear to be rare, but the cases that are known have occurred in families with a high prevalence of morbid obesity; again, leptin administration has ameliorated all the problems associated with leptin deficiency. As noted in previous sections, leptin participates in the control of food intake by acting on an intricate neuronal circuit involving hypothalamic and brainstem nuclei [19], where it integrates a variety of different orexigenic and anorexigenic signals.

Leptin therapy is not an effective treatment for morbid obesity that is not due to congenital deficiency of leptin or leptin receptors. In these noncongenital types of obesity, leptin concentrations are already high as a consequence of increased fat mass. The persistence of obesity in spite of high leptin levels suggests that high leptin levels can induce leptin resistance. This may occur due to a leptin-induced increase of SOCS3, which blocks intracellular transmission of the leptin signal [20], but our understanding of leptin resistance is still limited.

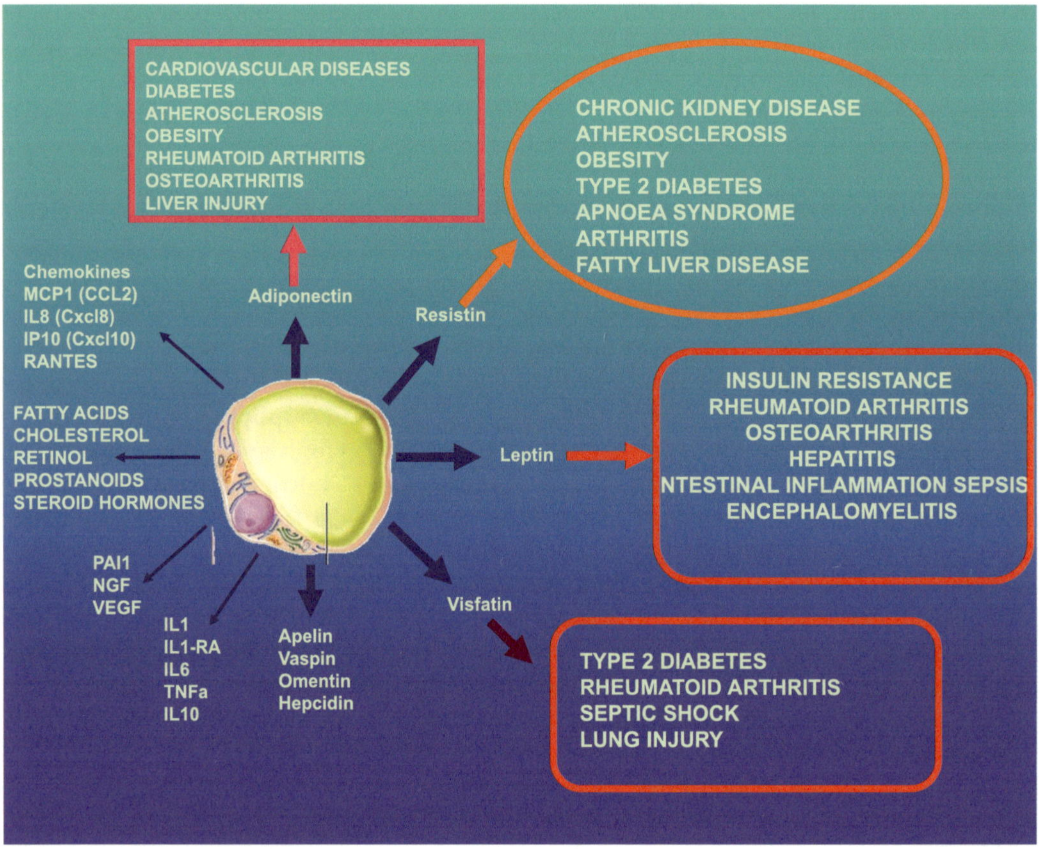

Fig. 1. A schematic representation of white adipose tissue (wat) functions. Besides to be the main energy store of the body and the site of synthesis of steroids and prostanoids, wat is also a source of a plethora of novel factors that modulate the immune/inflammatory response and promote atherosclerosis, vascular dysfunction and insulin resistance.

Db/db mice, which lack leptin receptors, suffer from thymus atrophy [21], and ob/ob mice, which lack leptin, are immunodeficient. Leptin must therefore play a role in immunity. This presumably explains why the murine immune system is depressed by acute starvation and reduced caloric intake, both of which result in low leptin levels [33], and why this depression is reverted by administration of exogenous leptin.

It promotes phagocyte function [24] and induces the synthesis of eicosanoids [25], nitric oxide [26] and several pro-inflammatory cytokines [26] in macrophages and monocytes. It increases IFNγ-induced production of nitric oxide synthase in murine macrophages [26]. It induces chemotaxis and the release of reactive oxygen species by neutrophils [27, 28]. It influences the proliferation, differentiation, activation and cytotoxicity of natural killer (NK) cells [29].

It may protect dendritic cells from apoptosis and promote their lipopolysaccharide-induced maturation and a cytokine production profile featuring low levels of IL10 and high levels of IL12, TNFα and costimulatory molecules, which favours the proliferation of allogeneic CD4+ T cells (whereas leptin receptor deficiency and sequestration of leptin have the opposite effects and result in depressed proliferation of allogeneic CD4+ T cells) [30]. Finally, it modifies T-cell balance, induces T-cell activation, and alters the pattern of T-cell cytokine production by directing T-cell differentiation towards a T_{H1} response [31, 32].

Leptin also prevents glucocorticoid-induced thymocyte apoptosis, and increases thymic cell counts [33]. The low circulating CD4+ T-cell counts, impaired T-cell proliferation and impaired release of T-cell cytokines exhibited by young human patients with morbid obesity due to congenital leptin deficiency are all ameliorated by administration of recombinant human leptin. The fact that several T-cell antigens are expressed aberrantly in both ob/ob and db/db mice suggests that leptin may influence the growth, differentiation and activation of T cells by interacting with T-cell co-stimulatory antigens such as CTLA4 and dipeptidyl peptidase IV [34]. It is possible, however, that in the thymus T cells are affected by leptin only indirectly, via other signalling molecules: fetal db/db thymi develop normally when transplanted into wild-type hosts; neither the thymus weight and cellularity nor the cellular and humoral immune responses of wild-type mice are affected by transplantation of bone marrow cells from db/db mice more than by transplantation from db/+ mice; and thymus weight and cellularity are decreased when bone marrow cells are transplanted from wild-type mice to db/db mice [47].

A salient aspect of the effects of leptin in the immune system is its action as a pro-inflammatory cytokine: it is produced by inflammatory cells [35], and leptin mRNA expression and circulating leptin levels are increased by a number of inflammatory stimuli, including IL1, IL6 and lipopolysaccharide (LPS) [36]. Leptin-deficient mice are less prone than non-leptin-deficient mice to develop inflammatory diseases, regardless of whether these involve innate or adaptive immunity; reported conditions include experimentally induced colitis, experimental autoimmune encephalomyelitis, type I diabetes and experimentally induced hepatitis [2]. In the innate case, a reported imbalance between pro- and anti-inflammatory cytokines [37] suggests that leptin is able to modify the cytokine secretion pattern of monocytes and macrophages through a STAT3-mediated mechanism [38]. In the adaptive case, resistance may be due to the above-noted influence of leptin deficiency on T_{H1}/T_{H2} balance [39]. When transferred to T-cell-deficient mice, murine CD4+ CD45RB^{high} T cells from db/db mice do not induce colitis as rapidly as do CD4^{+} CD45RB^{high} T cells from non-db/db mice, which feature leptin receptors [40]. Also, in rats with chemically induced intestinal inflammation, circulating leptin levels are elevated, and correlate with the degree of inflammation and the development of anorexia, during the first day following the induction of inflammation [41]. Serum leptin levels are likewise high in human patients with acute ulcerative colitis, in whom inflamed colonic epithelial cells secrete leptin into the intestinal lumen, where it is able to activate NFkB [42]. Thus leptin appears to play a significant role in intestinal inflammation as well as in the development of associated anorexia.

Mice in which experimental autoimmune encephalomyelitis (EAE) has been induced by inoculation of appropriate self-antigens constitute an animal model of human multiple sclerosis, a disease in which leptin levels in serum and cerebrospinal fluid are high and are negatively correlated with CD4+ CD25+ regulatory T cells [43]. Ob/ob mice do not develop EAE in response to EAE-inducing antigens, but this resistance is abolished by administration of leptin, and the abolition of resistance is accompanied by a switch from a T_{H2} to a T_{H1} pattern of cytokine release [44]. Also, the onset of EAE in wild-type mice is preceded by an increase in circulating leptin and is delayed by acute starvation [35]. Of particular interest is the finding that during the active phase of EAE leptin is secreted by both macrophages and T cells that have infiltrated the central nervous system (CNS), and that secretion by activated T cells appears to constitute an autocrine loop sustaining their proliferation [35]. By contrast, however, leptin secretion by T cells seems to have at most a marginal role in experimentally induced colitis and hepatitis, in which conditions no differences have been found between ob/ob and wild-type T cells regarding their ability to induce inflammation [45].

Serum leptin levels increase preceding not only the onset of EAE [35], but also the onset of diabetes in female non-obese diabetic (NOD) mice, in which leptin administration augments inflammatory infiltrates, increases interferon γ production by peripheral T cells, and speeds up the destruction of pancreatic β cells [46]. These latter findings suggest that leptin may promote the development of type 1 diabetes through a T_{H1} response.

Finally, leptin administration increases both inflammatory and platelet responses in humans during caloric deprivation [48], and in WAT-less mice increases T-cell–mediated hepatic inflammation [49]. Together with a number of other neuroendocrine messengers, leptin appears to play a major role in autoimmune diseases such as rheumatoid arthritis. In patients with rheumatoid arthritis, circulating leptin levels are high [51, 52], and leptin production is much higher in osteoarthritic cartilage than in normal cartilage [55].

Of all the connective tissues that compose a skeletal joint, articular cartilage is the most damaged by rheumatic disease. Under pathological conditions, control of the balance between synthesis and degradation of extracellular matrix by chondrocytes is lost, and the production of a host of inflammation mediators by these cells eventually leads to complete loss of cartilage structure [53, 54]. The finding that administration of exogenous leptin increases IGF1 and TGFβ1 production by rat knee joint cartilage has suggested that high circulating leptin levels in obese individuals may protect cartilage from osteoarthritic degeneration [55]. However, most of the evidence points the other way: in rheumatoid arthritis patients a fasting-induced fall in circulating leptin is associated with CD4+ lymphocyte hyporeactivity and increased IL4 secretion [50]; experimental antigen-induced arthritis is less severe in leptin-deficient ob/ob mice than in wild-type mice [39]; and in cultured chondrocytes type 2 nitric oxide synthase (NOS2) is activated by the combination leptin plus IFNγ (though by either without the other) [57], and NOS2 activation by IL1 is increased by leptin [58] (nitric oxide has well-documented pro-inflammatory effects on joint cartilage, triggering the loss of chondrocyte phenotype, chondrocyte apoptosis, and the activation of metalloproteases). Intracellularly, the joint action of IL1 and leptin involves JAK2, PI3K, MEK1 and p38.

A pro-inflammatory effect of leptin on cartilage would be in keeping with the fact that, in comparison with men, women have both higher circulating leptin levels and a greater propensity to develop osteoarthritis [56]. It would also explain association between obesity and inflammatory conditions, especially those related with alterations of cartilage homeostasis.

4. Adiponectin

Adiponectin, also called gelatin binding protein 28 (GBP28), adipose most abundant gene transcript 1(apM1), and 30 kDa adipocyte complement-related protein (Acrp30, AdipoQ), is a 244-residue protein that, as far as is known, is produced prevalently by WAT. It increases fatty acid oxidation and reduces the synthesis of glucose in the liver [61]. Ablation of the adiponectin gene has no dramatic effect on knock-out mice on a normal diet, but when placed on a high-fat, high-sucrose diet they develop severe insulin resistance and exhibit lipid accumulation in muscles [62]. Circulating adiponectin levels tend to be low in morbidly obese patients and increase with weight loss and with the use of thiazolidinediones, which enhance sensitivity to insulin [67].

Adiponectin acts mainly via two receptors, one (AdipoR1) found mainly in skeletal muscle and the other (AdipoR2) in liver (for a third route, see the next section). Transduction of the adiponectin signal by AdipoR1 and AdipoR2 involves the activation of AMPK, PPAR (α and γ) and presumably other signalling molecules also. Adiponectin exhibits structural homology with collagen VIII and X and complement factor C1q, and circulates in the blood in relatively large amounts in oligomeric forms (mainly trimers and hexamers, but also a 12-18-mer form [59]), constituting about 0.01% of total plasma protein. Whether the various oligomers have different activities, which would make the effect of adiponectin controlable through its oligomerization state, is somewhat controversial and may depend on target cell type: although authors working with myocytes reported that trimers activated AMP-activated protein kinase (AMPK) whereas higher oligomers activated NFκb, it has also been reported that 12-18-mers promote AMPK in hepatocytes [60].

Although adiponectin was discovered nearly at the same time as leptin, its role in protection against obesity and obesity-related disorders only began to be recognized some years later. It is now beginning to be recognized that, in addition, it has a wide range of effects in pathologies with inflammatory components, such as cardiovascular disease, type 2 diabetes, metabolic syndrome and rheumatoid arthritis. One indication of a relationship between adiponectin and inflammation is provided by the finding that its secretion by cultured adipocytes is inhibited by pro-inflammatory cytokines such as IL6 [65] and TNFα [66]. More recently, an explanation of how hypoadiponectinaemia might contribute to the development of inflammation-related diseases has been suggested by the finding that adiponectin promotes the phagocytosis of apoptotic cells (by interacting with calreticulin on the phagocyte surface), since the accumulation of apoptotic débris is known to be able to cause inflammation and immune system dysfunction [67]. In the remainder of this section we look at the relationship of adiponectin to inflammatory processes in several types of pathology.

Adiponectin has been described as a potent anti-atherogenic factor that protects vascular endothelium against atherogenic inflammation through multiple effects on the endothelium itself and other vascular structures [63]. It inhibits the adhesion of monocytes to endothelial cells, reduces the synthesis of adhesion molecules and tumor necrosis factor, and reduces NFκB levels [64]. Subnormal levels of adiponectin have been linked to inflammatory atherosclerosis in humans [69], and in animal models they are associated with increased vascular smooth cell proliferation in response to injury, increased free fatty acid levels, and insulin resistance [70]. The conjunction of pro-diabetic and pro-atherogenic effects of reduced adiponectin levels, as seen in metabolic syndrome, make adiponectin a link between obesity and inflammation.

In contrast to its protective role against obesity and vascular diseases, it appears that in skeletal joints adiponectin is pro-inflammatory and involved in matrix degradation. Plasma adiponectin levels in rheumatoid arthritis patients are higher than in healthy controls [51] (and adiponectin levels in synovial fluid are higher in rheumatoid arthritis patients than in patients with osteoarthritis [72]). In human synovial fibroblasts adiponectin selectively induces, via the p38 MAPK pathway, two of the main mediators of rheumatoid arthritis, IL6 and matrix metalloproteinase 1 [71]. Chondrocytes also present functional adiponectin receptors, activation of which leads to the induction of type 2 NOS via a signalling pathway that involves PI3 kinase; and adiponectin-treated chondrocytes similarly increase IL6, TNFα and MCP1 synthesis (but not release of prostaglandin E_2 or leukotriene B_4). Taken together, these results suggest that it may be worth considering adiponectin as a potential target of treatment for degenerative joint diseases. On the other hand, the high adiponectin levels of patients with rheumatoid arthritis can also be interpreted as an attempt to overcome the well-known pro-inflammatory effect of leptin, for example by counteracting the pro-inflammatory effects of TNFα and reducing the production of IL6 and CRP in rheumatoid arthritis [73].

In experimental models of liver injury, adiponectin has been reported to have anti-inflammatory effects: in rodents, adiponectin administration improves liver function in both alcoholic and non-alcoholic fatty liver disease as the result of TNF suppression, and in mice it reduces liver enzyme levels, hepatomegaly and steatosis [74], attenuates liver fibrosis [75], and protects against LPS-induced liver injury [76].

Finally, there is also evidence that adiponectin may influence the development of certain neoplasias and the course of wound healing [77, 78].

5. Resistin

Resistin is a dimeric protein that received its name from its apparent induction of insulin resistance in mice. It belongs to the FIZZ (found in inflammatory zones) family (now also known as RELMs, i.e. resistin-like molecules). The first member this family to be discovered, FIZZ1 (also known as RELMα), is a protein that is found in above-normal levels in the bronchoalveolar fluid of mice with experimentally induced asthma [79]. FIZZ2 (RELMβ) was discovered in the proliferating epithelium of intestinal crypt [80]. Resistin (FIZZ3) has been found in adipocytes, macrophages and other cell types. In rodents, a fourth FIZZ protein, RELMγ, has been identified in WAT and haematopoietic tissues [81].

As noted above, it has been postulated that resistin mediates insulin resistance, but this role may be limited to rodents. Initial enthusiasm for this theory, which provides a direct link between adiposity and insulin resistance [83], was quickly quenched by contradictory findings in both mice and humans. It nonetheless appears safe to assert that resistin levels depend upon both nutritional state and hormonal environment; that they are low during fasting and restored by refeeding; and that growth hormone, catecholamines and endothelin 1 are all able to increase resistin secretion [82].

5.1 Resistin and inflammation

That resistin is involved in inflammatory conditions in humans is suggested by its secretion in appreciable quantities by mononuclear cells. Also, resistin levels are correlated with those of cell adhesion molecules such as ICAM1 in patients with obstructive sleep apnoea [87], and in atherosclerotic patients are positively associated with other markers of inflammation, such as soluble TNF-R type II and lipoprotein-associated phospholipase A2 [88]. Furthermore, LPS has been reported to induce resistin gene expression in primary human and murine macrophages via a cascade involving the secretion of pro-inflammatory cytokines [86]; and in human peripheral blood mononuclear cells resistin appears both to induce [85] and be induced by [84] IL6 and TNFa (induction of these cytokines by resistin occurring via the NFκB pathway [85]). However, both TNFα and IL6 downregulate resistin or have no effect in adipocytes [84].

A pro-inflammatory role of resistin in atherosclerosis is suggested by reports that in vascular endothelial cells it induces the inflammation marker long pentraxin 3 [90] and promotes the release of endothelin 1 and production of VCAM1, ICAM1 and monocyte chemotactic protein 1 (MCP1) [89]. In murine models of atherosclerosis, resistin is present in sclerotic lesions at levels that are proportional to the severity of the lesion [92]. In humans resistin is associated with coronary artery calcification, a quantitative marker of atherosclerosis [91].

There are indications that resistin may also be involved in the pathogenesis of rheumatoid arthritis: resistin has been found in the plasma and the synovial fluid of rheumatoid arthritis patients [92], and injection of resistin into mice joints induces an arthritis-like condition, with leukocyte infiltration of synovial tissues, hypertrophy of the synovial layer and pannus formation [85]. However, plasma resistin levels in rheumatoid arthritis patients appear to be no different from those found in healthy controls [51,85]; and although in some studies of rheumatoid arthritis patients resistin levels were higher in synovial fluid than in serum (which shows that circulating levels of adipokines do not necessarily reflect the situation in the joint), the discrepancy may be due simply to the increased permeability of inflamed synovial membrane [93].

6. Other adipokines

6.1 Visfatin

Visfatin is an insulin-mimetic adipokine that was originally discovered in liver, skeletal muscle and bone marrow as a growth factor for B lymphocyte precursors (whence its alternative name, pre-B-colony enhancing factor, or PBEF). It is up-modulated in models of acute lung injury and sepsis. It was re-discovered by Fukuhara et al. [94] using a differential display technique to identify genes that are relatively specifically expressed in abdominal fat. Circulating visfatin levels are closely correlated with WAT accumulation, visfatin mRNA levels increase in the course of adipocyte differentiation, and visfatin synthesis is regulated by several factors, including glucocorticoids, TNFα, IL6 and growth hormone. In an experimental model of obesity-associated insulin resistance, circulating visfatin levels increased during the development of obesity, apparently due solely to secretion by abdominal WAT (since visfatin mRNA increased only in this tissue, not in subcutaneous WAT or liver). However, visfatin is not only produced by WAT, but also by endotoxin-challenged neutrophils, in which it prevents apoptosis through a mechanism mediated by caspases 3 and 8 [95]. Also, patients with inflammatory bowel diseases have increased circulating visfatin levels and increased levels of visfatin mRNA in their intestinal epithelium; and visfatin has been shown to induce chemotaxis and the production of IL1β, TNFα, IL6 and costimulatory molecules by CD14+ monocytes, and to increase their ability to induce alloproliferative responses in lymphocytes, effects which are mediated intracellularly by p38 and MEK1 [96]. Visfatin is therefore certainly pro-inflammatory in some circumstances. In addition, circulating visfatin is higher in patients with rheumatoid arthritis than in healthy controls [51]. Even though it is currently unclear what is visfatin physiological role or relevance in the context of rheumatoid arthritis, it may reflect modulation of the inflammatory or immune response by visfatin; or it may forms part of a compensatory mechanism that facilitates the accumulation of intra-abdominal fat so as to prevent rheumatoid cachexia; or it may simply be an epiphenomenon.

6.2 Apelin

Apelin is a bioactive peptide that was originally identified in bovine stomach extracts as the endogenous ligand of the orphan G protein-coupled receptor APJ [97]. It is derived from a 77-amino-acid prepropeptide that is cleaved into a 55-amino-acid fragment and then into shorter forms. The physiologically active form is thought to be apelin 36, although the pyroglutamylated form of apelin 13, which is also produced endogenously, is more potent. Boucher et al. [98] recently found that apelin is produced and secreted by mature human and murine adipocytes, and that the apelin mRNA levels found in these cells are similar to those found in the stroma-vascular fraction (which contains other cell types present in adipose tissue) and in organs such as kidney and heart [98]. In obese humans plasma apelin levels are significantly higher than in lean controls [98,100], and that this may be due to production by WAT is suggested by the finding that in several murine models of obesity above-normal plasma apelin levels are accompanied by above-normal apelin mRNA levels in adipocytes [98]. TNFα increases both apelin production in adipose tissue and blood plasma apelin levels when administered to mice by intraperitoneal injection [99]. Intriguingly, in mice with diet-induced obesity, macrophage counts and the levels of pro-inflammatory agents such as TNFα seem to rise progressively in adipose tissue before a rise in circulating insulin levels indicates the onset of insulin resistance [101]. So, it could be conceivable that in adipocytes there is a substantial regulation of apelin synthesis exerted by TNFα, leading to sustained apelin secretion in obesity.

Thus, one may envisage that over-production of apelin in the obese may be an adaptive response that attempts to forestall the onset of obesity-related disorders such as mild chronic inflammation, hypertension and cardiovascular dysfunctions. Accordingly, further elucidation of the role of apelin is of major interest.

6.3 Vaspin

Vaspin (visceral-adipose-tissue-derived serpin) was discovered by Hida et al. [102] as a serpin (serine protease inhibitor) that was produced in the visceral adipose tissue of Otsuka Long-Evans Tokushima Fatty rats at the age when obesity and plasma insulin concentrations reach a peak; thereafter, vaspin production decreased as diabetes worsened and body weight fell in untreated mice, but serum vaspin levels were maintained by treatment with insulin or pioglitazone. Administration of vaspin to obese mice improved glucose tolerance and insulin sensitivity, and reversed altered expression of genes that may promote insulin resistance.

Kloting et al. [103] reported that human vaspin mRNA is not detectable in the adipose tissue of normal, lean, glucose-tolerant individuals, but can be induced by increased fat mass, decreased insulin sensitivity, and impaired glucose tolerance. The regulation of vaspin gene expression seems to be fat depot-specific. The induction of vaspin by adipose tissue may constitute a compensatory mechanism in response to obesity, severe insulin resistance and type 2 diabetes.

7. Conclusions

It is now clear that adipokines play multiple important roles in the body, and the increasing research effort in this area is gradually revealing the intricate adipokine-mediated interplay among white adipose tissue, metabolic diseases and inflammatory (auto)immune illnesses. Although many issues remain foggy, in this section we outline several possible avenues for therapeutic action that this work has already opened.

There is now a huge amount of data on the promotion of inflammation by high circulating leptin levels. It might perhaps be possible to control the amount of bioavailable circulating leptin, and hence to prevent leptin-induced inflammation, by means of a soluble, high-affinity leptin-binding molecule analogous to the soluble TNFα receptors used to treat rheumatoid arthritis. Alternatively, it might be possible to block the leptin receptor with monoclonal humanized antibodies or mutant leptins that are able to bind to the receptor without activating it. An obvious proviso here is that receptors mediating the influence of leptin on food intake should not be blocked, lest the patient develop hyperphagia and obesity; but the fact that this influence is exerted in the brain, on the other side of the blood-brain barrier, would seem to make such discrimination possible. At present, little is known in this area because current anti-leptin agents were developed to control the adipostatic effects of leptin, and hence to cross the blood brain barrier.

The anti-atherosclerotic and vasoprotective effects of adiponectin are another source of inspiration for possible pharmacological approaches to inflammatory diseases. In particular, one strategy against diabetes and relevant cardiovascular and metabolic diseases might be to tackle the hypoadiponectinaemia associated with these conditions. Given the high levels of adiponectin in the blood, exogenous administration of the adipokine itself would probably have little effect; but drugs that specifically enhance endogenous adiponectin production, such as thiazolidinediones, might well prove to be effective. It should not be forgotten, of course, that the primary causes of obesity are generally nutritional and lifestyle factors such as overeating and physical inactivity, and that front line treatment of obesity-related hypoadiponectinemia and obesity-related hyperproduction of detrimental adipokines therefore essentially involves the correction of these factors.

8. Acknowledgements

Part of the research described in this chapter was supported by the Spanish Ministry of Health through the Fondo de Investigación Sanitaria, Instituto de Salud Carlos III and by the Xunta de Galicia. The work of Oreste Gualillo and Francisca Lago is funded by the Instituto de Salud Carlos III and the Xunta de Galicia (SERGAS) through a research staff stabilization contract.

We apologize to the authors of the many relevant papers, mention of which in this chapter has been prevented by shortage of space.

9. References

[1] Zhang Y, Proenca R, Maffei M, Barone M, Leopold L, Friedman JM. Positional cloning of the mouse obese gene and its human homologue. Nature. 1994; 372(6505):425-32.

[2] Otero M, Lago R, Lago F, Casanueva FF, Dieguez C, Gomez-Reino JJ, Gualillo O. Leptin, from fat to inflammation: old questions and new insights. FEBS Lett. 2005; 579(2):295-301.
[3] Trayhurn P, Wood IS. Adipokines: inflammation and the pleiotropic role of white adipose tissue. Br J Nutr. 2004; 92(3):347-55.
[4] Trayhurn P, Wood IS. Signalling role of adipose tissue: adipokines and inflammation in obesity. Biochem Soc Trans. 2005; 33(Pt 5):1078-81.
[5] Lau DC, Dhillon B, Yan H, Szmitko PE, Verma S. Adipokines: molecular links between obesity and atherosclerosis. Am J Physiol Heart Circ Physiol. 2005; 288(5):H2031-41.
[6] Hotamisligil GS, Shargill NS, Spiegelman BM. Adipose expression of tumor necrosis factor-alpha: direct role in obesity-linked insulin resistance. Science. 1993; 259(5091):87-91.
[7] Trayhurn P, Bing C, Wood IS. Adipose tissue and adipokines--energy regulation from the human perspective. J Nutr. 2006; 136(7):1935S-9S.
[8] Ahima RS, Prabakaran D, Mantzoros C, et al. Role of leptin in the neuroendocrine response to fasting. Nature 1996; 382: 250-252
[9] Chan JL, Heist K, DePaoli AM, Veldhuis JD, Mantzoros CS. The role of falling leptin levels in the neuroendocrine and metabolic adaptation to short-term starvation in healthy men. J Clin Invest. 2003; 111: 1409-21.
[10] Zakrzewska KE, Cusin I, Sainsbury A, Rohner-Jeanrenaud F, Jeanrenaud B. Glucocorticoids as counterregulatory hormones of leptin: toward an understanding of leptin resistance. Diabetes 1997; 46: 717-9.
[11] Boden G, Chen X, Kolaczynski JW, Polansky M. Effects of prolonged hyperinsulinemia on serum leptin in normal human subjects. J. Clin. Inv 1997; 100: 1107-13
[12] Sarraf P, Frederich RC, Turner EM, et al. Multiple cytokines and acute inflammation raise mouse leptin levels: potential role in inflammatory anorexia. J. Exp. Med. 1997; 185: 171-5.
[13] Gualillo O, Eiras S, Lago F, Dieguez C, Casanueva FF. Elevated serum leptin concentrations induced by experimental acute inflammation. Life Sci. 2000; 67: 2433-41.
[14] Blum WF, Englaro P, Hatsch S, et al. Plasma leptin levels in healthy children and adolescents: dependence on body mass index, body fat mass, gender, pubertal stage, and testosterone. Clin. Endocrinol. Metab. 1997; 82: 2904-10.
[15] Otero M, Lago R, Gomez R, Dieguez C, Lago F, Gomez-Reino J, Gualillo O. Towards a pro-inflammatory and immunomodulatory emerging role of leptin. Rheumatology (Oxford). 2006; 45(8):944-50
[16] Fruhbeck G. Intracellular signalling pathways activated by leptin. Biochem J. 2006; 393: 7-20
[17] Bates, S.H., Stearns, W.H., Dundon, T.A., Schubert, M., Tso, A.W., Wang, Y., Banks, A.S., Lavery, H.J., Haq, A.K., Maratos-Flier, E., Neel, B.G., Schwartz, M.W. and Myers Jr., M.G. STAT3 signalling is required for leptin regulation of energy balance but not reproduction. Nature 2003 , 421 (6925), 856–859.
[18] Gualillo O, Eiras S, White DW, Dieguez C, Casanueva FF. Leptin promotes the tyrosine phosphorylation of SHC proteins and SHC association with GRB2. Mol Cell Endocrinol. 2002; 190: 83-9.

[19] Prodi F, Obici S. The brain as a molecular target for diabetic therapy. Endocrinology 2006; 147(6): 2664-9.
[20] Bjorbaek C, Elmquist JK, Frantz JD, Flier JS. The role of SOCS3 in leptin signalling and leptin resistance. J Biol Chem 1999; 274: 30059-65.
[21] Kimura M, Tanaka S, Isoda F, Sekigawa K, Yamakawa T, Sekihara H. T lymphopenia in obese diabetic (db/db) mice is non-selective and thymus independent. Life Sci. 1998; 62: 1243-50
[22] Tilg H, Moschen AR. Adipocytokines: mediators linking adipose tissue, inflammation and immunity. Nature Reviews Immunology 2006; 6:772-783.
[23] Matarese G, Moschos S, Mantzoros CS. Leptin in immunology. J Immunol. 2005; 174: 3137-42.
[24] Zarkesh-Esfahani H, Pockley G, Metcalfe RA, et al. High-dose leptin activates human leukocytes via receptor expression on monocytes. J Immunol. 2001; 167: 4593-9
[25] Mancuso P, Canetti C, Gottschalk A, Tithof PK, Peters-Golden M. Leptin augments alveolar macrophage leukotriene synthesis by increasing phospholipase activity and enhancing group IVC iPLA2 (cPLA2gamma) protein expression. Am J Physiol Lung Cell Mol Physiol. 2004; 287: 497-502.
[26] Raso GM, Pacilio M, Esposito E, Coppola A, Di Carlo R, Meli R. Leptin potentiates IFN-gamma-induced expression of nitric oxide synthase and cyclo-oxygenase-2 in murine macrophage J774A.1. Br J Pharmacol. 2002; 137: 799-804
[27] Caldefie-Chezet F, Poulin A, Tridon A, Sion B, Vasson MP. Leptin: a potential regulator of polymorphonuclear neutrophil bactericidal action? J Leukoc Biol. 2001; 69: 414-8.
[28] Caldefie-Chezet F, Poulin A, Vasson MP. Leptin regulates functional capacities of polymorphonuclear neutrophils. Free Radic Res. 2003; 37: 809-14.
[29] Tian Z, Sun R, Wei H, Gao B. Impaired natural killer (NK) cell activity in leptin receptor deficient mice: leptin as a critical regulator in NK cell development and activation. Biochem Biophys Res Commun. 2002; 298: 297-302.
[30] Lam, Q. L. K., Liu, S., Cao, X. and Lu, L., Involvement of leptin signaling in the survival and maturation of bone marrow-derived dendritic cells. Eur. J. Immunol. 2006. 36(12): 3118-3130.
[31] Farooqi IS, Matarese G, Lord GM, et al. Beneficial effects of leptin on obesity, T cell hyporesponsiveness, and neuroendocrine/metabolic dysfunction of human congenital leptin deficiency. J Clin Invest. 2002;110: 1093-103.
[32] Lord GM, Matarese G, Howard JK, Baker RJ, Bloom SR, Lechler RI. Leptin modulates the T-cell immune response and reverses starvation-induced immunosuppression. Nature. 1998; 394: 897-901.
[33] Howard JK, Lord GM, Matarese G, et al. Leptin protects mice from starvation-induced lymphoid atrophy and increases thymic cellularity in ob/ob mice. J Clin Invest. 1999; 104: 1051-9.
[34] Ruter J, Hoffmann T, Demuth HU, Moschansky P, Klapp BF, Hildebrandt M. Evidence for an interaction between leptin, T cell costimulatory antigens CD28, CTLA-4 and CD26 (dipeptidyl peptidase IV) in BCG-induced immune responses of leptin- and leptin receptor-deficient mice. Biol Chem. 2004; 385:537-41.

[35] Sanna V, Di Giacomo A, La Cava A, et al. Leptin surge precedes onset of autoimmune encephalomyelitis and correlates with development of pathogenic T cell responses. J Clin Invest. 2003; 111: 241-50

[36] Faggioni R, Feingold KR, Grunfeld C. Leptin regulation of the immune response and the immunodeficiency of malnutrition. FASEB J. 2001; 14: 2565-71.

[37] Faggioni R, Fantuzzi G, Gabay C, et al. Leptin deficiency enhances sensitivity to endotoxin-induced lethality. Am J Physiol. 1999; 276: 136-42

[38] Williams L, Bradley L, Smith A, Foxwell B. Signal transducer and activator of transcription 3 is the dominant mediator of the anti-inflammatory effects of IL-10 in human macrophages. J Immunol. 2004; 172: 567-76.

[39] Busso N, So A, Chobaz-Peclat V, et al. Leptin signaling deficiency impairs humoral and cellular immune responses and attenuates experimental arthritis. J Immunol. 2002; 168: 875-82

[40] Siegmund B, Sennello JA, Jones-Carson J, et al. Leptin receptor expression on T lymphocytes modulates chronic intestinal inflammation in mice. Gut. 2004; 53: 965-72.

[41] Barbier M, Cherbut C, Aube AC, Blottiere HM, Galmiche JP. Elevated plasma leptin concentrations in early stages of experimental intestinal inflammation in rats. Gut 1998; 43: 783-790

[42] Tuzun A, Uygun A, Yesilova Z, et al. Leptin levels in the acute stage of ulcerative colitis. J Gastroenterol Hepatol. 2004; 19:429-32

[43] Matarese G, Carrieri PB, La Cava A, et al. Leptin increase in multiple sclerosis associates with reduced number of CD4(+)CD25+ regulatory T cells. Proc Natl Acad Sci. 2005; 102: 5150-5

[44] Matarese G, Di Giacomo A, Sanna V, et al. Requirement for leptin in the induction and progression of autoimmune encephalomyelitis. J Immunol. 2001; 166: 5909-16

[45] Fantuzzi G, Sennello JA, Batra A, et al. Defining the role of T cell-derived leptin in the modulation of hepatic or intestinal inflammation in mice. Clin Exp Immunol. 2005; 142: 31-8

[46] Matarese G, Sanna V, Lechler RI, et al. Leptin accelerates autoimmune diabetes in female NOD mice. Diabetes. 2002; 51: 1356-61

[47] Palmer G, Aurrand-Lions M, Contassot E, Talabot-Ayer D, Ducrest-Gay D, Vesin C, Chobaz-Peclat V, Busso N, Gabay C. Indirect effects of leptin receptor deficiency on lymphocyte populations and immune response in db/db mice. J Immunol. 2006 Sep 1;177(5):2899-907.

[48] Canavan B, Salem RO, Schurgin S, et al. Effects of physiological leptin administration on markers of inflammation, platelet activation, and platelet aggregation during caloric deprivation. J Clin Endocrinol Metab. 2005; 90: 5779-85.

[49] Sennello J.A,, Fayad R., Morris A.M., et al. Regulation of T cell-mediated hepatic inflammation by adiponectin and leptin. Endocrinology. 2005; 146: 2157-64

[50] Fraser DA, Thoen J, Reseland JE, Forre O, Kjeldsen-Kragh J. Decreased CD4+ lymphocyte activation and increased interleukin-4 production in peripheral blood of rheumatoid arthritis patients after acute starvation. Clin Rheumatol 1999; 18: 394–401.

[51] Otero M, Lago R, Gomez R, Lago F, Dieguez C, Gomez-Reino JJ, Gualillo O. Changes in fat-derived hormones plasma concentrations: adiponectin, leptin, resistin and visfatin in rheumatoid arthritis subjects. Ann Rheum Dis. 65(9):1198-201

[52] Bokarewa M, Bokarew D, Hultgren O, Tarkowski A. Leptin consumption in the inflamed joints of patients with rheumatoid arthritis. Ann Rheum Dis 2003; 62: 952–6

[53] Goldring MB. The role of the chondrocyte in osteoarthritis. Arthritis Rheum. 2000; 43: 1916-26.

[54] Goldring MB, Berenbaum F. The regulation of chondrocyte function by proinflammatory mediators: prostaglandins and nitric oxide. Clin Orthop Relat Res. 2004; 427: 37-46

[55] Dumond H, Presle N, Terlain, B, et al. Evidence for a key role of leptin in osteoarthritis. Arthritis Rheum. 2003; 48: 3118-29.

[56] Teichtahl AJ, Wluka AE, Proietto J, Cicuttini FM. Obesity and the female sex, risk factors for knee osteoarthritis that may be attributable to systemic or local leptin biosynthesis and its cellular effects. Med Hypotheses. 2005; 65: 312-5.

[57] Otero M, Gomez Reino JJ, Gualillo O. Synergistic induction of nitric oxide synthase type II: in vitro effect of leptin and interferon-gamma in human chondrocytes and ATDC5 chondrogenic cells. Arthritis Rheum. 2003; 48: 404-9.

[58] Otero M, Lago R, Lago F, Reino JJ, Gualillo O. Signalling pathway involved in nitric oxide synthase type II activation in chondrocytes: synergistic effect of leptin with interleukin-1. Arthritis Res Ther. 2005; 7: 581-591.

[59] Kadowaki T, Yamauchi T, Kubota N, Hara K, Ueki K, Tobe K. Adiponectin and adiponectin receptors in insulin resistance, diabetes, and the metabolic syndrome.J Clin Invest. 2006; 116(7):1784-1792.

[60] Ronti T, Lupattelli G, Mannarino E, The endocrine role of adipose tissue: an update. Clin Endocrinol 2006; 64:355-365.

[61] Berg AH, Scherer PE. Adipose tissue, inflammation, and cardiovascular disease.Circ Res. 2005; 96(9):939-49.

[62] Whitehead JP, Richards AA, Hickman IJ, MacDonald GA, Prins JB. Adiponectin, a key adipokine in the metabolic syndrome. Diabetes, Obesity and Metabolism 2006; 8:264-280.

[63] Kadowaki T, Yamauchi T. Adiponectin and adiponectin receptors. Endocrine Rev 2005 26: 439-451.

[64] Tan KC, Xu C, Chow WS, Lam MC, Ai VH, Tam SC, Lam KS. Hypoadiponectinemia is associated with impaired endothelium-dependent vasodilation. J Clin Endocrinol Metab 2004; 89: 765-760.

[65] Fasshuer M, Kralish S, Klier M, Lossner U, Bluher M, Klein J,Paschke R. Adiponectin gene expression and secretion is inhibited by IL-6 in 3T3-L1 adipocytes. Biochem Biophys Res Comm 2003; 301:1045-1050.

[66] Bruun JM, Lihn AS, Verdich C, Pedersen SB, Toubro S, Astrup A, Richelsen B. Regulation of adiponectin by adipose tissue derived cytokines: in vivo and in vitro investigations in humans. Am J Physiol Endocrinol Metab, 2003; 285: E527-E533.

[67] Takemura Y, Ouchi N, Shibata R, Aprahamian T, Kirber MT, Summer RS, Kihara S, and Walsh K. Adiponectin modulates inflammatory reactions via calreticulin

receptor–dependent clearance of early apoptotic bodies. J Clin Invest .Published January 25, 2007. 10.1172/JCI29709

[68] Maeda N, Takahashi M, Funahashi T, Kihara S, Nishizawa H, Kishida K,Nagaretani H, Matsuda M, Komuro R, Ouchi N, Kuriyama H, Hotta K, Nakamura T,Shimomura I, Matsuzawa Y. PPARgamma ligands increase expression and plasma concentrations of adiponectin, an adipose-derived protein.Diabetes. 2001; 50(9):2094-9.

[69] Funahashi T, Nakamura T, Shimomura I, Maeda K, Kuriyama H, Takahashi M, Arita Y, Kihara S, Matsuzawa Y. Role of adipocytokines on the pathogenesis of atherosclerosis in visceral obesity. Intern Med. 1999; 38(2):202-6.

[70] Pischon T, Girman CJ, Hotamisligil GS, Rifai N, Hu FB, Rimm EB. Plasma adiponectin levels and risk of myocardial infarction in men. JAMA. 2004; 291(14):1730-7.

[71] Ehling A, Schaffler A, Herfarth H, Tarner IH, Anders S, Distler O, Paul G, Distler J, Gay S, Scholmerich J, Neumann E, Muller-Ladner U. The potential of adiponectin in driving arthritis. J Immunol. 2006;176(7):4468-78.S

[72] Schaffler A, Ehling A, Neumann E, Herfarth H, Paul G, Tarner I, et al. Adipocytokines in synovial fluid. JAMA 2003; 290:1709–10.

[73] Fantuzzi G. Adipose tissue, adipokines, and inflammation. J Allergy Clin Immunol, 2005; 115 (5): 911-919.

[74] Xu A, Wang Y, Keshaw H, Xu LY, Lam KS, Cooper GJ. The fat-derived hormone adiponectin alleviates alcoholic and nonalcoholic fatty liver diseases in mice.J Clin Invest. 2003; 112(1):91-100.

[75] Kamada Y, Tamura S, Kiso S, Matsumoto H, Saji Y, Yoshida Y, Fukui K, Maeda N, Nishizawa H, Nagaretani H, Okamoto Y, Kihara S, Miyagawa J, Shinomura Y,Funahashi T, Matsuzawa Y. Enhanced carbon tetrachloride-induced liver fibrosis in mice lacking adiponectin. Gastroenterology. 2003; 125(6):1796-807

[76] Masaki T, Chiba S, Tatsukawa H, Yasuda T, Noguchi H, Seike M, Yoshimatsu H. Adiponectin protects LPS-induced liver injury through modulation of TNF-alpha in KK-Ay obese mice. Hepatology. 2004; 40(1):177-84.

[77] Housa D, Housova J, Vernerova Z, Haluzik M. Adipocytokines and cancer.Physiol Res. 2006; 55(3):233-44.

[78] Kato H, Kashiwagi H, Shiraga M, Tadokoro S, Kamae T, Ujiie H, Honda S,Miyata S, Ijiri Y, Yamamoto J, Maeda N, Funahashi T, Kurata Y, Shimomura I,Tomiyama Y, Kanakura Y. Adiponectin acts as an endogenous antithrombotic factor. Arterioscler Thromb Vasc Biol. 2006; 26(1):224-30.

[79] Holcomb IN, Kabakoff RC, Chan B, Baker TW, Gurney A, Henzel W, Nelson C, Lowman HB, Wright BD, Skelton NJ, Frantz GD, Tumas DB, Peale FV Jr, Shelton DL, Hebert CC. FIZZ1, a novel cysteine-rich secreted protein associated with pulmonary inflammation, defines a new gene family. EMBO J. 2000; 19(15):4046-55

[80] Rajala MW, Obici S, Scherer PE, Rossetti L. Adipose-derived resistin and gut-derived resistin-like molecule-beta selectively impair insulin action on glucose production. J Clin Invest. 2003;111(2):225-30.

[81] Gerstmayer B, Kusters D, Gebel S, Muller T, Van Miert E, Hofmann K, Bosio A. Identification of RELM gamma, a novel resistin-like molecule with a distinct expression pattern. Genomics. 2003; 81(6):588-95.

[82] Koerner A, Kratzsch J, Kiess W. Adipocytokines: leptin-the classical. Resistin- the controversical, adiponectin-the promising, and more to come. Best Pract Res Clin Endocrinol Metab 2005; 19: 525-546.
[83] Steppan CM, Bailey ST, Bhat S, Brown EJ, Banerjee RR, Wright CM, Patel HR, Ahima RS, Lazar MA. The hormone resistin links obesity to diabetes. Nature. 2001; 409(6818):307-12.
[84] Pang S, Le Y. Role of Resistin in inflammation and inflammation related diseases. Cell Mol Immunol, 2006; 3(1):29-34
[85] Bokarewa M, Nagaev I, Dahlberg L, Smith U, Tarkowski A. Resistin, an adipokine with potent proinflammatory properties. J Immunol. 2005; 174(9):5789-95.
[86] Lehrke M, Reilly MP, Millington SC, Iqbal N, Rader DJ, Lazar MA. An inflammatory cascade leading to hyperresistinemia in humans. PLoS Med. 2004; 1(2):e45.
[87] Harsch IA, Koebnick C, Wallaschofski H, Schahin SP, Hahn EG, Ficker JH,Lohmann T, Konturek PC. Resistin levels in patients with obstructive sleep apnoea syndrome--the link to subclinical inflammation? Med Sci Monit. 2004; 10(9):CR510-5.
[88] Reilly MP, Lehrke M, Wolfe ML, Rohatgi A, Lazar MA, Rader DJ. Resistin is an inflammatory marker of atherosclerosis in humans. Circulation. 2005; 111(7):932-9.
[89] Verma S, Li SH, Wang CH, Fedak PW, Li RK, Weisel RD, Mickle DA. Resistin promotes endothelial cell activation: further evidence of adipokine-endothelial interaction. Circulation. 2003; 108(6):736-40.
[90] Kawanami D, Maemura K, Takeda N, Harada T, Nojiri T, Imai Y, Manabe I, Utsunomiya K, Nagai R. Direct reciprocal effects of resistin and adiponectin on vascular endothelial cells: a new insight into adipocytokine-endothelial cell interactions. Biochem Biophys Res Commun. 2004; 314(2):415-9
[91] Burnett MS, Lee CW, Kinnaird TD, Stabile E, Durrani S, Dullum MK, Devaney JM, Fishman C, Stamou S, Canos D, Zbinden S, Clavijo LC, Jang GJ, Andrews JA,Zhu J, Epstein SE. The potential role of resistin in atherogenesis. Atherosclerosis.2005; 182(2):241-8.
[92] Senolt L, Housa D, Vernerova Z, Jirasek T, Svobodova R, Veigl D, Anderlova K, Muller-Ladner U, Pavelka K, Haluzik M. Resistin is abundantly present in rheumatoid arthritis synovial tissue,synovial fluid, and elevated serum resistin reflects disease activity. Ann Rheum Dis. 2006; [Epub ahead of print].
[93] Schaffler A, Ehling A, Neumann E, Herfarth H, Tarner I, Scholmerich J,Muller-Ladner U, Gay S. Adipocytokines in synovial fluid. JAMA. 2003; 290(13):1709-10.
[94] Fukuhara A, Matsuda M, Nishizawa M, Segawa K, Tanaka M, Kishimoto K, Matsuki Y, Murakami M, Ichisaka T, Murakami H, Watanabe E, Takagi T, Akiyoshi M, Ohtsubo T, Kihara S, Yamashita S, Makishima M, Funahashi T, Yamanaka S, Hiramatsu R,Matsuzawa Y, Shimomura I. Visfatin: a protein secreted by visceral fat that mimics the effects of insulin. Science. 2005; 307(5708):426-30.
[95] Jia SH, Li Y, Parodo J, Kapus A, Fan L, Rotstein OD, Marshall JC. Pre-B cell colony-enhancing factor inhibits neutrophil apoptosis in experimental inflammation and clinical sepsis. J Clin Invest. 2004; 113(9):1318-27.
[96] Moschen AR, Kaser A, Enrich B, Mosheimer B, Theurl M, Niederegger H, Tilg H.Visfatin, an adipocytokine with proinflammatory and immunomodulating properties.J Immunol. 2007 Feb 1; 178(3):1748-58.

[97] Tatemoto, K., Hosoya, M., Habata, Y., Fujii, R., Kakegawa, T., Zou, M. X., Kawamata, Y., Fukusumi, S., Hinuma, S., Kitada, C., et al., Isolation and characterization of a novel endogenous peptide ligand for the human APJ receptor. Biochem. Biophys. Res. Commun.1998; 251,471-476.

[98] Boucher, J., Masri, B., Daviaud, D., Gesta, S., Guigné, C., Mazzucotelli, A., Castan-Laurell, I., Tack, I., Knibiehler, B., Carpene, C., Audigier, Y., Saulnier-Blache, J. S., Valet, P. Apelin, a newly identified adipokine up-regulated by insulin and obesity. Endocrinology 2005; 146,1764-1771.

[99] Daviaud D, Boucher J, Gesta S, Dray C, Guigne C, Quilliot D, Ayav A, Ziegler O, Carpene C, Saulnier-Blache JS, Valet P, Castan-Laurell I. TNFalpha up-regulates apelin expression in human and mouse adipose tissue. FASEB J. 2006; 20(9):1528-30.

[100] Heinonen, M. V., Purhonen, A. K., Miettinen, P., Paakkonen, M., Pirinen, E., Alhava, E., Akerman, K., Herzig, K. H. Apelin, orexin-A and leptin plasma levels in morbid obesity and effect of gastric banding. Regul. Pept. 2005; 130:7-13.

[101] Xu, H., Barnes, G. T., Yang, Q., Tan, G., Yang, D., Chou, C. J., Sole, J., Nichols, A., Ross, J. S., Tartaglia, L. A., Chen, H. Chronic inflammation in fat plays a crucial role in the development of obesity-related insulin resistance. J. Clin. Invest. 2003; 112:1821-1830.

[102] K. Hida, J. Wada, J. Eguchi, H. Zhang, M. Baba, A. Seida, I. Hashimoto, T. Okada, A. Yasuhara, A. Nakatsuka, K. Shikata, S. Hourai, J. Futami, E. Watanabe, Y. Matsuki, R. Hiramatsu, S. Akagi, H. Makino and Y.S. Kanwar, Visceral adipose tissue-derived serine protease inhibitor: a unique insulin-sensitizing adipocytokine in obesity, Proc. Natl. Acad. Sci. USA 2005; 102: 10610–10615.

[103] Kloting N, Berndt J, Kralisch S, Kovacs P, Fasshauer M, Schon MR, Stumvoll M, Bluher M. Vaspin gene expression in human adipose tissue: association with obesity and type 2 diabetes.Biochem Biophys Res Commun. 2006; 339(1):430-6.

3

Glucokinase as a Glucose Sensor in Hypothalamus - Regulation by Orexigenic and Anorexigenic Peptides

Carmen Sanz, Isabel Roncero, Elvira Alvarez,
Verónica Hurtado and Enrique Blázquez
University Complutense of Madrid. Medical School and CIBERDEM,
Department of Cellular Biology and Department of Biochemistry and Molecular Biology,
Spain

1. Introduction

Glucose homeostasis requires hormonal and neural mechanisms in an attempt to get a normal functioning of the brain and of peripheral tissues. Blood glucose levels must be maintained within a physiological range depending of feeding and hormonal status, having the alterations of normoglycemic levels deleterious consequences. Hypothalamus plays a major role on feeding behaviour and energy homeostasis. It contains the called "satiety centre" and "hunger centre" located in ventromedial (VMH) and lateral hypothalamus (LH) respectively. These brain areas, besides others, may be altered by metabolic signals, such as changes in the electrical activity of neurons by direct application of glucose or by modifications of blood glucose levels. In this regard, glucose activates or inhibits neuronal activity, and both responses suggest the presence of glucose sensors in these brain areas.

Glucose sensors are molecular designs responsible for detecting and measuring glucose concentrations in the extracellular space. Thus, glucose sensor are presents in gut, endocrine pancreatic cells, portal vein, central nervous system and rare neuroendocrine cells, and they are responsible to avoid marked blood glucose oscillations, which permit to maintain glucose homeostasis.

First evidence of the existence of a glucose sensor system was reported in pancreatic beta-cells (Matschinsky 1990), constituted by glucokinase (GK). GK catalyses glucose phosphorylation with low afffinity and it is not inhibited by its product (glucose-6-phosphate), which allows increased glucose utilization as its concentration rises. Due to GK properties, the glucose catabolism rate is proportional to glucose levels in the extracellular space and for that reason GK is the major contributor to glucose sense, since catalyses the rate-limiting step of glucose catabolism. Interestingly, glucose transporter isoform 2 (GLUT-2) also with a high Km for glucose transport, has a different role since glucose transport occurs in both directions of the beta-cell membrane and glucose transport is 100-fold higher that the rates of glucose metabolism.

Our previous findings (Alvarez et al., 1996; Navarro et al., 1996) indicating the presence of GK together with GLUT-2 and glucagon-like peptide-1 receptor (GLP-1R) in the same cells

of hypothalamic areas implied in the control of feeding behaviour, suggest that a glucose sensor system may be present in those structures as discussed in the section 3.
GLP-1, together with others peptides, such as leptin, insulin, GLP-2, are anorexigenic peptides that acts in hypothalamic areas contributing to generate a state of satiety. By the contrary peptides orexigenic such as neuropeptide Y (NPY), orexin, galanin, ghrelin, etc, contribute to increase food intake. These effects may be the results of an accurate molecular crosstalk between the cells which secrete these peptides and the glucose sensing cells.
The importance of GK in the hypothalamic glucose sensing and its relation with anorexigenic and orexigenic peptides are discussed in this chapter.

2. Brain glucose sensor

Glucose is needed as an energy substrate but also as a signaling molecule in several processes. Glucoregulatory mechanisms are of primary functional concern to provide a continued glucose supply to the central neurons system and to face metabolic needs of peripheral tissues. Alterations of normoglycemic levels have deleterious consequences that increase the morbidity and mortality rates of the population.
In the 1950´s, the glucostatic hypothesis (Mayer 1953) postulated that glucose receptors exist in the hypothalamus and possibly in other central and peripheral regions involved in the regulation of food intake. Thus, glucose balance should be tightly regulated and taking into account the pancreatic glucose sensor concept, it would be reasonable to suggest the existence of a similar system in the brain that might modulate feeding behaviour and the release of counteregulatory hormones that defend against hypoglycemia. We proposed (Alvarez et al., 1996; Navarro et al., 1996) that the hypothalamus senses plasma glucose levels in a similar fashion to beta-cells, causing changes in the expression and secretion of neuropeptides (Yang et al., 2004). Our findings indicated that GK mRNA and protein are coexpressed together with GLUT-2 in the hypothalamus of human and experimental animals, mainly in areas involved in the control of food intake such as VMH and LH (Navarro et al., 1996; Roncero et al., 2000). Taking into account these studies, it have been addressed central role of GK as glucose sensor, reinforced by GLUT-2, the K^{+}_{ATP} channel subunits SUR1 and SUR2, as well as Kir6.2, in central glucose sensing (Jordan et al., 2010).
By analogy with the beta-cell, the general idea is that the glucose metabolism and variations in ratio ATP/ADP are the keys for neural sensing of glucose. However the ATP metabolism is a general mechanism for any electrical response, while neurons produce specific electrical responses. Others authors have proposed relationship between neuronal glucose-sensing and electrical responses (Figure 1). These hypothesis include electrogenic glucose entry, the existence of specific non-transporting detectors of extracellular glucose or glucose receptors and the possibility that glial cells would be responsible of glucose changes detection.
An example of electrogenic glucose entry to neuron is the mediated by the sodium-glucose co-transporters (SGLTs), where glucose is directly coupled to Na^{+} ion movement. That entry is directly conditioned by extracellular glucose concentration. This mechanism is used in the secretion of GLP-1 by intestinal cells in response to glucose (Gribble et al., 2003) and in the excitability of glucose-response neurons of VMH and arcuate nucleus (ARC) (Yang et al., 1999) that will comment below.
Diez-Sampedro suggest the existence of a "glucose receptor" that mediates the changes in electrical activitiy (Diez-Sampedro et al., 2003). Thus, in some peripheral neurons, have been identified a glucose transporter protein (SGLT3/SLC5A4) that not transport glucose into the

cell, instead, this protein acted as a sensing receptor, converting elevations of extracellular glucose into Na^+-dependent depolarization of the membrane (Figure 1).
An additional hypothesis (Pellerin & Magistretti 2004) is that astrocytes could be the primary physiological detectors of extracellular glucose changes. This model proposed that rise in extracellular glucose induce glial lactate production which is transported from glia and into the neurons by lactate transporter (MCT1) and trigger the depolarization and excitation of neurons by closing the K^+_{ATP} channels (Burdakov & Ashcroft 2002) (Figure 1).

2.1 Glucose-inhibited (GI) and glucose-excited (GE) neurons

Claude Bernard showed the earliest evidence that the brain is involved in glycemic control since the lesion of the hypothalamus in dog, induced hyperglycemia (Bernard 1849). Later, Jean Mayer (Mayer 1953) proposed that hypothalamic cells could monitor plasma glucose variations and postulated that these cells transduced variations of glucose concentrations into electrical or chemical signals that control feeding behavior. Electrophysiological studies carried out in hypothalamic slices, demonstrated the existence of neurons able to modulate their firing activity in response to changes in extracellular glucose levels (Anand et al., 1964). These are glucose-excited (GE; previously called glucose-responsive) neurons, which increase their firing rate with elevation of glucose concentrations in extracellular, or glucose-inhibited (GI; previously called glucose-sensitive) neurons, which are activated by a decrease in extracellular glucose concentration or by cellular glucoprivation (Routh 2002; Yang et al., 2004).

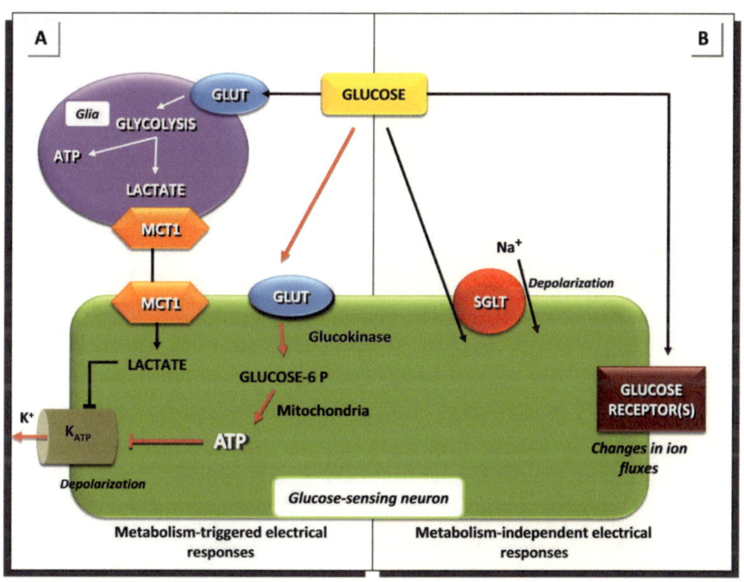

Fig. 1. Signalling pathways proposed to be involved in glucose sensing by hypothalamic neurons. A) Signalling pathways of glucose-metabolism-triggered electrical responses for neural sensing of glucose. Red lines indicate the canonical pathways share with beta-cell. Other signalling pathways could be mediate by previous glucose metabolization to lactate by glial cells. B) Pathways that triggers glucose metabolism-independent electrical responses. These pathways involved electrogenic glucose entry through sodium-glucose cotransporters (SGLT) or the presence of glucose receptors

Although both types of neurons are widely distributed in the brain, they are highly present in regions involved in the control of energy homeostasis and food intake such as hypothalamic nuclei and the brain stem (Adachi et al., 1995). Additionally it has been recently reported a novel glucose-sensing region in the medial amygdalar nucleus (Zhou et al., 2010).

The existence of glucose-regulated neurons has been studied by intravenous or intracerebroventricular injections of 2-deoxyglucose or 5-thio-glucose and posterior electrophysiological recordings or by the detection c-fos-like immunoreactivity (which is highly expressed in activated neurons). Using these approaches, responsive neurons have been found in the VMH, paraventricular (PVN) and LH, ARC, parabrachial nucleus (PBN), nucleus tractus solitarius (NTS), area postrema (AP), dorsal motor nucleus of the vagus (DMNX), and the region of the basolateral medulla (BLM) (Ritter & Dinh 1994; Dallaporta et al., 1999).

2.2 Electrophysiological pattern

Diverse signalling pathways are involved in the modulation of the electrical activity of hypothalamic neurons by glucose. On the one hand, glucose could alter neuronal electrical activity acting as energy substrate by influencing energy metabolism inside neuron and glia cells (Figure 1). On the other hand glucose could be considerer as an extracellular signalling messenger that could trigger specific glucose receptors controlling the membrane ion fluxes. Other possibility could be that glucose itself can be transported by electrogenic transporters (Figure 1). Which of these general mechanisms is dominant in different glucose-sensing neurons remains to be determined.

The mechanisms regulating GE cells have been more thoroughly understood and were assumed to employ a beta-cell glucosensing strategy. Thus, glucose enters the beta-cell via GLUT-2, facilitating its diffusion down a concentration gradient. Then GK phosphorylates glucose allowing for its entry into the glycolytic pathway that leads to an increase in the ATP. The consequent increase in the cytosolic ATP/ADP concentration ratio then closes the K^+_{ATP} channels. In the beta-cell, these channels are made up of Kir6.2/SUR1 subunits (Ashcroft & Rorsman 2004). Since open K^+_{ATP} channels generate hyperpolarization of the beta-cell and so dampen its excitability, their closure results in decreasing potassium outflow and depolarization with increased electrical activity. Actually, GK are the key glucose-sensing features of this scheme because they ensure that changes in extracellular glucose levels within the physiological range are converted to proportional changes in electrical excitability. This is due to the low affinity for glucose of GK, unlike the more ubiquitously expressed hexokinase I, and that GK is not inhibited by its product, glucose-6-phosphate.

The functional importance of GK in GE neurons was studied by pharmacological inhibition which decreased neuronal activity. *In vitro* studies on primary VMH cultures have shown that selective downregulation of GK leads to selective loss of glucose sensing and a decrease in cellular ATP concentration corresponding with an increase in K^+_{ATP} channel activation (Dunn-Meynell et al., 2002; Kang et al., 2006). This supports the model that inhibition of GK, in at least a proportion of GE neurons, reduces ATP production causing K^+_{ATP} channel opening and cell hyperpolarization. Recent findings indicate that although elements of canonical model used in beta-cell, are functional in some hypothalamic cells, this pathway is not universally essential for excitation of glucose-sensing neurons by glucose. In rats and humans, the expression of GLUT-2, GK (Navarro et al., 1996; Roncero et al., 2000) and Kir6.2 was found in some but not all GE neurons (Kang et al., 2004) and were also present in non-glucose-sensing neurons (Lynch et al., 2000). For example, glucose-induced excitation of ARC neurons was recently reported in mice lacking Kir6.2, and no significant increases in cytosolic ATP levels could be detected in hypothalamic neurons after changes in extracellular glucose. Thus, the molecular support for the idea that all GE neurons rely on the beta-cell tools to sense glucose is currently inconclusive and possible alternative glucose-sensing strategies could include electrogenic glucose entry, glucose-induced release of glial lactate, and extracellular glucose receptors (Pellerin & Magistretti 2004; Burdakov et al., 2005).

Much less is known about GI neurons and whether these neurons follow the same glucose sensing strategy remains unclear (Burdakov & Lesage 2010). It has been proposed to involve reduction in the depolarizing activity of the Na^+/K^+ pump, or activation of a hyperpolarizing Cl^- current. Although it has been suggested that the metabolic model of glucose sensing applies to GI neurons, there is convincing evidence for metabolism-independent neuronal glucose sensing in GI neurons. As it has been mentioned, Kang group's (Kang et al., 2004) showed that some but not all glucose sensing neurons of the VMN express GK and SUR1, suggesting that other regulatory mechanisms must control glucose sensing in some of these neurons. Furthermore, Gonzalez et al (Gonzalez et al., 2009), used direct electrophysiological measurements of glucose sensing orexin neurons to show that metabolism independent glucose sensing exists in GI neurons. They found that GK inhibitors do not block glucose sensing in these neurons. However, despite the evidence for metabolism-independent as well as dependent glucose sensing mechanisms, the nature of the glucose sensing machinery in GI neurons remains unclear.

2.3 Hypothalamic distribution of GE and GI neurons

Hypothalamic glucose-sensing neurons comprise subgroups of cells in PVN, LH, ARC, VMH hypothalamic regions, and can be either electrically inhibited or excited by elevations in extracellular glucose (Anand et al., 1964; Oomura et al., 1969; Routh 2002; Wang et al., 2004). The distribution of GE glucose response neurons in the hypothalamus are confinated mostly to the VMH, ARC, and PVN (Dunn-Meynell et al., 1998; Silver & Erecinska 1998; Wang et al., 2004). However, GI neurons are found mainly in the LH (Oomura et al., 1974), median ARC, and PVN.

There are two major subpopulations of neurons in the ARC of the hypothalamus implicated in the control of feeding. One population contains pro-opiomelanocortin (POMC) and α-melanocyte-stimulating hormone (α-MSH) that are anorexigenic peptides and inhibits food intake. The second population of neurons contains agouti-related protein (AgRP) and neuropeptide Y (NPY) orexigenic peptides that stimulate food intake (Cone et al., 2001). GI neurons are present in the VMN in the ARC and in the LH and partly overlap with the orexigenic NPY/AgRP and possibly orexin neurons. GE neurons correspond in part to POMC neurons in the VMN and possibly in the ARC and POMC neurons in the LH (Mountjoy & Rutter 2007).

2.4 Effect of glucose concentrations on the brain glucose sensors

Some of the glucose-sensing neurons in the LH, ARC and VMH hypothalamic regions electrically respond to changes in glucose within the physiological ranges of glucose (Wang et al., 2004; Burdakov et al., 2005; Song & Routh 2005). As a general rule, the extracellular concentration of glucose in the brain is 10–30% of that in the blood (Silver & Erecinska 1998). During euglycemia, brain glucose levels are 0.7-2.5 mM, and may be reached 5mM under severe plasma hyperglycemia. On the other hand, plasma hypoglycaemia can cause the brain glucose to fall to 0.2-0.5 mM. Changes in plasma glucose corresponding to meal-to-meal fluctuation (about 5–8mM) (Silver & Erecinska 1994) lead to changes in glucose concentration in the brain that it is expected to be in the range between 1 and 2.5mM (Routh 2002). It is also noteworthy that glucose-sensing neurons located near regions with a reduced blood–brain barrier for example, the median eminence region that neighbors the hypothalamic ARC (Elmquist et al., 1999), may be exposed to a much higher glucose concentrations than other brain cells, even approaching those present in the plasma. If this is the case, for glucose-sensing neurons of the ARC, high glucose concentrations (greater than 5 mM) may well comprise a physiologically relevant stimulus (Fioramonti et al., 2004) . In this way, it has been described in the ARC, the presence of GE and GI neurons responsive to glucose over either a low (0–5 mM) or a high glucose concentration range (5–20 mM); the latter are referred to as high GE (HGE) or high GI (HGI) neurons, respectively (Fioramonti et al., 2004; Penicaud et al., 2006).

More details about the effect of glucose oscillations in the glucose sensor GK will be discussed in the section 4 of this chapter.

3. Glucokinase as part of a hypothalamic glucose sensor system

GK is a member of the hexokinase family (ATP:D-hexose 6-phosphotransferase, EC 2.7.1.1) that catalyses the phosphorylation of glucose to glucose 6-phosphate. Hexokinases I, II and III have a high affinity for glucose, with low Km (Michaelis constant) values in the micromolar range. GK or hexokinase type IV has a low affinity for glucose; it is not inhibited by physiological concentrations of glucose 6-phosphate, and has a molecular mass of about 50 kDa (Iynedjian 1993)

For years, the liver and the pancreatic islets were considered to be the only tissues in which GK activity could be detected. Later on, GK mRNAs of appropriate sizes were found in the corticotroph anterior pituitary cell line AtT-20, in rat pituitaries (Hughes et al., 1991) and in brain and intestine of the rat, but no enzyme activity was reported in neither (Jetton et al., 1994; Alvarez et al., 1996; Navarro et al., 1996). However, Roncero et al 2000 described that GK gene expression in rat brain gave rise to a protein of 52 kDa, with a high Km phosphorylating activity. Brain GK showed kinetic properties similar to those previously reported for the enzyme of hepatic or pancreatic islet origin. It has a high apparent Km for glucose (8.9–15 mM) and displays no product inhibition by glucose 6-phosphate. The contribution of GK to the total glucose phosphorylating activity was 40–19% in different cerebral regions, measured with a radiometric assay, and of 25–14% as determined by a spectrophotometric method.

The presence of tissue-specific promoters in the GK gen allows differential regulation. The upstream promoter, now rightly called neuro-endocrine promoter to distinguish it from the hepatic promoter (Iynedjian et al., 1996; Levin et al., 2004), is functional in beta-cells and in the brain (Magnuson & Shelton 1989; Roncero et al., 2000), while the downstream promoter is used only in liver . GK levels in beta-cells appear to be controlled by glucose, probably through a post-transcriptional mechanism (Iynedjian 1993; Matschinsky et al., 1993). In contrast, the liver-specific promoter is mainly affected by insulin and glucagon, which explains the extraordinary transcriptional regulation by the nutritional state (Iynedjian 1993).

The short-term regulation of GK activity involves several mechanisms: Long-chain fatty acyl-CoAs have been shown to be allosteric competitive inhibitors in vitro of the liver enzyme (Tippett & Neet 1982) and human beta-cell GK (Moukil et al., 2000). Glucose regulates the activity of GK through a "mnemonic" mechanism, which increases the activity of liver GK in the presence of high levels of glucose and decreases it when the glucose level is low (Cornish-Bowden & Storer 1986). GK activity in the liver is also regulated by the GK regulatory protein (GKRP), which behaves as a competitive inhibitor of GK. In the presence of fructose 6-phosphate GKRP binds to GK and inhibits its activity, whereas fructose 1-phosphate prevents the formation of the complex GKRP-GK (Van Schaftingen 1989). GKRP is not only a protein that binds and inactivates GK, but also regulates the translocation of GK between the cytoplasm and the nucleus. When glycogenolysis and/or gluconeogenesis are activated, the concentration of fructose 6-phosphate increases in the liver and produces the inhibition of GK, which facilitates the release of glucose by the liver. When carbohydrates are present in the diet, fructose is phosphorylated to fructose-1 phosphate, which favours glucose utilization by the liver (Agius & Peak 1993; Toyoda et al., 1995; Shiota et al., 1999). Thus, in the liver, the subcellular translocation of GK regulates the enzyme activity in accordance with the metabolic needs of the cells. It is therefore accepted that translocation of GK to the nucleus at low glucose concentrations needs GKRP as an anchoring protein that allows transport through the nuclear pore complex. However, it is unclear whether the nuclear export of GK requires GKRP. In pancreatic islets, GK activity may also be regulated by a protein, in a similar way to that described in hepatocytes (Malaisse et al., 1990).
Subsequent research has also identified several GK binding proteins that could act as cytoplasmic binding proteins. They include a dual-specificity protein phosphatase, the glucokinase-associated phosphatase (Munoz-Alonso et al., 2000), and the bifunctional enzyme 6-phosphofructo-2-kinase/fructose-2,6-bisphosphatase (Baltrusch et al., 2001). Other studies indicate that a minor fraction of GK and GKRP may be integrated in a multienzyme complex, including the pro-apoptotic protein BAD, and become associates with mitochondria in hepatocytes (Arden et al., 2006). These data suggest the existence of different pools of cytoplasmic GK with specialized metabolic functions (Arden et al., 2006). It has also been reported that AMP-activated protein kinase (AMPK) inhibits GK translocation from the nucleus.
In pancreatic beta-cells GK is considered to be a true glucose sensor (Matschinsky 1990) involved in glucose-dependent insulin release. The GK glucose sensor concept is supported by the fact that GK mutations are responsible for some types of maturity-onset diabetes of the young-2 (MODY-2) (Vionnet et al., 1992) and for persistent hyperinsulinaemic hypoglycaemia in infancy (PHHI) (Christesen et al., 2002). In addition, as noted above, targeted disruption of the GK gene in the beta-cells of mice produces severe alterations in insulin release (Grupe et al., 1995).

3.1 Expression, activity and localization of hypothalamic GK and glucokinase regulatory protein (GKRP) in the hypothalamus

Several brain areas, such as the LH and VMH and the dorsomedial medulla oblongata, including the NTS and the motor nucleus of the vagus, modulate glucose homeostasis in the liver and pancreas (Oomura & Yoshimatsu 1984). As previously cited, glucose is mainly excitatory in the VMH and inhibitory in the LH and NTS (Oomura & Yoshimatsu 1984), suggesting the presence of glucose sensors in neurons of these brain areas. Indeed, stimulation of glucoreceptors present in the neurons of the VMH, promotes the release of the counter-regulatory hormones, catecholamines and glucagon, which defend the organism against glucopenia (Borg et al., 1995).

Our findings, indicate that GLUT-2, GK and GLP-1R are expressed in the same cells of the rat and human hypothalamus (Alvarez et al., 1996) (Figure 2), and are located in areas involved in the regulation of energy homeostasis, feeding behaviour and glucose metabolism. It is noteworthy that in the brain, GLP-1 contributes to reducing food intake (Navarro et al., 1996; Turton et al., 1996), and the co-localization of those three components in hypothalamic neurons suggests that a glucose sensor system may be involved in the transduction of signals required to produce a state of satiety.

As we previously cited, GK activity may also be regulated by GKRP, acting in accordance with the metabolic needs of the cells (Van Schaftingen et al., 1984; Shiota et al., 1999; Roncero et al., 2004). Interestingly, we reported the coexpression of GK and GKRP in both rat and human brains (Roncero et al., 2000; Alvarez et al., 2002; Roncero et al., 2004), as well as GKRP interacting with GK in the presence of fructose-6-phosphate, which suggests that both are active and both may participate in the glucosensing process in the central nervous system (Alvarez et al., 2002).

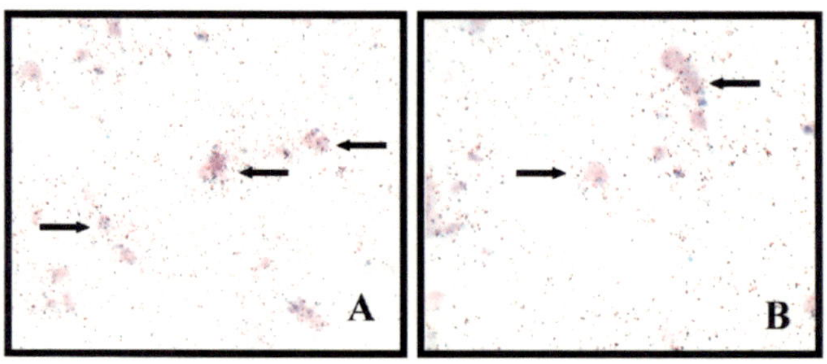

Fig. 2. In situ hybridization histochemistry of GLP-1R and GLUT-2 or GK mRNAs. **A** double-labeling of GLP-1R and GLUT-2 mRNAs in the VMH. **B** Double-labeling of GLP-1R and GK mRNAs in the VMH. Silver grains indicate the localization of either GLUT-2 or GK mRNAs. Blue reaction product indicates labelling of GLP-1R mRNAs. (Microphotographs suministrated by Dr. J. Chowen)

GK and GKRP have been found in foetal pancreas and liver (Vandercammen & Van Schaftingen 1993; Garcia-Flores et al., 2002). Also in foetal hypothalamus GK mRNA was present in day 18 of development (Sutherland et al., 2005). Our result concluded that GK and GKRP were functionally active before birth in the rat brain. Both proteins colocalised in the same cells of hypothalamus and the cerebral cortex of 21-day-old foetuses (F-21) (Roncero et al., 2009) (Figure 3).

The presence of GK mRNA was confirmed in approximately 50% of GE and GI neurons in the VMH. Some of these neurons also contained mRNAs for subunits of K^{+}_{ATP} channels (Kang et al., 2004). The use of specific small interfering RNA (siRNA) to knock-down GK in primary cultures of neurons from the rat VMH, abolished the responses to glucose (Kang et al., 2006). Together, these findings supported the idea that GK was the glucose sensor of at least a fraction of VMH neurons, functioning as the rate determining enzyme of glucose metabolism and controlling neuronal excitability. In the VMH, GK mRNA was shown to be expressed in neurons synthesizing POMC and NPY/AgRP, which play critical roles in neural pathways involved in the regulation of food intake and energy expenditure.

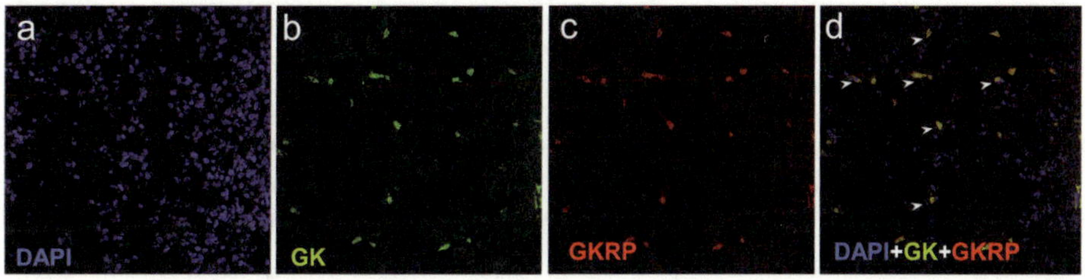

Fig. 3. GK and GKRP detection in the hypothalamus. Inmunofluorescent detection of GK (green b) or GKRP (red c) proteins in VMH from twenty-one-day old foetuses. Nuclear staining (a) was carried out in blue with 4,6-diamid-o-2-phenylindole (DAPI). The arrows (d) indicate the double positive cells for GK and GKRP.

4. Regulation of hypothalamic GK by glucose or regulatory peptides

The glucose-sensing neurons have receptors for orexigenic and anorexigenic neuropeptides that may modulate feeding behaviour through a glucose sensor system (Schuit et al., 2001).

The effects of orexigenic and anorexigenic peptides and glucose on GK gene expression were tested (Sanz et al., 2007) in GT1-7 immortalized hypothalamic neurons, which are glucose-sensing cells (Lee et al., 2005) able to respond to glucose deprivation or high-glucose levels, as well as having intrinsic GK activity. Neither the promoter activity of the GK gene in transfected GT1-7 cells nor the endogenous GK gene expression were modified by the action of different concentrations of glucose or GLP-1, leptin, or NPY in the extracellular space. However, GK enzyme activities were modified by these peptides.

Using hypothalamic slices in culture, instead cell line, which it is a better physiological model, the effect of glucose orexigenic and anorexigenic peptides on GK activities in VMH and LH areas were assayed. In the VMH there was a tendency for GK activities to increase as glucose rose in the extracellular media and high-GK activity was found at lower glucose concentrations in the LH. These findings could reflect a different type of behavior for the GE and GI neurons located in the VMH and the LH, when challenged by different concentrations of glucose. This would be in agreement with the tendency of GK activity to increase with rises in glucose in the range of 0.5–20 mM that was reported in the VMH (Sanz et al., 2007), while neurons in LH were not excited by the higher concentrations of glucose but by lower concentrations of this hexose, as happens with GK activities (Sanz et al., 2007). The observed changes in GK activity in response to glucose in certain hypothalamic areas suggest that such activity would not only be tissue-specific but also even cell-specific in defined brain areas. Interestingly, GK activities were thus significantly lower in LH than in VMH at high glucose concentrations, but this effect was reversed by the presence of insulin. This distinctive response observed in LH at high glucose may be related to different functional activities of these two areas, rather than to other kind of effects. The data obtained in these studies indicate a different response to glucose levels in the VMH and LH and also that some orexigenic and anorexigenic peptides might modulate GK activities in neurons of these areas. Additionally, it suggests that in most of the cases modifications of hypothalamic GK occur at the enzyme activity level rather than in transcriptional expression.

5. Role of hypothalamic GK on the control of feeding behaviour and body weight

Coexpression of GLUT-2, GK and GKRP in areas involved in feeding behaviour (Roncero et al., 2000; Roncero et al., 2004) might play a role in glucose sensing, in which GK and GKRP made possible a real sensor activity. Furthermore the effects of anorexigenic and orexigenic peptides through its receptors in this system should facilitate the transduction of signals required to produce a state of satiety. In fact, we have reported experimental evidences that GLP-1 is an anorexigenic peptide and controls the glucose metabolism in the human hypothalamus areas involved in the regulation of feeding behaviour (Alvarez et al., 2005) (Navarro et al., 1996).

5.1 Anorexigenic and orexigenic peptides

Early suggestions that hypothalamus plays a major role on feeding behaviour and energy homeostasis were obtained after brain lesion and stimulation studies. Remembering these observations, such as electrical stimulation of VMH suppress food intake and that bilateral lesions of these structures induce hyperphagia and obesity, VMH was named as the satiety centre, while alterations of LH induced the opposite set of responses and thus was called the hunger centre. Also, the dorsomedial medulla oblongata, including the NTS and the motor nucleus of the vagus, are implied in these processes. Now, we know the existence of specific subpopulations of neurons involved in energy homeostasis that are included in neuronal pathways with anorexigenic and orexigenic biomolecules (table 1), that generate integrated responses to afferent stimuli related to modifications in metabolites or in fuels storage.

The VMH is the responsible for integrating peripheral signals of nutrient status and adiposity. For example, the ARC contains neurons secreting the NPY and POMC. These neuropeptides have opposite effects on energy homeostasis, since NPY increases food intake and inhibit energy expenditure, while POMC exerts the contrary effects (Adage et al., 2001). Other studies suggest that some VMH neurons are GABAergic, although there is not a clear relationship to glucose-sensing capacity. More recent findings show that most VMH neurons express the protein steroidogenic factor-1 (SF-1) and that SF-1-positives neurons have key roles in glucose homeostasis (Tong et al., 2007; Tsuneki et al., 2010). The LH cells contain the peptides orexins/hypocretins, which are not expressed anywhere else in the brain (de Lecea et al., 1998; Sakurai et al., 1998). Lack of orexin/hypocretin produces hypophagia and late onset obesity among others effects (Hara et al., 2001).

A number of peptidic hormones, previously thought to be specific to the gastroenteropancreatic system and later found also in the mammalian brain, have been shown to modulate appetite, energy, and body weight. They play these physiological effects together with other biomolecules such as NPY, opioid peptides, galanin, vasopressin, and GHRH (Bray 1992). Thus, feeding behaviour is controlled by the antagonist effects of anorexigenic and orexigenic biomolecules. The complex mechanisms underlying the abundance of such variety of feeding behaviour-modulating substances can be understood on the basis of, the specific role for each molecule as a regulatory mechanism in energy balance status, the specifity of macronutrient intake (carbohydrate, fat or proteins) and meal size control, and the shifts in feeding behaviour related to hormonal status, gender, age, and circadian rhythms (Leibowitz 1992).

It is accepted that cells of several hypothalamic nuclei detect circulating satiety signals and transmit this information to other brain areas. Anorexigenic and orexigenic biomolecules are located in VMH, LH, PVN and ARC interacting one to others in a way that they may induce a characteristic feeding behaviour. Thus, peptide Y (Y3-36) is released from gastrointestinal tract postprandially, and acts on NPY Y_2 receptor in the ARC to inhibit feeding with a "long-term" effect (Batterham et al., 2002). On the contrary, other satiety signals induced by gut-brain peptides such as GLP-1, GLP-2 and CCK produced (Navarro et al., 1996; Turton et al., 1996; Rodriquez de Fonseca et al., 2000; Tang-Christensen et al., 2000) a "short-term" effect, while insulin and leptin (Batterham et al., 2002) inhibit the appetite by increasing the formation of POMC and reducing NPY action. In addition, ghrelin a peptide released by the stomach is stimulated before the meals to facilitate NPY action (Coiro et al., 2006).

ANOREXIGENIC		OREXIGENIC
CART	Leptin	AGRP
CCK	α-MSH	Galanin
CRH	Neurotensin	Ghrelin
GLP-1	Oxytocin	MCH
GHRH	Pro-opiomelanocortin	Noradrenaline
GLP-2	Peptide Y (Y 3-36)	NPY
IL-1β	TRH	Opioid peptides
Insulin	Serotonin	Orexin A and B
	Urocortin	

Table 1. Anorexigenic and orexigenic biomolecules implied in the control of feeding behaviour.

Intracerebroventricular or subcutaneous administration of GLP-1 produced a marked reduction of food intake and water ingestion. Exendin-4, proved to be a potent agonist of GLP-1R also decreased both food and water intake in a dose-dependent manner, while exendin (9-39) considered as an antagonist of the GLP-1R, reversed the inhibitory effects of GLP-1 or exendin-4 (Navarro et al., 1996; Turton et al., 1996; Rodriguez de Fonseca et al., 2000). Additionally, icv administration of GLP-1 to mice and rats produced a marked decrease of food intake but not of water ingestion. Surprisingly, this effect was avoided by the administration of exendin (9-39) (Tang-Christensen et al., 2000) .

5.2 Hypothalamic slices as a physiological model for the study of hypothalamic regulation by glucose and peptides

Some hypothalamic neuronal cell models have been generated from embryonic and adult animals to carry out molecular genetic analysis of hypothalamic neuronal function. Some examples are the GT1-7 and N1E-115 cell lines or the recently hypothalamic neuronal cell models generated by Belsham´s group (Dalvi et al., 2011). However, the use of organotypic slice cultures is an approach with many advantages. A broad range of studies shows that organotypic cultures retain many in vivo characteristics as regards, neuronal morphology, cellular and anatomical relations and network connections (Sundstrom et al., 2005). The advantages of the slices culture are the isolated and well defined environment of the in vitro preparations and in this way several brain areas have been studied (hippocampus, cerebellum, cortex, striatum, brain stem structures, spinal cord, retina and hypothalamus).

For these reasons, these cultures are increasingly been used as models to investigate mechanisms and treatment strategies for neurodegenerative disorders or exposure to neurotoxic compounds (Kristensen et al., 2003), traumatic brain injury (TBI) (Morrison et al., 2006) and neurogenesis (Lossi et al., 2009). Hypothalamic slices have also been frequently used for electrophysiological studies developed in vitro to evaluate the firing rate of specific neurons located in VMH and LH (Yang et al., 1999)

Most hypothalamic organotypic slice cultures have been derived from neonatal animals. In fact, slices of developing brain tissue can be grown for several weeks as so called organotypic slice cultures (Noraberg et al., 2005), but also adult rats have been used. In this sense our group have used short-term hypothalamic slices cultures, obtained from adult rat, to test the effect of different peptides on the gene expression and enzymatic activity in the VMH and LH areas (Sanz et al., 2007; Sanz et al., 2008). Thus, the hypothalamic organotypic cultures are a useful model for the study of the physiological effect of some peptides on specific hypothalamic nuclei, which could be dissected after the treatment and analyzed by enzymatic, molecular, biochemical or histological procedures.

5.3 Interactions between anorexigenic peptides and cerebral glucose metabolism in humans

By previous studies we know that GLP-1 is an anorexigenic peptide. The proglucagon gene is expressed mainly in the brainstem and hypothalamus, through a mRNA transcript identical to that produced in pancreas and intestine (Drucker & Asa 1988), which permits the formation of glucagon-related peptides in the brain. Furthermore, the hypothalamus and brainstem are the areas with the highest concentration of GLP-1 and its receptors (Uttenthal et al., 1992), suggesting that this peptide has a local function, as well as a more remote signalling role. The expression of GLP-1R gene gives rise to a protein with effects on the selective release of neurotransmitters (Mora et al., 1992), appetite and fluid homeostasis, as well as serves as a signal to reduce food intake (Navarro et al., 1996; Turton et al., 1996; Rodriquez de Fonseca et al., 2000). Also, the coexpression of GLP-1R with those of GLUT-2 and GK in the same cells suggest that these proteins play a role in glucose sensing (Navarro et al., 1996). A further step was to evaluate the GLP-1 effect on cerebral-glucose metabolism in control subjects by positron emission tomography (PET), using 2-F-18 deoxy-D-glucose (FDG). PET is an imaging technology in which compounds labelled with positron-emitting radioisotopes serve as molecular probes to identify and determine biochemical processes in vivo.

We used (Alvarez et al., 2005) intravenously injected FDG to trace the transport and phosphorylation of glucose in brain. FDG-6-phosphate is the end product of the process of glucose metabolism and it is not a substrate for subsequent metabolic reactions then it is retained in the cell proportionately to the rate of glycolysis. The activity measured reflects FDG transport and phosphorylation by the cells and, in the case of the hypothalamus and brainstem which contains cells expressing GLUT-2 and GK, may provide some information about brain glucose sensing.

PET imaging was sensitive to GLP-1 administration (Figure 4). Thus, this peptide significantly reduced cerebral glucose metabolism in the hypothalamus and brainstem as compared with the data obtained in normal control subjects without GLP-1 administration. These changes can be explained in terms of this peptide can enter the brain by binding to blood barrier-free organs such as the subfornical organ and the area postrema (Orskov et al., 1996). Also, it could be transported into the brain through the choroid plexus, which has a high density of GLP-1 receptors.

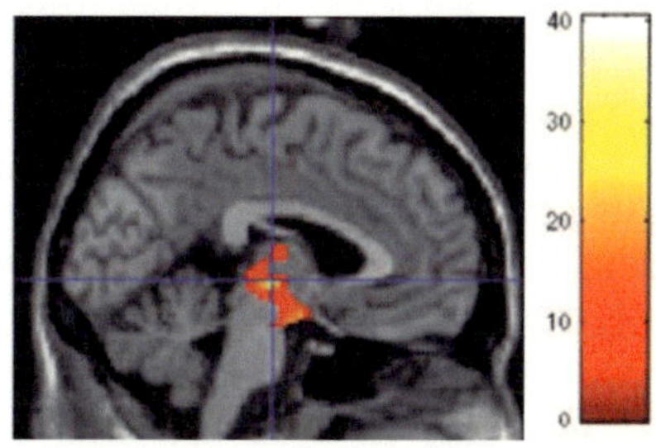

Fig. 4. PET of glucose metabolism in brains of human controls subjects, i.v. perfused with or without GLP-1 (0.75 pmol/Kg body weight for 30 minutes). The differences between both tests were of 6 months, and were projected on sagittal normalized brain MRI. PET imaging was sensitive to the peptide administration. Thus GLP-1 significantly reduced ($p<0.001$) cerebral glucose metabolism in the hypothalamus and brainstem as compared with the data obtained in normal control subjects without peptide administration.

Using PET technology we observed that iv administration of GLP-1 produced a significant reduction in carbohydrate metabolism in selective areas of the brain, including the hypothalamus and brainstem, both areas involved in feeding behaviour. Thus, the accumulation of FDG-6-phosphate into the cells serves to assess the facilitated transport and hexokinase phosphorylation of glucose, which, in the case of hypothalamus and brainstem cells containing GLUT-2 and GK, might facilitate the glucose-sensing process. These findings are of interest because glucoreceptive sites controlling food intake and blood glucose have been found in the medulla oblongata and mesencephalon of the rat (Ritter et al., 2000), in addition to those reported in the hypothalamus. Also, GLP-1 is expressed in human brain, and it most likely mediates the effect of GLP-1 on glucose metabolism in selective areas of hypothalamus and brainstem; it may also facilitate the process of glucose sensing in these areas. Because the reduced number of neurons involved in glucose sensing (Oomura et al., 1969; Ashford et al., 1990) , approximately 40% of cells in the VMH and 30% of cells in the LH, PET imaging offers a good procedure for identifying these cell signals in vivo more accurately compared with the more commonly used in vitro procedures.
These findings provide first evidences of the action of an anorexigenic peptide on glucose metabolism in the hypothalamus and brainstem, and might explain the satiety-induced effects of peripheral or central administration of GLP-1 and the central alterations produced by the iv administration of the peptide. Furthermore, open new doors for studying the effects of other regulatory peptides in subjects under control and pathophysiological situations.

6. Others hypothalamic metabolic sensors: AMPK structure and regulation

AMP-activated protein kinase (AMPK) functions as a cellular energy sensor being activated during energy depletion. The kinase is mainly activated by an increase AMP/ATP ratio. Activation of AMPK regulates a large number of downstream targets stimulating ATP-generating, catabolic pathways and inhibiting anabolic pathways (Hardie et al., 1998; Rutter et al., 2003).
AMPK is a heterotrimeric serine/threonine kinase consisting of a catalytic α-subunit encoded by 2 genes (α1 or α2), a β-subunit encoded by 2 genes (β1, β2) and a regulatory γ-subunit encoded by 3 genes (γ1, γ2, γ3). Different isoforms and alternative splicing of some

mRNAs encoding these subunits, give rise to large variety of heterotrimeric combinations (Hardie 2007; Viollet et al., 2009). It is known that some tissues can express several types of AMPK complexes.

AMPK can be regulated by an allosteric mechanism, through AMP binding to γ subunit, and by covalent phosphorylation at Thr^{172} located in the kinase domain of the α-subunit. The level of phosphorylation is also regulated by AMP through stimulation of upstream kinases and by inhibition of dephosphorylation by protein phosphatases. One of the identified upstream kinases of AMPK is the tumor-suppressor (Liver Kinase B1: LKB1). In neural and endothelial cells AMPK may be also activated by rises in cytosolic Ca^{2+} concentration. The calmodulin-dependent protein kinase kinase (CaMKK) can also activate AMPK by phosphorylation of Thr^{172}.

The AMPK is able to detect changes in cellular energy state that occur in response to variations in nutrient concentrations. Any cellular or metabolic stress that reduces ATP production or accelerates ATP consumption will increase the ratio of the ADP/ATP, which will be amplified by the action of adenylate kinase resulting in increased AMP/ATP with consequent activation of AMPK. Once activated, AMPK first directly affects the activity of key enzymes of glucose metabolism and fatty acids and at a second more long term regulates transcriptional control of the main elements involved in these metabolic pathways. The net result of the activation of AMPK will restore energy balance inhibiting anabolic pathways responsible for the synthesis of macromolecules. (Figure 5)

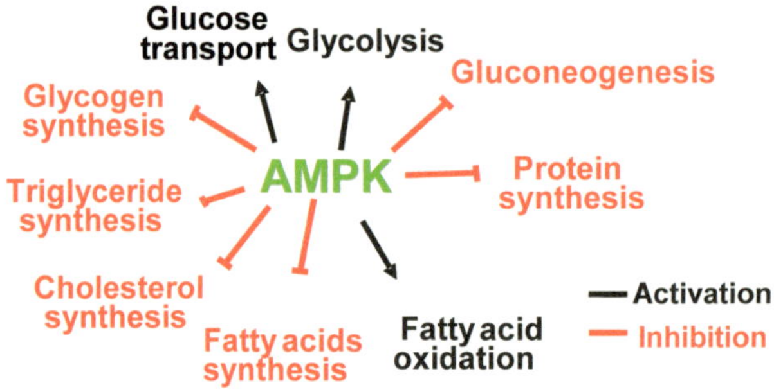

Fig. 5.AMPK regulation of downstream metabolic events. AMPK restores energy balance by activation of processes that produce energy and inhibition of those that consume energy.

6.1 Role of AMPK in hypothalamic glucose sensing

AMPK is broadly expressed throughout the brain with a mainly neuronal distribution (Turnley et al., 1999). Hypothalamic AMPK has been proposed to play a role in the central regulation of food intake and energy balance. In this way, fasting increases and re-feeding decreases AMPK activity in various hypothalamic nuclei (Minokoshi et al., 2004). Several studies have demonstrated that hypothalamic AMPK is regulated by blood glucose levels. Peripheral or central hyperglycaemia inhibits AMPK in several hypothalamic nuclei. Insulin-induced hypoglycaemia and inhibition of intracellular glucose utilization through the administration of 2-deoxyglucose both increased hypothalamic AMPK activity and food intake.

The use of catalytic subunit of AMPK knockout mice (AMPKα1$^{-/-}$ and AMPKα2$^{-/-}$) indicated that AMPKα1$^{-/-}$ mice has no metabolic alterations, whereas AMPKα2$^{-/-}$ mice showed insulin-resistance characterized by impaired insulin stimulated whole-body glucose utilization and skeletal muscle glycogen synthesis and reduced insulin secretion. However, they showed no apparent changes in body weight and food intake (Viollet et al., 2009).

In the last years AMPK has been proposed as a cellular energy sensor that is able to assemble many regulatory signals and nutritional environmental changes, also involved in maintaining whole body energy balance (Hardie et al., 2006). Regulation of AMPK activity in hypothalamic areas involved in the control of feeding behaviours have been also described as a mechanism to detect nutritional variations including glucose levels (Mountjoy & Rutter 2007). Neurons implied in the control of food intake have as well glucose sensor that respond to fluctuations in extracellular glucose levels.

In general most cells will express glucose transporters that have high affinity for glucose; therefore ATP synthesis by glucose metabolism only stops when glucose levels are pathologically low. However, cells that have a glucose sensor mechanism, express GLUT-2 and GK. The presence of these proteins of high Km for transport and metabolism of glucose will allow that ATP synthesis decreases when decreases the concentration of glucose in the physiological range and this allows that in these cells the AMPK can be activated by low levels of glucose and inhibited by high glucose levels in the physiological range.

The hypothalamic AMPK role has been studied in vivo by expression of AMPK mutants: Inhibition of hypothalamic AMPK suppresses neuronal NPY/AgRP signalling and inhibit food intake. However, elevated AMPK increases NPY/AgRP expression, food intake and body weight (Minokoshi et al., 2004).

The role of AMPK in the two major subpopulations of neurons involved in the regulation of feeding was later analyzed by knock out of AMPKα2 in specific neurons of mice. The results showed that genetic deletion of AMPKα2 in hypothalamic POMC neurons (POMC AMPKα2-KO) developed obesity. However, AMPKα2 specifically knocked in AgRP neurones (AgRP AMPKα2-KO) exhibited an age-related lean phenotype (Claret et al., 2007). Those mice do not respond to changes in extracellular glucose. The unexpected results suggest that absence of AMPK in orexigenic AgRP neurons reduced body weight, whereas lack of AMPK in anorexigenic POMC neurons increased body weight. These results suggest a role for AMPK as a common glucose-sensor in these neurons (Claret et al., 2007). It is important to emphasize that GE neurons do not overlap completely with POMC neurons in the ARC while the GI neurons do not completely overlap with NPY/AgRP neurons. Those findings indicated the complexity of the functions of hypothalamic AMPK.

6.2 Regulation by orexigenic and anorexigenic peptides

Several reports indicate that AMPK is also regulated by several orexigenic and anorexigenic signals (Minokoshi et al., 2004). Thus, hypothalamic AMPK activity was inhibited in ARC and PVN by anorexigenic peptides as leptin and insulin by contrast, orexigenic peptides (ghrelin) increased specifically α2AMPK activity

In other hand, other studies reported AMPK-independent pathways. The effect of leptin were maintained in POMC α2AMPK-KO neurons and insulin depolarised AgRP neurons in AgRP α2AMPK-KO (Claret et al., 2007). The different results may be explained, in addition to the different techniques and experimental setups, by the presence of distinct subpopulations of GE and GI neurons with different neuropeptide phenotypes, responses to hormonal stimuli and, in some cases, different glucose-sensing mechanisms.

The downstream pathways of AMPK in the hypothalamus may involve the acetyl-CoA carboxylase (ACC)-malonyl-CoA-carnitine palmitoyltransferase 1 (CPT1) pathway and the

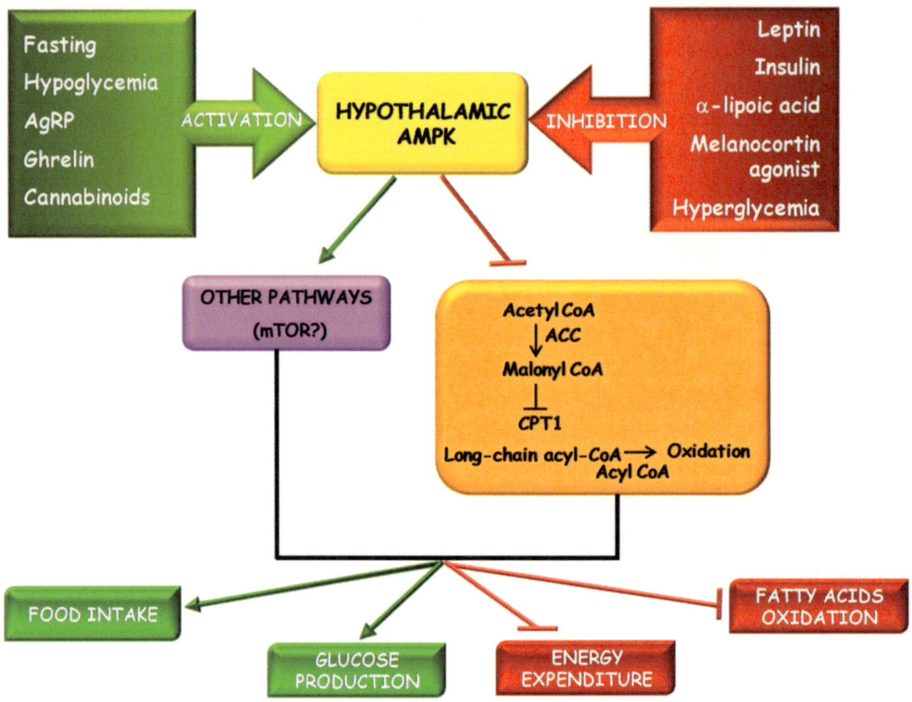

Fig. 6. Regulation of hypothalamic AMPK activity. Downstream targets involved in this signaling pathway. Several orexigenic and anorexigenic peptides regulate AMPK activity. Some of downstream targets of AMPK in the hypothalamus: ACC, acetyl-CoA carboxylase; CPT1, carnitine palmitoyltransferase 1. The effect of AMPK on the mammalian target of rapamycin (mTOR) pathway has not been directly proved in the hypothalamus.

mammalian target of rapamycin (mTOR) pathway. Activation of ACC, as a consequence of AMPK inhibition, would lead to increased intracellular malonyl-CoA levels, which would inhibit mitochondrial CPT1 and fatty acid oxidation.

The mTOR is another possible target of AMPK (Figure 6). AMPK inhibits mTOR signalling, thereby suppressing protein synthesis, which is an important pathway by which AMPK conserves cellular energy. The mTOR signalling pathway plays a crucial role in the regulation of food intake and body weight in the hypothalamus (Cota et al., 2006; Ropelle et al., 2008). The mTOR is colocalized with AgRP/NPY and POMC neurons in the ARC (Perrin et al., 2004). Fasting downregulates mTOR signalling, whereas re-feeding activates it.

Interestingly, hypothalamic AMPK also mediates the counter-regulatory response to hypoglycaemia, increasing the release of peripheral hormones such as corticosterone, catecholamines and glucagon (Han et al., 2005; McCrimmon et al., 2006). Thus AMPK is not only a peripheral or a central mediator, but also a key enzyme in coordinating the interaction between peripheral and central energy regulation.

It is generally accepted that in peripheral organs, fuel overabundance alters the activity of metabolic sensors (decreased AMPK and increased the mTOR and its down-stream target the S6Kinase (p70S6K)) causing insulin resistance (Kola et al., 2005).

AMPK and mTOR activity respond to changes in glucose and other nutrients in hypothalamic centres involved in control of feeding and deregulation of this signalling pathways might be implied in the develop of obesity and diabetes type 2. GLP-1 treatment to type 2 diabetic subjects normalizes fasting levels of blood glucose and decreases glucose levels after ingestion of a meal (Niswender 2010). GLP-1 is able to induce several effects that contribute to feeding behaviour. Preliminary data from our laboratory also suggest that, at least some of those effects, might mediate through regulation of AMPK and p70S6K in VMH and LH.

7. Conclusions

Glucoregulatory mechanisms are of primary functional concern to provide a continued glucose supply to the central nervous system and to face metabolic needs of peripheral tissues. Glucose sensors are molecular designs that accurately measure glucose concentrations in the extracellular space facilitating the mechanisms need to maintain glucose homeostasis. GK might be responsible of glucose sensing in some of hypothalamic GE and GI neurons (VMH, LH ARC, PVN and dorsomedial nucleus). GK properties of high-Km phosphorylation of glucose and that it is not inhibited by glucose-6-phosphate, enable that glucose catabolism be proportional to glucose levels in the extracellular space. Also, the functional coexpression of GK with GLUT-2, GKRP and GLP-1R in hypothalamic areas implied in feeding behaviour, could orchestrate regulatory signals to maintain body weight and energy balance. Glucose, orexigenic and anorexigenic peptides contribute to control GK, as well as other energetic sensors such as AMPK. The effect of nutrients occurs on GK and AMPK enzyme activities as required by a short-term response and in a distinctive pattern between VMH and LH. Also, GLP-1 produced a significant reduction of glucose metabolism in selective areas of human brain including hypothalamus and brainstem, both areas involved in feeding behaviour. These findings open new doors for studying the effects of others regulatory peptides in subjects under control and pathophysiological situations. In summary, this chapter has shown a view of the complexity of the network of regulatory signals, where GK, AMPK and regulatory peptides are involved, leading to an optimal energy balance and body weight.

8. Acknowledgment

This work was supported by the CIBER de Diabetes y Enfermedades Metabólicas Asociadas (CIBERDEM) of the Instituto de Salud Carlos III, Madrid, Spain; by grants from the Ministerio de Ciencia e Innovación, Fondo de Investigaciones Sanitarias, Spain and from the Fundación de Investigación Médica Mutua Madrileña, Spain and from Complutense University of Madrid-Santander Bank, Spain.

9. References

Adachi, A.; Kobashi, M. & Funahashi, M. (1995). Glucose-responsive neurons in the brainstem. *Obes Res,* Vol.3 Suppl 5, (Dec), pp. 735S-740S.

Adage, T.; Scheurink, A. J.; de Boer, S. F.; de Vries, K.; Konsman, J. P.; Kuipers, F.; Adan, R. A.; Baskin, D. G.; Schwartz, M. W. & van Dijk, G. (2001). Hypothalamic, metabolic, and behavioral responses to pharmacological inhibition of CNS melanocortin signaling in rats. *J Neurosci,* Vol.21, No.10, (May 15), pp. 3639-3645.

Agius, L. & Peak, M. (1993). Intracellular binding of glucokinase in hepatocytes and translocation by glucose, fructose and insulin. *Biochem J,* Vol.296 (Pt 3), (Dec 15), pp. 785-796.

Alvarez, E.; Martinez, M. D.; Roncero, I.; Chowen, J. A.; Garcia-Cuartero, B.; Gispert, J. D.; Sanz, C.; Vazquez, P.; Maldonado, A.; de Caceres, J.; Desco, M.; Pozo, M. A. & Blazquez, E. (2005). The expression of GLP-1 receptor mRNA and protein allows the effect of GLP-1 on glucose metabolism in the human hypothalamus and brainstem. *J Neurochem,* Vol.92, No.4, (Feb), pp. 798-806.

Alvarez, E.; Roncero, I.; Chowen, J. A.; Thorens, B. & Blazquez, E. (1996). Expression of the glucagon-like peptide-1 receptor gene in rat brain. *J Neurochem,* Vol.66, No.3, (Mar), pp. 920-927.

Alvarez, E.; Roncero, I.; Chowen, J. A.; Vazquez, P. & Blazquez, E. (2002). Evidence that glucokinase regulatory protein is expressed and interacts with glucokinase in rat brain. *J Neurochem,* Vol.80, No.1, (Jan), pp. 45-53.

Anand, B. K.; Chhina, G. S.; Sharma, K. N.; Dua, S. & Singh, B. (1964). Activity of Single Neurons in the Hypothalamic Feeding Centers: Effect of Glucose. *Am J Physiol,* Vol.207, (Nov), pp. 1146-1154.

Arden, C.; Baltrusch, S. & Agius, L. (2006). Glucokinase regulatory protein is associated with mitochondria in hepatocytes. *FEBS Lett,* Vol.580, No.8, (Apr 3), pp. 2065-2070.

Ashcroft, F. & Rorsman, P. (2004). Type 2 diabetes mellitus: not quite exciting enough? *Hum Mol Genet,* Vol.13 Spec No 1, (Apr 1), pp. R21-31.

Ashford, M. L.; Boden, P. R. & Treherne, J. M. (1990). Glucose-induced excitation of hypothalamic neurones is mediated by ATP-sensitive K+ channels. *Pflugers Arch,* Vol.415, No.4, (Jan), pp. 479-483.

Baltrusch, S.; Lenzen, S.; Okar, D. A.; Lange, A. J. & Tiedge, M. (2001). Characterization of glucokinase-binding protein epitopes by a phage-displayed peptide library. Identification of 6-phosphofructo-2-kinase/fructose-2,6-bisphosphatase as a novel interaction partner. *J Biol Chem,* Vol.276, No.47, (Nov 23), pp. 43915-43923.

Batterham, R. L.; Cowley, M. A.; Small, C. J.; Herzog, H.; Cohen, M. A.; Dakin, C. L.; Wren, A. M.; Brynes, A. E.; Low, M. J.; Ghatei, M. A.; Cone, R. D. & Bloom, S. R. (2002). Gut hormone PYY(3-36) physiologically inhibits food intake. *Nature,* Vol.418, No.6898, (Aug 8), pp. 650-654.

Bernard, C. (1849). Chiens rendus diabetiquex. *Compt End Soc Biol,* Vol.1, pp. 60

Borg, W. P.; Sherwin, R. S.; During, M. J.; Borg, M. A. & Shulman, G. I. (1995). Local ventromedial hypothalamus glucopenia triggers counterregulatory hormone release. *Diabetes,* Vol.44, No.2, (Feb), pp. 180-184.

Bray, G. A. (1992). Peptides affect the intake of specific nutrients and the sympathetic nervous system. *Am J Clin Nutr,* Vol.55, No.1 Suppl, (Jan), pp. 265S-271S.

Burdakov, D. & Ashcroft, F. M. (2002). Shedding new light on brain metabolism and glial function. *J Physiol,* Vol.544, No.Pt 2, (Oct 15), pp. 334.

Burdakov, D. & Lesage, F. (2010). Glucose-induced inhibition: how many ionic mechanisms? *Acta Physiol (Oxf),* Vol.198, No.3, (Mar), pp. 295-301.

Burdakov, D.; Luckman, S. M. & Verkhratsky, A. (2005). Glucose-sensing neurons of the hypothalamus. *Philosophical Transactions of the Royal Society B: Biological Sciences,* Vol.360, No.1464, (December 29, 2005), pp. 2227-2235.

Claret, M.; Smith, M. A.; Batterham, R. L.; Selman, C.; Choudhury, A. I.; Fryer, L. G.; Clements, M.; Al-Qassab, H.; Heffron, H.; Xu, A. W.; Speakman, J. R.; Barsh, G. S.; Viollet, B.; Vaulont, S.; Ashford, M. L.; Carling, D. & Withers, D. J. (2007). AMPK is essential for energy homeostasis regulation and glucose sensing by POMC and AgRP neurons. *J Clin Invest,* Vol.117, No.8, (Aug), pp. 2325-2336.

Coiro, V.; Saccani-Jotti, G.; Rubino, P.; Manfredi, G.; Melani, A. & Chiodera, P. (2006). Effects of ghrelin on circulating neuropeptide Y levels in humans. *Neuro Endocrinol Lett,* Vol.27, No.6, (Dec), pp. 755-757.

Cone, R. D.; Cowley, M. A.; Butler, A. A.; Fan, W.; Marks, D. L. & Low, M. J. (2001). The arcuate nucleus as a conduit for diverse signals relevant to energy homeostasis. *Int J Obes Relat Metab Disord,* Vol.25 Suppl 5, (Dec), pp. S63-67.

Cornish-Bowden, A. & Storer, A. C. (1986). Mechanistic origin of the sigmoidal rate behaviour of rat liver hexokinase D ('glucokinase'). *Biochem J,* Vol.240, No.1, (Nov 15), pp. 293-296.

Cota, D.; Proulx, K.; Smith, K. A.; Kozma, S. C.; Thomas, G.; Woods, S. C. & Seeley, R. J. (2006). Hypothalamic mTOR signaling regulates food intake. *Science,* Vol.312, No.5775, (May 12), pp. 927-930.

Christesen, H. B.; Jacobsen, B. B.; Odili, S.; Buettger, C.; Cuesta-Munoz, A.; Hansen, T.; Brusgaard, K.; Massa, O.; Magnuson, M. A.; Shiota, C.; Matschinsky, F. M. & Barbetti, F. (2002). The second activating glucokinase mutation (A456V): implications for glucose homeostasis and diabetes therapy. *Diabetes,* Vol.51, No.4, (Apr), pp. 1240-1246.

Dalvi, P. S.; Nazarians-Armavil, A.; Tung, S. & Belsham, D. D. (2011). Immortalized Neurons for the Study of Hypothalamic Function. *American Journal of Physiology - Regulatory, Integrative and Comparative Physiology,* Vol., pp.

Dallaporta, M.; Himmi, T.; Perrin, J. & Orsini, J. C. (1999). Solitary tract nucleus sensitivity to moderate changes in glucose level. *Neuroreport,* Vol.10, No.12, (Aug 20), pp. 2657-2660.

de Lecea, L.; Kilduff, T. S.; Peyron, C.; Gao, X.; Foye, P. E.; Danielson, P. E.; Fukuhara, C.; Battenberg, E. L.; Gautvik, V. T.; Bartlett, F. S., 2nd; Frankel, W. N.; van den Pol, A. N.; Bloom, F. E.; Gautvik, K. M. & Sutcliffe, J. G. (1998). The hypocretins: hypothalamus-specific peptides with neuroexcitatory activity. *Proc Natl Acad Sci U S A,* Vol.95, No.1, (Jan 6), pp. 322-327.

Diez-Sampedro, A.; Hirayama, B. A.; Osswald, C.; Gorboulev, V.; Baumgarten, K.; Volk, C.; Wright, E. M. & Koepsell, H. (2003). A glucose sensor hiding in a family of transporters. *Proc Natl Acad Sci U S A,* Vol.100, No.20, (Sep 30), pp. 11753-11758.

Drucker, D. J. & Asa, S. (1988). Glucagon gene expression in vertebrate brain. *J Biol Chem,* Vol.263, No.27, (Sep 25), pp. 13475-13478.

Dunn-Meynell, A. A.; Rawson, N. E. & Levin, B. E. (1998). Distribution and phenotype of neurons containing the ATP-sensitive K+ channel in rat brain. *Brain Research,* Vol.814, No.1-2, pp. 41-54.

Dunn-Meynell, A. A.; Routh, V. H.; Kang, L.; Gaspers, L. & Levin, B. E. (2002). Glucokinase is the likely mediator of glucosensing in both glucose-excited and glucose-inhibited central neurons. *Diabetes,* Vol.51, No.7, (Jul), pp. 2056-2065.

Elmquist, J. K.; Elias, C. F. & Saper, C. B. (1999). From lesions to leptin: hypothalamic control of food intake and body weight. *Neuron,* Vol.22, No.2, (Feb), pp. 221-232.

Fioramonti, X.; Lorsignol, A.; Taupignon, A. & Penicaud, L. (2004). A new ATP-sensitive K+ channel-independent mechanism is involved in glucose-excited neurons of mouse arcuate nucleus. *Diabetes,* Vol.53, No.11, (Nov), pp. 2767-2775.

Garcia-Flores, M.; Zueco, J. A.; Arenas, J. & Blazquez, E. (2002). Expression of glucose transporter-2, glucokinase and mitochondrial glycerolphosphate dehydrogenase in pancreatic islets during rat ontogenesis. *Eur J Biochem,* Vol.269, No.1, (Jan), pp. 119-127.

Gonzalez, J. A.; Reimann, F. & Burdakov, D. (2009). Dissociation between sensing and metabolism of glucose in sugar sensing neurones. *J Physiol,* Vol.587, No.Pt 1, (Jan 15), pp. 41-48.

Gribble, F. M.; Williams, L.; Simpson, A. K. & Reimann, F. (2003). A novel glucose-sensing mechanism contributing to glucagon-like peptide-1 secretion from the GLUTag cell line. *Diabetes,* Vol.52, No.5, (May), pp. 1147-1154.

Grupe, A.; Hultgren, B.; Ryan, A.; Ma, Y. H.; Bauer, M. & Stewart, T. A. (1995). Transgenic knockouts reveal a critical requirement for pancreatic beta cell glucokinase in maintaining glucose homeostasis. *Cell,* Vol.83, No.1, (Oct 6), pp. 69-78.

Han, S. M.; Namkoong, C.; Jang, P. G.; Park, I. S.; Hong, S. W.; Katakami, H.; Chun, S.; Kim, S. W.; Park, J. Y.; Lee, K. U. & Kim, M. S. (2005). Hypothalamic AMP-activated protein kinase mediates counter-regulatory responses to hypoglycaemia in rats. *Diabetologia,* Vol.48, No.10, (Oct), pp. 2170-2178.

Hara, J.; Beuckmann, C. T.; Nambu, T.; Willie, J. T.; Chemelli, R. M.; Sinton, C. M.; Sugiyama, F.; Yagami, K.; Goto, K.; Yanagisawa, M. & Sakurai, T. (2001). Genetic ablation of orexin neurons in mice results in narcolepsy, hypophagia, and obesity. *Neuron,* Vol.30, No.2, (May), pp. 345-354.

Hardie, D. G. (2007). AMP-activated/SNF1 protein kinases: conserved guardians of cellular energy. *Nat Rev Mol Cell Biol,* Vol.8, No.10, (Oct), pp. 774-785.

Hardie, D. G.; Carling, D. & Carlson, M. (1998). The AMP-activated/SNF1 protein kinase subfamily: metabolic sensors of the eukaryotic cell? *Annu Rev Biochem,* Vol.67, pp. 821-855.

Hardie, D. G.; Hawley, S. A. & Scott, J. W. (2006). AMP-activated protein kinase--development of the energy sensor concept. *J Physiol,* Vol.574, No.Pt 1, (Jul 1), pp. 7-15.

Hughes, S. D.; Quaade, C.; Milburn, J. L.; Cassidy, L. & Newgard, C. B. (1991). Expression of normal and novel glucokinase mRNAs in anterior pituitary and islet cells. *J Biol Chem,* Vol.266, No.7, (Mar 5), pp. 4521-4530.

Iynedjian, P. B. (1993). Mammalian glucokinase and its gene. *Biochem J,* Vol.293 (Pt 1), (Jul 1), pp. 1-13.

Iynedjian, P. B.; Marie, S.; Wang, H.; Gjinovci, A. & Nazaryan, K. (1996). Liver-specific enhancer of the glucokinase gene. *J Biol Chem,* Vol.271, No.46, (Nov 15), pp. 29113-29120.

Jordan, S. D.; Konner, A. C. & Bruning, J. C. (2010). Sensing the fuels: glucose and lipid signaling in the CNS controlling energy homeostasis. *Cell Mol Life Sci,* Vol.67, No.19, (Oct), pp. 3255-3273.

Kang, L.; Dunn-Meynell, A. A.; Routh, V. H.; Gaspers, L. D.; Nagata, Y.; Nishimura, T.; Eiki, J.; Zhang, B. B. & Levin, B. E. (2006). Glucokinase is a critical regulator of ventromedial hypothalamic neuronal glucosensing. *Diabetes,* Vol.55, No.2, (Feb), pp. 412-420.

Kang, L.; Routh, V. H.; Kuzhikandathil, E. V.; Gaspers, L. D. & Levin, B. E. (2004). Physiological and molecular characteristics of rat hypothalamic ventromedial nucleus glucosensing neurons. *Diabetes,* Vol.53, No.3, (Mar), pp. 549-559.

Kola, B.; Hubina, E.; Tucci, S. A.; Kirkham, T. C.; Garcia, E. A.; Mitchell, S. E.; Williams, L. M.; Hawley, S. A.; Hardie, D. G.; Grossman, A. B. & Korbonits, M. (2005). Cannabinoids and ghrelin have both central and peripheral metabolic and cardiac effects via AMP-activated protein kinase. *J Biol Chem,* Vol.280, No.26, (Jul 1), pp. 25196-25201.

Kristensen, B. W.; Noer, H.; Gramsbergen, J. B.; Zimmer, J. & Noraberg, J. (2003). Colchicine induces apoptosis in organotypic hippocampal slice cultures. *Brain Res,* Vol.964, No.2, (Feb 28), pp. 264-278.

Lee, K.; Li, B.; Xi, X.; Suh, Y. & Martin, R. J. (2005). Role of neuronal energy status in the regulation of adenosine 5'-monophosphate-activated protein kinase, orexigenic neuropeptides expression, and feeding behavior. *Endocrinology,* Vol.146, No.1, (Jan), pp. 3-10.

Leibowitz, S. F. (1992). Neurochemical-neuroendocrine systems in the brain controlling macronutrient intake and metabolism. *Trends Neurosci,* Vol.15, No.12, (Dec), pp. 491-497.

Levin, B. E.; Routh, V. H.; Kang, L.; Sanders, N. M. & Dunn-Meynell, A. A. (2004). Neuronal glucosensing: what do we know after 50 years? *Diabetes,* Vol.53, No.10, (Oct), pp. 2521-2528.

Lossi, L.; Alasia, S.; Salio, C. & Merighi, A. (2009). Cell death and proliferation in acute slices and organotypic cultures of mammalian CNS. *Prog Neurobiol,* Vol.88, No.4, (Aug), pp. 221-245.

Lynch, R. M.; Tompkins, L. S.; Brooks, H. L.; Dunn-Meynell, A. A. & Levin, B. E. (2000). Localization of glucokinase gene expression in the rat brain. *Diabetes,* Vol.49, No.5, (May 1, 2000), pp. 693-700.

Magnuson, M. A. & Shelton, K. D. (1989). An alternate promoter in the glucokinase gene is active in the pancreatic beta cell. *J Biol Chem,* Vol.264, No.27, (Sep 25), pp. 15936-15942.

Malaisse, W. J.; Malaisse-Lagae, F.; Davies, D. R.; Vandercammen, A. & Van Schaftingen, E. (1990). Regulation of glucokinase by a fructose-1-phosphate-sensitive protein in pancreatic islets. *Eur J Biochem,* Vol.190, No.3, (Jul 5), pp. 539-545.

Matschinsky, F.; Liang, Y.; Kesavan, P.; Wang, L.; Froguel, P.; Velho, G.; Cohen, D.; Permutt, M. A.; Tanizawa, Y.; Jetton, T. L. & et al. (1993). Glucokinase as pancreatic beta cell glucose sensor and diabetes gene. *J Clin Invest,* Vol.92, No.5, (Nov), pp. 2092-2098.

Matschinsky, F. M. (1990). Glucokinase as glucose sensor and metabolic signal generator in pancreatic beta-cells and hepatocytes. *Diabetes,* Vol.39, No.6, (Jun), pp. 647-652.

Mayer, J. (1953). Glucostatic Mechanism of Regulation of Food Intake. *New England Journal of Medicine,* Vol.249, No.1, pp. 13-16.

McCrimmon, R. J.; Fan, X.; Cheng, H.; McNay, E.; Chan, O.; Shaw, M.; Ding, Y.; Zhu, W. & Sherwin, R. S. (2006). Activation of AMP-activated protein kinase within the ventromedial hypothalamus amplifies counterregulatory hormone responses in rats with defective counterregulation. *Diabetes,* Vol.55, No.6, (Jun), pp. 1755-1760.

Minokoshi, Y.; Alquier, T.; Furukawa, N.; Kim, Y. B.; Lee, A.; Xue, B.; Mu, J.; Foufelle, F.; Ferre, P.; Birnbaum, M. J.; Stuck, B. J. & Kahn, B. B. (2004). AMP-kinase regulates food intake by responding to hormonal and nutrient signals in the hypothalamus. *Nature,* Vol.428, No.6982, (Apr 1), pp. 569-574.

Mora, F.; Exposito, I.; Sanz, B. & Blazquez, E. (1992). Selective release of glutamine and glutamic acid produced by perfusion of GLP-1 (7-36) amide in the basal ganglia of the conscious rat. *Brain Res Bull,* Vol.29, No.3-4, (Sep-Oct), pp. 359-361.

Morrison, B., 3rd; Cater, H. L.; Benham, C. D. & Sundstrom, L. E. (2006). An in vitro model of traumatic brain injury utilising two-dimensional stretch of organotypic hippocampal slice cultures. *J Neurosci Methods,* Vol.150, No.2, (Jan 30), pp. 192-201.

Moukil, M. A.; Veiga-da-Cunha, M. & Van Schaftingen, E. (2000). Study of the regulatory properties of glucokinase by site-directed mutagenesis: conversion of glucokinase to an enzyme with high affinity for glucose. *Diabetes,* Vol.49, No.2, (Feb), pp. 195-201.

Mountjoy, P. D. & Rutter, G. A. (2007). Glucose sensing by hypothalamic neurones and pancreatic islet cells: AMPle evidence for common mechanisms? *Exp Physiol,* Vol.92, No.2, (Mar), pp. 311-319.

Munoz-Alonso, M. J.; Guillemain, G.; Kassis, N.; Girard, J.; Burnol, A. F. & Leturque, A. (2000). A novel cytosolic dual specificity phosphatase, interacting with glucokinase, increases glucose phosphorylation rate. *J Biol Chem,* Vol.275, No.42, (Oct 20), pp. 32406-32412.

Navarro, M.; Rodriquez de Fonseca, F.; Alvarez, E.; Chowen, J. A.; Zueco, J. A.; Gomez, R.; Eng, J. & Blazquez, E. (1996). Colocalization of glucagon-like peptide-1 (GLP-1) receptors, glucose transporter GLUT-2, and glucokinase mRNAs in rat hypothalamic cells: evidence for a role of GLP-1 receptor agonists as an inhibitory signal for food and water intake. *J Neurochem,* Vol.67, No.5, (Nov), pp. 1982-1991.

Niswender, K. (2010). Diabetes and obesity: therapeutic targeting and risk reduction - a complex interplay. *Diabetes Obes Metab,* Vol.12, No.4, (Apr), pp. 267-287.

Noraberg, J.; Poulsen, F. R.; Blaabjerg, M.; Kristensen, B. W.; Bonde, C.; Montero, M.; Meyer, M.; Gramsbergen, J. B. & Zimmer, J. (2005). Organotypic hippocampal slice cultures for studies of brain damage, neuroprotection and neurorepair. *Curr Drug Targets CNS Neurol Disord,* Vol.4, No.4, (Aug), pp. 435-452.

Oomura, Y.; Ono, T.; Ooyama, H. & Wayner, M. J. (1969). Glucose and osmosensitive neurones of the rat hypothalamus. *Nature,* Vol.222, No.5190, (Apr 19), pp. 282-284.

Oomura, Y.; Ooyama, H.; Sugimori, M.; Nakamura, T. & Yamada, Y. (1974). Glucose inhibition of the glucose-sensitive neurone in the rat lateral hypothalamus. *Nature,* Vol.247, No.439, (Feb 1), pp. 284-286.

Oomura, Y. & Yoshimatsu, H. (1984). Neural network of glucose monitoring system. *J Auton Nerv Syst,* Vol.10, No.3-4, (May-Jun), pp. 359-372.

Orskov, C.; Poulsen, S. S.; Moller, M. & Holst, J. J. (1996). Glucagon-like peptide I receptors in the subfornical organ and the area postrema are accessible to circulating glucagon-like peptide I. *Diabetes,* Vol.45, No.6, (Jun), pp. 832-835.

Pellerin, L. & Magistretti, P. J. (2004). Neuroenergetics: calling upon astrocytes to satisfy hungry neurons. *Neuroscientist,* Vol.10, No.1, (Feb), pp. 53-62.

Penicaud, L.; Leloup, C.; Fioramonti, X.; Lorsignol, A. & Benani, A. (2006). Brain glucose sensing: a subtle mechanism. *Curr Opin Clin Nutr Metab Care,* Vol.9, No.4, (Jul), pp. 458-462.

Perrin, C.; Knauf, C. & Burcelin, R. (2004). Intracerebroventricular infusion of glucose, insulin, and the adenosine monophosphate-activated kinase activator, 5-aminoimidazole-4-carboxamide-1-beta-D-ribofuranoside, controls muscle glycogen synthesis. *Endocrinology,* Vol.145, No.9, (Sep), pp. 4025-4033.

Ritter, S. & Dinh, T. T. (1994). 2-Mercaptoacetate and 2-deoxy-D-glucose induce Fos-like immunoreactivity in rat brain. *Brain Res,* Vol.641, No.1, (Mar 28), pp. 111-120.

Ritter, S.; Dinh, T. T. & Zhang, Y. (2000). Localization of hindbrain glucoreceptive sites controlling food intake and blood glucose. *Brain Res,* Vol.856, No.1-2, (Feb 21), pp. 37-47.

Rodriguez de Fonseca, F.; Navarro, M.; Alvarez, E.; Roncero, I.; Chowen, J. A.; Maestre, O.; Gomez, R.; Munoz, R. M.; Eng, J. & Blazquez, E. (2000). Peripheral versus central effects of glucagon-like peptide-1 receptor agonists on satiety and body weight loss in Zucker obese rats. *Metabolism,* Vol.49, No.6, (Jun), pp. 709-717.

Roncero, I.; Alvarez, E.; Chowen, J. A.; Sanz, C.; Rabano, A.; Vazquez, P. & Blazquez, E. (2004). Expression of glucose transporter isoform GLUT-2 and glucokinase genes in human brain. *J Neurochem,* Vol.88, No.5, (Mar), pp. 1203-1210.

Roncero, I.; Alvarez, E.; Vazquez, P. & Blazquez, E. (2000). Functional glucokinase isoforms are expressed in rat brain. *J Neurochem,* Vol.74, No.5, (May), pp. 1848-1857.

Roncero, I.; Sanz, C.; Alvarez, E.; Vazquez, P.; Barrio, P. A. & Blazquez, E. (2009). Glucokinase and glucokinase regulatory proteins are functionally coexpressed before birth in the rat brain. *J Neuroendocrinol,* Vol.21, No.12, (Dec), pp. 973-981.

Ropelle, E. R.; Pauli, J. R.; Fernandes, M. F.; Rocco, S. A.; Marin, R. M.; Morari, J.; Souza, K. K.; Dias, M. M.; Gomes-Marcondes, M. C.; Gontijo, J. A.; Franchini, K. G.; Velloso, L. A.; Saad, M. J. & Carvalheira, J. B. (2008). A central role for neuronal AMP-activated protein kinase (AMPK) and mammalian target of rapamycin (mTOR) in high-protein diet-induced weight loss. *Diabetes,* Vol.57, No.3, (Mar), pp. 594-605.

Routh, V. H. (2002). Glucose-sensing neurons: Are they physiologically relevant? *Physiology & Behavior,* Vol.76, No.3, pp. 403-413.

Rutter, G. A.; Da Silva Xavier, G. & Leclerc, I. (2003). Roles of 5'-AMP-activated protein kinase (AMPK) in mammalian glucose homoeostasis. *Biochem J,* Vol.375, No.Pt 1, (Oct 1), pp. 1-16.

Sakurai, T.; Amemiya, A.; Ishii, M.; Matsuzaki, I.; Chemelli, R. M.; Tanaka, H.; Williams, S. C.; Richardson, J. A.; Kozlowski, G. P.; Wilson, S.; Arch, J. R.; Buckingham, R. E.; Haynes, A. C.; Carr, S. A.; Annan, R. S.; McNulty, D. E.; Liu, W. S.; Terrett, J. A.; Elshourbagy, N. A.; Bergsma, D. J. & Yanagisawa, M. (1998). Orexins and orexin receptors: a family of hypothalamic neuropeptides and G protein-coupled receptors that regulate feeding behavior. *Cell,* Vol.92, No.4, (Feb 20), pp. 573-585.

Sanz, C.; Roncero, I.; Vazquez, P.; Navas, M. A. & Blazquez, E. (2007). Effects of glucose and insulin on glucokinase activity in rat hypothalamus. *J Endocrinol,* Vol.193, No.2, (May), pp. 259-267.

Sanz, C.; Vazquez, P.; Navas, M. A.; Alvarez, E. & Blazquez, E. (2008). Leptin but not neuropeptide Y up-regulated glucagon-like peptide 1 receptor expression in GT1-7 cells and rat hypothalamic slices. *Metabolism,* Vol.57, No.1, (Jan), pp. 40-48.

Schuit, F. C.; Huypens, P.; Heimberg, H. & Pipeleers, D. G. (2001). Glucose sensing in pancreatic beta-cells: a model for the study of other glucose-regulated cells in gut, pancreas, and hypothalamus. *Diabetes,* Vol.50, No.1, (Jan), pp. 1-11.

Shiota, C.; Coffey, J.; Grimsby, J.; Grippo, J. F. & Magnuson, M. A. (1999). Nuclear import of hepatic glucokinase depends upon glucokinase regulatory protein, whereas export is due to a nuclear export signal sequence in glucokinase. *J Biol Chem,* Vol.274, No.52, (Dec 24), pp. 37125-37130.

Silver, I. A. & Erecinska, M. (1994). Extracellular glucose concentration in mammalian brain: continuous monitoring of changes during increased neuronal activity and upon limitation in oxygen supply in normo-, hypo-, and hyperglycemic animals. *J Neurosci,* Vol.14, No.8, (Aug), pp. 5068-5076.

Silver, I. A. & Erecinska, M. (1998). Glucose-induced intracellular ion changes in sugar-sensitive hypothalamic neurons. *J Neurophysiol,* Vol.79, No.4, (Apr), pp. 1733-1745.

Song, Z. & Routh, V. H. (2005). Differential effects of glucose and lactate on glucosensing neurons in the ventromedial hypothalamic nucleus. *Diabetes,* Vol.54, No.1, (Jan), pp. 15-22.

Sundstrom, L.; Morrison, B., 3rd; Bradley, M. & Pringle, A. (2005). Organotypic cultures as tools for functional screening in the CNS. *Drug Discov Today,* Vol.10, No.14, (Jul 15), pp. 993-1000.

Sutherland, V. L.; McReynolds, M.; Tompkins, L. S.; Brooks, H. L. & Lynch, R. M. (2005). Developmental expression of glucokinase in rat hypothalamus. *Brain Res Dev Brain Res,* Vol.154, No.2, (Feb 8), pp. 255-258.

Tang-Christensen, M.; Larsen, P. J.; Thulesen, J.; Romer, J. & Vrang, N. (2000). The proglucagon-derived peptide, glucagon-like peptide-2, is a neurotransmitter involved in the regulation of food intake. *Nat Med,* Vol.6, No.7, (Jul), pp. 802-807.

Tippett, P. S. & Neet, K. E. (1982). An allosteric model for the inhibition of glucokinase by long chain acyl coenzyme A. *J Biol Chem,* Vol.257, No.21, (Nov 10), pp. 12846-12852.

Tong, Q.; Ye, C.; McCrimmon, R. J.; Dhillon, H.; Choi, B.; Kramer, M. D.; Yu, J.; Yang, Z.; Christiansen, L. M.; Lee, C. E.; Choi, C. S.; Zigman, J. M.; Shulman, G. I.; Sherwin, R. S.; Elmquist, J. K. & Lowell, B. B. (2007). Synaptic glutamate release by ventromedial hypothalamic neurons is part of the neurocircuitry that prevents hypoglycemia. *Cell Metab,* Vol.5, No.5, (May), pp. 383-393.

Toyoda, Y.; Miwa, I.; Satake, S.; Anai, M. & Oka, Y. (1995). Nuclear location of the regulatory protein of glucokinase in rat liver and translocation of the regulator to the cytoplasm in response to high glucose. *Biochem Biophys Res Commun,* Vol.215, No.2, (Oct 13), pp. 467-473.

Tsuneki, H.; Wada, T. & Sasaoka, T. (2010). Role of orexin in the regulation of glucose homeostasis. *Acta Physiol (Oxf),* Vol.198, No.3, (Mar), pp. 335-348.

Turnley, A. M.; Stapleton, D.; Mann, R. J.; Witters, L. A.; Kemp, B. E. & Bartlett, P. F. (1999). Cellular distribution and developmental expression of AMP-activated protein kinase isoforms in mouse central nervous system. *J Neurochem,* Vol.72, No.4, (Apr), pp. 1707-1716.

Turton, M. D.; O'Shea, D.; Gunn, I.; Beak, S. A.; Edwards, C. M.; Meeran, K.; Choi, S. J.; Taylor, G. M.; Heath, M. M.; Lambert, P. D.; Wilding, J. P.; Smith, D. M.; Ghatei, M. A.; Herbert, J. & Bloom, S. R. (1996). A role for glucagon-like peptide-1 in the central regulation of feeding. *Nature,* Vol.379, No.6560, (Jan 4), pp. 69-72.

Uttenthal, L. O.; Toledano, A. & Blazquez, E. (1992). Autoradiographic localization of receptors for glucagon-like peptide-1 (7-36) amide in rat brain. *Neuropeptides,* Vol.21, No.3, (Mar), pp. 143-146.

Van Schaftingen, E. (1989). A protein from rat liver confers to glucokinase the property of being antagonistically regulated by fructose 6-phosphate and fructose 1-phosphate. *Eur J Biochem,* Vol.179, No.1, (Jan 15), pp. 179-184.

Van Schaftingen, E.; Bartrons, R. & Hers, H. G. (1984). The mechanism by which ethanol decreases the concentration of fructose 2,6-bisphosphate in the liver. *Biochem J,* Vol.222, No.2, (Sep 1), pp. 511-518.

Vandercammen, A. & Van Schaftingen, E. (1993). Species and tissue distribution of the regulatory protein of glucokinase. *Biochem J,* Vol.294 (Pt 2), (Sep 1), pp. 551-556.

Viollet, B.; Athea, Y.; Mounier, R.; Guigas, B.; Zarrinpashneh, E.; Horman, S.; Lantier, L.; Hebrard, S.; Devin-Leclerc, J.; Beauloye, C.; Foretz, M.; Andreelli, F.; Ventura-Clapier, R. & Bertrand, L. (2009). AMPK: Lessons from transgenic and knockout animals. *Front Biosci,* Vol.14, pp. 19-44.

Vionnet, N.; Stoffel, M.; Takeda, J.; Yasuda, K.; Bell, G. I.; Zouali, H.; Lesage, S.; Velho, G.; Iris, F.; Passa, P. & et al. (1992). Nonsense mutation in the glucokinase gene causes early-onset non-insulin-dependent diabetes mellitus. *Nature,* Vol.356, No.6371, (Apr 23), pp. 721-722.

Wang, R.; Liu, X.; Hentges, S. T.; Dunn-Meynell, A. A.; Levin, B. E.; Wang, W. & Routh, V. H. (2004). The regulation of glucose-excited neurons in the hypothalamic arcuate nucleus by glucose and feeding-relevant peptides. *Diabetes,* Vol.53, No.8, (Aug), pp. 1959-1965.

Yang, X. J.; Kow, L. M.; Funabashi, T. & Mobbs, C. V. (1999). Hypothalamic glucose sensor: similarities to and differences from pancreatic beta-cell mechanisms. *Diabetes,* Vol.48, No.9, (Sep), pp. 1763-1772.

Yang, X. J.; Kow, L. M.; Pfaff, D. W. & Mobbs, C. V. (2004). Metabolic pathways that mediate inhibition of hypothalamic neurons by glucose. *Diabetes,* Vol.53, No.1, (Jan), pp. 67-73.

Zhou, L.; Podolsky, N.; Sang, Z.; Ding, Y.; Fan, X.; Tong, Q.; Levin, B. E. & McCrimmon, R. J. (2010). The Medial Amygdalar Nucleus: A Novel Glucose-Sensing Region That Modulates the Counterregulatory Response to Hypoglycemia. *Diabetes,* Vol.59, No.10, (October 1, 2010), pp. 2646-2652.

4

'Exercise-Eating Linkage' Mediated by Neuro-Endocrine Axis and the Relevance in Regulation of Appetite and Energy Balance for Prevention of Obesity

Takahiro Yoshikawa
Department of Sports Medicine, Osaka City University Graduate School of Medicine, Osaka, Japan

1. Introduction

A significant number of modern people of all ages are affected by obesity epidemic in developed and parts of developing world, resulting in immense health and financial burden (Field, 2002; Ogden et al., 2006; Orsi et al., 2011). Obesity is thought to be an independent risk factor for development of various medical conditions, such as type 2 diabetes, hypertension, dyslipidemia, and cardiovascular disease (Daniels, 2009; Fontaine, 2003; Ginsberg, 2000; Kahn & Flier, 2000; National Institutes of health [NIH], 1998), necessitating weight management for prevention and treatment of these serious diseases. Obesity epidemic reflects modern growing trends to promote excess energy intake (EI) and to discourage energy expenditure (EE) (Egger et al., 2001; Food and Agriculture Organization of the United Nations [FAO], 2003; Hill et al., 2003). Thus, it is well recognized that lifestyle intervention, such as changes in behavior by combination of reductions in EI and increases in physical activity, can achieve ideal weight control (Bray, 2008). Nevertheless, it seems impossible for most of people to fight down consciously their impulses of overeating in modern societies where they have easy access to unlimited supply of highly palatable and energy-dense food (Cohen, 2008).

In such circumstance, appetite is receiving extensive attention for one of key factors to adjust or disrupt energy balance (EB). In particular, an important group of the intricate factors for the appetite control are gut hormone family, including ghrelin, peptide YY (PYY), glucagon-like peptide-1 (GLP-1), oxyntomodulin (OXM), and cholecystokinin (CCK) (Huda et al., 2006; Näslund & Hellström, 2007). Recent advances have been made in understanding the structures, sources, releasers, target organs and receptors, and how these gut hormones influence brain systems for the control of appetite and EI. In brief, these gut hormones are secreted from gastrointestinal organs in response to nutrient conditions and give signals to hypothalamic and brainstem nuclei both of which are in close anatomical proximity to a circumventricular organ with an incomplete blood-brain barrier (BBB), such as median eminence and area postrema. Ghrelin is only an orexigenic hormone and secreted shortly before meals, whereas other gut hormones are all anorectic and released into circulation postprandially in proportion to calorie intake.

While these gut hormones have been well-studied for over a decade, numerous studies have so far investigated a possible association of lifestyle habit, such as exercise, with appetite and EI (King, 1999). Interestingly, recent studies, including ours, have revealed inhibitory effects of exercise on the sensation of hunger and satiety and amount of EI associated with the gut hormone release in various population (Broom et al., 2009; Martins et al., 2007; Ueda et al., 2009a, 2009b), suggesting the presence of an 'exercise-eating linkage' mediated by neuro-endocrine axis in human body. The evidence also suggest an intriguing possibility that physical activity has an impact not simply on EE but also on variations in appetite, leading to negative EB.

The present review provides an overview of 1) changes in sensation of hunger and satiety and amount of EI by various types of exercise and next highlights 2) association of exercise with blood kinetics of gut hormones and its relevance in regulation of appetite and EB. Lastly, 3) future perspective of this research field will be discussed.

2. 'Exercise-eating linkage', is it real?

So far, there has been considerable research on changes in subjective appetite parameters and amount of EI by various types of exercise. Exercise is generally assumed to induce a transient energy deficit and subsequent automatic drive in hunger and EI for energy compensation. However, a majority of previous studies failed to show that a single bout of exercise increase hunger or EI. Such discrepancy between EE and EI can be observed in a wide range of population, irrespective of age, gender, body weight, dietary restraint and exercise intensity. For instance, acute high-intensity exercise (about 70% VO_2 max) is unlikely to cause the subsequent increase in EI in unrestraint males with normal body weight, favoring negative EB (Imbeault et al., 1997; Thompson et al., 1988). Similarly, poor compensation was observed in response to energy deficit by a single bout of high-intensity exercise (cycling 50 min, 70% VO_2 max) in restrained young females with normal body weight (Lluch et al., 1998). Although unrestrained female counterparts rated a range of foods to be more palatable after similar type of exercise, it had no significant short-term effect on energy or macronutrient intake (King et al., 1996). Moderate physical activity (a single bout of 20-min brisk walking) suppressed appetite in middle-aged obese women who were not on special diet (i.e. unrestrained eaters) (Tsofliou, 2003). Similar to acute effects of exercise on appetite, a graded increase in EE by 7-day repeated exercise regimens did not show any significant increases in subjective feeling of hunger and food consumption in lean individuals, generating considerable negative EB (Stubbs et al., 2002a, 2002b). Given the evidence above, 'exercise-eating linkage' is, if any, unlikely to benefit the maintenance of EB, at least short term. Rather, 'exercise-eating linkage' might give rise to transient appetite suppression after exercise. However, it is known that various metabolic and behavioral responses i.e. decrease in EE and increase in appetite and EI after exercise, automatically or volitionally, operate in a long-term process of compensation for the exercise-induced energy deficit, minimizing the negative EB and body weight reduction, and the compensatory responses considerably vary among individuals (King et al., 2007, 2008). And it is assumed that such accurate adjustments of EI to an increase in EE seem to take matter of weeks (Whybrow et al., 2008).

In this regard, however, caution should be exercised when interpreting the findings from these studies. Unlike other animals, internal physiological signals for energy repletion and depletion were not sufficient for the control of appetite and eating behavior in humans. It is well recognized that human eating behavior is a multifactorial process where various external stimuli, including sensory, cognitive, environmental (e.g. social and habitual) variables might play important roles as well as internal signals arising peripherally from gastric distension and energy imbalance (De Castro, 1996). Thus, it is reasonable that eating behavior after exercise can be largely affected by these external factors (British Nutrition Foundation, 1999) and the findings might depend on the background, such as each study setting and subject characteristics. In most previous studies in which association of (short- or long-term) exercise with EI were investigated, test meals were given to subjects *ad libitum*, where the subjects can recognize how much they have eaten, and the subject characteristics (gender, body type and taste) are inconsistent among studies and psychological condition (stress), habitual factors (binge eating) and cognitive factors (reward and preoccupation with food), such as 'food is a reward for exercise' (King, 1999), were often uncontrolled, thus often leading to mixed findings among studies.

3. Exercise and gut hormones: implication for 'exercise-eating linkage'

3.1 Ghrelin

An increasing amount of research has investigated the possibilities that exercise stimulates various gut hormone release into circulation. And, some of recent studies focused on the impact of the exercise-induced gut hormone release on subsequent appetite and EI. In particular, evidence is accumulating for the effect of exercise on the plasma ghrelin levels, but somewhat inconsistent. A single bout of exercise at fasted condition has been shown not to induce significant changes in plasma levels of total ghrelin in normal weight subjects (Kraemer et al., 2004; Zoladz et al., 2005), whereas similar exercise at premeal condition can raise the circulating ghrelin concentrations in moderately overweight postmenopausal women (Borer et al., 2005). Total ghrelin levels were not affected by aerobic exercise intervention for 5 days without body weight reduction (Mackelvie et al., 2007), whereas the plasma levels gradually increased during the 12-weeks aerobic and resistance exercise with significant decreases in body weight and fat (Kim et al., 2008), suggesting that exercise has only a limited impact on the fasting total ghrelin levels unless the body weight of subjects is reduced. Changes in the fasting plasma levels of total ghrelin are likely to depend not on the duration but on the intensity of exercise (Erdmann et al., 2007). Total ghrelin is classified into two categories; orexigenic acylated ghrelin (AG) and anorectic desacyl ghrelin (DG). In contrast to the total ghrelin, orexigenic AG is suppressed by a single bout of exercise at fasted state, resulting in the negative energy balance (Broom et al., 2007). And the postexercise reduction in AG was observed in the lean as well as obese subjects (Marzullo et al., 2008). The effects of long-term exercise training on plasma AG / DG levels seem to be dependent on the duration of exercise. The longer the exercise is performed, the more decrease in AG/DG is observed in favor of body weight reduction (Kim et al., 2008).

3.2 Satiety hormones

Similar to ghrelin, it is only in the last few years that studies have focused on the effects of exercise-induced changes in plasma levels of satiety hormones on appetite regulation and most of these studies have been performed mainly in normal weight individuals. Majority of the early studies focused on plasma PP levels in various setting of exercise preprandially (Hilsted et al., 1980; Sullivan et al., 1984), and postprandially (Greenberg et al., 1986). PP release is likely to be exercise intensity-dependent (Holmqvist et al., 1986). Early studies measured the circulating PP levels as the index of sympathetic activity rather than its physiological roles for appetite regulation (Holmqvist et al., 1986). Plasma GLP-1 levels have been shown to change by exercise in a small number of studies, most of which investigated the association of high intensity exercise with the fasting plasma levels in athletes (O'Connor et al., 1995, 2006). While a single bout of aerobic exercise at fasted state for 10hrs enhanced a response of plasma PYY levels to a test meal after the exercise, such changes were not shown by resistance exercise (Broom 2009).

In most of these studies, the nutrient stimuli are simply replaced by those of exercise, that is, preprandial exercise. However, because these satiety gut hormones are basically released after nutrient intake, it seems worthwhile to examine whether the postprandial plasma levels of these hormones can be affected by exercise and these hormonal changes could affect the subsequent appetite regulation. Recently, some studies, including ours, have investigated kinetics in postprandial release of gut hormones into circulation by a single bout of exercise (Martins et al., 2007; Ueda et al., 2009a, 2009b). One of these studies has demonstrated the postprandial increase in plasma levels of PYY and GLP-1 during and after 1hr exercise at the intensity of 60% of maximal HR. In particular, the time course changes in plasma PYY concentration seem to be mirror image to those in hunger ratings, suggesting that postprandial release of PYY suppress the hunger feeling during and after exercise (Martins et al., 2007). We also investigated acute effect of a single bout of 1 hr aerobic cycling exercise (50% $\dot{V}O_2max$) on the postprandial plasma levels of gut hormones after standard breakfast in overweight and normal young males and determined the involvement of the hormonal changes in regulation of EB in subjects with normal body weight and overweight (Ueda et al., 2009a, 2009b). We assessed the total release of individual gut hormone during and after the exercise as the area under the curve (AUC) of the time course curve of each hormone. In both body type groups, the aerobic exercise significantly increased subsequent release of PYY and GLP-1 in plasma, while plasma levels of acylated ghrelin were not significantly altered. Of note, exercise-induced suppression of relative EI (absolute EI minus absolute EE) in overweight subjects was significantly larger than in control subjects despite lack of significant difference in PYY and GLP-1 levels between two subject groups. The discrepancy might stem from variability of cognitive and sensory factors between two body type groups. In line with this, when the data were analyzed separately in overweight and normal body type group, a significant linear correlation between the increase in AUC values of plasma PYY and GLP-1 levels by exercise and the concurrent decrease in relative EI was observed within each subject group (unpublished data). Collectively, one could argue that neuro-endocrine axis consisting of satiety gut hormones and brain appetite center could play some important roles in 'exercise-eating linkage' of exercise-induced appetite suppression for a while after a single bout of exercise.

Based on the long-term compensation of exercise-induced energy deficit described above, it seems to be necessary to examine whether sustained exercise training also have an impact on the circulating levels of satiety gut hormone and appetite control through the hormonal axis as well as a single bout exercise. The point is important for planning programs in practice for better appetite and weight control. And a few studies have only recently addressed the issue. A significant rise in fasting plasma levels of PYY was shown in overweight adolescent males and females after 32 weeks of exercise training (60-85% peak VO_2, 45min/day, and 3days/week) (Jones et al., 2009). However, neither effects on ratings of appetite feelings nor those on EB were examined. Another study showed that, while postprandial suppression of plasma AG levels seems to be enhanced, postprandial plasma levels of PYY and GLP-1 also tend to be higher after 12 weeks of exercise intervention (75% maximal heart rate, 500kcal energy deficit/day, and 5days/week) while the subjective feelings of hunger increased paradoxically after a test meal (Martins et al., 2010). Although these findings might suggest the possibility that long-term exercise might modify the profiles of orexigenic and satiety gut hormones in circulation, available data are still scarce, particularly as to whether these hormonal changes could suppress superfluous appetite. Further information will be needed for understanding how these gut hormones could affect the long-term regulation of appetite and EI.

4. Future perspectives

As described above, findings of recent studies to date indicate the presence of 'exercise-eating linkage' via neuro-endocrinal axis. Now the following important questions remain unanswered.

Does the responsiveness vary among different intensity and style of exercise or among different body weight types? Does the responsiveness of hypothalamus to the gut hormones fluctuate during exercise? Interestingly, a single bout of 6hr exercise improves the responsiveness of hypothalamus to leptin and appetite control in male rats (Flores et al., 2006; Ropelle et al., 2008). Another study demonstrated that habitual exercise influence appetite and EI in response to covert preload energy manipulation (Long et al., 2002; van Walleghen et al., 2007). In particular, Long SJ *et al.* raised the possibility that exercise may enhance the accuracy of appetite control by the exercise-induced improvement in insulin sensitivity (Aldred et al., 1995; Haber et al., 1977; Holt et al., 1992; Poehlman et al., 2000). Insulin exerts appetite-inhibiting effects via hypothalamus activation (Schwartz 2000). It is still unknown whether the response to satiety gut hormones also can be altered by exercise. Based on previous studies in which these peptides are dosed peripherally, obesity *per se* does not seem to affect the responsiveness to some satiety gut hormones, such as PYY (Batterham et al., 2003).

Does the change in gut hormone levels with exercise have significant effects on other physiological systems as well as appetite regulation? Interestingly, PYY administration decreases respiratory quotient (RQ) and reduces adiposity in diet-induced obese mice (Adams et al., 2006). In human study, high fasting and postprandial peak PYY was observed in subjects with low resting metabolic rate (RMR) (daily EE) and low RQ (Guo et al., 2006). The findings raise an intriguing possibility that exercise might induce PYY secretion and regulate not only the appetite but also EE and fuel partitioning in favour of fat oxidation, providing the additional evidence of advantage of exercise intervention for weight and body fat reduction.

Possible association of the fluctuating gut hormone levels with subsequent appetite and EB are intriguing. However, more important question is how much effect we can expect such intrinsic signal of exercise-induced hormonal changes to modulate the overall appetite system in which other diverse extrinsic factors are largely involved. Hypothalamus is one of pivotal entry points of the peripheral internal signals into central pathways mediating brain appetite regulation along with nucleus tractus solitarius (NTS) in brainstem. There are reciprocal connections between these two entry points and these areas communicate with higher centers such as brain reward centers (e.g. ventrotegmental area, nucleus accumbens, ventral pallidum, and orbitofrontal cortex) which play a role in integration of various sensory information and hedonic signals (Wynne et al., 2005). One of recent neurophysiological studies revealed that the sensory inputs produced by sight, smell, taste and texture of food converge at specific brain regions, such as orbitofrontal cortex, and interact with peripheral hunger/satiety signals at hypothalamus, including autonomic nerve activation and gut hormones, and finally determine eating behavior (Rolls, 2005, 2006). In addition, taste information is also sent to the reward system, which mediates the motivation of eating of palatable food, and finally transfers the signals to the hypothalamus (Yamamoto, 2008). While human intrinsic appetite control systems remain unchanged in recent few decades, the excess food stimuli override appetite suppressive responses, such as humoral and neural satiety signals arising from gastrointestinal organs, resulting in overeating and subsequent obesity. Exercise might partly correct the disparity between the primitive appetite control systems and the current expanding food consumption by upregulating the peripheral satiety signals. Interestingly, a recent human study using brain functional MRI demonstrated that, after intravenous infusion of PYY at physiological plasma concentrations, mimicking the fed state, hypothalamic neural activity was not correlated with caloric intake, while the changes in neural signals within higher center, the orbitofrontal cortex, correlated with caloric intake, suggesting that brain activity predicting caloric intake appeared to switch from hypothalamus to higher center, orbitofrontal cortex in the presence of PYY (Batterham et al., 2007). Based on this observation, the exercise-induced increase in the plasma PYY levels might cause some possible effects on the neural

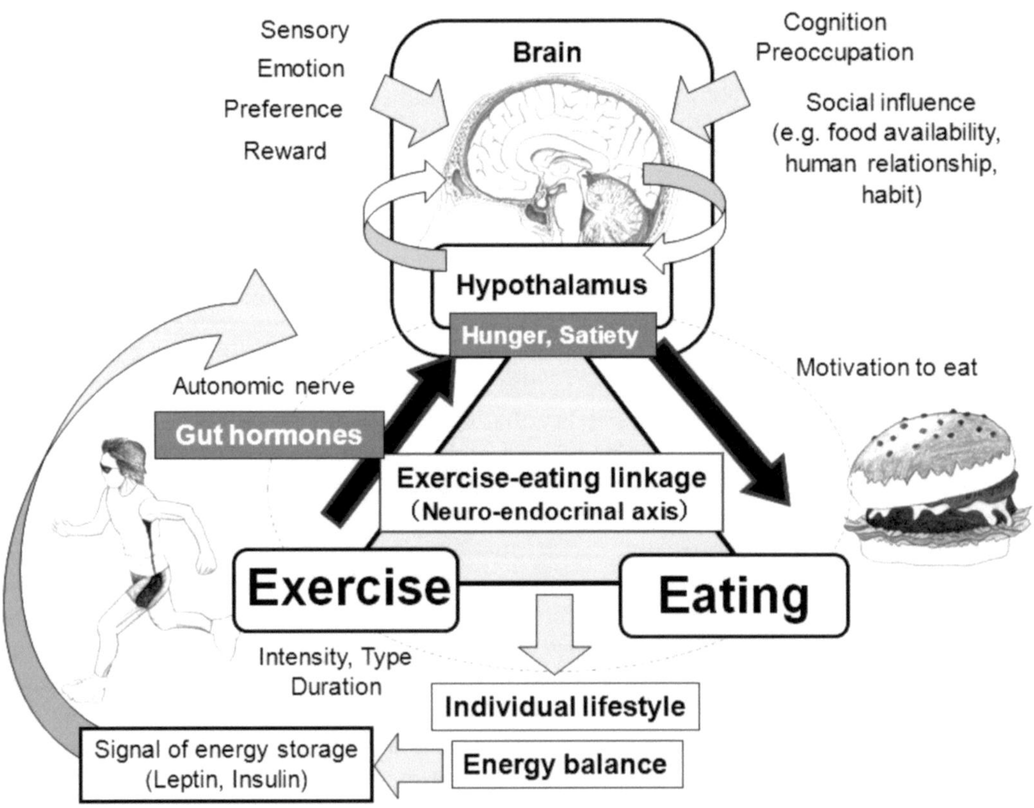

Fig. 1. Overview of exercise-eating linkage via neuro-endocrinal axis

activity in higher centers for appetite control. In addition to the changes in gut hormones, exercise also influences brain dopaminergic, GABAergic, noradrenergic and serotonergic systems (Meeusen & De Meirleir, 1995). In rat models, changes in synthesis and metabolism of these neurotransmitters and receptors during exercise were observed in distinct brain regions including hypothalamus (Kramer et al., 2000). Although it is beyond the scope of this review to include these neurophysiological findings, we should keep in mind the large general picture of these control systems before we consider the implication for the association of exercise with appetite, EB and gut hormones. Future studies will be needed to investigate the effects of (acute or long-term) exercise on the overall appetite regulatory systems (exercise-eating linkage) based on the crosstalk interactions between peripheral endocrine system and central appetite centers (neuro-endocrinal axis) (Figure). Furthermore, the understanding might give us clues to reveal the reasons why there is inter-individual variability in ratings of hunger and amount of food ingested after exercise (King et al., 2007), leading to tailored strategies of preventive programs and treatment for overeating and obesity.

In conclusion, The evidence of exercise-induced changes in satiety gut hormones with suppression of hunger feeling and subsequent relative EI provides considerable support for the value of exercise not only in a measure of expenditure but also in preventing from overeating and obesity. Understanding of this area in endocrinology combined with neurophysiology of eating behaviour in higher brain centers might facilitate the development of promising approach to maintain better dietary life with appropriate exercise and healthy body weight.

5. References

Adams SH, Lei C, Jodka CM, Nikoulina SE, Hoyt JA, Gedulin B, Mack CM, Kendall ES. PYY[3-36] administration decreases the respiratory quotient and reduces adiposity in diet-induced obese mice. *J Nutr.* 2006;136:195-201.

Aldred HE, Hardman AE, Taylor S. Influence of 12 weeks of training by brisk walking on postprandial lipemia and insulinemia in sedentary middle-aged women. *Metabolism.* 1995;44:390-7.

Batterham RL, Cohen MA, Ellis SM, Le Roux CW, Withers DJ, Frost GS, Ghatei MA, Bloom SR. Inhibition of food intake in obese subjects by peptide YY3-36. *N Engl J Med.* 2003;349:941-8.

Batterham RL, ffytche DH, Rosenthal JM, Zelaya FO, Barker GJ, Withers DJ, Williams SC. PYY modulation of cortical and hypothalamic brain areas predicts feeding behaviour in humans. *Nature.* 2007;450:106-9.

Borer KT, Wuorinen E, Chao C, Burant C. Exercise energy expenditure is not consciously detected due to oro-gastric, not metabolic, basis of hunger sensation. *Appetite.* 2005;45:177-81.

Bray GA. Lifestyle and pharmacological approaches to weight loss: efficacy and safety. *J Clin Endocrinol Metab.* 2008;93(11 Suppl 1):S81-8.

British Nutrition Foundation. *Obesity.* Blackwell Science: Oxford, 1999.

Broom DR, Stensel DJ, Bishop NC, Burns SF, Miyashita M. Exercise-induced suppression of acylated ghrelin in humans. *J Appl Physiol.* 2007;102:2165-71.

Broom DR, Batterham RL, King JA, Stensel DJ. Influence of resistance and aerobic exercise on hunger, circulating levels of acylated ghrelin, and peptide YY in healthy males. *Am J Physiol Regul Integr Comp Physiol.* 2009;296:R29-35.

Cohen DA. Neurophysiological pathways to obesity: below awareness and beyond individual control. *Diabetes*. 2008;57:1768-73.

Daniels SR. Complications of obesity in children and adolescents. *Int J Obes (Lond)*. 2009;33:S60-5.

De Castro JM. How can eating behavior be regulated in complex environments of free-living humans? *Neurosci Biobehav Rev*. 1996;20:119-31.

Egger GJ, Vogels N, Westerterp KR. Estimating historical changes in physical activity levels Med J Aust. 2001;175(11-12):635-6.

Erdmann J, Tahbaz R, Lippl F, Wagenpfeil S, Schusdziarra V. Plasma ghrelin levels during exercise - effects of intensity and duration. *Regul Pept*. 2007;143:127-35.

Field AE, Epidemiology and health and economic consequences of obesity. In: Wadden TA, Stunkard AJ, editors. Handbook of obesity treatment. New York: Guilford Press; 2002. p3-18.

Flores MB, Fernandes MF, Ropelle ER, Faria MC, Ueno M, Velloso LA, Saad MJ, Carvalheira JB. Exercise improves insulin and leptin sensitivity in hypothalamus of Wistar rats. *Diabetes*. 2006;55:2554-61.

Fontaine KR, Years of life lost due to obesity. JAMA. 2003;289:187-193.

Food and Agriculture Organization of the United Nations (FAO). Global and regional food consumption pattern and trends; http://www.fao.org/DOCREP/005/AC911E/ac911e05.htm

Ginsberg HN. Insulin resistance and cardiovascular disease. *J Clin Invest*. 2000;106:453-8.

Greenberg GR, Marliss EB, Zinman B. Effect of exercise on the pancreatic polypeptide response to food in man. *Horm Metab Res*. 1986;18:194-6.

Guo Y, Ma L, Enriori PJ, Koska J, Franks PW, Brookshire T, Cowley MA, Salbe AD, Delparigi A, Tataranni PA. Physiological evidence for the involvement of peptide YY in the regulation of energy homeostasis in humans. *Obesity (Silver Spring)*. 2006;14:1562-70.

Haber GB, Heaton KW, Murphy D, Burroughs LF. Depletion and disruption of dietary fibre. Effects on satiety, plasma-glucose, and serum-insulin. *Lancet*. 1977;2:679-82.

Hill JO, Wyatt HR, Reed GW, Peters JC. Obesity and the environment: where do we go from here? *Science*. 2003;299:853-5.

Hilsted J, Galbo H, Sonne B, Schwartz T, Fahrenkrug J, de Muckadell OB, Lauritsen KB, Tronier B. Gastroenteropancreatic hormonal changes during exercise. *Am J Physiol*. 1980;239:G136-40.

Holmqvist N, Secher NH, Sander-Jensen K, Knigge U, Warberg J, Schwartz TW. Sympathoadrenal and parasympathetic responses to exercise. *J Sports Sci*.1986;4:123-8.

Holt S, Brand J, Soveny C, Hansky J. Relationship of satiety to postprandial glycaemic, insulin and cholecystokinin responses. *Appetite*. 1992;18:129-41.

Huda MS, Wilding JP, Pinkney JH. Gut peptides and the regulation of appetite. *Obes Rev*. 2006;7:163-82.

Imbeault P, Saint-Pierre S, Alméras N, Tremblay A. Acute effects of exercise on energy intake and feeding behaviour. *Br J Nutr*. 1997;77:511-21.

Jones TE, Basilio JL, Brophy PM, McCammon MR, Hickner RC. Long-term exercise training in overweight adolescents improves plasma peptide YY and resistin. *Obesity (Silver Spring)*. 2009;17:1189-95 .

Kahn BB, Flier JS. Obesity and insulin resistance. J Clin Invest. 2000;106:473-481.

Kim HJ, Lee S, Kim TW, Kim HH, Jeon TY, Yoon YS, Oh SW, Kwak H, Lee JG. Effects of exercise-induced weight loss on acylated and unacylated ghrelin in overweight children. *Clin Endocrinol (Oxf)*. 2008;68:416-22.

King NA, Snell L, Smith RD, Blundell JE. Effects of short-term exercise on appetite responses in unrestrained females. *Eur J Clin Nutr*. 1996;50:663-7.

King NA. What processes are involved in the appetite response to moderate increases in exercise-induced energy expenditure? *Proc Nutr Soc*. 1999;58:107-13.

King NA, Caudwell P, Hopkins M, Byrne NM, Colley R, Hills AP, Stubbs JR, Blundell JE. Metabolic and behavioral compensatory responses to exercise interventions: barriers to weight loss. *Obesity (Silver Spring)*. 2007;15:1373-83.

King NA, Hopkins M, Caudwell P, Stubbs RJ, Blundell JE. Individual variability following 12 weeks of supervised exercise: identification and characterization of compensation for exercise-induced weight loss. *Int J Obes (Lond)*. 2008;32:177-84.

Kraemer RR, Durand RJ, Acevedo EO, Johnson LG, Kraemer GR, Hebert EP, Castracane VD. Rigorous running increases growth hormone and insulin-like growth factor-I without altering ghrelin. *Exp Biol Med*. 2004;229:240-6.

Kramer JM, Plowey ED, Beatty JA, Little HR, Waldrop TG. Hypothalamus, hypertension, and exercise. *Brain Res Bull*. 2000;53:77-85.

Lluch A, King NA, Blundell JE. Exercise in dietary restrained women: no effect on energy intake but change in hedonic ratings. *Eur J Clin Nutr*. 1998;52:300-7.

Long SJ, Hart K, Morgan LM. The ability of habitual exercise to influence appetite and food intake in response to high- and low-energy preloads in man. *Br J Nutr*. 2002;87:517-23.

Mackelvie KJ, Meneilly GS, Elahi D, Wong AC, Barr SI, Chanoine JP. Regulation of appetite in lean and obese adolescents after exercise: role of acylated and desacyl ghrelin. *J Clin Endocrinol Metab*. 2007;92:648-54.

Martins C, Morgan LM, Bloom SR, Robertson MD. Effects of exercise on gut peptides, energy intake and appetite. *J Endocrinol*. 2007;193:251-8.

Martins C, Kulseng B, King NA, Holst JJ, Blundell JE. The effects of exercise-induced weight loss on appetite-related peptides and motivation to eat. *J Clin Endocrinol Metab*. 2010;95:1609-16.

Marzullo P, Salvadori A, Brunani A, Verti B, Walker GE, Fanari P, Tovaglieri I, De Medici C, Savia G, Liuzzi A. Acylated ghrelin decreases during acute exercise in the lean and obese state. *Clin Endocrinol (Oxf)*. 2008;69:970-1.

Meeusen R, De Meirleir K. Exercise and brain neurotransmission. *Sports Med*. 1995;20:160-88.

National Institutes of health (NIH). Clinical guidelines on the identification, evaluation, and treatment of overweight and obesity in adults: the evidence report. *Obes Res*. 1998;6:51S-210S.

Näslund E, Hellström PM. Appetite signaling: from gut peptides and enteric nerves to brain. *Physiol Behav*. 2007;92:256-62.

O'Connor AM, Johnston CF, Buchanan KD, Boreham C, Trinick TR, Riddoch CJ. Circulating gastrointestinal hormone changes in marathon running. *Int J Sports Med*. 1995;16:283-7.

O'Connor AM, Pola S, Ward BM, Fillmore D, Buchanan KD, Kirwan JP. The gastroenteroinsular response to glucose ingestion during postexercise recovery. *Am J Physiol Endocrinol Metab*. 2006;290:E1155-61.

Ogden CL, Carroll MD, Curtin LR, McDowell MA, Tabak CJ, Flegal KM. Prevalence of overweight and obesity in the United States, 1999-2004. *JAMA*. 2006;295:1549-55.

Orsi CM, Hale DE, Lynch JL. Pediatric obesity epidemiology. *Curr Opin Endocrinol Diabetes Obes*. 2011;18:14-22.

Poehlman ET, Dvorak RV, DeNino WF, Brochu M, Ades PA. Effects of resistance training and endurance training on insulin sensitivity in nonobese, young women: a controlled randomized trial. *J Clin Endocrinol Metab.* 2000;85:2463-8.

Rolls ET. Taste, olfactory, and food texture processing in the brain, and the control of food intake. *Physiol Behav.* 2005;85:45-56.

Rolls ET. Brain mechanisms underlying flavour and appetite. *Philos Trans R Soc Lond B.* 2006;361:1123-36.

Ropelle ER, Fernandes MF, Flores MB, Ueno M, Rocco S, Marin R, Cintra DE, Velloso LA, Franchini KG, Saad MJ, Carvalheira JB. Central exercise action increases the AMPK and mTOR response to leptin. *PLoS One.* 2008;3:e3856.

Schwartz MW, Woods SC, Porte D Jr, Seeley RJ, Baskin DG. Central nervous system control of food intake. *Nature.* 2000;404:661-71.

Stubbs RJ, Sepp A, Hughes DA, Johnstone AM, Horgan GW, King N, Blundell J. The effect of graded levels of exercise on energy intake and balance in free-living men, consuming their normal diet. *Eur J Clin Nutr.* 2002a;56:129-40.

Stubbs RJ, Sepp A, Hughes DA, Johnstone AM, King N, Horgan G, Blundell JE. The effect of graded levels of exercise on energy intake and balance in free-living women. *Int J Obes Relat Metab Disord.* 2002b;26:866-9.

Sullivan SN, Champion MC, Christofides ND, Adrian TE, and Bloom SR. Gastrointestinal regulatory peptide responses in long-distance runners. *Phys Sports Med.* 1984;12:77–82.

Thompson DA, Wolfe LA, Eikelboom R. Acute effects of exercise intensity on appetite in young men. *Med Sci Sports Exerc.* 1988;20:222-7.

Tsofliou F, Pitsiladis YP, Malkova D, Wallace AM, Lean ME. Moderate physical activity permits acute coupling between serum leptin and appetite-satiety measures in obese women. *Int J Obes Relat Metab Disord.* 2003;27:1332-9.

Ueda SY, Yoshikawa T, Katsura Y, Usui T, Nakao H, Fujimoto S. Changes in gut hormone levels and negative energy balance during aerobic exercise in obese young males. *J Endocrinol.* 2009a;201:151-9.

Ueda SY, Yoshikawa T, Katsura Y, Usui T, Fujimoto S. Comparable effects of moderate intensity exercise on changes in anorectic gut hormone levels and energy intake to high intensity exercise. *J Endocrinol.* 2009b;203:357-64.

van Walleghen EL, Orr JS, Gentile CL, Davy KP, Davy BM. Habitual physical activity differentially affects acute and short-term energy intake regulation in young and older adults. *Int J Obes (Lond).* 2007;31:1277-85.

Whybrow S, Hughes DA, Ritz P, Johnstone AM, Horgan GW, King N, Blundell JE, Stubbs RJ. The effect of an incremental increase in exercise on appetite, eating behaviour and energy balance in lean men and women feeding ad libitum. *Br J Nutr.* 2008;100:1109-15.

Wynne K, Stanley S, McGowan B, Bloom S. Appetite control. *J Endocrinol.* 2005;184:291-318.

Yamamoto T. Central mechanisms of roles of taste in reward and eating. *Acta Physiol Hung.* 2008;95:165-86.

Zoladz JA, Konturek SJ, Duda K, Majerczak J, Sliwowski Z, Grandys M, Bielanski W. Effect of moderate incremental exercise, performed in fed and fasted state on cardio-respiratory variables and leptin and ghrelin concentrations in young healthy men. *J Physiol Pharmacol.* 2005;56:63-85.

5

Estrogen Receptors in Glucose Homeostasis

Malin Hedengran Faulds and Karin Dahlman-Wright
Karolinska Institutet
Sweden

1. Introduction

Metabolic diseases affect more than 230 million people worldwide with an expectancy to increase to around 350 million in the coming 25 years. It is currently the fourth leading cause of death by disease. The metabolic syndrome refers to a group of interrelated metabolic abnormalities that include disturbed glucose homeostasis, insulin resistance (IR), increased body weight and abdominal fat accumulation, mild dyslipidemia and hypertension. Individuals with the metabolic syndrome have an increased risk of cardiovascular disease (CVD) and Type 2 diabetes (T2D).

Estrogens have traditionally been connected with female reproduction, however, the importance of these hormones in tissues outside of the reproductive system including the liver, bone, the cardiovascular system and brain have since been established (Gruber et al., 2002). Estrogen and the estrogen receptors (ERs) are well-known regulators of glucose homeostasis and several epidemiological and prospective studies associate estrogen to various aspects of the metabolic syndrome (Louet et al., 2004). Postmenopausal women develop visceral obesity, IR and are at high risk for T2D. Treatment of healthy postmenopausal women with estrogen has been shown to improve insulin sensitivity and to lower blood glucose (Crespo et al., 2002). Furthermore, hormone replacement therapy (HRT) in postmenopausal women with coronary artery disease was associated with a 35% reduction in the incidence of T2D (Kanaya et al., 2003). Male aromatase-deficient patients, as well as a male patient with loss of ERα function, display impaired glucose metabolism, IR and hyperinsulinemia (Zirilli, et al. 2008). In addition, the aromatase deficient patients showed impaired liver functions, hepatic steatosis, and altered lipid profile (Maffei, et al. 2004). Additional observations in rodents support the notion that estrogen mediates anti-diabetic effects. For example, female rodents are protected against hyperglycemia, unless they are ovariectomized, in spontaneous rodent models of T2D.

Studies in knock-out mouse models have shed light on the role of estrogen and its receptors in rodent obesity and glucose tolerance. Mice with functional knock-out of the aromatase enzyme (ArKO mice) are unable to synthesize endogenous estrogen and display an obese and insulin resistant phenotype (Fisher et al., 1998). A similar phenotype was observed in mice lacking ERα (ERαKO) but not in mice lacking ERβ (ERβKO), indicating that ERα is the major mediator for the estrogenic effects on insulin sensitivity and body weight (Heine et al., 2000). Although ERα appears to be more important in relation to body weight and insulin sensitivity, it remains possible that ERβ also contributes in this context, particularly in older mice and under specific metabolic conditions (Foryst-Ludwig et al., 2008).

2. Carbohydrate metabolism

Carbohydrate catabolism starts with digestion in the small intestine where monosaccharides derived from food are absorbed into the circulation. The most important carbohydrate is glucose, which is metabolized by most organisms. Circulating levels of glucose are controlled by two hormones; insulin and glucagon. When circulating levels of glucose are raised, insulin is secreted by the pancreatic β cells to stimulate glucose uptake in liver, muscles and white adipose tissue (WAT), where excess glucose is stored as glycogen by the process of glycogenesis. When blood glucose levels decrease, glucagon is secreted from the pancreatic α cells to stimulate the breakdown of glycogen to glucose through glycogenolysis (see figure 1).

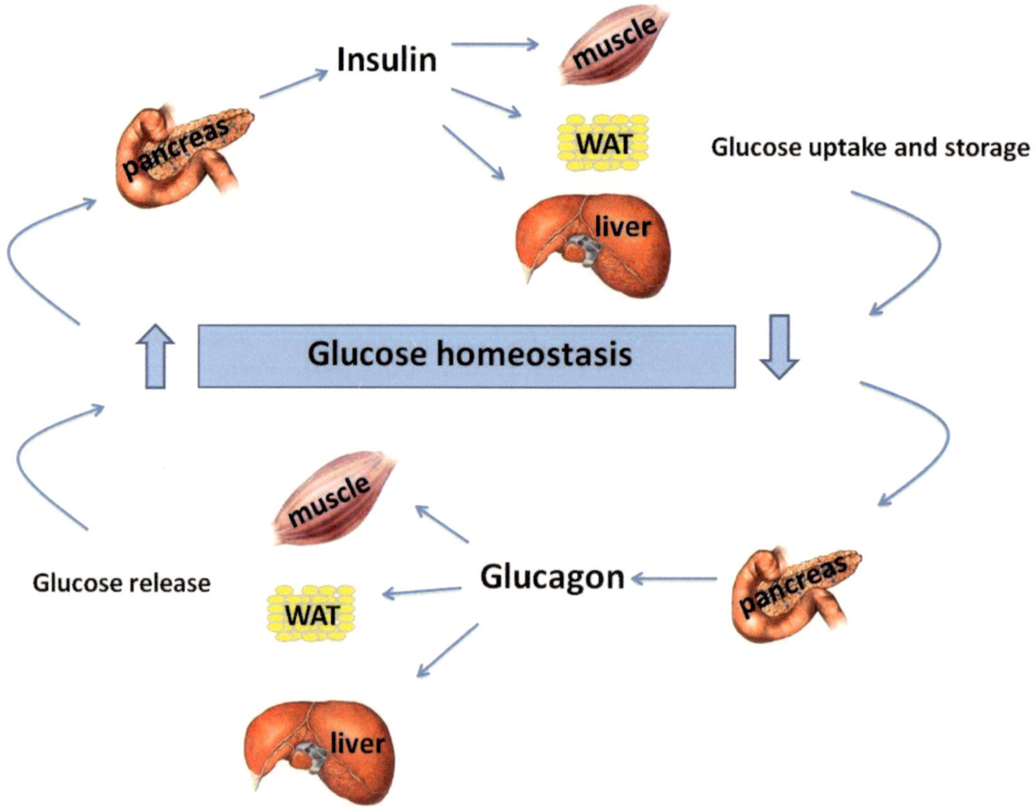

Fig. 1. **Regulation of glucose homeostasis.** In response to glucose excess, insulin is secreted by the pancreatic β cells to stimulate glucose uptake and storage in muscles, liver and white adipose tissue (WAT). When glucose levels decrease, glucagon is secreted to stimulate glucose release into circulation.

The β cells in the pancreatic islets of Langerhans release insulin in two phases. The first is a rapid response to increase blood glucose levels and the second phase is a slow release that is triggered independently of glucose. There are several substances apart from glucose known to stimulate insulin release, including amino acids from dietary proteins, acetylcholine released from vagus nerve endings, gastrointestinal hormones and glucose-dependent insulinotropic peptides (reviewed by (Kieffer et al., 1996)).
The hormone glucagon is secreted from the α cells in the pancreatic islets of Langerhans and promotes conversion of hepatic glycogen into glucose, which is subsequently released into the blood. The output of glucagon is triggered by low levels of circulating glucose (Nussey & Whitehead, 2001).
IR is a physiological condition where insulin is less effective in lowering circulating glucose. IR in muscle and WAT reduces glucose uptake whereas hepatic IR results in reduced glycogen synthesis and storage and a failure of insulin to suppress glucose production and subsequent release into the blood (reviewed by (Benito, 2011)). IR commonly refers to the reduced glucose lowering effects of insulin as described above. However, other functions of insulin are also affected. For example, IR in adipocytes results in reduced uptake of circulating lipids and increased hydrolysis of stored triglycerides, which leads to elevated levels of circulating free fatty acids (Savage et al., 2007). High plasma levels of insulin, glucose and lipids due to IR are major components of the metabolic syndrome, which could develop into T2D.

3. Estrogen signaling and estrogen receptors

Estrogens are sex steroids, which stem from the common pre-cursor cholesterol. The last step in the synthesis of estrogen from androgens is catalyzed by the P450 enzyme aromatase. The three major physiological estrogens include 17β-estradiol (E2), estrone (E1) and estriol. The major physiological estrogen in fertile females is E2, which has a similar affinity for both ERs. In addition, ERs are activated by a range of synthetic ligands including selective estrogen receptor modulators (SERMs) such as raloxifen and tamoxifen, the ERα selective agonist propyl-pyrazole-triol (PPT) and the ERβ-selective agonist diarylpropionitrile (DPN) (Heldring et al., 2007).
Estrogens exert their physiological effects through the two ER subtypes, ERα and ERβ, which are members of the superfamily of nuclear receptors. The human ESR1 gene, which is encoding for ERα, is located on the chromosome 6, at 6q25.1, and includes 8 exons. The ERβ encoding gene, ESR2, is located on chromosome 14 at 14q22–24. ERα is mainly expressed in reproductive tissues, kidney, bone, WAT and liver, while ERβ is expressed in the ovary, prostate, lung, gastrointestinal tract, bladder and the central nervous systems (CNS) (Matthews & Gustafsson, 2003).
Genetic associations have been described for polymorphisms of the ESR1 gene and several pathological conditions related to metabolism in general, including cardiovascular diseases, T2D, myocardial infarction, hypertension and venous thromboembolism (Schuit et al., 2004; Shearman et al., 2003; Yoshihara et al., 2009). Polymorphisms of the ESR1 gene can also affect lipoprotein metabolism (Lamon-Fava et al., 2010).
ESR2 polymorphisms have been associated with anorexia nervosa, bulimic disease and premature coronary artery disease (Eastwood et al., 2002; Nilsson et al., 2004; Peter et al., 2005).
ERs share a common structure with the other members of the nuclear receptor family. The N-terminal A/B domain is the most variable region with less than 20% amino acid identity between the two ERs and confers subtype specific actions on target genes. This region

harbors the activation function-1 (AF-1), which is ligand-independent and shows promoter- and cell-specific activities. The centrally located C-domain harbors the DNA binding domain (DBD), which is involved in DNA binding and receptor dimerization. This domain is highly conserved between ERα and ERβ with 97% amino acid identity. The D-domain is referred to as the hinge domain and displays low conservation between ERα and ERβ (30%). This domain has been shown to contain a nuclear localization signal. The C-terminal E-domain contains the ligand-binding domain (LBD) and the two subtypes display 56% conservation in this region. The LBD contains a hormone-dependent activation function (AF-2) and also includes functions responsible for ligand binding and receptor dimerization. The F-domain has less than 20% amino acid identity between the two ER subtypes and the functions of this domain remain undefined (Zhao et al., 2008).

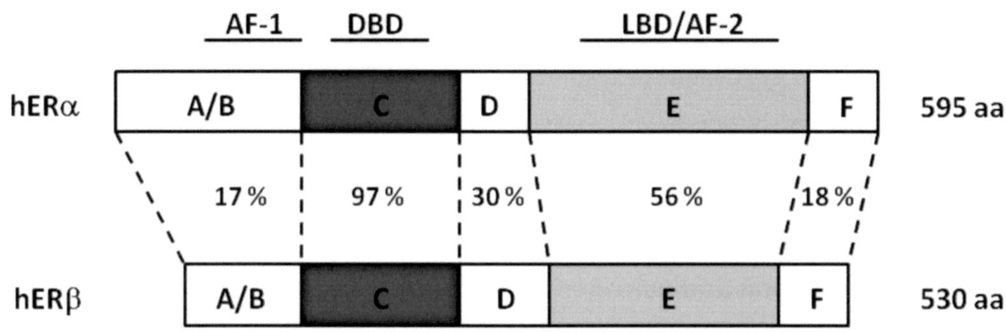

Fig. 2. **Structure and homology between human ERα and ERβ.** The A/B domain is referring to the ligand independent transcription activation function-1 (AF-1). The C domain is mediating DNA binding and the D domain represents the hinge domain, which harbors nuclear localization signals. The E domain is involved in ligand binding and contains the ligand dependent AF-2 function, which is involved in ligand binding. Depicted is also the homology in percent between the various domains between the two subtypes.

Like other nuclear receptors, ligand-bound ERs act as dimers to regulate transcriptional activation. Full transcriptional activity of the ERs is mediated through a synergistic action between the two activation domains, AF-1 and AF-2. Both ERα and ERβ contain a potent AF-2 function, but unlike ERα, ERβ seems to have a weaker corresponding AF-1 function and depends more on the ligand-dependent AF-2 for its transcriptional activation function (Dahlman-Wright et al., 2006). In their unliganded state, ERs are associated with protein complexes of heat shock proteins, which inhibit their functions.

The classical estrogen signaling occurs through a direct binding of ligand activated ER dimers to estrogen-responsive elements (EREs) in the regulatory regions of estrogen target genes followed by activation of the transcriptional machinery at the transcription start sites of regulated genes. Estrogen also modulates gene expression by a second mechanism in which ERs interact with other DNA bound transcription factors, such as activating protein-1 (AP-1) and stimulating protein-1 (Sp-1) to regulate gene expression, through a process referred to as transcription factor cross-talk. Estrogen may also elicit effects through non-genomic mechanisms, which involve the activation of downstream signaling cascades like protein kinase A (PKA), protein kinase C (PKC) and mitogen-activated protein (MAP) kinase via membrane-localized ERs.

Recently, an orphan G protein-coupled receptor (GPR) 30 in the cell membrane was reported to mediate non-genomic and rapid estrogen signaling (Revankar et al., 2005; Thomas et al., 2005). GPR30 is structurally unrelated to ERα and ERβ and the rapid effects from stimulation of this receptor include release of intracellular Ca^{2+} and subsequent activation of calcium-calmodulin-dependent kinases or activation of MAP kinase and phosphoinositide 3-kinase pathways. Human GPR30 is located on chromosome 7p22.3, and is composed of three exons. Exon3 constitutes the amino acid coding region of GPR30. Based on genetic linkage analysis, the region of the chromosome containing GPR30 is thought to be related to familial hypertensive disease in humans (Lafferty et al., 2000). The mRNA for GPR30 appears to be expressed in most tissues.

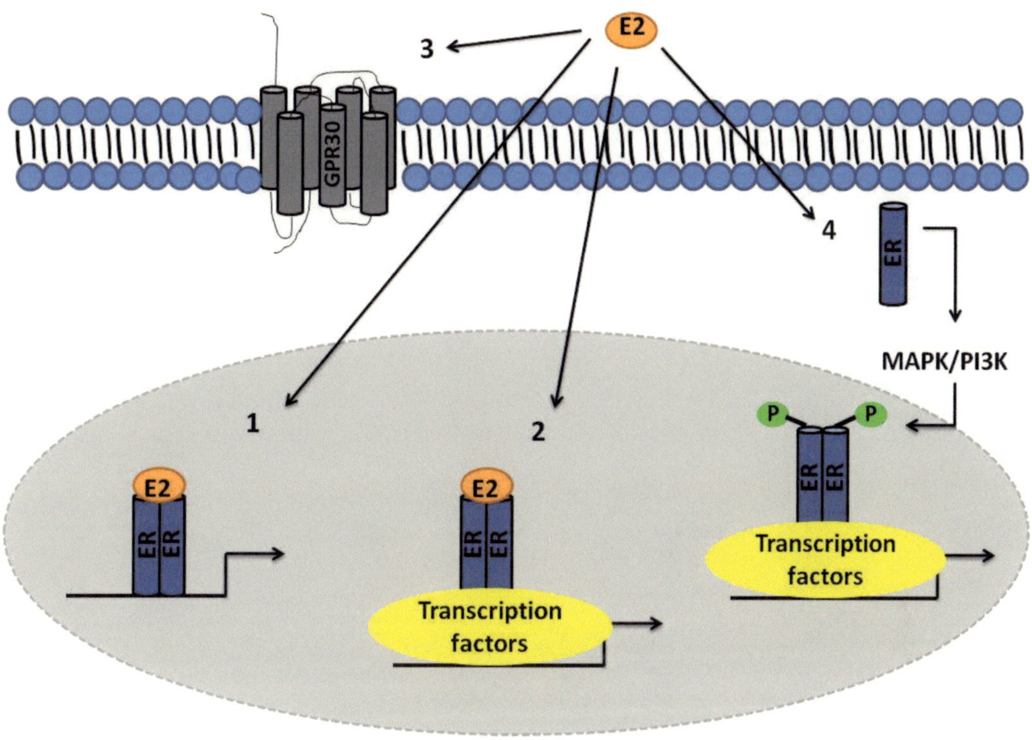

Fig. 3. **Estrogen signaling mechanisms.** I. Classical pathway involving activation of the ERs followed by DNA binding. II. Non-classical pathway involving interactions with transcription factors and subsequent indirect DNA binding. III. Non-genomic pathway involving GPR30. IV. Ligand-independent pathway involving kinase cascades and subsequent ER phosphorylation.

4. Estrogen signaling in glucose homeostasis

Estrogen and estrogen signaling have long been known to be important regulators of glucose homeostasis and are implicated in maintaining normal insulin sensitivity. Fluctuations in estrogen levels below the physiological range, as a consequence of menopause or ovariectomy, may promote IR and T2D. In humans, the most consistent effects of oral contraceptives or HRT are decreased levels of fasting plasma glucose and improved glucose tolerance. Absence of estrogen signaling in men, due to deficiency of the aromatase enzyme or ERα, results in impaired glucose metabolism. It has also been shown that polymorphisms in the ERα gene are associated with development of the metabolic syndrome and T2D (Yoshihara et al., 2009).

Estrogens further display inhibitory effects on maltase, sucrose and lactase activities in the intestine. Estrogen supplements have been shown to manifest a range of disaccharidase and lipase inhibitory actions that help to delay the absorption of dietary carbohydrates in the intestine, which will lead to suppression of the increased glucose levels observed after meals (Hamden et al., 2011).

Several rodent studies link estrogen to glucose regulatory effects. Female rodents are protected against hyperglycemia, unless they are ovariectomized, in spontaneous rodent models of T2D and ArKO mice display severe IR (Jones et al., 2000). ERα and ERβ have both been suggested to be involved in blood glucose homeostasis. ERαKO mice are insulin resistant and ERα has been shown to be involved in regulation of glucose metabolism by acting in different tissues including liver, skeletal muscle, adipose tissue, endocrine pancreas and the central nervous system (CNS) as depicted in figure 4. Although ERα appears to be more important in relation to body weight and insulin sensitivity, it remains possible that ERβ also contributes in this context, particularly in older mice and under specific metabolic conditions.

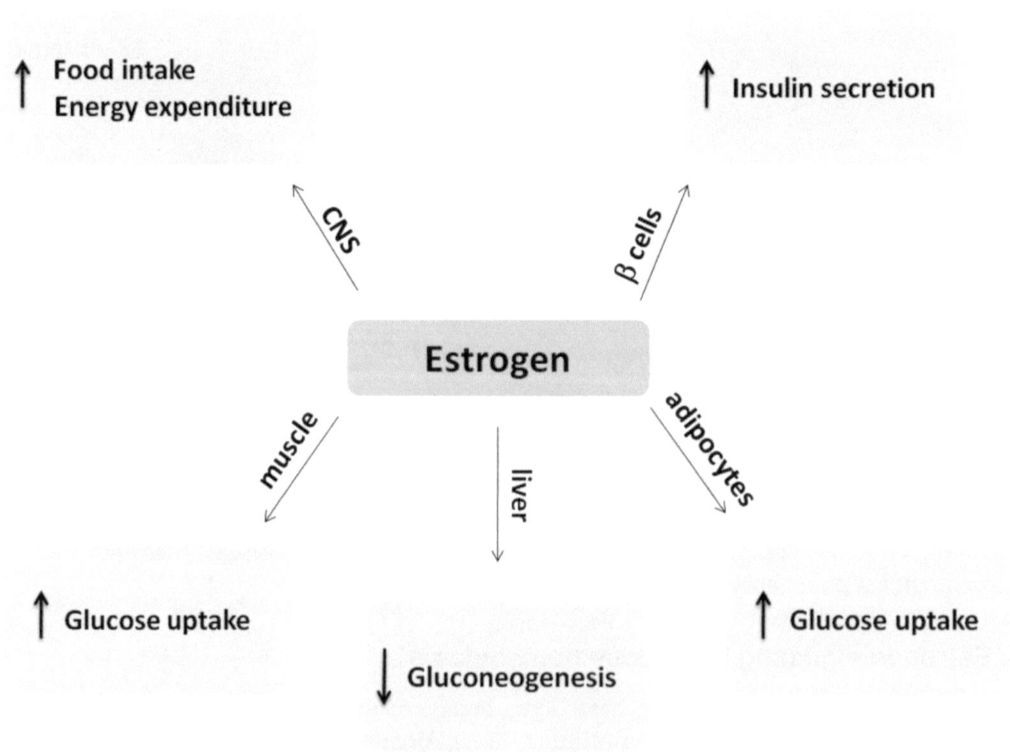

Fig. 4. **Estrogen influences glucose metabolism in the central nervous system (CNS), pancreatic β cells, muscles, liver and adipocytes.**

4.1 ERs and the role of the central nervous system in glucose homeostasis

The first finding supporting that the central nervous system (CNS) was involved in the regulation of glucose homeostasis was that ruptures in the fourth ventricle resulted in glucosuria. This initial study was followed by numerous other studies and it is now firmly established that the CNS regulates glucose homeostasis through the hormones insulin, leptin and glucagon-like peptide (GLP)-1, as well as by glucose and fatty acids (FA). A series of complex systems regulate energy homeostasis in order to keep energy levels and body weight stable (Miller, 1982). Glucose is the vital energy source for the brain. There are several glucose sensing neurons in the hypothalamus, which have been established to be essential components in the regulation of feeding behavior and hypoglycemic counter-regulatory responses (reviewed in (Marty et al., 2007)). The hypothalamus is subdivided into interconnecting nuclei, including the arcuate nucleus (ARC), paraventricular nucleus (PVN), ventromedial nucleus (VMN), dorsomedial nucleus (DMN) and lateral hypothalamic area (LHA) (Simpson et al., 2009). These central brain circuits receive signals from the periphery, which indicate satiety, energy levels and energy stores (Morton et al, 2006) and process these afferent signals to modulate food intake and energy expenditure.

The actions of insulin have also been shown to play a direct role in the CNS since neuron-specific insulin receptor deficient (NIRKO) mice develop mild IR and display elevated circulating insulin levels (Bruning et al., 2000). Injections of insulin directly into the third cerebral ventricle have been shown to suppress hepatic glucose production without effecting body weight or circulating levels of insulin (Obici et al., 2002). Further, inhibition of insulin or its downstream signaling pathway in the CNS, i.e. the insulin receptor and phosphatidylinositol-3 kinase (PI3K), impaired the ability of increased levels of insulin to suppress gluconeogenesis. Targeted deletion of insulin receptor expression selectively in the hypothalamus elicited IR in rats, which is in accordance with the results in NIRKO mice. These studies show that the CNS regulates glucose homeostasis through the action of insulin and requires intact insulin signaling pathways involving the binding of insulin to its receptor and subsequent activation of down-stream mediators.

Estrogen is known to be highly relevant for the regulation of satiety, energy expenditure and body weight. Ovariectomy and menopause are associated with increased food intake, which can be reversed with estrogen replacement therapy (Eckel, 2004; Tchernof et al., 2000). The anorectic effects of estrogen are partially mediated through actions in the hypothalamus as demonstrated by studies showing that direct E2 injections into the PVN area or the ARC/VMN of the hypothalamus effectively reduced food intake (Butera & Beikirch, 1989; Nunez et al., 1980). The same study also showed that the hypothalamic neurons, which regulate energy homeostasis, were affected by E2 administration. Energy homeostasis and feeding behavior controlled by the hypothalamus also follow the menstrual cycle and food intake in women varies across the cycle with the lowest daily food intake during the peri-ovulatory period when estrogen levels are peaking (Asarian & Geary, 2006).

ERα and ERβ are both expressed in the different areas of the hypothalamus (Gillies & McArthur, 2010). ERα appears to be the major mediator of the estrogenic effects on central regulation of body weight by estrogens but whether this is regulated by food intake or actions on energy expenditure is controversial. Total ERα knockout mice are obese with increased fat accumulation in the absence of increased food intake. Targeted disruption of ERα in the VMN areas in the hypothalamus of female mice leads to weight gain, increased visceral adiposity, hyperphagia, hyperglycemia and impaired energy expenditure (Musatov et al., 2007). ERβ knockout mice, on the other hand, display similar food consumption patterns as wild-type mice (Foryst-Ludwig et al., 2008).

4.2 ERs and the role of pancreatic β cells in glucose homeostasis

The endocrine pancreas is an adapting tissue with the capacity to quickly respond to variations in the metabolic status of the organism. The β cells in the islets of Langerhans readily adapt to peripheral IR by increasing their secretory response, as well as their cell mass. If β cells fail to compensate, blood glucose concentration will rise to pathological levels and frank T2D will develop.

Estrogenic effects on various physiological aspects of the islet of Langerhans have been known for a long time and estrogens are established regulators of pancreatic β cell functions. In humans, E2 reverses the effect of menopause on glucose and insulin metabolism, resulting in increased pancreatic insulin secretion, as well as improved insulin sensitivity (Brussaard et al., 1997; Stevenson et al., 1994). Plasma insulin levels are increased in pregnant rats in response to the increased levels of estrogen. Studies in mice have suggested that long-term exposure to E2 increased insulin content, insulin gene expression and insulin release without changing β cell mass. E2 has also been shown to acutely enhance glucose stimulated insulin secretion at physiological concentrations through the action of ERα both *in vitro* and *in vivo* (Alonso-Magdalena et al., 2008; Nadal et al., 1998).

ERα has been identified as the functional predominant receptor isoform in the murine pancreas. E2-dependent insulin release in cultured pancreatic islets was reduced in ERα-deficient mice, when compared to islets derived from either ERβ-deficient or wild-type mice (Alonso-Magdalena et al., 2008). Also, E2, acting mainly through ERα, has been shown to protect pancreatic β cells from apoptosis induced by oxidative stress in mice.

Even though ERα seems to be the dominant subtype to convey the estrogenic response in the pancreas, the role of ERβ might also be of importance. ERβ-deficient mice have been shown to display a mild islet hyperplasia and delayed first phase insulin release (Barros et al., 2009).

The membrane bound estrogen-responsive GPR30 is also expressed in rodent pancreas. Studies using adult female GPR30-deficient mice reveal that these mice do not exhibit E2-induced release of insulin, which is consistent with experiments using isolated pancreatic islet cells *in vitro* (Martensson et al., 2009). There are not any differences in expression of glucose-related genes, such as the glucose transporter (GLUT) 2 and glucokinase, in GPR30 knockout mice when compared with wild-type mice (Martensson et al., 2009). Thus, GPR30 may act as a regulator of insulin release after E2 stimulation. Consistent with this, GPR30 mRNA is expressed in secretory gland cells, which may indicate that GPR30 is involved in insulin secretion pathways (Levin & Weissman, 2009).

4.3 ERs and the role of the liver in glucose homeostasis

The liver is the largest organ in the body and possesses purifying and metabolizing functions. One of its most important tasks is to store glucose in the form of glycogen. The liver is capable of containing up to 10% of its volume as glycogen. The liver releases glycogen when nutrients are scarce. Liver glycogen is converted into circulating glucose in response to pancreatic signals; in hypoglycemic conditions glucagon is released to stimulate a release of hepatic glycogen. In a hyperglycemic state, the pancreas releases insulin to stimulate the liver to release less glucose. The maintenance of glucose homeostasis is

depending on whole body glucose uptake and glucose production by glycogenolysis and gluconeogenesis in the liver.
Hepatic IR is impairment of insulin action in the liver, however, the mechanisms behind this is not completely elucidated. Hepatic IR is found in both obese non-diabetic, obese T2D patients and patients with non-alcoholic fatty livers. Early manifestations of hepatic IR are increased fasting gluconeogenesis.
Liver abnormalities are common outcomes of obesity-related IR. Hepatic steatosis is primarily caused by increased hepatic free fatty acids (FFA) released from insulin resistant adipocytes. Due to hepatic IR, hyperinsulinemia and hyperglycemia induce *de novo* lipogenesis. Fat accumulation in adipocytes is typically followed by fat deposition in the liver and skeletal muscle and by subsequent development of IR in these tissues. There are indications showing that obesity-related IR can cause fatty liver while, vice versa, excessive intra-hepatic fat accumulation may promote IR and weight gain.
Estrogens regulate liver glucose homeostasis mainly by acting via ERα as shown by studies in ERα-deficient mice. Euglycaemic-hyperinsulinaemic clamp analysis revealed that ERα deficiency was associated with a pronounced hepatic IR as determined by the inability of insulin to suppress liver glucose production (Bryzgalova et al., 2008). Global gene expression analysis of hepatic tissue isolated from ERα-deficient and control mice revealed that ERα-deficiency was associated with increased expression of key genes involved in hepatic lipid biosynthesis

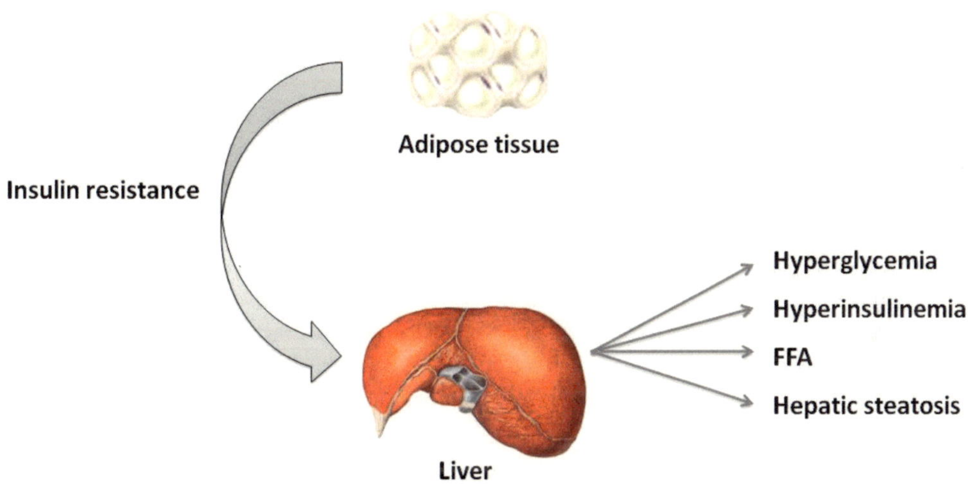

Fig. 5. **Schematic overview of hepatic IR.** The liver responds to IR in adipose tissue with increased release of glucose and free fatty acids (FFAs), as well as an increased accumulation of triglycerides, which will cause hyperinsulinemia and hepatic steatosis.

4.4 ERs and the role of skeletal muscle in glucose homeostasis

Skeletal muscle accounts for 40–60% of the human body mass and is the major site of glucose disposal, thereby regulating whole body glucose homeostasis. Insulin-stimulated disposal of circulating glucose is mediated through glucose transport across the muscle cell surface and this step is one of the rate-limiting steps for glucose clearance. Glucose crosses the plasma membranes and enters the skeletal muscle through the GLUT proteins by facilitated transport. Glucose clearance in response to postprandial insulin secretion is mainly mediated by skeletal muscle. The insulin signaling pathways inducing glucose uptake in skeletal muscle are well studied and involve insulin receptor, insulin receptor substrate (IRS), phosphatidylinositol-3 kinase (PI3-K) and AKT kinase subsequently leading to translocation of GLUT-4 to the cell membrane. IR in skeletal muscle is thought to be a primary defect in T2D (see fig. 6 for overview).

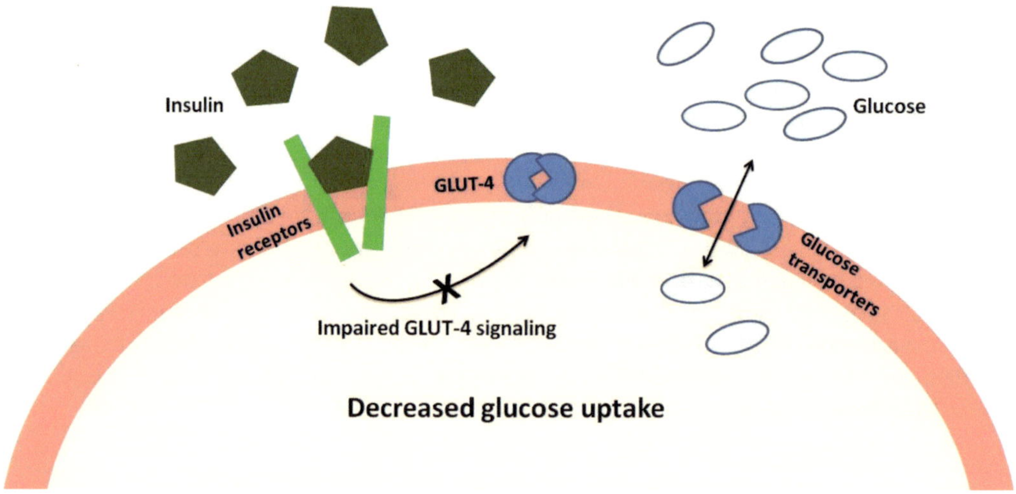

Fig. 6. **Insulin resistance in skeletal muscle cells.** When insulin binds to its receptors, translocation of GLUT-4 to the cell membrane is triggered and glucose can readily cross the cell membrane by facilitated transport and be stored in the skeletal muscles. Under insulin resistant states, the GLUT-4 signaling is impaired, leading to decreased glucose uptake by the muscles.

ERα and ERβ receptors seem to have opposing effects on the expression of GLUT-4 transporters. ERα was shown to induce and ERβ seems to inhibit GLUT-4 expression in skeletal muscle (Barros et al., 2006). Recent studies indicate that tamoxifen-treated ERα knockout mice displayed increased GLUT-4 expression in skeletal muscle, which indicates a pro-diabetogenic effect of ERβ (Barros et al., 2009). It appears that both ER isoforms determine the metabolic estrogen actions in skeletal muscle with ERα mediating protective actions and ERβ deleterious.

4.5 ERs and the role of adipose tissue in glucose homeostasis

Adipose tissue is formed by mature adipocytes, pre-adipocytes, immune cells, extracellular matrix and vascular endothelium. Under normal physiologic conditions, insulin concentrations control within a narrow range the balance between fatty acid storage as triglycerides and their release into the circulation during fasting state. Adipose tissue is very sensitive to insulin concentrations and insulin inhibits lipolysis at concentrations that are much lower than those needed to inhibit hepatic glucose production or stimulate muscle glucose uptake. Although insulin-dependent postprandial glucose disposal *in vivo* is believed to occur mainly by uptake into skeletal muscle, insulin-enhanced glucose uptake into adipose tissue also contributes to whole-body glucose homeostasis.

There are well-documented sex differences in the pathophysiology of obesity and metabolic disorders. Women tend to accumulate more subcutaneous fat whereas men accumulate more visceral fat (Bonds et al., 2006; Crespo et al., 2002; Nuutila et al., 1995). The prevalence of early IR and impaired glucose tolerance seem to be higher in men than in women.

E2 is considered an important regulator of adipose tissue development and lipid deposition in humans, rodents and other species. The deficiency of estrogen hormones after menopause or in experimental models, causes an increase in body mass and intra-abdominal adipose tissue leading to an android feature. The effects observed as a consequence of deficiency of sex steroids can be reversed by hormone replacement therapy.

Changes in adipose tissue distribution in women have been associated with increased risk of diseases and metabolic disturbances, including coronary artery disease, IR and glucose intolerance (Bonds et al., 2006). In obesity and T2D, there is a marked adipocyte resistance to the anti-lipolytic effects of insulin and the circulating FFA concentrations are typically elevated (Kissebah et al., 1976). Chronic over feeding induces metabolic stress and the adipocytes become hypertrophic and fail to proliferate and differentiate in a sufficient manner.

Sex hormone programming in animals has also been shown to affect adipose tissue. A single postnatal injection of estradiol benzoate resulted in the development of IR, increased adipose tissue mass and adipocyte size in adult female rats, suggesting that postnatal ER activation exerts strong programming effects on metabolic processes (Alexanderson et al., 2010).

Stromal cells from adipose tissue have been shown to locally produce estrogens (Simpson et al., 2009). It is well confirmed that there is a decrease in steroid hormone-binding globulins in obese states in both pre- and post-menopausal women. In post-menopausal women, there is a direct association between estrogen levels and body mass index (BMI) (Cleary & Grossmann, 2009; Lukanova et al., 2004). E2 is mainly produced by the adipocytes after menopause through conversion of androgens or estrone and this production is not regulated by feedback mechanisms (Siiteri, 1987). It is suggested that this adipose-derived E2 may participate in the ERα-mediated enrichment of insulin biosynthesis (Alonso-Magdalena et al., 2008) and in the induction of glucose stimulated insulin secretion to help the pancreatic β-cells adapt to the higher demand of insulin during obesity.

5. Concluding remarks

Lifestyle evolution and the higher intake of high calorie diets largely contribute to the worldwide growing incidence of metabolic diseases. In addition to the most common preventive strategy based on physical activity and reduced calorie intake, identification of new molecular targets able to limit the development of metabolic disturbances represents one of the most important public health challenges.

Estrogens have emerged as important regulators of glucose homeostasis during the last decades, corroborating data from clinical and experimental studies. Insulin sensitivity has been demonstrated to be higher in women before menopause than in age-matched men and postmenopausal women, which supports a beneficial effect of estrogens on insulin action and glucose homeostasis. It is also highly recognized that menopause promotes visceral fat accumulation and IR, which will ultimately lead to significantly higher risk of developing T2D. In addition, HRT has been reported to reverse the symptoms and to dampen the

incidence of T2D in postmenopausal women by 21–35% compared to women not given HRT.
Effects of estrogen signaling on glucose homeostasis have been further demonstrated by studies showing that patients bearing genetic mutations and, thus, lack either ERα or aromatase expression, develop obesity, IR and impaired glucose tolerance. Genetically engineered mice models have confirmed these clinical observations, as ERα or aromatase gene deficiency similarly promotes several features of the metabolic syndrome. Taken together, ERα seems to play a protective role in insulin and glucose metabolism, with actions on the liver, adipose tissue, muscle and pancreatic β cells. In addition, ERα regulates food intake and energy expenditures through actions on the CNS. ERβ seems to have an opposing role with the potential to negatively influence insulin and glucose metabolism by impairing the function of adipose tissue and inhibiting the expression of GLUT4 in the muscle.
Established and novel ER subtype selective ligands are valuable tools for deciphering the specific roles of ERα and ERβ in physiology and disease. The development of novel treatment regimes for metabolic disease targeting ERα is hampered by the uterotrophic and mammotrophic effects of ERα with the major concern being the risk of developing hormone-dependent cancer. Further studies are needed to identify and develop novel compounds that target estrogen signaling in selective metabolic tissues but lack the mitogenic effects in others, like ovaries and the breast.

6. References

Alexanderson, C., Stener-Victorin, E., Kullberg, J., Nilsson, S., Levin, M., Cajander, S., et al. (2010) A single early postnatal estradiol injection affects morphology and gene expression of the ovary and parametrial adipose tissue in adult female rats. *J Steroid Biochem Mol Biol, 122*(1-3), 82-90.

Alonso-Magdalena, P., Ropero, A. B., Carrera, M. P., Cederroth, C. R., Baquie, M., Gauthier, B. R., et al. (2008). Pancreatic insulin content regulation by the estrogen receptor ER alpha. *PLoS One, 3*(4), e2069.

Asarian, L., & Geary, N. (2006). Modulation of appetite by gonadal steroid hormones. *Philos Trans R Soc Lond B Biol Sci, 361*(1471), 1251-1263.

Barros, R. P., Gabbi, C., Morani, A., Warner, M., & Gustafsson, J. A. (2009). Participation of ERalpha and ERbeta in glucose homeostasis in skeletal muscle and white adipose tissue. *Am J Physiol Endocrinol Metab, 297*(1), E124-133.

Barros, R. P., Machado, U. F., Warner, M., & Gustafsson, J. A. (2006). Muscle GLUT4 regulation by estrogen receptors ERbeta and ERalpha. *Proc Natl Acad Sci U S A, 103*(5), 1605-1608.

Benito, M. Tissue specificity on insulin action and resistance: past to recent mechanisms. (2011) *Acta Physiol (Oxf), 201*(3), 297-312.

Bonds, D. E., Lasser, N., Qi, L., Brzyski, R., Caan, B., Heiss, G., et al. (2006). The effect of conjugated equine oestrogen on diabetes incidence: the Women's Health Initiative randomised trial. *Diabetologia, 49*(3), 459-468.

Bruning, J. C., Gautam, D., Burks, D. J., Gillette, J., Schubert, M., Orban, P. C., et al. (2000). Role of brain insulin receptor in control of body weight and reproduction. *Science, 289*(5487), 2122-2125.

Brussaard, H. E., Gevers Leuven, J. A., Frolich, M., Kluft, C., & Krans, H. M. (1997). Short-term oestrogen replacement therapy improves insulin resistance, lipids and fibrinolysis in postmenopausal women with NIDDM. *Diabetologia, 40*(7), 843-849.

Bryzgalova, G., Lundholm, L., Portwood, N., Gustafsson, J. A., Khan, A., Efendic, S., et al. (2008). Mechanisms of antidiabetogenic and body weight-lowering effects of estrogen in high-fat diet-fed mice. *Am J Physiol Endocrinol Metab, 295*(4), E904-912.

Butera, P. C., & Beikirch, R. J. (1989). Central implants of diluted estradiol: independent effects on ingestive and reproductive behaviors of ovariectomized rats. *Brain Res, 491*(2), 266-273.

Cleary, M. P., & Grossmann, M. E. (2009). Minireview: Obesity and breast cancer: the estrogen connection. *Endocrinology, 150*(6), 2537-2542.

Crespo, C. J., Smit, E., Snelling, A., Sempos, C. T., & Andersen, R. E. (2002). Hormone replacement therapy and its relationship to lipid and glucose metabolism in diabetic and nondiabetic postmenopausal women: results from the Third National Health and Nutrition Examination Survey (NHANES III). *Diabetes Care, 25*(10), 1675-1680.

Dahlman-Wright, K., Cavailles, V., Fuqua, S. A., Jordan, V. C., Katzenellenbogen, J. A., Korach, K. S., et al. (2006). International Union of Pharmacology. LXIV. Estrogen receptors. *Pharmacol Rev, 58*(4), 773-781.

Eastwood, H., Brown, K. M., Markovic, D., & Pieri, L. F. (2002). Variation in the ESR1 and ESR2 genes and genetic susceptibility to anorexia nervosa. *Mol Psychiatry, 7*(1), 86-89.

Eckel, L. A. (2004). Estradiol: a rhythmic, inhibitory, indirect control of meal size. *Physiol Behav, 82*(1), 35-41.

Fisher, C. R., Graves, K. H., Parlow, A. F., & Simpson, E. R. (1998). Characterization of mice deficient in aromatase (ArKO) because of targeted disruption of the cyp19 gene. *Proc Natl Acad Sci U S A, 95*(12), 6965-6970.

Foryst-Ludwig, A., Clemenz, M., Hohmann, S., Hartge, M., Sprang, C., Frost, N., et al. (2008). Metabolic actions of estrogen receptor beta (ERbeta) are mediated by a negative cross-talk with PPARgamma. *PLoS Genet, 4*(6), e1000108.

Gillies, G. E., & McArthur, S. (2010) Estrogen actions in the brain and the basis for differential action in men and women: a case for sex-specific medicines. *Pharmacol Rev, 62*(2), 155-198.

Gruber, C. J., Tschugguel, W., Schneeberger, C., & Huber, J. C. (2002). Production and actions of estrogens. *N Engl J Med, 346*(5), 340-352.

Hamden, K., Jaouadi, B., Zarai, N., Rebai, T., Carreau, S., & Elfeki, A. (2011). Inhibitory effects of estrogens on digestive enzymes, insulin deficiency, and pancreas toxicity in diabetic rats. *J Physiol Biochem, 67*(1), 121-128.

Heine, P. A., Taylor, J. A., Iwamoto, G. A., Lubahn, D. B., & Cooke, P. S. (2000). Increased adipose tissue in male and female estrogen receptor-alpha knockout mice. *Proc Natl Acad Sci U S A, 97*(23), 12729-12734.

Heldring, N., Pike, A., Andersson, S., Matthews, J., Cheng, G., Hartman, J., et al. (2007). Estrogen receptors: how do they signal and what are their targets. *Physiol Rev, 87*(3), 905-931.

Jones, M. E., Thorburn, A. W., Britt, K. L., Hewitt, K. N., Wreford, N. G., Proietto, J., et al. (2000). Aromatase-deficient (ArKO) mice have a phenotype of increased adiposity. *Proc Natl Acad Sci U S A, 97*(23), 12735-12740.

Kanaya, A. M., Vittinghoff, E., Shlipak, M. G., Resnick, H. E., Visser, M., Grady, D., et al. (2003). Association of total and central obesity with mortality in postmenopausal women with coronary heart disease. *Am J Epidemiol, 158*(12), 1161-1170.

Kieffer, T. J., Heller, R. S., Unson, C. G., Weir, G. C., & Habener, J. F. (1996). Distribution of glucagon receptors on hormone-specific endocrine cells of rat pancreatic islets. *Endocrinology, 137*(11), 5119-5125.

Kissebah, A. H., Alfarsi, S., Adams, P. W., & Wynn, V. (1976). Role of insulin resistance in adipose tissue and liver in the pathogenesis of endogenous hypertriglyceridaemia in man. *Diabetologia, 12*(6), 563-571.

Lafferty, A. R., Torpy, D. J., Stowasser, M., Taymans, S. E., Lin, J. P., Huggard, P., et al. (2000). A novel genetic locus for low renin hypertension: familial hyperaldosteronism type II maps to chromosome 7 (7p22). *J Med Genet, 37*(11), 831-835.

Lamon-Fava, S., Asztalos, B. F., Howard, T. D., Reboussin, D. M., Horvath, K. V., Schaefer, E. J., et al. (2010). Association of polymorphisms in genes involved in lipoprotein metabolism with plasma concentrations of remnant lipoproteins and HDL subpopulations before and after hormone therapy in postmenopausal women. *Clin Endocrinol (Oxf), 72*(2), 169-175.

Levin, P. D., & Weissman, C. (2009). Obesity, metabolic syndrome, and the surgical patient. *Anesthesiol Clin, 27*(4), 705-719.

Louet, J. F., LeMay, C., & Mauvais-Jarvis, F. (2004). Antidiabetic actions of estrogen: insight from human and genetic mouse models. *Curr Atheroscler Rep, 6*(3), 180-185.

Lukanova, A., Lundin, E., Zeleniuch-Jacquotte, A., Muti, P., Mure, A., Rinaldi, S., et al. (2004). Body mass index, circulating levels of sex-steroid hormones, IGF-I and IGF-binding protein-3: a cross-sectional study in healthy women. *Eur J Endocrinol, 150*(2), 161-171.

Maffei, L., Murata, Y., Rochira, V., Tubert, G., Aranda, C., Vazquez, M., Clyne, C.D., Davis, S., Simpson, E.R. & Carani, C. (2004) Dysmetabolic syndrome in a man with a novel mutation of the aromatase gene: effects of testosterone, alendronate, and estradiol treatment. *J Clin Endocrinol Metab, 89*, 61-70.

Martensson, U. E., Salehi, S. A., Windahl, S., Gomez, M. F., Sward, K., Daszkiewicz-Nilsson, J., et al. (2009). Deletion of the G protein-coupled receptor 30 impairs glucose tolerance, reduces bone growth, increases blood pressure, and eliminates estradiol-stimulated insulin release in female mice. *Endocrinology, 150*(2), 687-698.

Marty, N., Dallaporta, M., & Thorens, B. (2007). Brain glucose sensing, counterregulation, and energy homeostasis. *Physiology (Bethesda), 22*, 241-251.

Matthews, J., & Gustafsson, J. A. (2003). Estrogen signaling: a subtle balance between ER alpha and ER beta. *Mol Interv, 3*(5), 281-292.

Miller, D. S. (1982). Factors affecting energy expenditure. *Proc Nutr Soc, 41*(2), 193-202.

Morton, G. J., Cummings, D. E., Baskin, D. G., Barsh, G. S., & Schwartz, M. W. (2006). Central nervous system control of food intake and body weight. *Nature, 443*(7109), 289-295.

Musatov, S., Chen, W., Pfaff, D. W., Mobbs, C. V., Yang, X. J., Clegg, D. J., et al. (2007). Silencing of estrogen receptor alpha in the ventromedial nucleus of hypothalamus leads to metabolic syndrome. *Proc Natl Acad Sci U S A, 104*(7), 2501-2506.

Nadal, A., Rovira, J. M., Laribi, O., Leon-quinto, T., Andreu, E., Ripoll, C., et al. (1998). Rapid insulinotropic effect of 17beta-estradiol via a plasma membrane receptor. *Faseb J, 12*(13), 1341-1348.

Nilsson, M., Naessen, S., Dahlman, I., Linden Hirschberg, A., Gustafsson, J. A., & Dahlman-Wright, K. (2004). Association of estrogen receptor beta gene polymorphisms with bulimic disease in women. *Mol Psychiatry, 9*(1), 28-34.

Nunez, A. A., Gray, J. M., & Wade, G. N. (1980). Food intake and adipose tissue lipoprotein lipase activity after hypothalamic estradiol benzoate implants in rats. *Physiol Behav, 25*(4), 595-598.

Nussey, S., & Whitehead, S. (2001).

Nuutila, P., Maki, M., Laine, H., Knuuti, M. J., Ruotsalainen, U., Luotolahti, M., et al. (1995). Insulin action on heart and skeletal muscle glucose uptake in essential hypertension. *J Clin Invest, 96*(2), 1003-1009.

Obici, S., Zhang, B. B., Karkanias, G., & Rossetti, L. (2002). Hypothalamic insulin signaling is required for inhibition of glucose production. *Nat Med, 8*(12), 1376-1382.

Peter, I., Shearman, A. M., Vasan, R. S., Zucker, D. R., Schmid, C. H., Demissie, S., et al. (2005). Association of estrogen receptor beta gene polymorphisms with left ventricular mass and wall thickness in women. *Am J Hypertens, 18*(11), 1388-1395.

Revankar, C. M., Cimino, D. F., Sklar, L. A., Arterburn, J. B., & Prossnitz, E. R. (2005). A transmembrane intracellular estrogen receptor mediates rapid cell signaling. *Science, 307*(5715), 1625-1630.

Savage, D. B., Petersen, K. F., & Shulman, G. I. (2007). Disordered lipid metabolism and the pathogenesis of insulin resistance. *Physiol Rev, 87*(2), 507-520.

Schuit, S. C., Oei, H. H., Witteman, J. C., Geurts van Kessel, C. H., van Meurs, J. B., Nijhuis, R. L., et al. (2004). Estrogen receptor alpha gene polymorphisms and risk of myocardial infarction. *Jama, 291*(24), 2969-2977.

Shearman, A. M., Cupples, L. A., Demissie, S., Peter, I., Schmid, C. H., Karas, R. H., et al. (2003). Association between estrogen receptor alpha gene variation and cardiovascular disease. *Jama, 290*(17), 2263-2270.

Siiteri, P. K. (1987). Adipose tissue as a source of hormones. *Am J Clin Nutr, 45*(1 Suppl), 277-282.

Simpson, K. A., Martin, N. M., & Bloom, S. R. (2009). Hypothalamic regulation of food intake and clinical therapeutic applications. *Arq Bras Endocrinol Metabol, 53*(2), 120-128.

Stevenson, J. C., Crook, D., Godsland, I. F., Collins, P., & Whitehead, M. I. (1994). Hormone replacement therapy and the cardiovascular system. Nonlipid effects. *Drugs, 47 Suppl 2*, 35-41.

Tchernof, A., Poehlman, E. T., & Despres, J. P. (2000). Body fat distribution, the menopause transition, and hormone replacement therapy. *Diabetes Metab, 26*(1), 12-20.

Thomas, P., Pang, Y., Filardo, E. J., & Dong, J. (2005). Identity of an estrogen membrane receptor coupled to a G protein in human breast cancer cells. *Endocrinology, 146*(2), 624-632.

Yoshihara, R., Utsunomiya, K., Gojo, A., Ishizawa, S., Kanazawa, Y., Matoba, K., et al. (2009). Association of polymorphism of estrogen receptor-alpha gene with circulating levels of adiponectin in postmenopausal women with type 2 diabetes. *J Atheroscler Thromb, 16*(3), 250-255.

Zhao, C., Dahlman-Wright, K., & Gustafsson, J. A. (2008). Estrogen receptor beta: an overview and update. *Nucl Recept Signal, 6*, e003.

Zirilli, L., Rochira, V., Diazzi, C., Caffagni, G., & Carani, C. (2008) Human models of aromatase deficiency. *J Steroid Biochem Mol Biol, 109*, 212-218.

6

Expression of Neuropeptide Y of GIFT Tilapia (*Oreochromis sp.*) in Yeast *Pichia Pastoris* and Its Stimulatory Effects on Food Intake and Growth

Guangzhong Wang, Caiyun Sun, Haoran Lin and Wensheng Li*
State Key Laboratory of Biocontrol,
Institute of Aquatic Economic Animals and
Guangdong Provincial Key Laboratory for Aquatic Economic Animals,
School of Life Sciences, Sun Yat-Sen University, Guangzhou,
P. R. China

1. Introduction

Neuropeptide Y (NPY), a peptide with 36 amino acid residues which was first isolated from porcine brain (Tatemoto et al., 1982), is most highly expressed in the hypothalamic arcuate nucleus (ARC) (Lin et al., 2004). NPY is a member of the NPY family which consists of NPY, peptide YY (PYY), pancreatic polypeptide (PP) and peptide Y (PY)(Cerda-Reverter and Larhammar, 2000a). There are three NPY-related peptides were expressed in fish. They are NPY, peptide YY and peptide Y(Cerda-Reverter et al., 2000b; Sundstrom et al., 2008). Currently, NPY peptides or cDNA sequences have been obtained from many fish species including catfish, goldfish, sea bass, Atlantic cod, flounder, rainbow trout, zebrafish(Volkoff, 2006). As other low molecular weight secreted peptide, NPY is synthesized as larger peptide precursor which consists of a hydrophobic signal peptide, the mature peptide, the amidation-proteolytic site, and the carboxy-terminal extended peptide (Cerda-Reverter and Larhammar, 2000a). A partial cDNA coding for the mature peptide of NPY of tilapia (red tilapia, *Oreochromis sp.*) has been cloned and reported. The size of the sequence is of 192bp, which encodes a 28 a.a. signal peptide and the 36 a.a. mature peptide, while the sequence encoding carboxy-terminal extension aside the C-terminal of mature peptide has not been reported yet (Carpio et al., 2006).

NPY is well known to be involved in many physiological functions, such as cardiovascular regulation, affective disorder, memory retention, neuroendocrine control and feeding in mammals(Pedrazzini, 2004). In fact, NPY has been considered as the most potent orexigenic peptide in mammals (Halford et al., 2004; Kalra et al., 1999; Valassi et al., 2008; Woods et al., 1998). Many studies have proved that NPY is also an important energy metabolism regulator of vertebrates. When fed with a high-carbohydrate diet; diabetic rats exhibit increased gene expression of the NPY in the hypothalamic ARC, and high-fat diet suppressed NPY expression(Chavez et al., 1998). Intraventricular administration of NPY has been shown to enhance carbohydrate and fat utilization in rats which leads to a significant increase in energy consumption and body weight (Kiris GA, 2007). NPY executes these functions mainly through its receptor Y1, Y2 and Y5 (Aldegunde and Mancebo, 2006; Pedrazzini et al., 2003).

NPY is one of the most highly conserved neuroendocrine peptides in vertebrates(Blomqvist et al., 1992). The NPY peptides of fish species also showed remarkable sequence homology with mammals, suggesting the similar functions of NPY in fish and mammals(Cerda-Reverter et al., 2000b; Sundstrom et al., 2005).As its mammalian counterpart, NPY is also a very important regulator of food intake and energy metabolism in fish(Volkoff, 2006; Volkoff et al., 2005). For example, both central and peripheral injections of mammalian or fish NPY significantly stimulated food intake in a dose dependent manner in goldfish (Lopez-Patino et al., 1999; Narnaware et al., 2000). NPY mRNA levels increased substantially a few hours before feeding goldfish, which was fed at fixed time, and then declined after feeding; Fasting could also upgrade the expression of goldfish NPY, while re-feeding restored the NPY mRNA levels (Narnaware and Peter, 2001a). In addition, NPY expression was regulated by high glucose or high fat diet but not affected by the protein composition of food (Narnaware and Peter, 2002). The relationship between NPY and feeding promotion were also found in other fish species. Ventricle injection with porcine NPY significantly promoted the feeding of rainbow trout within 2-3 hours(Aldegunde and Mancebo, 2006). Brain NPY mRNA level of Atlantic cod changed before and after diet, and reached the highest level at feeding time(Kehoe and Volkoff, 2007). The short-term changes of NPY level were all related to temporary feeding regulation. Similar to mammals, NPY is a long-term energy metabolism regulation factor, long-term treatment of NPY could also significantly change the growth and feeding behavior of fish species. Recombinant protein expressed in *Escherichia coli.* of tilapia NPY significantly promoted the growth and food intake of tilapia by injection(Carpio et al., 2006). Immersion bath with the same prokaryotic expression of NPY three times a week significantly increased the body weight and body length of catfish (Carpio Y, 2007). NPY either administered by i.p. injection or through feed stimulated food intake as well as growth of *Oreochromis niloticus* (Kiris GA, 2007).

Yeast has been used in food and feed additive production for a long time. Because of the lower toxicity and higher environmental security, the yeast culture supernatant of yeast expression system for foreign genes expression can be directly used as feed of animal without purification. In addition to the advantages of molecular and genetic manipulations sharing with *Saccharomyces*, *Pichia pastoris* has higher protein expression efficiency and is easier for high-density fermentation. Moreover, as a eukaryote, *Pichia pastoris* has advantages in post-translational processing of higher eukaryotic expression systems such as protein processing, protein folding, and posttranslational modification that *E. Coli.* systems can not carry out, while being as easy to manipulate as *E. Coli* or *Saccharomyces cerevisiae*. It is faster, easier, and lower cost than other eukaryotic expression systems and generally gives higher expression levels. *Pichia pastoris* itself secrete little proteins into the culture medium, such facilities the secretion and purification of recombinant proteins. In addition, single or multiple copies of foreign genes were easy to integration into the genome of *Pichia pastoris* in specific site, which makes the recombinant strains to be genetically stable. These features make *Pichia* a very useful protein expression system suitable for industrial production (Faber et al., 1995; Romanos et al., 1992).

Treating fish with hormones or peptides to induce the food intake and growth by injections is definitely not a realistic method in aquaculture because they would require expensive, time-consuming injection in individual fish. To feed fish with capsules or feed containing agonists/antagonists of appetite-regulating factors might represent a viable solution (Gelineau, 2001; Volkoff et al., 2010). Previous experiments have shown that trout fed with CCK antagonists eat significantly more than their mean daily intake on the other days of the experiment (Gelineau, 2001). Tilapia, commonly known as the African carp, belongs to *Perciformes, Perciformes Suborder, Cichlidae.* Now, tilapia is one of the most important fish species used in aquaculture in the world. Because of its low cost, tilapia has been thought as the 21st century protein for poor people. In the present study, under purpose of developing new environmental friendly feed additives for fish, we isolated the ORF of NPY from GIFT tilapia and established the *Pichia* strains of pPICZαA-TiNPY1-X-33 and pPICZαA-TiNPY2-X-33 to express recombinant NPY proteins. Administration of the purified NPY to GIFT tilapia showed that long-term treatment of the recombinant peptide can stimulate food intake, promote growth and reduce feed conversion ratio. Moreover, this recombinant peptide obviously stimulated pituitary GH mRNA expression, while inhibit NPY and orexin mRNA expressions in hypothalamus.

2. Material and methods

2.1 Animals

All fish used in the present experiment are GIFT Strain tilapia (*Oreochromis niloticus*), and were obtained from local Panyu tilapia breeding fishery of Guangzhou, China. A male tilapia with body weight of 1.5kg was used for molecular cloning of NPY cDNA. Juvenile fish with the body weight ranging from 65 to 80g were selected for NPY feeding experiments. Since the tilapia at this stage was "prepubertal" and sexual dimorphism was not apparent, fish of mixed sexes were used for in vivo study. All fish were kept alive in well aerated freshwater under a 12L:12D photoperiod at 26 to 28°C. Fish for feeding experiment were cultured in a 150L tank with the density of 12 fish per tank and were acclimated to a constant flow of filtered water for two weeks before the feeding experiment. During the acclimation period, all fish were fed with normal extruded floating pellets twice a day. After finish the experiment, all fish were sacrificed by anesthesia in 0.05% MS222 (Sigma, St. Louis, MO) followed by spinosectomy according to the regulation of animal use at Sun Yat-Sen University.

2.2 Reagents and test substrates

TRIzol reagent, DNAse I, SuperScript II, T/A clone TM PCR Product Cloning Kit, Platinum Taq DNA Polymerase, Zeocin, and Real-time PCR Master Mix (SYBR Green) were purchased from Invitrogen (Carlsbad, CA). E.Z.N.A Gel Extraction Kit and E.Z.N.A Plasmid Extraction Kit were obtained from Omega Bio-Tek (USA). Anti-Neuropeptide Y Rabbit pAb was purchased from Calbiochem (U.S.A). Sheep anti-rabbit secondary antibody IgG-HRP was purchased from Boster Biological Engineering Co., Ltd., (China). His•Bind Columns was bought from Novagen (USA). Trpton, Yeast extract and Dextrose were purchased from OXIOID (Britain). The membrane of PVDF (0.2μm) was obtained from Pall life sciences (U.S.A). Protein Marker is BIO-RAD kaleidoscope Prestained Standards.

2.3 Molecular cloning of GIFT tilapia NPY

Specific primers for amplification of tilapia NPY cDNA were designed based on the reported NPY sequence of red tilapia (GenBank Accession No. AY779047). The forward primer was F1 (5′-ATGCATCCTAACTTGGTGAGC-3′) and the reverse primer was R1 (5′-GGCCACGCGTCGACTAGTAC-3′, AUAP). PCR was performed using the RT sample prepared from the hypothalamus as the template to pull out GIFT NPY cDNA. Briefly, total RNA was extracted from the hypothalamus of GIFT tilapia using TRIzol®reagent method. 1μg total RNA was reverse transcribed to first strand cDNA by SuperScript First-Strand Synthesis System for RT-PCR (Invitrogen) and Oligo(dT)12-18 primer (Invitrogen Adapter Primer). 5μl of the above 20μl reverse transcription reaction mixture was used to amplify a NPY fragment with the size of 650 bp, which include the open reading frame (ORF) and the 3′ untranslation region. The total volume of PCR reaction is 100μl containing with 0.5μl Platinum Taq DNA Polymerase and the corresponding PCR buffer, 200 μM of each dNTP, 30 μM $MgCl_2$ and 200 pmole of F1 and AUAP primers. PCR reactions were conducted for 36 cycles with the denaturation at 94 °C for 15 sec, annealing at 53°C for 15 sec and extension at 72°C for 1 min. The PCR products were size-fractionated in 1.5% agarose gel and purified by using E.Z.N.A® Gel Extraction Kit. The purified PCR product was then ligated into cloning T plasmid vector (pTZ57R/T plasmid vector). The recombinant pTZ57R/T vector was transformed into DH5a (Escherichia coli), after screening and identification, plasmids of positive colonies were extracted using E.Z.N.A® Plasmid Extraction Kit and sequenced using M13F primer.

2.4 Construction of pPICZaA-TiNPY1and pPICZaA-TiNPY2 expression vectors

Three gene specific primers for amplification of the mature peptide of tilapia NPY were designed based on the sequence obtained to establish two different expression vectors. A forward primer (F2: 5′-CGGCCTCGAGAAAAGAGAGGCTGAAGCTTACCCAGTGAA ACCA-3′) contains an *Xho I* site and the sequence encoding partial signal peptide which could be digested by *Xho I* on yeast secretory expression vector pPICZαA(Invitrogen). The reverse primers were R2 (5′-TGCTCTAGATACCTCTGTCTTGT-3′) which contains an *Xba I* site and R3 (5′-TGATCTAGATCAATGATGATGATGATGATGATACCTCTGTCTTGT-3′). Besides the *Xba I* site, R3 also contains the sequence encoding 6× his tag and a stop codon. Using the NPY cDNA we obtained as template, two fragments with the size of 201bp (NPY1) and 226bp (NPY2) were amplified by using primer pairs of F2/R2 and F2/R3, respectively. PCR reactions were conducted for 36 cycles with the denaturation at 94 °C for 15 sec, annealing at 65°C for 15 sec and extension at 72°C for 30 sec. The PCR products were size-fractionated in 1.5% agarose gel and purified by using E.Z.N.A® Gel Extraction Kit. The purified PCR product and *Pichia pastoris* expression vector pPICZαA were digested by *Xho I* and *Xba I,* respectively. After purification, the digested PCR products were ligated with the linearized pPICZαA. After sequencing confirmation, two recombinant expression vectors, pPICZαA-TiNPY1 and pPICZαA-TiNPY2, were established. The NPY gene of interest is cloned in frame with a C-terminal peptide containing the c-myc epitope and a polyhistidine (6× His) tag as in pPICZαA- TiNPY1, or with only the polyhistidine (6× His) tag as in pPICZαA- TiNPY2. The recombinant NPY proteins are expressed as fusions to an N-terminal signal peptide, a-factor secretion signal of the *Saccharomyces cerevisiae.* Both vectors would give high expression level of the interest gene in *Pichia pastoris* when induced by methanol.

2.5 Establishment of *Pichia X-33* strains of pPICZαA-TiNPY1 and pPICZαA-TiNPY2

The competent cells of *Pichia X-33* strain were prepared according to the manual of the Easyselect™ Pichia Expression Kit (Invitrogen). Two recombinant expression vectors of pPICZαA-TiNPY1 and pPICZαA-TiNPY2 were linearized by the digestion of PmeI (NEB) within the 5'AOX 1 region and then transformed into the competent cell of *Pichia X-33* by electroporation. The linearized pPICZαA-TiNPY1 or pPICZαA-TiNPY2 was directly integrated within the 5′ AOX1 region of Pichia host genome (*Pichia X-33* strain purchased from Invitrogen) by gene insertion. The two transformation mixtures were respectively spread onto YPDS plates (Yeast Extract Peptone Dextrose Medium), which contained 1% yeast extract, 2% peptone, 2% dextrose (glucose), 1 M sorbitol, 2% agar and 200 μg/ml Zeocin™(or 100 μg/ml Zeocin, and then screening on 200/500/1000 μg/ml Zeocin YPDS for multi-copy integrants). These plates then were incubated at 28-30°C for about 4 days until the positive single colonies of *Pichia X-33* were observed. In a parallel study, the PICZαA blank vectors were introduced into the competent cells of *Pichia X-33* strain and which acts as a negative control. At this point, two recombinant *Pichia X-33* strains were constructed, they were pPICZαA-TiNPY1-X-33 and pPICZαA-TiNPY2-X-33 , which could express recombinant TiNPY1 (tilapia NPY mature peptide with a C-terminal peptide containing the c-myc epitope and 6× His tag, total 58 a.a.) or TiNPY2 (tilapia NPY mature peptide with only the 6× His tag, total 42 a.a.) respectively.

2.6 Induction of recombinant protein expression of TiNPY1 and TiNPY2

Single colonies of genetically engineered *Pichia pastoris* strains pPICZαA-Ti NPY1-X-33, pPICZαA-TiNPY2-X-33 and pPICZαA-X-33 (as a negative control NC_0) were picked and cultured in 5ml BMGY medium(1% yeast extract, 2% peptone, 100 mM potassium phosphate, pH 6.0, 1.34% YNB, 4×10^{-5}% biotin, 1% glycerol) at 30°C in a shaking incubator (250rpm)for 24h. When the OD600 of the culture is within the range from 4.0 to 6.0, 200μl culture of each colony was stocked in 15% glycerol at -80 °C.

The remained cells were harvested by centrifuging at 1500 g for 5 minutes at 4°C. Discard the supernatant and resuspend the cell pellet into BMMY medium (1% yeast extract, 2% peptone, 100 mM potassium phosphate, pH 6.0, 1.34% YNB, 4×10^{-5}% biotin, 0.5% methanol) to induce NPY protein expression at 28-30°C with the shaking speed of 250rpm. The media of one of PICZαA-TiNPY1-X-33 or pPICZαA-TiNPY2-X-33 was not be replaced and maintained in BMGY medium to act as negative control of NC_1 and NC_2.

1ml cultures of each tube were sampled and cultured in BMMY medium with 0.5% methanol to maintain induction every 24 hours. In a parallel study, instead of replacing the culture medium, one culture of PICZαA-TiNPY1-X-33 or pPICZαA-TiNPY2-X-33 remained to be cultured in BMGY and act as negative control of NC_1 and NC_2. Sampled cultures were centrifuged to collect supernatant respectively, and the supernatants were stored at -20°C or directly concentrated and analyzed by Tricine-SDS-PAGE gel and western blot. The expressed recombinant protein by pPICZαA-TiNPY1-X-33 and pPICZαA-TiNPY2-X-33 were named TiNPY1 and TiNPY2.

2.7 Analysis of recombinant NPY proteins by Tricine-SDS-PAGE and western blot

The harvested supernatants with recombinant proteins were concentrated and analyzed by Tricine-SDS-PAGE gel electrophoresis according to the standard procedure. Samples were first run under 50V for 1h and then change the voltage to 75V for another 1h. After electrophoresis, the gel was stained with Coomassie blue for 20 min, and then analyzed whether the recombinant proteins TiNPY1 (with a molecular weight about 6.9KD) and TiNPY2 (with a molecular weight about 5.1KD) were present or not.

After analysis by Tricine- SDS-PAGE gel electrophoresis, samples induced with different time were analyzed by western blot. After separation by Tricine-SDS-PAGE gel electrophoresis, proteins were electro-transferred from the gel to a PVDF membrane. The recombinant protein was recognized with a rabbit polyclonal antibody against porcine NPY (purchased from Calbiochem Corporation, USA) with a dilution of 1:1000, which was recognized by sheep anti-rabbit secondary antibody IgG-HRP (purchased from Boster Biological Engineering Co., Ltd., China). Western blot results were detected by chemiluminescence detection system.

2.8 Expression kinetics of NPY

Since the protein banding patterns of TiNPY1 and TiNPY2 in supernatant were varying with different induction time, it is necessary to study the kinetics of NPY expression. In the present study, NPY1 expression was taken as a model to study the relationship of induction time and TiNPY1 protein expression pattern. Four colonies of pPICZαA-TiNPY1-X-33 were used to express recombinant protein of NPY. The supernatants were harvested for Tricine-SDS-PAGE gel electrophoresis and western blot at the time point of 12h, 24h and 48h after 0.5% methanol induction.

2.9 Purification of the recombinant NPY proteins

Since Recombinant protein TiNPY1 and TiNPY2 were conjugated with 6× His tag, His•Bind Column (NOVAGEN) could be used to purify these proteins. pH of supernatants of methanol-induced culture were adjusted to 7.9 by NaOH and then all samples were loaded into the His•Bind Column which was equilibrated with 15ml binding buffer(0.5 M NaCl, 20mM Tris-HCl, 5mM imidazole, pH 7.9) before use. The column was washed by 10ml wash buffer (0.5M NaCl, 60mM imidazole, 20mM Tris-HCl, pH 7.9) to remove unbound proteins. The recombinant protein was eluted by elute buffer with different concentration of imidazole (150/250/500mM imidazole, 0.5M NaCl, 20mM Tris-HCl, pH 7.9).Each fraction was eluted with one milliliter elution. Tricine-SDS-PAGE gel electrophoresis was conducted to analyze the purification with comparisons of before and after purified supernatants.

2.10 Sequencing of N-terminal amino acid of NPY

The purified TiNPY1 protein bands were electro-transferred from the gel to a PVDF membrane, and the sequencing of N-terminal amino acid of TiNPY1 was performed by using Sequencing instrument PROCISE491 (Applied Biosystemes Company, USA) with EDMEN degradation method.

2.11 Diet preparation and feeding experiment with juvenile tilapia

Five different diets for feeding experiments were prepared by homogeneously spraying three kinds of yeast culture supernatants directly onto the surface of ordinary commercial extruded floating feed. The concentrations of the recombinant proteins of NPY1 in three diets are 0.15, 0.3 and 0.6μg TiNPY1/g feed, respectively. A diet contains the recombinant protein TiNPY2 to a level of 0.3μg TiNPY2/g feed. A diet without any addition of recombinant protein acts as a negative control feed. All diets were stored at −20 °C before use.

After finishing two week's acclimation, 180 fish of GIFT Strain tilapia, with a body weight ranging from 60 to 80g (73.09±3.58 g) and length ranging from 12.0 to 14.0cm were randomly assigned to 15 aquariums and 12 fish were cultured in an aquarium. All 15 aquariums were divided into five groups with three aquariums (three replicates, n=12) per group. One group was fed with a kind of diet. Group1, 2, 3 were fed with diets containing 0.15, 0.3 and 0.6μg TiNPY1/g feed, respectively. Group 4 took the control feed and group 5 was fed with 0.3μg TiNPY2/g feed. The feeding experiment was taken for 50 days. All fishes were cultured at 28 °C under a 12 L: 12D photoperiod. Fish were fed with the pellet feed two times daily to satiation at 09:00 and 18:00 (animals didn't take any feed within one hour after the beginning of feeding). The remained feeds were removed one hour after each feeding operation and dried to calculate food intake of fish in each tank. Every 10 days, all fish in each aquarium were caught and dried briefly with towel, and then the weight for each fish was measured. The fish were not fed with anything within 24h before measurement. The body length of each fish was also measured at the beginning and the end of feed experiment. The whole feeding experiment lasted for 50 days.

After finishing the feeding experiment, all fish were sacrificed and their tissues were removed for the following experiments: pituitaries and hypothalamuses were used for RNA extraction and RT-PCR; Livers and all guts were weighed to determine the hepatosomatic index (HSI) and visceral body weight, which were calculated as 100× liver weight/body weight and 100× gut weight/body weight. The mRNA expression of growth hormone (GH), NPY and orexin were detected by using Real-time PCR technique. Fish dorsal white muscle of each group was sampled for moisture, crude protein and total lipid content were analyzed according to the method of Kjeldahl (AOAC, 1984) and Soxhlet extraction method, respectively.

2.12 Data transformation and statistical analysis

For feeding experiment, feeding conversion ratio (SGR) was calculated in terms of the number of grams of feed that are used to produce one gram of whole fish. For real-time PCR measurement of GH, NPY and orexin mRNA, 18S mRNA acts as an internal control to normalized with mRNA of the target gene. Data were presented as means ± SEM and analyzed with one-way ANOVA followed by Fisher's Least Significance Difference (LSD) test. Differences between groups were considered as significant at $P < 0.05$.

3. Results

3.1 Molecular cloning of cDNA encoding the NPY of GIFT tilapia and construction of the expression vectors of pPICZaA-TiNPY1and pPICZaA-TiNPY2

The ORF and 3' untranslation region (UTR) of GIFT tilapia NPY was cloned (Fig.1). The partial cDNA of NPY is 659bp in size with a 359bp 3'UTR and 300bp ORF encoding a 99 a.a. precursor protein. A putative signal peptide of 28 a.a. is located in the N-terminal of NPY. And a 36 a.a. mature peptide is highly conserved with that of human NPY (89% identity). The remained 35 a.a. is the C-terminal of NPY.

Two different expression vectors of GIFT tilapia were established and they were named as pPICZaA-TiNPY1 and pPICZaA-TiNPY2 (Fig.2) The insert size of pPICZaA-TiNP1 is 201bp which encodes 36 a.a. NPY mature peptide and a C-terminal peptide with a c-myc epitope and a polyhistidine (6× His) tag. The insert size of pPICZaA-TiNPY2 is 226bp which encodes NPY mature peptide and a polyhistidine (6× His) tag.

ATGCATCCTAACTTGGTGAGCTGGCTGGGGACTCTGGGGTTCCTGCTGTGGGCGCTGGTC 60

M H P N L V S W L G T L G F L L W A L V

TGCTTGGGCGCCTTGACGGAGGCATACCCAGTGAAACCAGAGAACCCCGGGGAGGACGCC 120

C L G A L T E A **Y P V K P E N P G E D A**

CCCGCGGAGGAGCTGGCCAAGTACTACTCAGCCCTGAGACATTACATCAACCTCATTACA 180

P A E E L A K Y Y S A L R H Y I N L I T

AGACAGAGGTATGGGAAGAGATCCAGTCCTGAGATTCTGGACACACTGGTCTCAGAGCTG 240

R Q R Y G K R S S P E I L D T L V S E L

CTGCTGAAGGAAAGCACAGACACGCTTCCACAGTCAAGATATGACCCATCAATGTGGTGA 300

L L K E S T D T L P Q S R Y D P S M W ★

TGCTGCCATCACTCTCGTCTCGCTCACTGCTGTCCCGCCAGCGCTGACATTCTGACCTCT 360

ACACGTCCGTCACTTACCTCCTACACCAAACGAACACCACGCCTCTGCCCTCCTTTCGCC 420

TCCATGAGCCGCAACGTATATATCCAACCCCTCTTCCTTACGCATCAGCCACACCCAACA 480

CTGCTTGAAGTCTGTGCCATAAAACTGTAAATACTTTATTCTGAGTCGTCATCTGTGCAA 540

CATGATCGTAAAGTGGAGGAGGGGGGGTCTGCTGATTGTATTGTATATTTGTGCTATTAA 600

AGATTCACTGTTTGAAAAAAAAAAAAAAAA 630

Fig. 1. Nucleotides and deduced amino acid (a.a.) sequence of tilapia NPY. The a.a. sequence underlined with the black dotted line is the predicted signal peptide. The mature peptide of NPY is highlight in grey box.

A

pPICZaA-TiNPY1: 5′ -CTCGAGAAAAGAGAGGCTGAAGCT

TACCCAGTGAAACCAGAGAACCCCGGGGAGGACGCCCCCGCGGAGGAGCTGGCC

Y P V K P E N P G E D A P A E E L A

AAGTACTACTCAGCCCTGAGACATTACATCAACCTCATTACAAGACAGAGGTATCTA

K Y Y S A L R H Y I N L I T R Q R Y **L**

GAACAAAAACTCATCTCAGAAGAGGATCTGAATAGCGCCGTCGACCATCATCATCAT

E Q K L I S E E D L N S A V D **H H H H**

CATCATTGA-3′

H H ★

B

pPICZaA-TiNPY2: 5′ -CTCGAGAAAAGAGAGGCTGAAGCT

TACCCAGTGAAACCAGAGAACCCCGGGGAGGACGCCCCCGCGGAGGAGCTGGCC

Y P V K P E N P G E D A P A E E L A

AAGTACTACTCAGCCCTGAGACATTACATCAACCTCATTACAAGACAGAGGTATCAT

K Y Y S A L R H Y I N L I T R Q R Y **H**

CATCATCATCATCATTGATCTAGATCAACAAAAACTCATCTCAGAAGAGGATCTGAA

H H H H H ★

TAGCGCCGTCGACCATCATCATCATCATCATTGA-3′

Fig. 2. Nucleotide and deduced amino acid sequences of NPY1 (A) and NPY2 (B) that were subcloned into pPICZaA to establish the expression vectors. The mature peptide of NPY is highlight in grey box, and the "H" in bold are 6XHis tags.

3.2 Establishment of the recombinant *Pichia X-33* stains of PICZαA-TiNPY1 and pPICZαA-TiNPY2

To get the high-yield strains of recombinant TiNPY1 and TiNPY2 produced by engineered *Pichia pastoris*, pPICZaA-TiNPY1 and pPICZaA-TiNPY2 were introduced into *Pichia X-33* strains by electroporation, respectively. After selection by using different concentration of Zeocin, the strains with the integration of TiNPY1, TiNPY2 and pPICzaA blank vector into the genome of *Pichia pastoris X-33*(Fig.3) were selected for our study. These strains with high Zeocin-resistance were named as pPICZαA-TiNPY1-X-33, pPICZαA-TiNPY2-X-33 and pPICZαA-X-33. pPICZαA-TiNPY1-X-33 can express a 58 a.a. peptide with 36 a.a. NPY mature peptide and a C-terminal peptide containing the c-myc epitope and 6× His tag, while the strain of pPICZαA-TiNPY1-X-33 can express a 42 a.a. peptide with NPY mature peptide and a 6× His tag.

3.3 Expression of recombinant NPY1 and NPY2 in *Pichia X-33* stains

To study the expression pattern of recombinant NPY1 and NPY2 in *Pichia pastoris* , pPICZαA-TiNPY1-X-33, pPICZαA-TiNPY2-X-33 were induced by using 5% methanol with the time points of 24h, 48h and 72h. The results of SDS-PAGE and Commassie blue staining of recombinant NPY at different times of methanol induction showed that six clones of each recombinant strain of pPICZαA-TiNPY1-X-33 and pPICZαA-TiNPY2-X-33 could express tilapia TiNPY1and TiNPY2, respectively. For pPICZαA-TiNPY2-X-33 after 24h methanol induction, in addition to a band with the size of 5-6KD was observed in all six colonies,

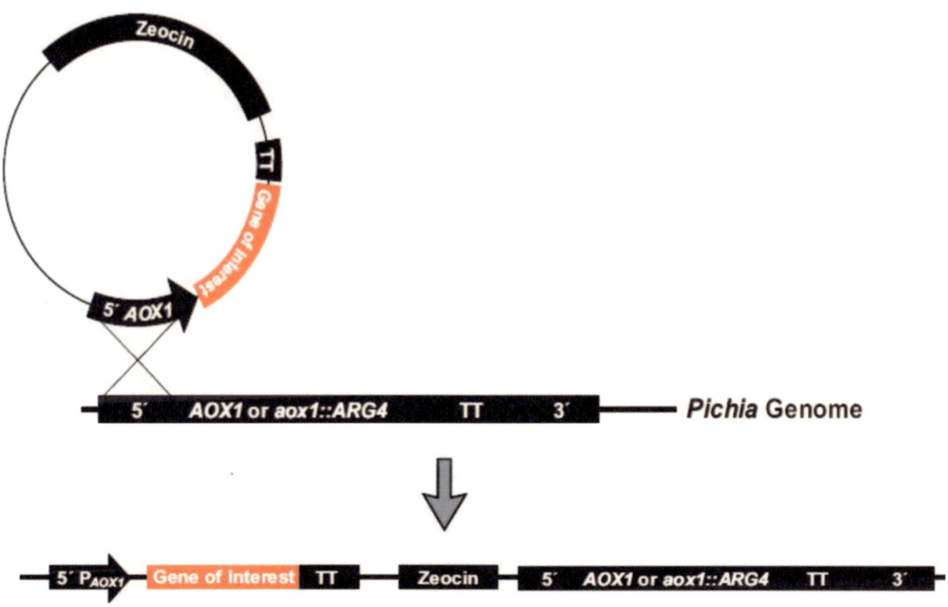

Fig. 3. Integration of TiNPY1, TiNPY2 and pPICza-A blank vector into the genome of Pichia pastoris X-33. The pPICzaA blank vector, pPICzaA-TiNPY-1 and pPICzaA-TiNPY-2 were transformed into Pichia pastoris X-33 by electroporation. After selection by using different concentration of Zeocin, three colonies of Pichia pastoris X-33 with high Zeocin resistance and high copy number were obtained, namely pPICZaA-TiNPY1-X-3, pPICZaA-TiNPY2-X-33 and pPICZaA-X-33.

there is a band with the size of 6-7KD expressed in colonies 1,2,3 and 4(Fig.4). After 48h induction, the band with the size of 5-6KD is still appear in all six colonies, but the expression level of the band is significantly lower than that of 24h-induction, while a band with a small size (2-4KD) was observed in all colonies(Fig.5). All bands almost disappeared except for colony 3 after methanol induction for 72h (Fig.6). Among the six colonies, only colony 3 has a stable expression pattern when induced by 5% methanol for 24h to 72h. Similar phenomenon was also observed in the strain of pPICZαA-TiNPY1-X-33. All six colonies selected expressed a peptide with the size of 7-9KD after 24h induction(Fig.4), but when the induction time increased to 48h, the band observed is about 5-6KD(Fig.5) and this band is still the major band after induction for 72h (Fig.6). In a parallel study, the pPICZαA - X-33 with methanol induction acts as negative control (NC0). The stains of pPICZαA-TiNPY1-X-33 and pPICZαA-TiNPY2-X-33 without methanol induction were also employed as negative controls (NC1 and NC2). No matter how long of the induction time, there is no band was present in the three negative controls.
Western blot was carried out to test the immunological characteristics of recombinant TiNPY1 and TiNPY2. These proteins were size-fractionated in 10% SDS-PAGE and transblotted onto the PVDF membrane. The recombinant proteins were recognized by a

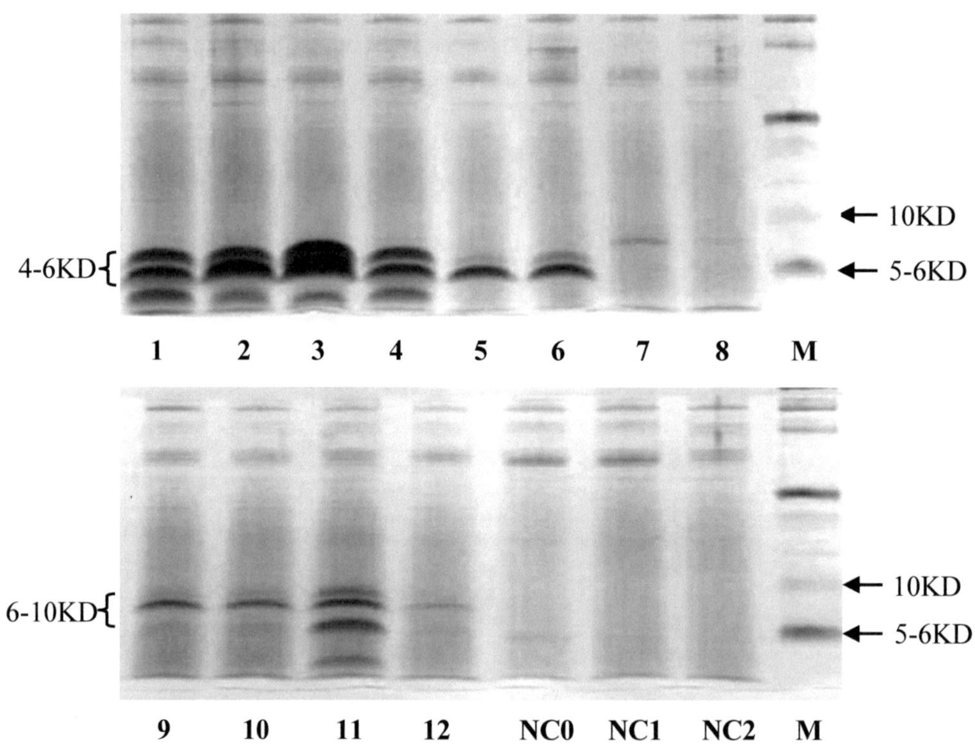

Fig. 4. SDS-PAGE detection of the expression of TiNPY1 and TiNPY2 after methanol induction for 24 hours.1-6:TiNPY2; 7-12:TiNPY1; NC0: pPICZaA-X-33 blank vector (negative control); NC1: pPICZaA-TiNPY1-X-33 without induction; NC2: pPICZaA-TiNPY2-X-33 without induction; M: protein marker. The size of TiNPY1 and TiNPY 2 is 6-9KD and 4-6KD, respectively.

rabbit polyclonal antibody against porcine NPY at a dilution 1:1000, which was recognized by sheep anti-rabbit secondary antibody IgG-HRP. 1μg of synthesized tilapia NPY with a molecular weight of 4.104KD was used as a positive control. The size of the NPY is smaller than both TiNPY1 and TiNPY2 because it lacks conjugated tags. The protein concentration of TiNPY1 and TiNPY2 in culture supernatants, when up-scale expressed in 1L shake-flask , were determined by scanning densitometry of dyed Tricine-SDS-PAGE gel and compared with the positive control (Fig.7,A). Western blot results showed that different from the SDS-PAGE detection that all colonies selected expressed the recombinant TiNPY1, only four colonies (No.2, 3, 4 and 6) were recognized by NPY antibodies (Fig.7,B). For TiNPY-2, SDS-PAGE showed that two of three colonies examined express two kinds of NPY with the molecular weight of 6-7KD and 5-6KD, while colony 3 only expressed the band with the size of 5-6KD (Fig.8,A). All these bands could be recognized by NPY antibody (Fig.8, B).

3.4 Time course study of the recombinant protein expression of TiNPY1

As the size and number of specific protein bands of TiNPY1 and TiNPY2 in supernatant were varying with different induction time, the expression kinetics of NPY1 was performed by inducing the expression of four pPICZαA-TiNPY1-X-33 colonies which came from the

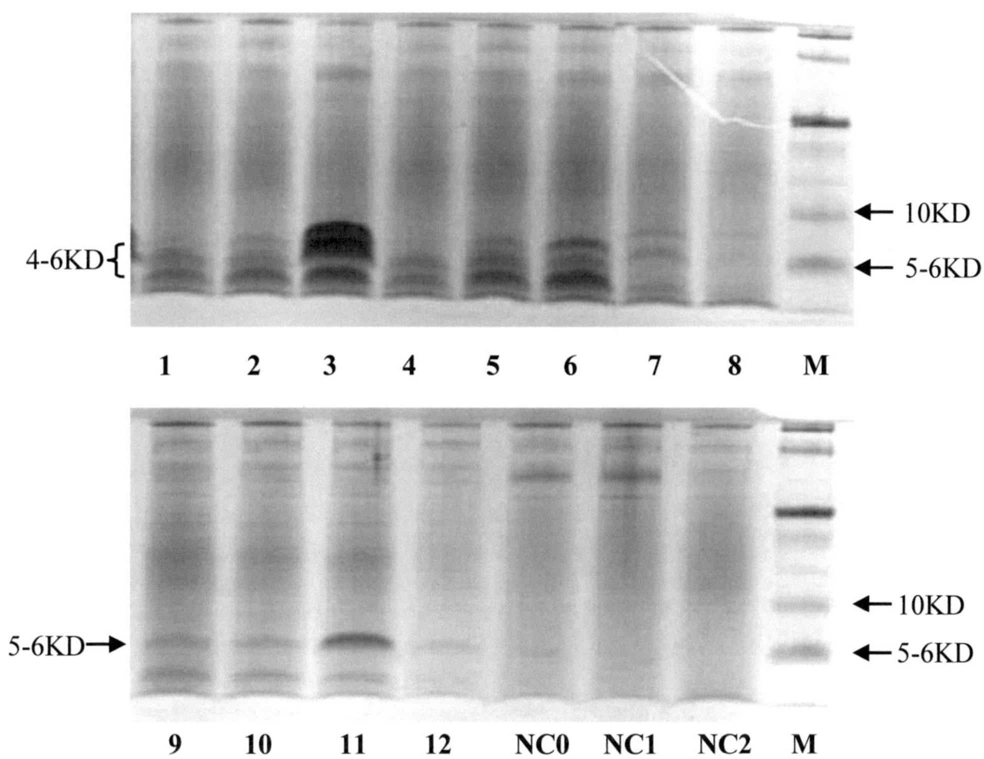

Fig. 5. SDS-PAGE detection of the expression of TiNPY1 and TiNPY2 after methanol induction for 48 hours.1-6:TiNPY2; 7-12:TiNPY1; NC0: pPICZaA-X-33 blank vector (negative control); NC1: pPICZaA-TiNPY1-X-33 without induction; NC2: pPICZaA-TiNPY2-X-33 without induction; M: protein marker. The size of TiNPY1 and TiNPY2 is 5-6KD and 4-6KD, respectively.

same colony (Fig.4, colony 11) and could express recombinant protein TiNPY1 efficiently. Tricine-SDS-PAGE result showed that when induced by methanol for 12h and 24h, the recombinant protein that pPICZαA-TiNPY1-X-33 expressed is about 10-12KD and 7-9KD. With the induction time increased to 48h, the molecular weight of TiNPY1 decreased to 6-7KD (Fig.9). Western blot result demonstrated that NPY antibody could only recognize the two protein bands induced by methanol for 12h as well as 24h. While after 48h induction, nothing could be observed in the membrane and two bands appeared before were missing, (Fig.10).

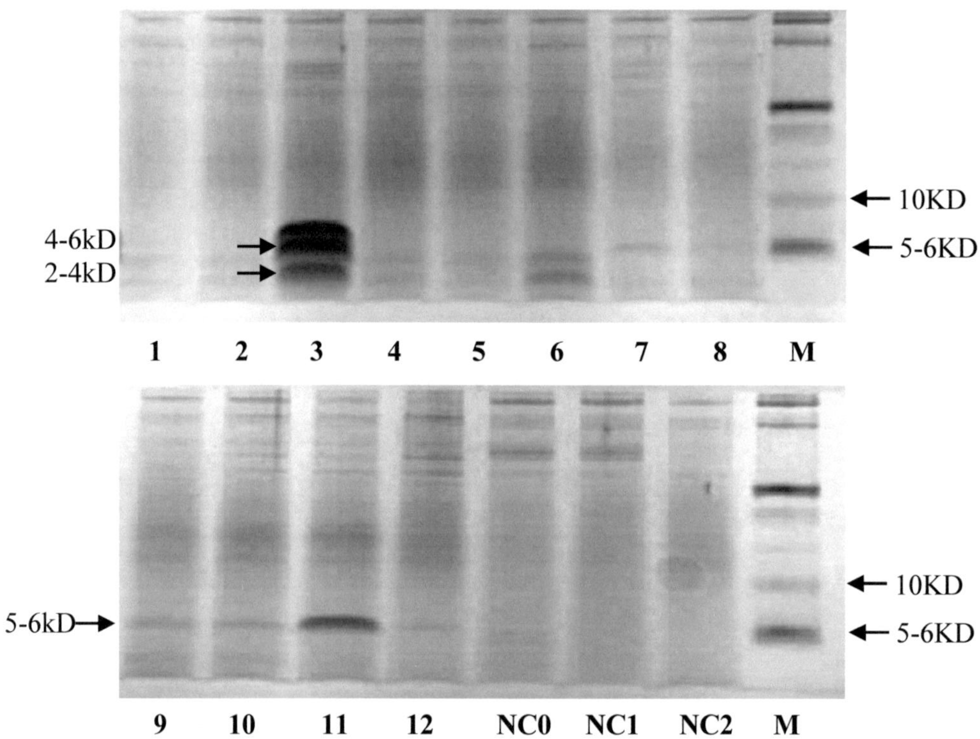

Fig. 6. SDS-PAGE detection of the expression of TiNPY1 and TiNPY2 after methanol induction for 72 hours. 1-6:TiNPY2; 7-12:TiNPY1; NC0: pPICZaA-X-33 blank vector (negative control); NC1: pPICZaA-TiNPY1-X-33 without induction; NC2: pPICZaA-TiNPY2-X-33 without induction; M: protein marker. The size of TiNPY1 and TiNPY2 is 5-6KD and 2-4kD, 4-6KD, respectively.

3.5 Purification of the recombinant tilapia NPY and sequencing of its N-terminal amino acid

As TiNPY1 and TiNPY2 were conjugated with 6× His tag, they could be purified with His•Bind Column by affinity chromatography. Samples from each fraction were size-fractionated by Tricine-SDS-PAGE with comparisons of supernatants before and after purification (Fig.11 and 12). The binding of the fusion recombinant proteins to the His•Bind Column (Ni-NTA column) was highly efficient as seen in Fig.11 (TiNPY1) and Fig.12 (TiNPY2). All of the three protein bands of TiNPY1 induced by methanol for 24 hours (Fig.

11) and two bands of TiNPY2 induced for 12 hours (Fig. 12) were eluted by 150mM imidazole. During the process of purification of TiNPY2, wash buffer was checked after washing to confirm that there were no recombinant proteins were washed out.

Two protein bands with larger molecular weight of TiNPY1 were purified and the 1-8th amino acids of their N-terminal were sequenced by instrument PROCISE491 (Applied Biosystemes Company, USA) with EDMEN degradation method. There are three kinds of proteins with different N-terminal a.a. (1-8th) were observed in the band with the largest molecular weight of TiNPY1. The protein with the N-terminal of N-EAYPVKPE is the major form which occupies 60-70% of TiNPY1. Proteins with the N-terminal of N-EAEAYPVK and N-YPVKPENP constitute of 20-30% and 5-10% of TiNPY1, respectively. The second band of TiNPY1 protein consists of two proteins with N-terminal of N-YPVKPENP (above 90%) and N-VKPENPGE (minority).

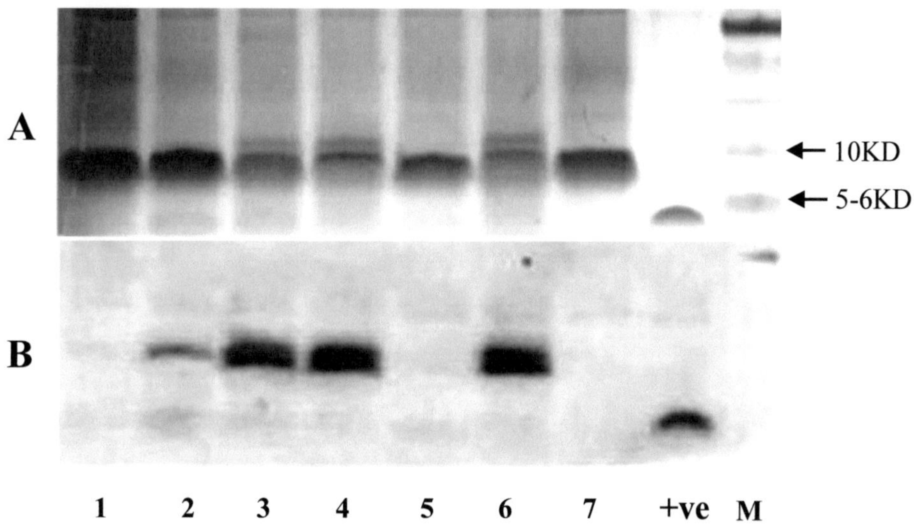

Fig. 7. SDS-PAGE to detect the expression of TiNPY1 (A) and western blot to confirm the immunological activity of recombinant TiNPY1. Samples (No.1-7) used in these experiments are recombinant TiNPY1 expressed by PICZaA-TiNPY1-X-33 after induction for different time. The synthesized tilapia NPY without His tags was used as positive control (4.104KD); M: protein marker

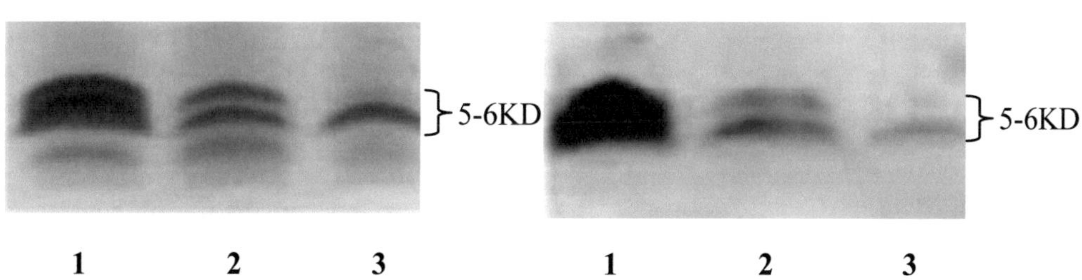

Fig. 8. SDS-PAGE to detect the expression of TiNPY2 (left) and western blot (right) to confirm the immunological activity of recombinant TiNPY2. Samples (No.1-3) used in these experiments are recombinant TiNPY2 expressed by PICZaA-TiNPY2-X-33.

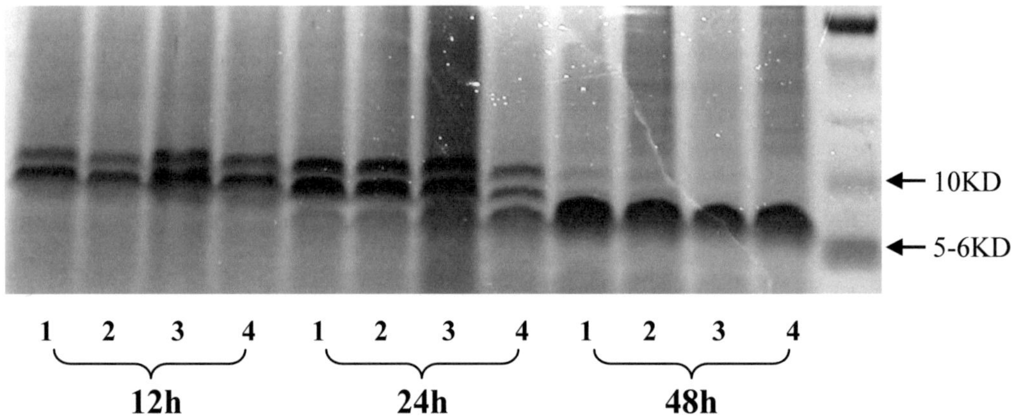

Fig. 9. Time course study of TiNPY1 expression induced by methanol. Four single colonies of pPICZaA-TiNPY1-X-33 with stable expression of TiNPY were used in the experiment. After induction of the expression by 0.5% methanol for 12h, 24h and 48h, the samples were harvested for SDS-PAGE.

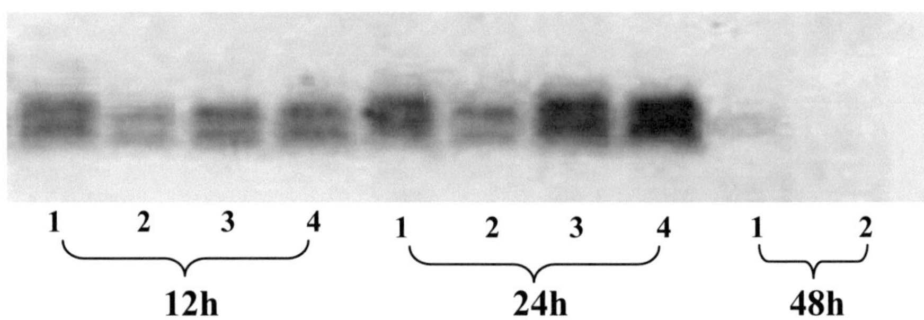

Fig. 10. Time course study of TiNPY1 expression by Western blot. The same samples used in SDS-PAGE study were used in this experiment. Two samples of 48h were the sample 3 and 4 in SDS-PAGE, respectively. Only TiNPY1 expressed after 12h and 24h induction were recognized by polyclonal antibody of NPY.

3.6 Effects of recombinant TiNPY on food intake and growth of the juveniles of GIFT tilapia

The results of in vivo study showed that the recombinant proteins of NPY could significantly stimulated food intake and body growth of GIFT tilapia. Compared to the control group (group 4), the percentages of average body weight increased in the group fed with 0.15μgTiNPY1/g feed (group 1), 0.3μgTiNPY1/g feed (group 2) or 0.6μgTiNPY1/g feed (group 3) were 29.65%, 32.11% and 12.60%, respectively. And the body weight of tilapia fed with 0.3μgTiNPY2/g feed was increased to 43.05% which gained the highest growth speed. The specific growth rates (SGR) and the final mean body lengths of all experimental groups [group 1 ($P<0.001$), group 2 ($P<0.001$), group 3 ($P<0.05$) and group 5 ($P<0.001$)] were significantly higher than the control group (group 4) after 50 days (Table 1). There were no obvious difference in initial mean weight of the 5 groups, but after 50 days' experiment, the final mean weight of group 1, group 2 and group 5 were significantly higher than group 4 by 15.31% (P<0.001), 16.59% (P<0.001) and 22.45% (P<0.001), respectively. The final mean weight of group 3 was 6.29% higher than the control group but with no significant difference (Table 1 and Fig.13). The possible detrimental effects of high levels of NPY on tilapia were studied through evaluation of HSI and gut weight ratio. No significant difference was found between groups fed with recombinant tilapia NPY and control group (Table 1). In the present study, we also analyzed the contents of moisture, crude protein, total lipid and ash of the dorsal white muscle of tilapia in each groups and no significant differences were observed except for the lipid content of group 5 compared to the control (P<0.01) (Table 2).

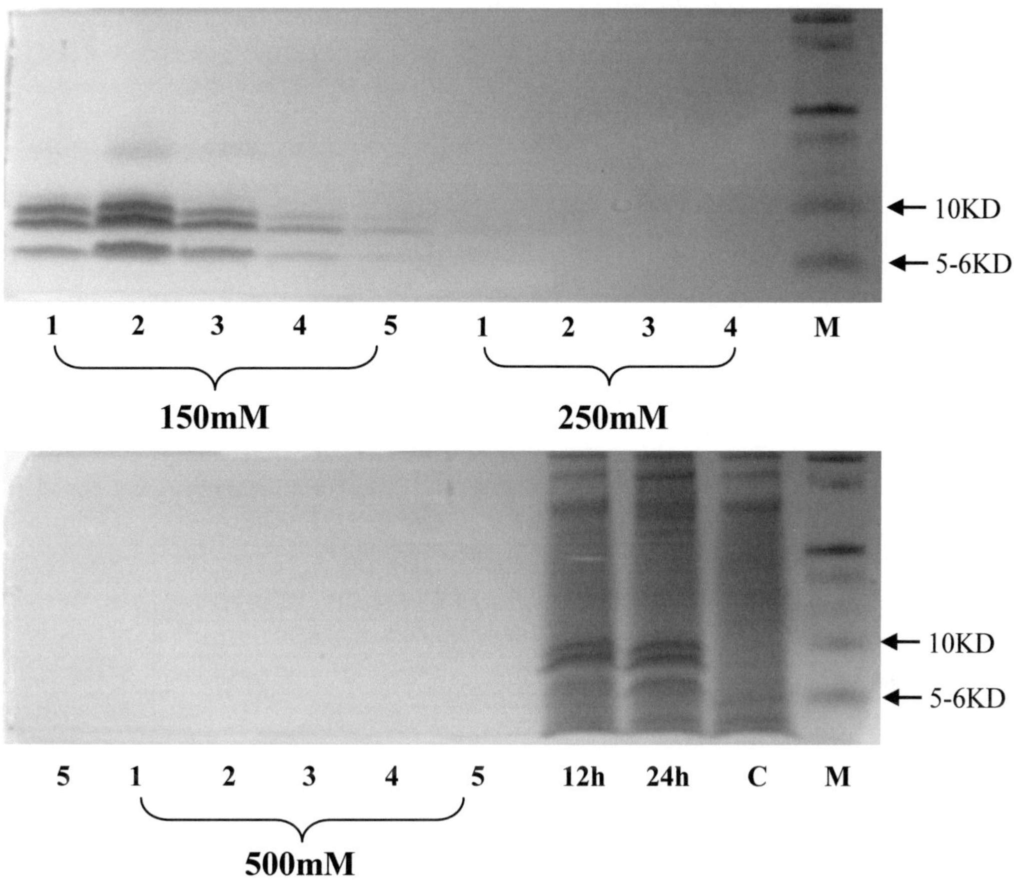

Fig. 11. Isolation and purification of TiNPY1 by His•Bind Column. TiNPY1 secreted by pPICZaA-TiNPY1-X-33 were isolated by His•Bind Column, and then were eluted by different concentration of imidazole (150mM, 250mM and 500mM). M: protein Marker; C: yeast culture supernatant flowing through His•Bind column; 12h and 24h: yeast culture supernatant induct for 12 and 24 hours.

After 50 days' feeding experiment, food consumptions in group 1 (0.15µgTiNPY1/g feed), 2 (0.3µgTiNPY1/g feed) and 5 (0.3µgTiNPY2/g feed) were significantly higher than the control group by18.03% (P<0.01), 20.80 %(P<0.01) and 30.22% (P<0.001) respectively, but there was no obvious difference between group3 (0.6µgTiNPY1/g feed) and control group (table 1). Consistent with the results of food consumption, feed conversion ratio (SGR) of group1 (1.72±0.017), group2 (1.73±0.017) and group5 (1.73±0.031) were significantly lower than the control group which with a FCR of 1.89±0.02. Again, no apparent distinction was observed between group3 and control group in FCR (Table 1 and Fig 14)

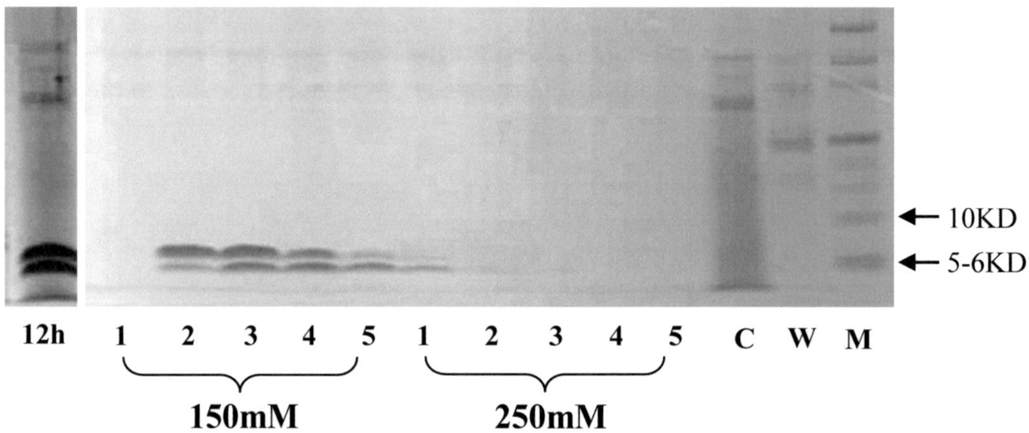

Fig. 12. Isolation and purification of TiNPY2 by His•Bind Column. TiNPY2 secreted by pPICZaA-TiNPY2-X-33 were isolated by His•Bind Column, and then eluted by different concentration of imidazole (150mM, 250mM). M: protein Marker; C: yeast culture supernatant flowing through His•Bind column; W: washing buffer. 12h: yeast culture supernatant induced for 12 hour.

Treatment	Group 1	Group 2	Group 3	Group 4	Group 5
Initial MBW(g)	72.94±0.49^{a}	72.88±0.11^{a}	73.03±0.30^{a}	73.69±0.41^{a}	72.94±0.27^{a}
Final MBW(g)	181.78±1.77^{c}	183.80±2.56^{c}	167.56±6.12^{a}	157.64±2.64^{a}	193.04±3.82^{c}
Initial MBL(cm)	13.01±0.06^{a}	13.00±0.01^{a}	12.99±0.06^{a}	13.04±0.07^{a}	13.00±0.07^{a}
Final MBL(cm)	17.45±0.10^{bc}	17.69±0.07c	17.32±0.10^{b}	17.02±0.11^{a}	17.69±0.07^{c}
SGR	1.83±0.023^{c}	1.85±0.027^{c}	1.66±0.075^{b}	1.52±0.037^{a}	1.95±0.036^{c}
Feed comsuption(g)	187.84±3.32^{bc}	192.26±4.91^{c}	174.13±5.26^{b}	159.15±6.45^{a}	207.24±2.94^{c}
FCR	1.72±0.017^{b}	1.73±0.017^{b}	1.85±0.065^{a}	1.89±0.020^{a}	1.73±0.031^{b}
HSI	2.92±0.088^{a}	2.76±0.072^{a}	2.85±0.103^{a}	2.90±0.101^{a}	2.81±0.080^{a}
Gut weight ratio	7.61±0.27^{a}	7.61±0.26^{a}	7.58±0.20^{a}	7.74±0.23^{a}	7.71±0.07^{a}

Table 1. Summary of the indexes related to the growth and feeding of tilapia treated with TiNPY1 and TiNPY2. Values are means ± SEM of three replicates, n=12 per replicate. Values with different superscripts are significantly different from each other (b indicated P <0.05 or c indicated P <0.001). MBW means body weight; MBL means body length; SGR (%/d) = (lnWt-lnW0)/d×100, Wt: final weights (g), W0: initial weights (g), d: experimental days; FCR = feed consumption (g)/fish weight gain (g); HIS=liver weight (g)/body weight (g); gut weight ratio= gut weight (g)/body weight (g). Group 1, 2, 3 were fed with 0.15, 0.3, 0.6μgTiNPY1/g feed; Group 4 fed with negative control diet; group 5 fed with 0.3μgTiNPY2/g feed.

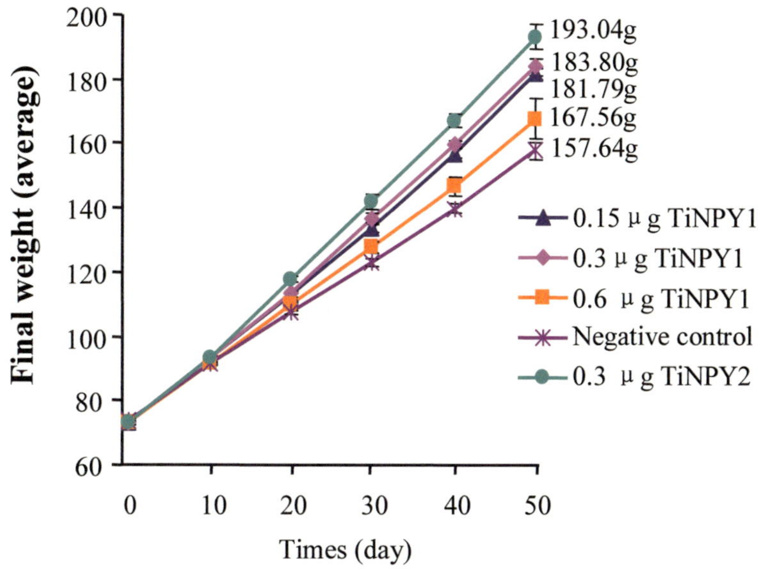

Fig. 13. Average individual body weight of tilapia fed with TiNPY1 or TiNPY2 in different days. Values are means ± SEM of three replicates (n=12 per replicate). The group fed with control diet acts as negative control.

Index	Group 1	Group 2	Group 3	Group 4	Group 5
Water (%)	76.40±0.31^{a}	76.56±0.21^{a}	76.34±0.20^{a}	76.29±0.037^{a}	76.48±0.20^{a}
Protein (%)	21.10±0.36^{a}	21.06±0.27^{a}	21.15±0.15^{a}	21.17±0.09^{a}	21.11±0.13^{a}
Lipid (%)	0.84±0.05^{ab}	0.88±0.06^{ab}	0.82±0.12^{ab}	0.72±0.12^{a}	0.98±0.05^{b}
Ash (%)	1.35±0.05^{a}	1.35±0.01^{a}	1.36±0.02^{a}	1.41±0.07^{a}	1.33±0.04^{a}

Table 2. White muscle composition of tilapia fed with TiNPY1 and TiNPY2 after 50 days. Values are means ± SEM of three replicates (n=12 per replicate). Values with different superscripts are significantly different from each other ($P<0.05$). Group 1, 2, 3 were fed with 0.15, 0.3, 0.6μgTiNPY1/g feed, respectively; Group 4 was fed with control diet and acts as a negative control. Group 5 was fed with 0.3μgTiNPY2/g feed.

3.7 Regulation of recombinant TiNPY on mRNA expressions of growth hormone, NPY and orexin in GIFT tilapia

Using real-time PCR technique, the effects of recombinant TiNPY on mRNA expressions of GH, NPY and orexin of tilapia were investigated. The results showed that 0.3μgTiNPY2/g feed could significantly stimulate pituitary GH mRNA expression. In contrast to TiNPY2, 0.15 and 0.3μgTiNPY1/g feed obviously inhibited GH mRNA expression and 0.6μgTiNPY1/g feed showed no effect on GH mRNA level (Fig.15).NPY and orexin are potent stimulators of food intake in teleosts and mainly expressed in hypothalamus of vertebrates. In this experiment, our study showed that 0.3μgTiNPY2/g feed significantly reduced mRNA expression of NPY as well as orexin and only 0.15 μgTiNPY1/g feed has similar inhibitory effect on NPY mRNA level (Fig.16 and 17). While 0.3, 0.6μgTiNPY1/g feed showed no effect on NPY mRNA expression (Fig.16) and all treatments of TiNPY1 haven't any obvious effect on orexin mRNA level (Fig.17).

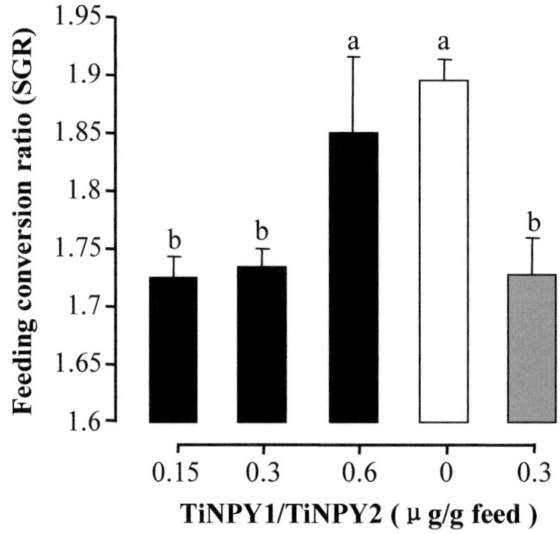

Fig. 14. Average feed conversion ratio (FCR) of tilapia fed with TiNPY1 (0.15, 0.3 and 0.6 μg/g feed, black columns) and TiNPY2 (0.3μg/g feed, grey column) after 50 days. The group fed with control diet acts as negative control (white column). Values presented are expressed as means ± SEM of three replicates (n=12 per replicate) and groups denoted by different letters represent a significant difference at $P < 0.05$(ANOVA followed by Fisher's LSD test).

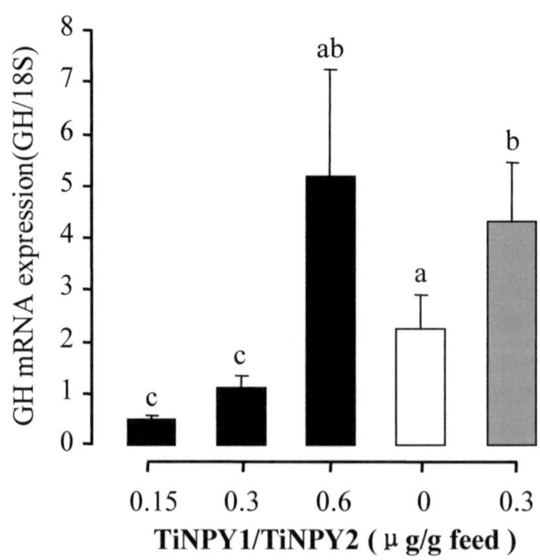

Fig. 15. Growth hormone (GH) mRNA expression of tilapia fed with TiNPY1 (0.15, 0.3 and 0.6μg/g feed, black columns) or TiNPY2 (0.3μg/g feed, grey column) after 50 days. The pituitaries of tilapia were homogenized for RNA extraction and RT-PCR. Then, Real-time PCR was used to detect the expression level of GH. The group fed with control diet acts as negative control (white column). Values presented are expressed as means ± SEM of three replicates (n=12 per replicate) and groups denoted by different letters represent a significant difference at $P<0.05$(ANOVA followed by Fisher's LSD test).

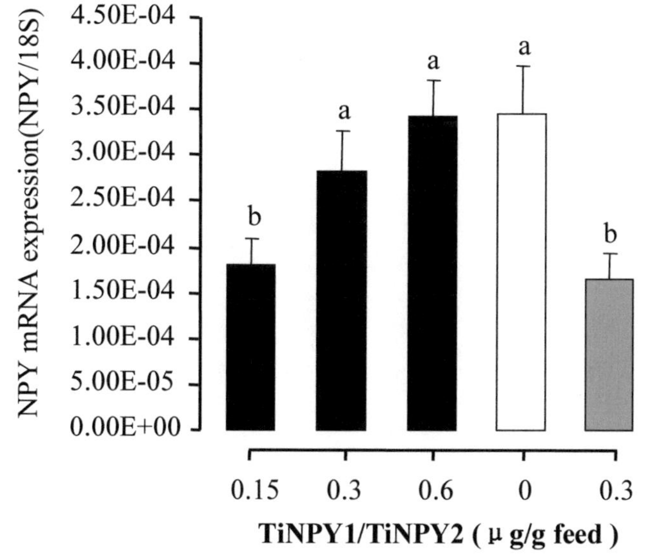

Fig. 16. NPY mRNA expression of tilapia fed with TiNPY1 (0.15, 0.3 and 0.6 μg/g feed, black columns) or TiNPY2 (0.3μg/g feed, grey column) after 50 days. The hypothalamuses of tilapia were homogenized for RNA extraction and RT-PCR. Then, Real-time PCR was used to detect the expression level of NPY. The group fed with control diet acts as negative control (white column). Values presented are expressed as means ± SEM of three replicates (n=12 per replicate) and groups denoted by different letters represent a significant difference at $P < 0.05$(ANOVA followed by Fisher's LSD test).

4. Discussion

Regulation of food intake is very important for the survival and growth of animals. As in mammals, NPY is also the most potent orexigenic peptide in fish (Matsuda, 2009; Volkoff, 2006; Volkoff et al., 2005). GIFT tilapia is a hybrid of Nile tilapia (*Oreochromis niloticus*) and it is a major fish species widely used in aquaculture of China. As the first step to study the functions of recombinant NPY protein in food intake regulation of GIFT tilapia, a cDNA for GIFT tilapia NPY was isolated by molecular cloning. The deduced a.a. sequence of GIFT tilapia NPY revealed that this peptide is the precursor of NPY that comprises the signal peptide, a region coding for the 36 a.a. mature peptide and a C-terminal domain. Sequence alignment of amino acids showed that the NPY mature peptide of GIFT tilapia is the identity of that red tilapia (GenBank: AAV49168) and highly homologous to human NPY with the identity of 86%. This result again clearly proved that NPY is the most highly conserved neuropeptide in vertebrates(Blomqvist et al., 1992).

In the study of protein function, *E. coli* is commonly used to express large quantities of protein. However, there are several obvious deficiencies exists in the *E. coli* expression system. Firstly, the recombinant proteins expressed using this system are intracellular types and are easy to form inclusion bodies of expressions. Secondly, the system lacks post-

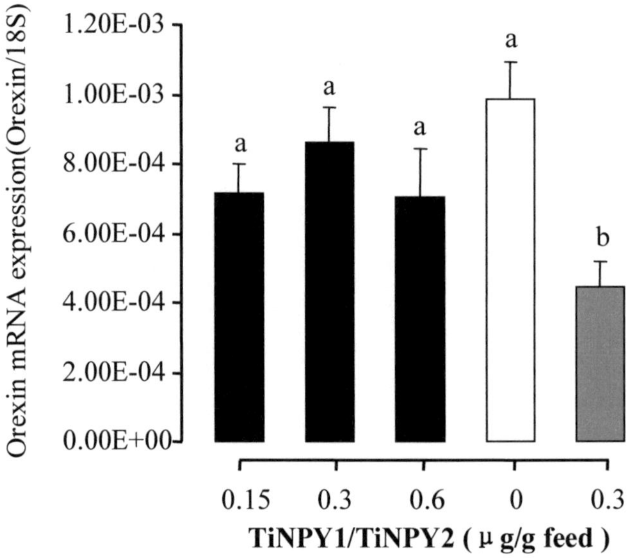

Fig. 17. Orexin mRNA expression of tilapia fed with TiNPY1 (0.15, 0.3 and 0.6 μg/g feed, black columns) or TiNPY2 (0.3μg/g feed, grey column) after 50 days. The hypothalamuses of tilapia were homogenized for RNA extraction and RT-PCR. Then, Real-time PCR was used to detect the expression level of orexin. The group fed with control diet acts as negative control (white column). Values presented are expressed as means ± SEM of three replicates (n=12 per replicate) and groups denoted by different letters represent a significant difference at $P<0.05$(ANOVA followed by Fisher's LSD test).

translational modification for foreign proteins. Thirdly, the immunogenic sources of *E. coli* such as exotoxin are often mixed with the products during cell fragmentation. Moreover, *E. coli* itself is an important source of water contamination. Therefore, these deficiencies limit its application in protein expression studies. As a eukaryote, yeast *Pichia pastoris*, a useful system for the expression of milligram-to-gram quantities of proteins for both basic laboratory research and industrial manufacture, owns advantages of higher eukaryotic expression systems such as protein processing, protein folding, and posttranslational modification, while being as easy to manipulate as *E. coli* or *Saccharomyces cerevisiae* (Carpio et al., 2009; Cregg et al., 2000).

Expression of target protein in *Pichia pastoris* can be either intracellular or secreted, and secretion requires a signal sequence on the expressed protein to target it to the secretory pathway. Although several different secretion signals have been used successfully, including the native signal peptide of the heterologous proteins, the secretion signal sequence from the *Saccharomyces cerevisiae* α factor prepro-peptide has been used with the most success(Cregg et al., 2000). The major advantage of expressing heterologous proteins as secreted proteins is that *Pichia pastoris* secretes very low levels of native proteins (Cregg et al., 2000), which facilitates the purification and acquisition of a large scale recombinant heterologous proteins. Additionally, it has recently been demonstrated that the culture supernatant proteins of *P. pastoris* can have beneficial effects on fish larval growth and innate immunity (Carpio et al., 2009). These characteristics make *P. pastoris* a very useful heterologous proteins expression system in production of recombinant proteins for aquaculture purposes. The processing of the α-factor mating signal sequence in pPICZα occurs in two steps: the preliminary cleavage of the signal sequence by the KEX2 gene product, with the final Kex2 cleavage occurring between arginine and glutamine in the sequence Glu-Lys-Arg * Glu-Ala-Glu-Ala, where * is the site of cleavage; and the Glu-Ala repeats are further cleaved by the STE13 gene product (user manual of EasySelect™ Pichia Expression Kit, Catalog no. K1740-01).

After obtained the ORF of GIFT tilapia NPY, two recombinant Pichia X-33 stains of PICZαA-TiNPY1 and pPICZαA-TiNPY2 were established and they can efficiently express recombinant TiNPY1 and TiNPY2, respectively. The two recombinant proteins were supposed to be expressed homogenously with no glycosylation, and comprise only one protein band in Tricine-SDS-PAGE and western blot analysis, respectively. However, three bands with different molecular weight of each recombinant NPY were observed after methanol induction for more than 12 hours, and all of them could be isolated and purified by Ni-NTA His•Bind Column, which means all of them conjugated with 6× His tag designed in our study. Interestingly, only the upper two bands (with larger molecular weight) could be recognized by rabbit polyclonal antibody against porcine NPY. Our hypothesis is that the N-terminal signal peptide from the α factor was not completely cut off and Glu-Ala repeats were left on the N-terminus of the expressed protein of the first band (with largest molecular weight), the second band contained mainly recombinant protein with native N-terminus of tilapia NPY; and the third band, with a smallest molecular weight and couldn't be recognized by NPY antibody, was the degradation of recombinant NPY with the degradation of native N-terminus and the preservation of C-terminus. This speculation was verified by N-terminal a. a. sequence with Edman stepwise degradation.

Oral delivery of peptide and protein has been proved to be the most suitable route and least intrusive for delivery to fish in the aquaculture industry (Kiris GA, 2007; Ledger et al., 2002). As mentioned above, NPY is the most important factor in regulating food intake and energy metabolism in vertebrates. To test the physiological functions of recombinant TiNPY and TiNPY2 of GIFT tilapia, yeast culture supernatants with different dosages of the two proteins were directly sprayed on the surface of ordinary commercial extruded floating feed and acts as daily diets to feed to the juvenile tilapia. As expected, both TiNPY1 and TiNPY2 could significantly stimulate the food intake of juvenile tilapia. Compared to the control group, the food intake of tilapia fed with 0.15 or 0.3μgTiNPY1/g feed, or fed with 0.3μgTiNPY2/g feed was increased to 18.03%, 20.80% and 30.22%, respectively. This result demonstrated again that NPY does not lose its feeding stimulatory effect when passed through the alimentary canal of fish as was found in the red tilapia (Kiris GA, 2007). Similar stimulated food intake results were found when Juvenile tilapia received intraperitoneal injection of recombinant neuropeptide Y expressed by *Escherichia coli* (1 μg/g of body weight) (Carpio et al., 2006), or i.p. injection (0.6 μg /g of body weight) or orally given (0.25 μg/g of feed) of human NPY (Kiris GA, 2007). And this result is also highly consistent with those reported in other fish species. For example, injections of mammal NPY or fish NPY promoted food intake of goldfish (Narnaware et al., 2000; Peng et al., 1993a) and rainbow trout (Aldegunde and Mancebo, 2006). Moreover, our study also showed that the FCRs of tilapia fed with 0.15 or 0.3μg/g feed of TiNPY1 and fed with 0.3μg/g feed of TiNPY2 were significantly lower than the control group, which perhaps suggests some significance in the aquaculture of tilapia. However, FCR was not altered in tilapia treated with recombinant NPY expressed by *Escherichia coli* (1 μg/g of body weight) (Carpio et al., 2006).

More food intake and low FCR often lead to faster growth. In the present study, the percentage of weight gain in the tilapia fed with 0.15μg/g feed, 0.3μg/g feed or 0.6μg/g feed of recombinant TiNPY1 were 29.65%, 32.11% or 12.60% respectively higher than the control group, which was fed with the control diet. The feed with 0.3μgTiNPY2/g feed made the highest growth speed, with a mean body weight gain of 43.05% higher than the control group. The similar fasted growth results were found in other studies. NPY injection significantly induced energy consumption and body weight of goldfish (Narnaware and Peter, 2001a; Narnaware and Peter, 2001b) and tilapia (Carpio et al., 2006; Kiris GA, 2007); 18 and 30 days after immersion baths with recombinant NPY expressed by *Escherichia coli* three times a week, body weight and body length of catfish were significantly higher than the control (Carpio Y, 2007); Both injection and oral administration with human NPY significantly promoted the growth and body weight of tilapia(Kiris GA, 2007).

The effect of NPY on food intake and growth seems dosage and species specific and too high or too low dosage could not elevate food intake in fish and shrimp (Kiris GA, 2007; Narnaware and Peter, 2001b), The growth and food intake of tilapia *Oreochromis niloticus* were both significantly higher at dosage of 0.25μg/g feed compared to the control, but lower dosage of 0.125 μg/g feed only stimulated food intake(Kiris GA, 2007); Although the group of red tilapia injected with 0.1mg/gbw of recombinant NPY showed a weight increase of 26% when compared to the control group, it is still not statistically significant (Carpio et al., 2006). In our study, weight increase of tilapia fed with a dosage of 0.6μgTiNPY1/g feed was 12.60% higher than control, but with no statistical significance, and significantly lower than fish fed with lower dosages of 0.15 and 0.3 TiNPY1μg/g feed. The tilapia fed with 0.3 μg TiNPY2/g feed obtained the fastest growth rate compared with groups fed with TiNPY1 and the control diet.

Some studies have reported that NPY is involved in the neuroendocrine regulation of growth hormone. For example, NPY stimulates GH secretion in vitro and in vivo in goldfish (Peng et al., 1993b; Peng et al., 1993a) and catfish (Mazumdar et al., 2006). Similar as in mammals, NPY also interacts with a number of appetite factors, e.g. orexin, leptin and CART, to regulate food intake in fish (Volkoff, 2006; Volkoff et al., 2005). In the present study, we also investigated the effects of recombinant proteins of TiNPY1 and TiNPY2 on mRNA expressions of GH in pituitary and NPY as well as orexin in hypothalamus. The results showed that TiNPY2 (0.3μg/g feed) significantly induced GH mRNA expression. In contrast to TiNPY2, low dosages of TiNPY1 (0.15 and 0.3μg/g feed) obviously inhibited GH mRNA expression and high dosage of TiNPY1 (0.6μg/g feed) showed no effect on GH mRNA level. For NPY and orexin, the same dosage of TiNPY2 significantly inhibited mRNA expression of NPY as well as orexin to 50% compared to the control group and only 0.15 μg TiNPY1/g feed has similar inhibitory effect on NPY mRNA level. In contrast, 0.3 and 0.6μgTiNPY1/g feed showed no effect on NPY mRNA expression and all treatments of TiNPY1 haven't any obvious effect on orexin mRNA level. These results, taken together, suggested that long-term feeding of tilapia with recombinant NPY proteins could upregulate GH mRNA expression and down-regulate the gene expressions of NPY and orexin. Further experiments are needed to test our hypothesis. In the whole experiment, we noticed that the effects of recombinant protein of TiNPY2 are much significant than that induced by TiNPY1. As the two forms of recombinant tilapia NPY expressed by yeast are only different in conjugated tags for identification and purification. The conjugated tag of TiNPY1, which was added a sequence with the molecular weight of 2.2KD to the recombinant protein, contains c-myc, 6× His tag and the amino-acid residues between them. While, the conjugated tag of TiNPY2, which was added to a sequence with the molecular weight of 0.8KDa to the recombinant protein, only contains six amino-acid residues of 6× His. The difference of their effects on the food intake and mRNA expression of GH, NPY and orexin may come from the difference of the conjugated tag attached with them .These results perhaps indicated that a larger conjugated tag of recombinant NPY would interfere its absorption or transportation across the blood-brain barrier. The function of recombinant NPY were also perhaps disturbed by the tags, as lipid content of the white muscle was higher in tilapia fed with TiNPY2 than those feed with TiNPY1 or control diet.

5. Conclusion

We obtained the cDNA encoding the precursor of NPY from GIFT tilapia. The deduced amino acids sequence of the mature peptide of GIFT tilapia is the same as that of red tilapia and it is highly conserved with human NPY. Two Pichia X-33 stains of PICZαA-TiNPY1 and pPICZαA-TiNPY2 were established and they can express the recombinant proteins of TiNPY1 and TiNPY2, respectively. Long-term feeding tilapia with TiNPY1 and TiNPY2 could significantly stimulate the food intake and growth of tilapia and at the same time to reduce the feeding conversion ratio of feed. Moreover, TiNPY2 can induce GH mRNA expression in the pituitary of tilapia and while potently suppressed mRNA expressions of hypothalamic NPY and orexin. For TiNPY1, lower dosages of which could inhibit GH and NPY mRNA expression. All dosages of TiNPY1 used in our experiment showed no effect on orexin mRNA expression. The present study clearly demonstrated that the recombinant protein of NPY expressed from the yeast *Pichia pastoris* has biological activity and oral delivery of NPY is a useful method in the aquaculture industry.

6. Acknowledgment

This work was supported by the National Basic Research Program (2010CB126302), the China Agriculture Research System (CARS-49), the Agriculture Research Special Funds of 3-49, the National High Technology Research Program (2007AA10Z165) and the Fundamental Research Funds for the Central Universities awarded to Professor Wensheng Li.

7. References

Aldegunde, M., Mancebo, M., (2006). Effects of neuropeptide Y on food intake and brain biogenic amines in the rainbow trout (Oncorhynchus mykiss). Peptides. 27, 719-27.

Blomqvist, A. G., et al., (1992). Strong evolutionary conservation of neuropeptide Y: sequences of chicken, goldfish, and Torpedo marmorata DNA clones. Proc Natl Acad Sci U S A. 89, 2350-4.

Carpio, Y., et al., (2006). Cloning, expression and growth promoting action of Red tilapia (Oreochromis sp.) neuropeptide Y. Peptides. 27, 710-8.

Carpio, Y., et al., (2009). Regulation of body mass growth through activin type IIB receptor in teleost fish. Gen Comp Endocrinol. 160, 158-67.

Carpio Y, L. K., Acosta J, Morales R, Estrada MP., (2007). Recombinant tilapia Neuropeptide Y promotes growth and antioxidant defenses in African catfish (Clarias gariepinus) fry. . Aquaculture 272 649-655.

Cerda-Reverter, J. M., Larhammar, D., (2000a). Neuropeptide Y family of peptides: structure, anatomical expression, function, and molecular evolution. Biochem Cell Biol. 78, 371-92.

Cerda-Reverter, J. M., et al., (2000b). Molecular evolution of the neuropeptide Y (NPY) family of peptides: cloning of three NPY-related peptides from the sea bass (Dicentrarchus labrax). Regul Pept. 95, 25-34.

Chavez, M., et al., (1998). Effect of a high-fat diet on food intake and hypothalamic neuropeptide gene expression in streptozotocin diabetes. J Clin Invest. 102, 340-6.

Cregg, J. M., et al., (2000). Recombinant protein expression in Pichia pastoris. Mol Biotechnol. 16, 23-52.

Faber, K. N., et al., (1995). Review: methylotrophic yeasts as factories for the production of foreign proteins. Yeast. 11, 1331-44.

Gelineau, A., Boujard, T., (2001). Oral administration of cholecystokinin receptor antagonists increase feed intake in rainbow trout. J. Fish Biol. . 58, 716–724.

Halford, J. C., et al., (2004). The pharmacology of human appetite expression. Curr Drug Targets. 5, 221-40.

Kalra, S. P., et al., (1999). Interacting appetite-regulating pathways in the hypothalamic regulation of body weight. Endocr Rev. 20, 68-100.

Kehoe, A. S., Volkoff, H., (2007). Cloning and characterization of neuropeptide Y (NPY) and cocaine and amphetamine regulated transcript (CART) in Atlantic cod (Gadus morhua). Comp Biochem Physiol A Mol Integr Physiol. 146, 451-61.

Kiris GA, K. M., Dikel S., (2007). Stimulatory effects of neuropeptide Y on food intake and growth of Oreochromis niloticus. Aquaculture. 264, 383-389.

Ledger, R., et al., (2002). The metabolic barrier of the lower intestinal tract of salmon to the oral delivery of protein and peptide drugs. J Control Release. 85, 91-103.

Lin, S., et al., (2004). NPY and Y receptors: lessons from transgenic and knockout models. Neuropeptides. 38, 189-200.

Lopez-Patino, M. A., et al., (1999). Neuropeptide Y has a stimulatory action on feeding behavior in goldfish (Carassius auratus). Eur J Pharmacol. 377, 147-53.

Matsuda, K., (2009). Recent advances in the regulation of feeding behavior by neuropeptides in fish. Ann N Y Acad Sci. 1163, 241-50.

Mazumdar, M., et al., (2006). Involvement of neuropeptide Y Y1 receptors in the regulation of LH and GH cells in the pituitary of the catfish, Clarias batrachus: an immunocytochemical study. Gen Comp Endocrinol. 149, 190-6.

Narnaware, Y. K., Peter, R. E., (2001a). Effects of food deprivation and refeeding on neuropeptide Y (NPY) mRNA levels in goldfish. Comp Biochem Physiol B Biochem Mol Biol. 129, 633-7.

Narnaware, Y. K., Peter, R. E., (2001b). Neuropeptide Y stimulates food consumption through multiple receptors in goldfish. Physiol Behav. 74, 185-90.

Narnaware, Y. K., Peter, R. E., (2002). Influence of diet composition on food intake and neuropeptide Y (NPY) gene expression in goldfish brain. Regul Pept. 103, 75-83.

Narnaware, Y. K., et al., (2000). Regulation of food intake by neuropeptide Y in goldfish. Am J Physiol Regul Integr Comp Physiol. 279, R1025-34.

Pedrazzini, T., (2004). Importance of NPY Y1 receptor-mediated pathways: assessment using NPY Y1 receptor knockouts. Neuropeptides. 38, 267-75.

Pedrazzini, T., et al., (2003). Neuropeptide Y: the universal soldier. Cell Mol Life Sci. 60, 350-77.

Peng, C., et al., (1993b). Neuropeptide-Y stimulates growth hormone and gonadotropin-II secretion in the goldfish pituitary: involvement of both presynaptic and pituitary cell actions. Endocrinology. 132, 1820-9.

Peng, C., et al., (1993a). Actions of goldfish neuropeptide Y on the secretion of growth hormone and gonadotropin-II in female goldfish. Gen Comp Endocrinol. 90, 306-17.

Romanos, M. A., et al., (1992). Foreign gene expression in yeast: a review. Yeast. 8, 423-88.

Sundstrom, G., et al., (2005). Ray-fin fish tetraploidization gave rise to pufferfish duplicates of NPY and PYY, but zebrafish NPY duplicate was lost. Ann N Y Acad Sci. 1040, 476-8.

Sundstrom, G., et al., (2008). Evolution of the neuropeptide Y family: new genes by chromosome duplications in early vertebrates and in teleost fishes. Gen Comp Endocrinol. 155, 705-16.

Tatemoto, K., et al., (1982). Neuropeptide Y--a novel brain peptide with structural similarities to peptide YY and pancreatic polypeptide. Nature. 296, 659-60.

Valassi, E., et al., (2008). Neuroendocrine control of food intake. Nutr Metab Cardiovasc Dis. 18, 158-68.

Volkoff, H., (2006). The role of neuropeptide Y, orexins, cocaine and amphetamine-related transcript, cholecystokinin, amylin and leptin in the regulation of feeding in fish. Comp Biochem Physiol A Mol Integr Physiol. 144, 325-31.

Volkoff, H., et al., (2005). Neuropeptides and the control of food intake in fish. Gen Comp Endocrinol. 142, 3-19.

Volkoff, H., et al., (2010). Influence of intrinsic signals and environmental cues on the endocrine control of feeding in fish: potential application in aquaculture. Gen Comp Endocrinol. 167, 352-9.

Woods, S. C., et al., (1998). NPY and food intake: discrepancies in the model. Regul Pept. 75-76, 403-8.

7

Hormones and Metabolism in Poultry

Colin G. Scanes
University of Wisconsin Milwaukee, USA

1. Introduction

Poultry are domesticated species of birds. Birds were domesticated for eggs (chickens, ducks and geese), meat (chickens, ducks, geese, turkeys, ostriches, emus, pigeons and game birds) or other uses including feathers (ostriches, ducks and geese), leather (ostriches), specific oils (ostriches, emus), cock-fighting (chickens) and homing (pigeons). Table 1 summarizes the approximate time when and the location where the species were domesticated.

Poultry by global production	Domestication			Production in 2009	
	Species	When	Location(s)	Meat million metric tons	Eggs million metric tons
Chickens	Gallus gallus	5000 Before Common Era (BCE)	North East China	79.6	62.4
Turkeys	Meleagris gallopavo	200-2500 BCE	Meso-America	5.3	< 1.0
Ducks	Anas platyrinchos	3000 BCE	Fertile Crescent and East Asia/China	3.8	5.0[b]
Geese	Anser anser/Anser cynoides	3000 BCE	Fertile Crescent and East Asia/China	2.4[a]	
Pigeons	Columbia livia	3000 BCE	Fertile Crescent	< 1.0	< 1.0
Ostriches	Struthio camelus	1857	South Africa	< 1.0	< 1.0
Emus	Dromaius novaehollandiae	within last 100 years	Australia	< 1.0	< 1.0

[a] Goose and guinea fowl combined; [b] Eggs other than chicken - predominantly duck and goose

Table 1. Poultry - Their Domestication and Production (based on Scanes, 2011 and data from the Food and Agricultural Organization)

Investigations of the hormonal control of growth and/or metabolism in poultry have predominantly been performed using chickens (reviewed Scanes, 2009). Not only have such studies focused on the chicken as an important agricultural animal but also the chick embryo has long been a model for developmental biology. Moreover, the chicken is the model species for birds. There are numerically many fewer studies in turkeys, ducks and ostriches together with a substantial body of research in Japanese quail as another avian model species.

Research approaches have included ablation and replacement studies, assay of circulating hormone concentrations or gene expression in response to physiological perturbations, genetic models associated with a singe gene such a dwarf or obese chickens and genetic models produced by multi-generation selection for specific phenotypes such as fast or slow growth. There have been limited transgenic studies on the hormonal control of growth or metabolism. There is presently not a robust knock-out model in poultry.

2. Glucose homeostasis

Steady state or basal circulating concentrations of glucose are much higher in poultry than in mammals. Indeed the circulating concentrations of glucose reported in poultry species would be considered grossly hyperglycemic or symptomatic of diabetes mellitus in mammals. For instance, circulating concentrations of glucose were reported in chickens as being between 190 to 220 mg/dL (reviewed by Hazelwood, 1986) or more recently based on 15 studies as 234 ±11.8 (SEM) mg/dL [13 ± 0.7 mM](Scanes, 2008).

Physiological state	Change in circulating concentration of glucose mM	Reference
Fasting (24hours)	No change or - 1.2	Belo et al., 1976; Harvey et al., 1976; Hazelwood & Lorenz, 1959
Insulin Administration	- 6 mM	Harvey et al., 1976;
Glucagon administration	+ 12 mM	Harvey et al., 1976;

Table 2. Changes in circulating concentrations of glucose in chickens with physiological state or perturbation

Despite the difference in set point, circulating concentrations are maintained within tight limits by a series of homeostatic mechanisms (see table 2). The physiological mechanisms are discussed below. Table 3 summarizes changes in various metabolites during fasting in chickens.

3. Hormones controlling circulating concentrations of glucose and metabolism

Circulating concentrations are maintained within tight limits by a series of physiological mechanisms. Synthesis of fatty acid and triglycerides in poultry are anatomically separated in poultry. Lipogenesis occurs predominantly in the liver of poultry while adipose tissue is the site of triglyceride synthesis and breakdown or lipolysis. These processes are under the

Physiological state	Change in circulating concentration of glucose	Reference
Glucose	No change or -4mM or -1.2 mM	Belo et al., 1976; Harvey et al., 1976; Hazelwood & Lorenz, 1959
Beta Hydroxy butyrate	+1.2 µM	Belo et al., 1976
Alanine	+110 µM	Belo et al., 1976
Serine	+250 µM	Belo et al., 1976
Glycine	-150 µM	Belo et al., 1976
Heart Glycogen	- 8.3 µmoles per g	Hazelwood & Lorenz, 1959
Liver Glycogen	- 85 µmoles per g	Hazelwood & Lorenz, 1959

Table 3. Changes in circulating concentrations of glucose, other metabolites and tissue glycogen in chickens when fasted

control of metabolic hormones with pancreatic glucagon, arguably, the most important. The role of glucagon and glucagons-like peptides of intestinal origin has received less attention. When circulating concentrations of glucose are elevated, there is a rapid increase in the rate of secretion of insulin from the pancreatic islet beta (β) cells and a concomitant rise in the circulating concentrations of insulin. The effects of insulin include the following:

- Increase in glucose uptake by muscle, liver and adipose tissue with glucose accumulating as glycogen together with increases in triglyceride in adipose tissue
- Increase in lipogenesis

When circulating concentrations of glucose are depressed, there is rapid increases secretion of glucagon from the pancreatic islet alpha (α) or A cells and a concomitant rise in the circulating concentrations of glucagon. The effects of glucagon include the following:

- Increased lipolysis in adipose tissue
- Decreased muscle and liver glycogen
- Decreased glucose utilization
- Increased gluconeogenesis
- Decrease in lipogenesis.

Other important hormones controlling metabolism in poultry include the avian adrenal glucocorticoid, corticosterone, and the thyroid hormone, triiodothyronine (T_3).

3.1 Insulin

The structure of chicken pro-insulin is long established (Perler et al., 1980). The amino-acid sequence for ostrich and chicken insulin are identical (Evans et al., 1988). The structure of insulin is identical in Pekin ducks, Muscovy ducks and domestic geese (Chevalier et al., 1996). Duck insulin has a lower potency and binding affinity to the mammalian insulin receptor compared to chicken insulin (Constans et al., 1991).

Insulin is released at times of surplus glucose, for instance following post prandial absorption of nutrients from the small intestine (DeBeer et al., 2009). The factors controlling insulin secretion are summarized in table 4. Insulin secretion from chicken pancreas *in situ* is increased by elevated glucose concentrations; this being potentiated by glucagon (King & Hazelwood, 1976). Similarly, elevated glucose concentrations increase insulin from chicken B islets *in vitro* (Datar et al., 2006). The stimulatory effect of glucagon is unlikely to be physiological as circulating concentrations of glucagon are very low when high insulin secretion is evident as, for instance, is seen following feeding (DeBeer et al., 2008). Circulating concentrations of insulin increased by the glucocorticoid, dexamethasone (Song et al., 2011). Similarly in ducks, insulin secretion is increased by glucose or arginine or oleic acid or glucagon (Foltzer & Miahle, 1980).

Stimulus	Insulin	Glucagon	Reference
Glucose	↑↑↑	↓↓	Chicken: Lanslow et al., 1970; King & Hazelwood, 1976; Honey et al., 1980 Duck: Foltzer & Miahle, 1980
Arginine	↑	↑	Chicken: King & Hazelwood, 1976; Honey et al., 1980 Duck: Foltzer & Miahle, 1980
Oleic Acid	↑	?	Chicken: Lanslow et al., 1970; King & Hazelwood, 1976; Duck: Foltzer & Miahle, 1980
Insulin	Not applicable	--	Chicken: Honey & Weir, 1979 Duck: Sitbon & Mialhe, 1978.
Glucagon	↑ in the presence of high glucose	Not applicable	Chicken: King & Hazelwood, 1976; Duck: Foltzer & Miahle, 1980
Somatostatin	↓	↑	Duck: Strosser et al., 1980
Corticosterone	↑↑	?	Chicken: Song et al., 2011
Epinephrine	↓	?	Chicken: Lanslow et al., 1970;

Table 4. Control of insulin and glucagon secretion in chickens and ducks

Despite the very high ambient circulating concentrations of glucose in poultry, insulin still plays an important role in the control of carbohydrate and to some extent also lipid metabolism. Insulin acts to increase energy storage as glycogen (liver and muscles) and triglyceride in adipose tissue (see figure 1). The physiological role of insulin in poultry is supported by the elevated circulating concentrations of glucose observed after fed chickens receive antisera against insulin (Simon et al., 2000).

3.1.1 Carbohydrate metabolism

Insulin evokes a movement of glucose from the blood. For instance, when administered to chickens insulin will induce a decline in circulating concentrations of glucose, albeit to levels that would be considered hyperglycemic in mammals (Hazelwood & Lorenz, 1959).

Chickens respond to insulin with a depression in circulating concentrations of glucose (Hazelwood & Lorenz, 1959) but are relatively insensitive to insulin (Vasilatos-Younken, 1986; Edwards et al., 1999). Insulin increases glucose uptake by skeletal muscle (M. fibularis longus) *in vitro* as indicated 2 deoxy--D-[1,2-3H]-glucose uptake (Zhao et al., 2009). In ducks, insulin increase in glucose uptake by skeletal muscle sarcolemmal vesicles while also inducing translocation of GLUT-4 like proteins from intracellular pools to the sarcolemma (Thomas-Delloye et al., 1999).

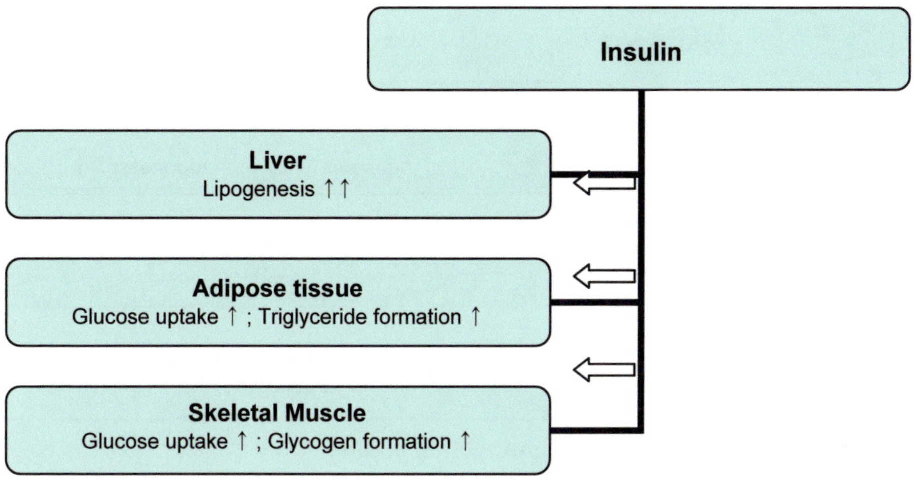

Fig. 1. Schema of physiological role of insulin in poultry

3.1.2 Lipid metabolism

Insulin can influence lipid metabolism but the physiological significant of these effects is uncertain. Fatty acid synthesis occurs predominantly in the liver of poultry and is under the control of metabolic hormones. Lipogenesis is increased *in vitro* in the presence of insulin together with T_3 (Goodridge, 1973; Wilson et al., 1986). Insulin also stimulates free fatty acid uptake by duck hepatocytes (Gross and Mialhe, 1984). However, insulin does not suppress the lipolytic effects of glucagon on chicken adipose tissue (Langslow & Hales, 1969).

3.2 Glucagon

In poultry, the major role of glucagon is to modulate carbohydrate and lipid metabolism to provide readily utilizable energy, at times of nutritional restriction. Ostrich glucagon is identical to duck glucagon (Ferreira et al., 1991).

Glucagon effects the mobilization of glucose and fatty acids from storage into the circulation together with decreasing glucose utilization (see figure 2). As might be expected, in the absence of feeding, as in regimens where chickens are fed on alternative days, there are large increases in the circulating concentrations of glucagons between meals (DeBeer et al., 2009). Surprisingly in view of its release during fasting, glucagon decreases food intake when administered centrally to chicks (Honda et al., 2007). The factors controlling glucagon secretion are summarized in table 4. Broadly, glucagon secretion is inhibited by glucose but stimulated by amino-acids. For instance, in ducks, glucagon secretion is increased by the amino-acid, arginine (Foltzer & Miahle, 1980).

3.2.1 Carbohydrate metabolism

Glucagon administration increases the circulating concentration of glucose (see table 2)(chicken: Harvey et al. 1978; turkey: McMurtry et al., 1996; ducks: Foltzer & Miahle, 1980). This is due to increases in hepatic glycogenolysis and gluconeogenesis together with decreased glucose utilization, for instance for fatty acid synthesis (Wilson et al., 1986). Glucagon has been found to stimulate gluconeogenesis, for instance, in the perfused chicken liver (Sugano et al., 1982).

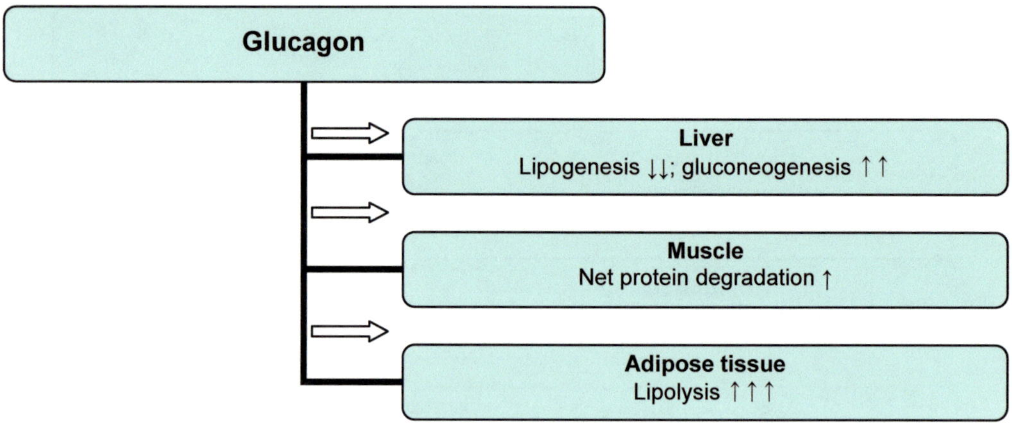

Fig. 2. Schema of physiological role of glucagon in poultry

3.2.2 Lipid metabolism

Glucagon suppresses lipogenesis in chicken hepatocytes in vitro (Wilson et al., 1986). Glucagon is the major lipolytic hormone in birds (Langslow & Hales, 1969) with its effect decreased in the presence of GH (e.g. Campbell & Scanes, 1987).

3.3 Protein metabolism

Glucagon increases gluconeogenesis and presumably net protein degradation in stores such as muscle. In ducks, glucagon increases both circulating concentrations of amino-acids (Foltzer & Miahle, 1980).

3.4 Thyroid hormones

As in mammals, the thyroid glands produce thyroxine (T_4). This is converted to the active Form, T_3. There is further deiodination and inactivation of T_3 by the T_3-degrading type III deiodinase. This enzyme is decreased in the presence of growth hormone (GH) (Darras et al., 1993). Metabolic effects of T_3 chickens include the following:

- T_3 increases heat production. Exposure of chickens to cool environmental temperatures has been reported to increase circulating concentrations of T_3, heat production and expression of uncoupling proteins (UCPs) (Collin et al., 2003). Thyroid hormones increase thermogenesis by a mechanism involving UCPs. Expression of UCPs in chickens is related to circulating concentrations of thyroid hormones, particularly T_3 (Collin et al., 2005).
- The amount of adipose tissue in chickens is related to thyroid status with increased adipose tissue in hypothyroid chickens treated with methimazole and reduced adipose

tissue in hyperthyroid chickens, receiving T_3 administration chronically (Decuypere et al., 1987)

- T_3, together with insulin, elevates the rate of lipogenesis in chicken hepatocytes *in vitro* (Wilson et al., 1986)
- Thyroid hormones influence metabolism in the small intestine with T_4 *in vitro* for 72 hours increasing glucose active transport in the duodenum of chick embryos (Black, 1988)
- T_3 decreasing the expression of genes related to obesity including brain-derived neurotrophic factor (BDNF), leptin receptor (LEPR), pro-opiomelanocortin (POMC), thyrotropin releasing hormone (TRH), and agouti-related protein (AGRP) in chicken hypothalamic neurons in vitro (Byerly et al., 2009).

3.5 Corticosterone

Corticosterone is the major glucocorticoid in birds. It has marked effects on carbohydrate, lipid and protein metabolism. Production of corticosterone is stimulated by ACTH and other hormones including calcitonin (e.g. Nakagawa-Mizuyachi et al., 2009). The glucocorticoid receptor (GR) is expressed in multiple tissues in the chicken including the liver and anterior pituitary gland (Porter at al., 2007). The activation of receptor and its translocation into the nucleus is stimulated by corticosterone and this is blocked by the specific glucocorticoid antagonist, ZK98299, when the chicken GR is expressed in Cos-7 cells (Proszkowiec-Weglarz & Porter, 2010). Hepatic expression of the glucocorticoid receptor in chickens is reported to be inversely correlated with circulating concentrations of corticosterone (Marelli et al., 2010) suggesting the corticosterone down regulates expression of its own receptor..

3.5.1 Carbohydrate metabolism

Effects of corticosterone on carbohydrate metabolism include the following:

- Increasing circulating concentrations of glucose (Lin et al., 2007; Jiang et al., 2008; Yuan et al., 2008; Zhao et al., 2009) although depressed circulating concentrations of glucose have also been reported (Gao et al., 2008)
- Increasing circulating concentrations of insulin (Jiang et al., 2008; Yuan et al., 2008; Zhao et al., 2009)
- Increasing glucose uptake as indicated 2 deoxy--D-[1,2-3H]-glucose uptake by fibularis longus muscle *in vitro* (Zhao et al., 2009)
- Decreasing glucose uptake response to either insulin or nitric oxide as indicated 2 deoxy--D-[1,2-3H]-glucose uptake by fibularis longus muscle in vitro (Zhao et al., 2009)
- Decreasing circulating concentrations of nitric oxide (Zhao et al., 2009)
- Increased breast muscle glycogen (Lin et al., 2007) but lower levels have also been reported (Gao et al., 2008).

Despite the marked effects on glucose metabolism, circulating concentrations of lactate are unchanged in chickens receiving glucocorticoid administration (Lin et al., 2007).

There is a growing viewpoint that corticosterone acts via induction of insulin resistance. Evidence for corticosterone inducing insulin resistance comes from the consistent increasing in circulating concentrations of both glucose and insulin (see above e.g. Yuan et al., 2008) and the decreased glucose uptake evoked by insulin as indicated 2 deoxy--D-[1,2-3H]-glucose uptake by fibularis longus muscle in vitro (Zhao et al., 2009)

3.5.2 Protein metabolism

The effects on corticosterone on protein metabolism include the following effects reported in chickens:

- Depressing body weight, and particularly breast muscle weight, following chronic administration of corticosterone (Lin et al., 2006)
- Increasing net breakdown of muscle protein due to both decreased synthesis and increased degradation (discussed in more detail under corticosterone and growth)
- Decreasing circulating concentrations of total amino-acids (Gao et al., 2008) and increased concentrations of urate (Lin et al., 2007). These are indicative of both increases in deamidation of amino-acids and consequently of gluconeogenesis (Lin et al., 2007)
- Increasing gluconeogenesis by perfused liver (Kobayashi et al., 1989)
- Reductions in super-oxide dismutase activity (Lin et al., 2009).

3.5.3 Lipid metabolism

Corticosterone has marked effects on lipid metabolism including:

- Increased liver weight (Jiang et al., 2008)
- Increased hepatic lipogenesis (Lin et al., 2006; Yuan et al., 2008)
- Increased abdominal and subcutaneous adipose weight (Bartov, 1982; Buyse et al., 1987; Jiang et al., 2008; Yuan et al., 2008)
- Increased circulating concentrations of non-esterified fatty acids (NEFA) (Jiang et al., 2008; Yuan et al., 2008)
- Increased circulating concentrations of triglyceride and very low density lipoprotein (VLDL) (Jiang et al., 2008)
- Increased adipose lipo-protein lipase (LPL) (Jiang et al., 2008; Yuan et al., 2008).

3.5.4 Immune effects of corticosterone

Administration of corticosterone to chicken results in reductions in the weights (and weights as a percentage of body weight) of the bursa Fabricius and spleen (Shini et al., 2008) Other effects include an initial transitory improvement of the antibody response to infectious bronchitis virus (IBV) vaccination followed by a marked impairment of the response to IBV (Shini et al., 2008)/ Other effects including increasing the heterophil to lymphocyte (H/L) ratio in the circulation (Shini et al., 2009). Corticosterone increases expression interleukins -1beta, IL-6, IL-10, IL-12alpha and IL-18 while decreasing that of chemokine C-C motif ligand (CCL)16 and transforming growth factor-beta4 in heterophils in the circulation of chickens (Shini et al., 2010).

3.5.5 Other metabolic effects of corticosterone

Other metabolic effects of corticosterone in chickens include the following:

- Increasing expression sodium and glucose co-transporter 1 (SGLT-1 vitamin D-dependent calcium-binding protein-28,000 molecular weight (CaBP-D28k), and peptide transporter 1 (PepT-1) mRNA in the duodenum (Hu et al., 2010)
- Increasing expression of genes related to obesity in the chicken hypothalamus including brain-derived neurotrophic factor (BDNF), neuropeptide Y and agouti-related protein (AGRP) (Byerly et al., 2009)
- Depressing adenosine deaminase activity in all regions of the chicken gastro-intestinal tract except the proventriculus (Bhattacharjee et al., 2009).

3.6 Other hormones and metabolism

3.6.1 Estrogen and metabolism

Estrogen has some effects on metabolism. Estrogen increases adiposity in poultry. For instance, synthetic estrogens increase adipose tissue in chickens (Carew & Hill, 1967; Snapir et al., 1983). Moreover, the anti-estrogen, tamoxifen, decreases adiposity in female chickens (Rozenboim et al., 1989; 1990). In addition, estrogens are responsible for the dramatic increase in the hepatic synthesis of the yolk lipo-proteins (Reviewed: Scanes et al., 2004).

3.6.2 Ghrelin and metabolism

Lipogenesis in the chicken liver is increased by ghrelin as indicated by expression of fatty acid synthase (Buyse et al., 2009). Moreover, ghrelin reduces the respiratory quotient in young chickens (Geelissen et al., 2006).

3.6.3 Growth Hormone (GH) and metabolism

Both native and biosynthetic growth hormone (GH) *per se* can stimulate lipolysis *in vitro* (Campbell & Scanes, 1985). Moreover, GH inhibits glucagon stimulated lipolysis (Campbell & Scanes, 1986).

3.6.4 Somatostatin and metabolism

The major gastro-intestinal hormone, somatostatin is reported to be a potent inhibitor of glucagon stimulated lipolysis with chicken adipose tissue (Di Scala et al., 1985).

4. Hormonal control of growth

In poultry, the two major hormones required for the full expression of growth are GH and T_3. Both require the anterior pituitary gland. GH is directly synthesized by somatotrophs in the caudal lobe of the anterior pituitary gland in poultry. T_3 is produced by monodeiodination of the thyroid hormones, thyroxine (T_4). In turn, secretion of T_4 is stimulated by the anterior pituitary hormone, thyrotropin (thyroid stimulating hormone TSH). Moreover, the circulating concentrations of T_3 are maintained by GH reducing deactivation by T3-degrading type III deiodinase (Darras et al., 1993).
Evidence for the importance of anterior pituitary hormones in the growth of poultry (see figure 3) comes from ablation and replacement therapy studies. In young chickens, hypophysectomy depressed growth (body weight or skeletal growth) with growth rate being partially restored with either GH or T_3 replacement therapy (King & Scanes, 1986; Scanes et al., 1986). Similarly in young turkeys, hypophysectomy reduced growth rate but no effects of GH are observed (Proudman et al., 1994).

4.1 Growth Hormone (GH) and Growth

Dwarf chickens exhibit markedly reduced growth (Scanes et al., 1983) due to lack of GH receptors (Burnside et al., 1991; Agarwal et al., 1994) and the reduced circulating concentrations of T_3 (Scanes et al., 1983). While GH may be essential for growth, additional exogenous GH have either no (chickens: Cogburn et al. 1989, Cravener et al., 1989; Rosebrough et al., 1991; turkeys: Bacon et al., 1995) or only a small positive effect on poultry growth (Leung et al., 1986; Vasilatos-Younken et al., 1988; Scanes et al., 1990) with the latter potentially transitory. Instead, it may be hypothesized that the set points for GH/IGF-I

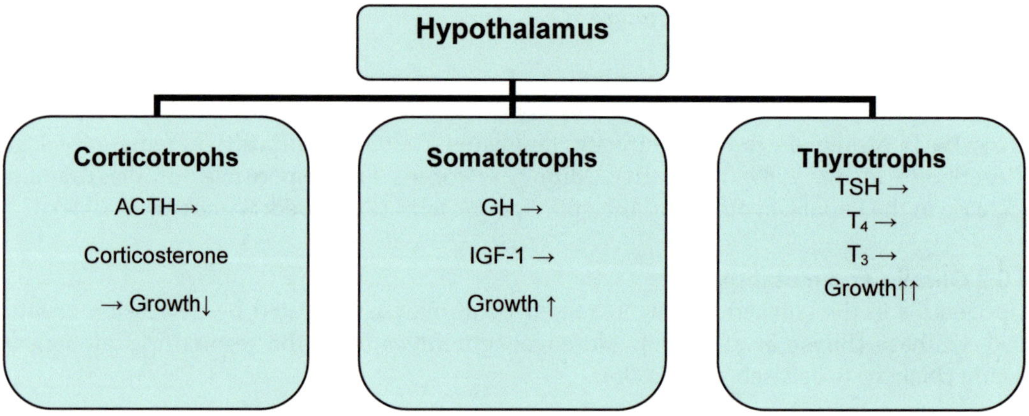

Fig. 3. Schema of physiological role of growth hormone in poultry

mediated growth are tightly controlled to insure optimal growth. It is argued that excess weight/size would be selected heavily against birds because of the energy requirements for flight.

GH acts specifically on the growth of immune tissues in birds. In birds, there is special separation between T and B cells during development in respectively the thymus and bursa Fabricius. In young chickens, hypophysectomy depresses thymus growth with GH partially overcoming this effect (King and Scanes, 1986; Johnson et al., 1993).

4.1.1 Control of GH synthesis and release

Release of GH from somatotrophs in the chicken pituitary is controlled by the following:

- The number of somatotrophs;
- The amount of GH available to be released, which is in turn dependant on GH gene expression and translation (GH synthesis);
- Stimulatory control by hypothalamic peptides such as GH releasing hormone (GHRH), thyrotropin releasing hormone (TRH), ghrelin and pituitary adenylate cyclase-activating peptide (PACAP) together with possibly leptin;
- Inhibitory control by the hypothalamic and peripheral somatostatin, together with negative feedback by hormones whose release/synthesis are increased by GH, namely insulin-like growth factor 1 (IGF-1) and triiodothyronine (T_3);
- The stimulatory and inhibitory effects depend upon both the concentrations of the stimulator or inhibitor and the responsiveness of somatotrophs to them. Not all chicken somatotrophs respond to all secretagogues; some respond to both GHRH and PACAP (85%), or to GHRH and TRH (73%) or to GHRH and leptin (51%) or to GHRH and ghrelin (21%) (Scanes et al., 2007).

Expression of the GH gene is inhibited by T_3 or IGF-1 in chickens (Radecki et al., 1994; Scanes et al., 1999).

4.2 Thyroid hormones and growth

In poultry, normal growth rate requires critical or optimal concentrations of T_3 and perhaps T_4 also. Administration of T_3 to dwarf chicks to restore normal circulating concentrations of T_3 produces some increase in growth rate (Marsh et al., 1984; Bowen et al., 1987). However, T_3 administration to chickens with circulating concentrations within the normal range

Environment, T_3 → **HYPOTHALAMUS** ← Nutritional status, IGF-1

↓

Releasing Factors

Stimulatory → ↓ ← Inhibitory

GHRH, TRH, Somatostatin,

PACAP ↓

Ghrelin

↓

Anterior Pituitary Gland

[Somatotrophs]

↓

Growth Hormone (GH)

↓

Liver

↓

Insulin - Like Growth factor - 1

Fig. 4. The hypothalamic growth hormone - insulin-like growth factor 1 - growth axis in poultry

depresses growth rate (Marsh et al., 1984; Bowen et al., 1987). Thyroid ablation by the goitrogen methimazole results in markedly lower growth rates (Chaisson et al., 1979; Decuypere et al., 1987) and circulating concentrations of IGF-1(Decuypere et al., 1987; Rosebrough et al., 2003). Growth rates of chickens are depressed by T3 administration and to a less extent T4 (Decuypere et al., 1987). This would support the concept that normal growth rate in poultry depends on a physiological "set- point".
Other growth related effects of thyroid hormones include the following:

- T_3 increases the growth rate of young hypophysectomised chickens (Scanes et al., 1986);
- Thyroid hormones induce development of the small intestine with thyroxine *in vitro* for 72 hours increasing microvillar growth and the rate of mitosis in the epithelia in chick embryo duodena (Black, 1978) and glucose active transport in the duodenum of chick embryos (Black, 1988);
- T3 decreases GH secretion by effects at both the levels of the anterior pituitary and the hypothalamus. For instance, T3 increases the expression of both type 2 and 5 somatostatin receptor sub-types (De Groef et al., 2007) and reduces the expression of thyrotropin releasing hormone (TRH) both in vivo and in vitro in chicken hypothalamic neurons (Byerly et al., 2009).

4.3 Insulin like growth factor-1 and growth

There is strong evidence that the effects of GH and thyroid hormones are mediated by hepatic production of insulin-like growth factor-1 (IGF-1). Circulating concentrations of IGF-

1are markedly decreased in hypophysectomized young chickens with GH partially reversing this effect (Huybrechts et al., 1985; Lazarus and Scanes, 1988). GH also elevates plasma IGF-1 in intact adult chickens (Scanes et al., 1999). Moreover, IGF-I release from chicken hepatocytes *in vitro* is elevated in the presence of GH and synergistically with GH and insulin (Houston & O'Neill, 1991). Circulating concentrations of IGF-1 are reduced by chronic methimazole administration with concentrations partially restored by T3 administration (Rosebrough and McMurtry, 2003). Chicks treated with the goitrogens, propylthiouracil, have depressed growth rate, circulating concentrations of IGF-I and hepatic expression of IGF-I (Tsukada et al., 1998) and T_4 administration partially restoring these parameters (Tsukada et al., 1998).

There is a report that the administration of IGF-I stimulate growth rate in chickens (Tomas et al., 1998). Moreover, there are increases in skeletal muscle mass and elevated rates of protein synthesis (Conlon & Kita, 2002) and depressed rates of degradation (Tomas et al., 1998). The effect of IGF-1 on chick growth has not been observed in other studies (McGuinness & Cogburn, 1991; Huybrechts et al., 1992; Tixier-Boichard et al., 1992). One mechanism by which, glucocorticoid hormones depress growth is by depressing IGF-1; circulating concentrations of IGF-1 have recently been observed to be decreased by the glucocorticoid, dexamethasone, in chickens (Song et al., 2011).

4.4 Other hormones and growth

Other hormones such as the adrenal cortical hormone, corticosterone, estradiol and testosterone can have marked effects on growth.

4.4.1 Corticosterone and growth

Glucocorticoids including the endogenous avian steroid, corticosterone, and the synthetic dexamethasone depress growth in chickens (Li et al., 2009; Hu et al., 2010; Song et al., 2011).

- Decreased skeletal muscle weight (Yuan et al., 2008; Song et al., 2011)
- Increased protein degradation as indicated by increases in the concentrations of 3-methyl histidine in both pectoralis and femoris muscles (Dong et al., 2007)
- Increases muscle proteolysis (Gao et al., 2008)
- Reduced skeletal protein synthesis as indicated by the RNA:protein ratio (Dong et al., 2007) Decreasing the growth of the small intestine in chickens although the effect is of a small magnitude than that with overall growth as weight of the small intestine relative to body weight is increased (Hu et al., 2010)
- Increases expression of myostatin (Song et al., 2011).
- Depressing duodenal and jejunal villus height and crypt depth (Hu et al., 2010)

Corticosterone plays the pivotal role in inducing functioning somatotropes during late embryonic development (Dean and Porter, 1999; Porter et al., 2001).

4.4.2 Estrogen and growth

Estrogen has effects on the growth of specific organs being responsible for the massive growth of the oviduct during sexual maturation (reviewed: Scanes et al., 2004). Estrogens play an important role in the formation of the calcium storing tissue, medullary bone, at the time of sexual maturation. Formation of medullary bone matrix is stimulated by estradiol and testosterone in immature male quail chicks with mineralization requiring vitamin D3 (Takahashi et al., 1983). Estradiol, in combination with testosterone, is has found to stimulate proliferation of chicken medullary osteoblasts and inhibit their apoptosis (Chen et al., 2010). Moreover, medullary bone formation is suppressed when aromatase, critical for estradiol synthesis, is inhibited (Deng et al., 2010).

4.4.3 Glucagon-like peptide 2 (GLP-2) and growth

Glucagon-like peptide 2 increases growth in chickens (Hu et al., 2010).

4.4.4 Testosterone and growth

The major circulating androgen in birds is testosterone. Testosterone acting via conversion to 5α Dehydro-testosterone (DHT) depresses growth in chickens (Fennell & Scanes, 1992a) while stimulating that of turkeys (Fennell & Scanes, 1992b).Androgens in combination with estrogens induce the formation of medullary bone at the time of sexual maturation (e.g. Chen et al., 2010).

5. References

Agarwal, S.K., Cogburn, L.A. & Burnside, J. (1994). Dysfunctional growth hormone receptor in a strain of sex-linked dwarf chickens: evidence for a mutation in the intra-cellular domain. *Journal of Endocrinology,* Vol.142, No.3, pp. 427-434, ISSN 0022-0795

Bacon, W.L., Long, D.W. & Vasilatos-Younken, R. (1995). Responses to exogenous pulsatile turkey growth hormone by growing 8-week-old female turkeys. *Comparative Biochemistry and Physiology A Molecular Biology,* Vol.111, No.3, pp. 471-482, ISSN 1095-6433.

Bartov, I. (1982). Corticosterone and fat deposition in broiler chicks: effect of injection time, breed, sex and age. *British Poultry Science,* Vol. 23, No. 2, pp.161-170, ISSN 0007-1668.

Belo, P. S., Romsos, D. R. & Leveille, G. A. (1976). Blood metabolites and glucose metabolism in the fed and fasted chicken. *Journal of Nutrition,* Vol. 106, No.8, pp. 1135–1143, ISSN 0022-3166.

Bhattacharjee, P. & Sharma, R. (2009). Antithetical effects of corticosterone and dibutyryl cAMP on adenosine deaminase in the gastrointestinal tract of chicken during postnatal development. *Molecular and Cellular Biochemistry,* Vol. 327, No. 1-2, 79-86, ISSN 0300-8177.

Black, B.L. (1978) Morphological development of the epithelium of the embryonic chick intestine in culture: influence of thyroxine and hydrocortisone. *American Journal of Anatomy,* Vol.153, No. 4, pp. 573-599, ISSN 1097-0177.

Black, B.L. (1988) Development of glucose active transport in embryonic chick intestine. Influence of thyroxine and hydrocortisone. *Comparative Biochemistry and Physiology A Comparative Physiology,* Vol. 90, No. 3, pp.379-386, ISSN 1095-6433.

Bowen, S.J., Huybrechts, L.M., Marsh, J.A. & Scanes, C.G. (1987). Influence of triiodothyronine and growth hormone on growth of dwarf and normal chickens: interactions of hormones and genotype. *Comparative Biochemistry and Physiology A Comparative Physiology,* Vol. 86, No. 1, pp. 137-142, ISSN 1095-6433.

Burnside, J., Liou, S.S. & Cogburn, L.A. (1991). Molecular cloning of the chicken growth hormone receptor complementary deoxyribonucleic acid: mutation of the gene in sex-linked dwarf chickens. *Endocrinology,* Vol. 128, No. 6, pp. 3183-3192, ISSN 0013-7227.

Buyse, J., Decuypere, E., Sharp, P.J., Huybrechts, L.M., Kühn, E.R. & Whitehead, C. (1987). Effect of corticosterone on circulating concentrations of corticosterone, prolactin, thyroid hormones and somatomedin C and on fattening in broilers selected for high or low fat content. *Journal of Endocrinology,* Vol. 112, No. 2, pp. 229-237, ISSN 0022-0795.

Buyse, J., Janssen, S., Geelissen, S., Swennen, Q., Kaiya, H., Darras, V.M. & Dridi, S. (2009). Ghrelin modulates fatty acid synthase and related transcription factor mRNA levels in a tissue-specific manner in neonatal broiler chicks. *Peptides,* Vol. 30, No. 7, pp.1342-1347, ISSN 0196-9785.

Byerly, M.S., Simon, J., Lebihan-Duval, E., Duclos, M.J., Cogburn, L.A. & Porter, T.E. (2009). Effects of BDNF, T3, and corticosterone on expression of the hypothalamic obesity gene network in vivo and in vitro. *American Journal of Physiology Regulatory Integrative Comparative Physiology,* Vol. 296, No. 4, pp. R1180-1189, ISSN 0363-6143.

Campbell, R.M. & Scanes, C.G. (1985). Lipolytic activity of purified pituitary and bacterially derived growth hormone on chicken adipose tissue *in vitro. Proceedings of the Society of Experimental Biology and Medicine,* Vol. 180, No. 3, pp. 513-517, ISSN 0037-9727.

Campbell, R.M. & Scanes, C.G. (1987). Growth hormone inhibition of glucagon and cAMP-induced lipolysis by chicken adipose tissue *in vitro. Proceedings of the Society of Experimental Biology and Medicine* Vol.184, No. 4, pp. 456-460, ISSN 0037-9727.

Carew, L.B. & Hill, F.W. (1967). Effect of diethylstilbestrol on energy and protein utilization by chicks fed a diet high in fat content. *Journal of Nutrition,* Vol. 92, No. 3, pp. 393-398, ISSN 0022-3166.

Chaisson, R.B., Sharp, P.J., Klandorf, H., Scanes, C.G. & Harvey, S. (1979). The effect of rapeseed meal and methimazole on levels of plasma hormones in growing broiler cockerels. *Poultry Science,* Vol. 58, No. 3, pp. 1575-1583, ISSN 1537-0437.

Chen, X., Deng, Y., Zhou, Z., Tao, Q., Zhu, J., Li, X., Chen, J. & Hou, J. (2010). 17beta-estradiol combined with testosterone promotes chicken osteoblast proliferation and differentiation by accelerating the cell cycle and inhibiting apoptosis in vitro. *Veterinary Research Communications,* Vol. 34, No. 2, pp. 143-152, ISSN 0165-7380.

Chevalier, B., Anglade, P., Derouet, M., Mollé, D. & Simon, J. (1996). Isolation and characterization of Muscovy (Cairna moschata) duck insulin. *Comparative Biochemistry and Physiology A Comparative Physiology, B Molecular Biology,* Vol. 114, No. 1, pp.19-26, ISSN 1095-6433.

Cogburn, L.A., Liou, S.S., Rand, A.L. & McMurtry, J.P. (1989). Growth, metabolic and endocrine responses of broiler cockerels given a daily subcutaneous injection of natural or biosynthetic chicken growth hormone. *Journal of Nutrition,* Vol. 119, No. 8, pp. 1213-1222, ISSN 0022-3166.

Collin A, Buyse J, van As P, Darras VM, Malheiros RD, Moraes, V.M., Reyns, G.E., Taouis, M. & Decuypere, E. (2003). Cold-induced enhancement of avian uncoupling protein expression, heat production, and triiodothyronine concentrations in broiler chicks. *General and Comparative Endocrinology,* Vol. 130, No. 1, pp. 70-77, ISSN 0016-6480.

Collin A, Cassy, S., Buyse, J., Decuypere, E. & Damon, M. (2005). Potential involvement of mammalian and avian uncoupling proteins in the thermogenic effect of thyroid hormones. *Domestic Animal Endocrinology*, Vol. 29, No.1, pp. 78-87, 0739-7240.

Conlon, M.A. & Kita, K. (2002). Muscle protein synthesis rate is altered in response to a single injection of insulin-like growth factor-I in seven-day-old Leghorn chicks. *Poultry Science*, Vol. 81, No. 10, pp. 1543-1547, ISSN 1537-0437.

Constans, T., Chevalier, B., Derouet, M., Simon, J. (1991). Insulin sensitivity and liver insulin receptor structure in ducks from two genera. A *American Journal of Physiology*, Vol. 261, No. 4, pp. R882-R890, ISSN 0363-6143.

Cravener, T.L., Vasilatos-Younken, R. & Wellenreiter, R.H. (1989). Effect of subcutaneous infusion of pituitary-derived chicken growth hormone on growth performance of broiler pullets. *Poultry Science*, Vol. 68, No. 8, pp. 1133-1140, ISSN 1537-0437.

Darras, V.M., Rudas, P., Visser, T.J., Hall, T.R., Huybrechts, L.M., Vanderpooten, A., Berghman, L.R., Decuypere, E. & Kühn, E.R. (1993). Endogenous growth hormone controls high plasma levels of 3,3',5-triiodothyronine (T3) in growing chickens by decreasing the T3-degrading type III deiodinase activity. *Domestic Animal Endocrinology*, Vol. 10, No. 1, pp. 55-65, ISSN 0739-7240.

Dean, C.E. & Porter, T.E. (1999). Regulation of somatotroph differentiation and growth hormone (GH) secretion by corticosterone and GH-releasing hormone during embryonic development. *Endocrinology*, Vol. 140, No. 3, pp. 1104-1110, ISSN 0013-7227.

De Beer, M., McMurtry, J.P., Brocht, D.M. & Coon, C.N. (2008). An examination of the role of feeding regimens in regulating metabolism during the broiler breeder grower period. 2. Plasma hormones and metabolites. *Poultry Science*, Vol. 87, No. 2, pp. 264-275, ISSN 1537-0437.

Decuypere, E., Buyse, J., Scanes, C.G., Huybrechts, I. & Kuhn, E.R. (1987). Effects of hyper- or hypothyroid status on growth, adiposity and levels of growth hormone, somatomedin C and thyroid metabolism in broiler chickens. *Reproduction Nutrition Développement*, Vol. 27, No.2B, pp. 555-565, ISSN 0926-5287.

De Groef, B., Grommen, S.V. & Darras, V.M. (2007). Feedback control of thyrotropin secretion in the chicken: thyroid hormones increase the expression of hypophyseal somatostatin receptor types 2 and 5. *General and Comparative Endocrinology*, Vol. 152, No. 2-3, pp.178-182, ISSN 0016-6480.

Deng, Y.F., Chen, X.X., Zhou, Z.L. & Hou, J.F. (2010). Letrozole inhibits the osteogenesis of medullary bone in prelay pullets. *Poultry Science*, Vol. 89, No. 5, pp. 917-023, ISSN 1537-0437.

Di Scala-Guenot, D., Strosser, M.T. & Mialhe, P. (1985). The biological activity of duck 'big' somatostatin on chicken adipose tissue. *Biochimica et Biophysica Acta*, Vol. 845, No. 2, pp. 261-264, ISSN 0005-2736.

Dong, H., Lin, H., Jiao, H.C., Song, Z.G., Zhao, J.P. & Jiang, K.J. (2007). Altered development and protein metabolism in skeletal muscles of broiler chickens (Gallus gallus domesticus) by corticosterone. *Comparative Biochemistry and Physiology A Molecular and Integrative Physiology*, Vol. 147, No. 1, pp.189-195, ISSN 1095-6433.

Edwards, M.R., McMurtry, J.P. & Vasilatos-Younken, R. (1999). Relative insensitivity of avian skeletal muscle glycogen to nutritive status. *Domestic Animal Endocrinology,* Vol. 16, No. 4, pp. 239-247, ISSN 0739-7240.

Evans, T.K., Litthauer, D. & Oelofsen, W. (1988). Purification and primary structure of ostrich insulin. *International Journal of Peptide and Protein Research,* Vol. 31, No. 5, pp. 454-462, *ISSN* 0367-8377.

Farhat, A. & Chavez, E.R. (2000). Comparative performance, blood chemistry, and carcass composition of two lines of Pekin ducks reared mixed or separated by sex. *Poultry Science,* Vol. 79, No. 4, pp. 460-465, ISSN 1537-0437.

Fennell, M.J. & Scanes, C.G. (1992a). Inhibition of growth in chickens by testosterone, 5a-dihydrotestosterone, and 19-nortestosterone. *Poultry Science,* Vol. 71, No. 2,pp. 357-366, ISSN 1537-0437.

Fennell, M.J. & Scanes, C.G. (1992b). Effects of androgen (testosterone, 5a-dihydrotestosterone, and 19-nortestosterone in turkeys. *Poultry Science,* Vol. 71, No. 3, pp. 539-549, ISSN 1537-0437.

Ferreira, A., Litthauer, D., Saayman, H., Oelofsen, W., Crabb, J. and Lazure, C. 1991. Purification and primary structure of glucagon from ostrich pancreas splenic lobes. *International Journal of Peptide and Protein Research,* Vol. 38, No. 4, pp. 90-95, *ISSN* 0367-8377.

Foltzer, C. & Mialhe, P. (1980). Pituitary and adrenal control of pancreatic endocrine function in the duck. III. Effects of glucose, oleic acid, arginine, insulin and glucagon infusions in hypophysectomized or normal ducks. Diabetes & Metabolism, Vol. 6, No. 4, pp. 257-63, ISSN 1262-3636.

Food and Agricultural Organization Agricultural Statistics. http://faostat.fao.org/site/569/default.aspx#ancor Accessed March 13, 2011

Gao, J., Lin, H., Song, Z.G. & Jiao, H.C. (2008). Corticosterone alters meat quality by changing pre-and postslaughter muscle metabolism. *Poultry Science,* Vol. 87, No. 8, pp. 1609-1617, ISSN 1537-0437.

Geelissen, S.M., Swennen, Q., Geyten, S.V., Kühn, E.R., Kaiya, H., Kangawa, K., Decuypere, E., Buyse, J. & Darras, V.M. (2006). Peripheral ghrelin reduces food intake and respiratory quotient in chicken. *Domestic Animal Endocrinology,* Vol. 30, No. 2, pp. 108-116, ISSN 0739-7240.

Goodridge, A.G. (1973). Regulation of fatty acid synthesis in isolated hepatocytes preparaed from livers of neonatal chicks. *Journal of Biological Chemistry,* Vol. 248, No. 6, pp. 1924-1931, ISSN 0021-9258.

Gross, R. & Mialhe, P. (1987). Glucose, beta adrenergic effects, and pancreatic endocrine function in the isolated perfused duck pancreas. *Acta endocrinologica,* Vol. 115, No. 1, pp. 105-111. ISSN:0001-5598

Gross, R. and Mialhe, P. 1984. Effect of insulin on free fatty acid uptake by hepatocytes in the duck. *Journal of Endocrinology,* Vol. 102, No. 3, pp. 381-386, ISSN 0022-0795.

Harvey, S., Scanes, C.G., Chadwick, A. & Bolton, N.J. (1978). Influence of fasting, glucose and insulin on the levels of growth hormone and prolactin in the plasma of the domestic fowl (Gallus domesticus). *Journal of Endocrinology.* Vol. 76, No. 3, pp. 501-506, ISSN 0022-0795.

Hazelwood, R.L. & Lorenz, F.W. (1959). Effects of fasting and insulin on carbohydrate metabolism of the domestic fowl. *American Journal of Physiology,* Vol. 197, Vol. 1, pp. 47-51, ISSN 0363-6143.

Hazelwood, R.L. (1986). Carbohydrate metabolism. In: *Avian Physiology* (Ed. P. D. Sturkie) pp.303-325. ISBN-13: 9780387961958, Springer Verlag, New York,

Honda, K., Kamisoyama, H., Saito, N., Kurose., Y., Sugahara, K. & Hasegawa, S. (2007). Central administration of glucagon suppresses food intake in chicks. *Neuroscience Letters,* Vol. 416, No. 2, pp. 198-201.*ISSN: 0304-3940.*

Honey, R.N. & Weir, G.C. (1979). Insulin stimulates somatostatin and inhibits glucagon secretion from the perfused chicken pancreas-duodenum. *Life Science,* Vol. 24, No. 19, pp. 1747-1750, ISSN 0024-3205.

Honey, R.N., Schwartz, J.A., Malhe, J. & Weir, G.C. (1980). Insulin, glucagons and somatostatin secretion from isolated perfused rat and chicken pancreas-duodenum. *American Journal of Physiology,* Vol. 238, No.2, pp. E150-E156, ISSN 0363-6143.

Houston, B. & O'Neill, I.E. (1991). Insulin and growth hormone act synergistically to stimulate insulin-like growth factor-I production by cultured chicken hepatocytes. *Journal of Endocrinology,* Vol. 128, No. 3, pp. 389-393, ISSN 0022-0795.

Hu, X.F. , Guo, Y.M. , Huang, B.Y. , Bun, S. , Zhang, L.B. , Li, J.H. , Liu, D. , Long, F.Y. , Yang, X. & Jiao, P. (2010). The effect of glucagon-like peptide 2 injection on performance, small intestinal morphology, and nutrient transporter expression of stressed broiler chickens. *Poultry Science,* Vol. 89, No. 9, pp. 1967-1974, ISSN 1537-0437.

Huybrechts, L.M., King, D.B., Lauterio, T.J., Marsh, J. & Scanes, C.G. (1985). Plasma concentrations of somatomedin-C in hypophysectomized, dwarf and intact growing domestic fowl as determined by heterologous radioimmunoassay. *Journal of Endocrinology,* Vol. 104, No. 2, pp. 233-239, ISSN 0022-0795.

Huybrechts, L.M., Decuypere, E., Buyse, J., Kühn, E.R. & Tixier-Boichard, M. (1992). Effect of recombinant human insulin-like growth factor-I on weight gain, fat content, and hormonal parameters in broiler chickens. *Poultry Science,* Vol. 71, No. 1, pp. 181-187, ISSN 1537-0437.

Jiang, K.J., Jiao, H.C., Song, Z.G., Yuan, L., Zhao, J.P. & Lin, H. (2008). Corticosterone administration and dietary glucose supplementation enhance fat accumulation in broiler chickens. *British Poultry Science,* Vol. 49, No. 5, pp. 625-631, ISSN 0007-0437.

Johnson, B.E., Scanes, C.G., King, D.B. & Marsh, J.A. (1993). Effect of hypophysectomy and growth hormone on immune development in the domestic fowl. Developmental and Comparative Immunology, Vol. 17, No. 4, pp. 331-339, ISSN 0145-305X.

King, D.B. & Scanes, C.G. (1986). Effects of mammalian growth hormone and prolactin on the growth of hypophysectomized chickens. *Proceedings of the Society of Experimental Biology and Medicine,* Vol. 182, No. 2, pp. 201-207, ISSN 0037-9727.

King, D.L. and Hazelwood, R.L. 1976. Regulation of avian insulin secretion by isolated perfused chicken pancreas. *American Journal of Physiology,* Vol. 231, No. 6, pp. 1830-1839, ISSN 0363-6143.

Kobayashi, T., Iwai, H., Uchimoto, R., Ohta, M., Shiota, M. & Sugano, T. (1989). Gluconeogenesis in perfused livers from dexamethasone-treated chickens. *American Journal of Physiology,* Vol. 256, No. 4, pp. R907-R914, ISSN 0363-6143.

Langslow, D.R. & Hales, C.N. (1969). Lipolysis in chicken adipose tissue *in vitro. Journal of Endocrinology*, Vol. 43, No. 2, pp. 243-260, ISSN 0022-0795.

Langslow, D.R., Butler, E.J., Hales, C.N. & Pearson, A.W. (1970). The response of plasma insulin, glucose and non-esterified fatty acids to various hormones, nutrients and drugs in the domestic fowl. *Journal of Endocrinology*, Vol. 46, No. 2, pp. 243-260, ISSN 0022-0795.

Lazarus, D.D. & Scanes, C.G. (1988). Acute effects of hypophysectomy and administration of pancreatic and thyroid hormones on circulating concentrations of somatomedin-C in young chickens: relationship between growth hormone and somatomedin C. *Domestic Animal Endocrinology*, Vol. 5, No. 4, pp. 283-289, ISSN 0739-7240.

Leung, F.C. & Taylor, J.E. (1983). In vivo and in vitro stimulation of growth hormone release in chickens by synthetic human pancreatic growth hormone releasing factor (hpGRFs). *Endocrinology*, Vol. 113, No. 5, pp. 1913-1915, ISSN 0013-7227.

Lin, H., Sui, S.J., Jiao, H.C., Buyse, J. & Decuypere, E. (2006). Impaired development of broiler chickens by stress mimicked by corticosterone exposure. *Comparative Biochemistry and Physiology A Molecular and Integrative Physiology*, Vol. 143, No. 3, pp. 400-405, ISSN 1095-6433.

Lin, H., Sui, S.J., Jiao, H.C., Jiang, K.J.., Zhao, J.P. & Dong, H . (2007). Effects of diet and stress mimicked by corticosterone administration on early postmortem muscle metabolism of broiler chickens. *Poultry Science*, Vol. 86, No. 3, pp. 545-554, ISSN 1537-0437.

Lin, H., Gao, J., Song, Z.G. & Jiao, H.C. (2009). Corticosterone administration induces oxidative injury in skeletal muscle of broiler chickens. *Poultry Science*, Vol. 88, No. 5, pp. 1044-1051, ISSN 1537-0437.

Marelli, S.P., Terova, G., Cozzi, M.C., Lasagna, E., Sarti, F.M. & Cavalchini, L.G . (2010). Gene expression of hepatic glucocorticoid receptor NR3C1 and correlation with plasmatic corticosterone in Italian chickens. *Animal Biotechnology*, Vol. 21, No. 2, pp. 140-148, ISSN: 1049-5398.

Marsh, J.A., Lauterio, T.J. & Scanes, C.G. (1984). Effects of triiodothyronine treatments on body and organ growth and development of immune function in dwarf chickens. *Proceedings of the Society of Experimental Biology and Medicine*, Vol. 117, No.1, pp. 82-91, ISSN 0037-9727.

McGuinness, M.C. & Cogburn, L.A. (1991). Response of young broiler chickens to chronic injection of recombinant-derived human insulin-like growth factor-I. *Domestic Animal Endocrinology*, Vol. 8, No. 4, pp. 611-620, ISSN 0739-7240.

McMurtry, J.P., Tsark, W., Cognurn, L., Rosebrough, R. & Brocht, D. (1996). Metabolic responses of the turkey hen (Meleagris gallopavo) to an intravenous injection of chicken or porcine glucagon. *Comparative Biochemistry and Physiology C Pharmacology, Toxicology and Endocrinology*, Vol. 114, No. 2, pp. 159-163, ISSN 1095-6433.

Nakagawa-Mizuyachi, K., Takahashi, T. & Kawashima, M. (2009). Calcitonin directly increases adrenocorticotropic hormone-stimulated corticosterone production in the hen adrenal gland. *Poultry Science*, Vol. 88, No. 10, pp. 2199-2205, ISSN 1537-0437.

Perler F., Efstratiadis A., Lomedico P., Gilbert W., Kolodner R. & Dodgson J.B. (1980). The evolution of genes: the chicken preproinsulin gene. *Cell*, Vol. 20, No.2, pp. 555-566, ISSN: 0092-8674.

Porter, T.E., Dean, C.E., Piper, M.M., Medvedev, K.L., Ghavam, S. & Sandor, J. (2001). Somatotroph recruitment by glucocorticoids involves induction of growth hormone gene expression and secretagogue responsiveness. *Journal of Endocrinology*, Vol. 169, No. 3, pp. 499-509, ISSN 0022-0795.

Porter, T.E., Ghavam, S., Muchow, M., Bossis, I. & Ellestad, L. (2007). Cloning of partial cDNAs for the chicken glucocorticoid and mineralocorticoid receptors and characterization of mRNA levels in the anterior pituitary gland during chick embryonic development. *Domestic Animal Endocrinology*, Vol. 33, No. 2, pp. 226-239, ISSN 0739-7240.

Proszkowiec-Weglarz, M. & Porter, T.E. (2010). Functional characterization of chicken glucocorticoid and mineralocorticoid receptors. *American Journal of Physiology Regulatory Integrative Comparative Physiology, Vol.* 298, No. 5, pp. R1257-1268, ISSN 0363-6143.

Proudman, J.A., McGuinness, M.C., Krishnan, K.A. & Cogburn, L.A. (1994). Endocrine and metabolic responses of intact and hypophysectomized turkey poults given a daily injection of chicken growth hormone. *Comparative Biochemistry and Physiology C Pharmacology, Toxicology and Endocrinology*, Vol. 109, No. 1, pp. 47-56, ISSN 1095-6433.

Radecki, S.V., Deaver D.R. & Scanes, C.G. (1994). Triiodothyronine reduces growth hormone secretion and pituitary growth hormone mRNA in the chicken, *in vivo* and *in vitro*. *Proceedings of the Society of Experimental Biology and Medicine*, Vol. 205, No. 4, pp. 340-346, ISSN 0037-9727.

Rosebrough, R.W. & McMurtry, J.P. (2003). Methimazole and thyroid hormone replacement in broilers. *Domestic Animal Endocrinology*, Vol. 24, No. 3, pp. 231-242, ISSN 0739-7240.

Rosebrough, R.W., McMurtry, J.P. & Vasilatos-Younken, R. (1991). Effect of pulsatile or continuous administration of pituitary-derived chicken growth hormone (p-cGH) on lipid metabolism in broiler pullets. *Comparative Biochemistry and Physiology A Comparative Physiology*, Vol. 99, No. 1-2, pp. 207-214, ISSN 1095-6433.

Rozenboim, I., Robinzon, B., Arnon, E. & Snapir, N. (1989). Effect of embryonic and neonatal administration of tamoxifen on adiposity in the broiler chicken. *British Poultry Science*, Vol. 30, No. 3, pp. 607-612, ISSN 0007-1668.

Rozenboim, I., Robinzon, B., Ron, B., Arnon, E. & Snapir, N. (1990) The response of broilers' adiposity to testosterone after embryonic exposure to androgen and tamoxifen. *British Poultry Science*, Vol. 31, No. 3, pp. 645-650, ISSN 0007-1668.

Scanes, C. G. (2008). Perspectives on Analytical Techniques and Standardization. *Poultry Science*, Vol. 87, No. 11, pp. 2175-2177, ISSN 1537-0437.

Scanes, C.G. (2009) Perspectives on the endocrinology of poultry growth and metabolism. *General and Comparative Endocrinology*, Vol. 163, No. 1-2, pp. 24-32, ISSN 0016-6480.

Scanes, C.G. (2011). *Fundamentals of Animal Science*. Delmar Cengage, ISBN-10: 1428361278, Clifton Park, NY.

Scanes, C.G., Marsh, J., Decuypere, E. & Rudas, P. (1983). Abnormalities in the plasma concentration of thyroxine, triiodothyronine and growth hormone in sex-linked dwarf and autosomal dwarf white leghorn domestic fowl (*Gallus domesticus*). *Journal of Endocrinology*, Vol. 97, No. 1, pp. 127-135, ISSN 0022-0795.

Scanes, C.G., Duyka, D.R., Lauterio, T.J., Bowen, S.J., Huybrechts, L.M., Bacon, W.L. & King, D.B. (1986). Effect of chicken growth hormone, triiodothyronine and hypophysectomy in growing domestic fowl. *Growth*, Vol. 50, No. 1, 12-31, ISSN 1440-169X.

Scanes, C.G., Proudman, J.A. & Radecki, S.V. (1999). Influence of Continuous Growth Hormone or Insulin-Like Growth Factor I Administration in Adult Female Chickens. *General and Comparative Endocrinology*, Vol. 114, No. 3, pp. 315-323, ISSN 0016-6480.

Scanes, C.G., Brant, G. & Ensminger, M.E. (2004). *Poultry Science*. ISBN 0-13-113375-6. Pearson Prentice, Upper Saddle River, NJ.

Scanes, C. G., Glavaski-Joksimovic, A., Johannsen, S. A., Jeftinija, S. & Anderson, L.L. (2007). Subpopulations of Somatotropes with Differing Intracellular Calcium Concentration Responses to Secretagogues. *Neuroendocrinology*, Vol. 85, No. 4, pp. 221-231, ISSN 0028-3835

Snapir, N., Robinzon, B. & Shalita, B. (1983). The involvement of gonads and gonadal steroids in the regulation of food intake, body weight and adiposity in the white Leghorn cock. Pharmacology Biochemistry and Behavior, Vol. 19, No. 4, pp. 617-624, ISSN: 0091-3057.

Shini, S., Kaiser, P., Shini, A. & Bryden, W.L. (2008). Biological response of chickens (Gallus gallus domesticus) induced by corticosterone and a bacterial endotoxin. *Comparative Biochemistry and Physiology B Biochemistry and Molecular Biology*, Vol.149, No. 2, pp. 324-333, ISSN 1095-6433.

Shini, S., Shini, A. & Huff, G.R. (2009). Effects of chronic and repeated corticosterone administration in rearing chickens on physiology, the onset of lay and egg production of hens. Physiology & Behavior, Vol. 98, No. 1-2, pp. 73-77, ISSN: 0031-9384.

Shini, S., Shini, A. & Kaiser, P. (2010). Cytokine and chemokine gene expression profiles in heterophils from chickens treated with corticosterone. *Stress*, Vol. 13, No. 3, pp. 185-194, ISSN 1025-3890.

Simon, J., Derouet, M. & Gespach, C. (2000). An anti-insulin serum, but not a glucagon antagonist, alters glycemia in fed chickens. Hormone and metabolic research, Vol. 32, No. 4, pp. 139-141,ISSN:0018-5043.

Sitbon, G. & Mialhe, P. (1978). Pancreatic hormones and plasma glucose: regulation mechanism in the goose under physiological conditions; 3. Inhibitory effects of insulin on glucagons secretion. *Hormones and Metabolic Research*, Vol. 10, No. 6, pp. 473-477, *ISSN* 0018-5043.

Song, Z., Zhang, X., Zhu, L., Jiao, H. & Lin, H. (2011). Dexamethasone Alters the Expression of Genes Related to the Growth of Skeletal Muscle in Chickens (Gallus gallus domesticus). *Journal of Molecular Endocrinology* Feb 16. [Epub ahead of print]

Strosser, M., Chen, T.L., Harvey, S. & Mialhe, P. (1980). Somatostatin stimulates glucagons secretion in ducks. *Diabetologia*, Vol. 18, No. 4, pp. 319-322. *ISSN* 0012-186X.

Sugano, T., Shiota, M., Khono, H. & Shimada, M. (1982). Stimulation of gluconeogenesis by glucagon and norepinephrine in the perfused chicken liver. Journal of Biochemestry, Vol. 92, No. 1, pp. 111-120, ISSN 0021-924X.

Takahashi, N., Shinki, T., Abe, E., Horiuchi, N., Yamaguchi, A., Yoshiki, S. & Suda, T. (1983). The role of vitamin D in the medullary bone formation in egg-laying Japanese quail and in immature male chicks treated with sex hormones. Calcified Tissue International, Vol. 35, No. 4-5, pp. 465-471, ISSN: 0171-967X

Tixier-Boichard, M., Huybrechts, L.M., Decuypere, E., Kühn, E.R., Monvoisin, J.L., Coquerelle, G., Charrier, J. & Simon, J. (1992). Effects of insulin-like growth factor-I (IGF-I) infusion and dietary tri-iodothyronine (T3) supplementation on growth, body composition and plasma hormone levels in sex-linked dwarf mutant and normal chickens. *Journal of Endocrinology*, Vol.133, No. 1, pp. 101-110, ISSN 0022-0795.

Thomas-Delloye, V., Marmonier, F., Duchamp, C., Pichon-Georges, B., Lachuer, J., Barré, H. and Crouzoulon, G. 1999. Biochemical and functional evidences for a GLUT-4 homologous protein in avian skeletal muscle. *Journal of Physiology*, Vol. 277, No. 6, pp. R1733-R1740, ISSN 0363-6143.

Tomas, F.M., Pym, R.A., McMurtry, J.P. & Francis, G.L. (1998). Insulin-like growth factor (IGF)-I but not IGF-II promotes lean growth and feed efficiency in broiler chickens. *General and Comparative Endocrinology*, Vol. 110, No. 3, pp. 262-275, ISSN 0016-6480.

Tsukada, A., Ohkubo, T., Sakaguchi, K., Tanaka, M., Nakashima, K., Hayashida, Y., Wakita, M. & Hoshino, S. (1998). Thyroid hormones are involved in insulin-like growth factor-I (IGF-I) production by stimulating hepatic growth hormone receptor (GHR) gene expression in the chicken. Growth Hormone & IGF Research, Vol. 8, No. 3, pp. 235-242, ISSN: 1096-6374.

Vasilatos-Younken, R., Cravener, T.L., Cogburn, L.A., Mast, M.G. & Wellenreiter, R.H. (1988). Effect of pattern of administration on the response to exogenous pituitary-derived chicken growth hormone by broiler-strain pullets. *General and Comparative Endocrinology*, Vol. 71, No. 2, pp. 268-283, ISSN 0016-6480.

Vasilatos-Younken, R. (1986). Age-related changes in tissue metabolic rates and sensitivity to insulin in the chicken. *Poultry Science*, Vol. 65, No. 7, pp.1391-1399, ISSN 0016-6480.

Wilson, S.B., Back, D.W., Morris, S.M., Swierczynski, J. & Goodridge, A.G. (1986). Hormonal regulation of lipogenic enzymes in chick embryo hepatocytes in culture. Expression of the fatty acid synthase gene is regulated at both translational and pretranslational steps. Journal of Biological Chemistry, Vol. 261, No. 32, pp. 15179-15182, ISSN 0021-9258.

Yuan, L., Lin, H., Jiang, K.J., Jiao, H.C. & Song, Z.G. (2008). Corticosterone administration and high-energy feed results in enhanced fat accumulation and insulin resistance in broiler chickens. *British Poultry Science,* Vol. 49, No. 4, pp. 487-495, ISSN 0007-1668.

Zhao, J.P., Lin, H., Jiao, H.C. & Song, Z.G. (2009). Corticosterone suppresses insulin- and NO-stimulated muscle glucose uptake in broiler chickens (*Gallus gallus domesticus*). *Comparative Biochemistry and Physiology C Pharmacology, Toxicology and Endocrinology,* Vol. 149, No. 3, pp. 448-454, ISSN 1095-6433.

8

Metabolic Control Targets for Patients with Type 1 Diabetes in Clinical Practice

María Gloria Baena-Nieto, Cristina López-Tinoco,
Jose Ortego-Rojo and Manuel Aguilar-Diosdado
Endocrinology & Nutrition Service, Puerta del Mar Hospital, Cadiz, Spain

1. Introduction

Diabetes and its micro- and macro-vascular complications constitute one of the principal social-health problems world-wide. It has high impact on the quality of life and prognosis of the individuals affected, as well as high direct and indirect economic costs to the Public Health Service. Following the publication of benchmark studies in the 1990s which indicated that the maintenance of glycaemia levels as close as possible to normality is associated with a lower incidence, progression and severity of the complications, the optimisation of metabolic control has been converted to a core therapeutic objective (DCCT, 1993; Herman, 1999; UKPDS, 1998). The tools for the management of diabetes have advanced spectacularly in these past few years, not only for the control of glycaemia but also for its measurement. As such, currently, there is a wide variety of drugs available with different mechanisms of action which, alone or in combination, enable a reasonable metabolic control in the majority of cases. Although insulin has been used for >80 years, the biggest advances in the mode of use have been over the last two decades. This change has been due, in great part, to: 1) development of new sources of insulin (analogues of insulin) together with the development and fine-tuning of different forms of its administration (continuous subcutaneous insulin infusion; CSII) in search of profiles of activity closer to the normal physiologic state; 2) change in philosophy in the therapeutic planning of diabetes, such that the strategies of co-responsibility and flexibility of life-style have become fundamental aspects; 3) introduction of self-control using capillary glycaemia (SCCG) in daily practice (De Witt & Hirsch, 2003); 4) recent incorporation in clinical practice of the use of glucose sensors, continuous glucose monitoring systems (CGMS) that generate the maximum information on modifications of glucose levels in plasma along the course of the whole day.

This review centres on the importance, in clinical practice, of the metabolic control targets for patients with DM type 1. Difficulties in achieving glycaemia goals using multiple insulin injection with new insulin analogues, and modern technologies such as CGMS and CSII are extensively analysed.

2. Importance of glycaemia control in the treatment of diabetes

Traditionally, the conventional therapy has been orientated towards achieving acceptable levels of glycaemia and stable clinical status in the asymptomatic patient. Intensive treatment of diabetes, according to the protocol of the Diabetes Control and Complications Trial (DCCT), consists in a therapeutic design orientated towards achieving almost normal levels of glycaemia. Included are: a rigorous educative plan with frequent actions for a life-style change, an insulin regimen with three or more daily injections (multiple doses of insulin), or CIIS and programme of SCCG four of more per day (DCCT, 1995).

Over the past few years there have been several studies evaluating the effect on the appearance and progression of the micro-vascular complications of diabetes using a strict control of glycaemia with intensive treatment (Herman, 1999). The most significant was the DCCT study published in 1993 (DCCT, 1993). Included were more than 1000 patients with DM type I and the results demonstrated that maintaining the levels of glucose within a range closest to normality, tended to reduce the appearance of retinopathy by 76%, nephropathy by 56% and neuropathy by 60%. The DCCT established the targets of glycaemia control and of glycosylated haemoglobin (HbA1c) in patients with DM type 1, together with the need to perform measurement of capillary glycaemia as part of the intensive treatment regimen.

In DM type 2, the Kumamoto study (Shichiri et al., 2000) with a design similar to the DCCT, demonstrated that intensive treatment (target of HbA1c <7%) reduced the risk of retinopathy by 69% and nephropathy by 70%. The United Kingdom Prospective Diabetes Study (UKPDS) published in 1998, demonstrated that intensive long-term treatment of the hyperglycaemia also reduced the appearance of micro-vascular complication in patients recently diagnosed with DM type 2 (UKPDS, 1998).

These studies demonstrated definitively that the better the control of glycaemia the tighter the association with the decrease in the rates of micro-vascular complications (retinopathy and nephropathy). Follow-up studies of the DCCT (DCCT-EDIC; 2000; Martin et al., 2006) and of the UKPDS (Holman et al., 2008) have highlighted that once the intensive treatment is established in the two groups with evidence of their benefits, those that had been performed earlier retain their benefits as the product of a "metabolic legacy".

Despite that many epidemiologic studies and meta-analyses (Selvin et al., 2004; Stettler et al., 2006) having clearly demonstrated a direct relationship between HbA1c and the incidence of cardiovascular disease (CVD), the potential of intensive control of glycaemia to reduce CVD has not been delineated, as yet. In the DCCT, no differences were observed between the groups with respect to the appearance of CVD events. However, at 8 years of conclusion of the study, the patients who had been assigned to the intensive treatment group had a 42% reduction in CVD and a 57% reduction in the risk of non-fatal myocardial infarction, stroke or death, compared to those who had been assigned to the standard treatment arm of the trial (Nathan et al., 2005). It has been demonstrated recently that, as with DM type 2, the benefit of intensive glycaemia control in patients with DM type 1 persists over decades (DCCT-EDIC, 2009).

In the UKPDS, a reduction was observed of 16% in the risk of CVD in the intensive treatment group, although this difference did not reach statistical significance. However, at 10 years of follow-up, a reduction in non-fatal acute myocardial infarction and in all-cause mortality of 13 and 27%, respectively (Holman et al., 2008) was demonstrated in the participants initially assigned to intensive control of glycaemia, compared to those assigned to conventional control. Nevertheless, the results of three large studies (ACCORD, Ismail-Beigi et al., 2010; ADVANCE, Patel et al., 2008; VADT, Duckworth at al., 2009) that had investigated the effect of glycaemia control in DM type 2, were unable to demonstrate that the intensive control of glycaemia achieved any reduction in the CVD, even though the patients were DM type 2 of long duration and with high risk of CVD.

Maintaining levels of glycaemia that are practically normal carries a series of notable risk. Among these is the increase in episodes of slight as well as of severe hypoglycaemia. The investigators in the EDIC study (Nathan et al., 2005) observed CVD benefits associated with intensive glycaemia control, but not in those with a level of HbA1c <6.5%. In the initial publications of the ACCORD study, the greater rates of mortality were produced in the 2 extreme categories of HbA1c, independently of the regimen of treatment. Also, the decreases in survival in the patients with lower HbA1c levels were related, at least in part, to the appearance of hypoglycaemia. As such, episodes of severe hypoglycaemia in patients with advanced disease need to be prevented, and not with the intention of achieving normal, or near normal, levels of HbA1c (<6.5%) in those in whom achieving normal levels safely do not appear probable.

2.1 Objectives of glycaemia control

The recommendations for glycaemia control targets in adults, in pregnant and in non-pregnant women are shown in Table 1. The recommendations are based on the blood levels of glucose which correlate with levels of HbA1c at 7%. The targets need to be individualised for each patient, and it is necessary to be assured of achieving them. In young and healthy patients that know the symptoms of hypoglycaemia and recover from them relatively easily, the targets need to approximate to the levels of glycaemia observed in persons without diabetes. However, the objectives of control are more strict during gestation, and more permissive for persons who have difficulties noting the symptoms of hypoglycaemia as well as those who present with severe hypoglycaemia or for those whose episodes of hypoglycaemia can be particularly dangerous (for example, patients with heart disease, cerebrovascular pathology or autonomic neuropathy). As such, in adults with limited life expectancy or advanced vascular disease, it would be more appropriate to have less strict targets. Post-prandial hyperglycaemia is defined as values of glycaemia >140 mg/dL at two hours after a meal. It is a frequent phenomenon that is unnoticed in the determination of HbA1c and basal glycaemia since it is already present when the levels of HbA1c are optimum. Several studies have shown that the levels of post-prandial glycaemia are strongly related to the CVD risk (Cavalot et al., 2006; Ceriello, 2005; European Diabetes Epidemiology Group, 1999;). Curiously, the contribution of post-prandial glycaemia appears to be more evident in patients with well-controlled diabetes (contribution of about 70% to the HbA1c when it is <7% and about 40% when it is >7.3%). However, the targets of post-prandial glycaemia using SCCG are controversial. In some epidemiology studies, values of elevated glucose following oral glucose load test have been associated with an increased risk of CVD, independently of the fasting plasma glucose level. Also, the phenomenon appears intimately linked with CVD such as endothelial dysfunction which is aggravated by post-prandial hyperglycaemia (Ceriello et al., 2002). The majority of authors recommend values of HbA1c <7% as the appropriate metabolic control objective (American Diabetes Association, 2011)

Achieving a good metabolic control in DM type 1 is not an easy issue. Results reported in international studies on the degree of metabolic control in 13,612 patients from Sweden (Katarina et al., 2007) and 27,035 from Austria and Germany (Gerstl et al., 2008) showed that only 21.2% and 27%, respectively, of type 1 DM patients have HbA1c <7%. We studied a cohort of patients with type 1 DM (n = 489) followed-up from 2005 to 2007. During the study period, the mean HbA1c decreased from 7.78% to 7.36% and the frequency of patients with HbA1c <7% increased from 24.6% to 27.1% and those with a mean HbA1c of >8% decreased from 42.6% to 38.7% (Baena et al., 2008).

HbA1c	< 7%
Pre-prandial plasma glucose	70-130 mg/dL
Post-prandial plasma glucose	<180 mg/dL
The objectives need to be individualised based on: • Duration of the diabetes • Life expectancy • Associated co-morbidities • Known CVD or advanced micro-vascular complications • Severe hypoglycaemia, or inadvertent To improve objectives of post-prandial glucose if HbA1c was beyond the target despite pre-prandial glucose levels	
In pregnancy: HbA1c Pre-prandial plasma glucose Post-prandial plasma glucose	 6% 60-99 mg/dL 100-129 mg/dL

Table 1. Recommended objectives for glycaemia control, in patients with diabetes

3. Glucose monitoring in patients with diabetes

SCCG is an essential component of intensive treatment, and the core of the DCCT publication is the enormous increase in its diffusion and utilisation. As a result of this, the new technologies applied to these systems have evolved rapidly, giving rise to successive new measures on the market.

HbA1c is the reference pattern to assess long-term glycaemia control and, together with the measured glucose, determines the guidelines for adjustments in treatment of diabetes by the attending physician.

As we have stated earlier, in the past few years there has been in increase in the evidence showing the influence of post-prandial hyperglycaemia and glycaemia control, on the development of diabetic complications (Ceriello, 2003).

SCCG consists of determining the capillary blood glucose of the patient, using the glucometer. It carries information complementary to HbA1c levels, such as fasting and post-prandial glucose, detection of hypoglycaemia, information on the daily glucose variability, etc. This enables optimisation of treatment, above all in patients receiving intensive therapy. However, the information provided by the glucometer refers to a specific moment in time. For greater and better information on glycaemic changes there needs to be continuous glucose monitoring systems (CGMS) that perform several measurements per hour and, as such, produce averaged information over the course of the day.

3.1 Indications for self-monitoring of glycaemia in patients with DM type 1

Type 1 diabetes is characterised by frequent fluctuation in glycaemia. SCCG is the method-of-choice and the timing is decided according the needs of the individual patient as well as the targets of the therapeutic regimen. There are no studies that demonstrate the efficacy of SCCG alone in improving the glycaemia control in patients with DM type 1, but they are an integral part of the treatment. The results of the DCCT study demonstrated that intensive treatment is the most appropriate option for the majority of patients with DM type 1. The two modalities of intensive treatment (multiple doses of insulin and continuous subcutaneous infusion of insulin) involved targets of glycaemia control close to normality, with a higher risk of hypoglycaemia (DCCT, 1993). To prevent episodes of asymptomatic hypoglycaemias and hyperglycaemias and, as such, to perform an appropriate adjustment of the insulin dose, it is necessary to frequently supervise the glycaemic levels. In the DCCT study there was a need for at least 4 SCCG measurements per day (pre-prandial and at bedtime) and post-prandial measurements were performed when the levels of HbA1c were not appropriate despite the values of the pre-prandial SCCG values being within the pre-established control targets. Further, a SCCG measurement was indicated at 3:00 a.m. once a week.

It is not clear what would be the optimum frequency of the capillary glucose measurements in patients with DM type 1, although there are various studies that have demonstrated that the increase in the self-control of glycaemia improves the metabolic control in these patients

Currently, the majority of patients with DM type 1 and with gestational diabetes treated with insulin need to have at least 3 SCCG per day (ADA, 2011) (grade A evidence), which should be individualised according to the characteristics of the patient and the therapeutic targets. In general, it is recommended that measurements regularly before meals and, on occasions, one or two hours after, and at night-time, provide information that is very useful for therapeutic optimisation (Bergenstal & Gavin, 2005).

The latest clinical practice guide of the American Diabetes Association (ADA) establishes the following recommendations based on the scientific evidence (ADA, 2011):

- Achieving a strict glycaemia control requires SCCG as an integral part of the therapeutic strategy (grade A evidence).
- The patients treated with multiple doses of insulin need to perform SCCG 3 or more times a day (grade A evidence).
- In patients treated with les than 3 doses of insulin, oral agents or single diabetic treatment, the SCCG is useful in achieving glycaemia control targets within the context of a specific educative program (grade E evidence).
- To achieve the targets of post-prandial glycaemia control there needs to post-prandial SCCG performed (grade E evidence).
- There is a need to instruct the patient on the usefulness of the SCCG, and to evaluate the technique and its use regularly so that the data obtained can be used in treatment adjustment (grade E evidence).

3.2 Modalities of self-monitoring of glycaemia

3.2.1 Self-monitoring the level of blood sugar using the glucometer

SCCG requires a capillary blood sample obtained, usually, from finger-prick using a micro-lancet and using a glucose meter. The majority of glucose meters currently available generate plasma values by the device reader, or directly in plasma, or by multiplying the whole blood value by 1.12 so that the value is comparable with that from the laboratory (Valeri et al., 2004).

The measurement of glucose using the modern enzymatic methods (hexokinase or glucose oxidase) generates a rapid, reliable and precise measurement. The strips impregnated with these enzymes collect the blood sample and are read by the device in a short period of time (Goldstein et al., 2004).

The majority of machines have a memory to save the previous results, and some even have the option of downloading to a computer and with printer graphics to enable the analysis of the data and to optimise the metabolic self-monitoring. Some devices enable patients to record data such as the medication dose or the presence of symptoms. The most recent are smaller sized and require less quantity of blood for the analysis. For patients with impaired sight, there are devices that can adapt to voice synthesizer to deliver an audible version of the result. Most results can be obtained within about 5 seconds, depending on the characteristics of the apparatus (Bode et al., 2001).

In some countries such as the USA, there are currently available certain glucometers that use other different sites than that of the finger to obtain the blood sample, in an attempt to reduce the discomfort of the finger-prick. In a study performed on one of these devices that obtained blood from the arm it is noted that reliable results were obtained that were less painful than the finger prick (Fineberg et al., 2001).

3.2.2 Continuous monitoring of glucose - glucose sensors

Over the last decade the SCCG system has been the only measurement available for the monitoring of glycaemia levels. Despite its unquestioned usefulness, it is an invasive technique, tedious for the patient, generates limited information at any specific time, and without additional information to establish trends.

The concentration of glucose in the interstitial tissues is reflected in its concentration in capillary and venous blood, since the glucose diffuses into interstitial tissue to equilibrate both compartments. Based on this, the CGMS measures the glucose concentration in the interstitial liquid of the subcutaneous cellular tissue in a minimally invasive manner, using a sensor subcutaneously located. The CGMS can detect glycaemia oscillations continuously, such that maximum information can be generated on the direction, magnitude, duration, frequency and possible causes of the fluctuations of glycaemia over the long-term course of the day. Hence, it is very useful in optimising the treatment of patients with diabetes (Maran et al., 2005) (Garg, 2009). It precludes the limitations of information of the CGMS system of intensive treatment in the cases of detection in periods of inadvertent hypo- and hyperglycaemia (Klonoff, 2005). However, the sensors currently available do not have the precision of capillary glucometers and, hence, the use is approved as a complement, and not as a substitution, for SCCG.

The invasive intravascular sensors measure plasma glucose directly and has been used to monitor hospitalised patients. However, there have not been any studies published on their functioning and usefulness in extended groups of patients (Klonoff, 2005).

3.2.2.1 Types of glucose sensors

Continuous monitoring of glucose was introduced in the 1970s, with a complex system termed biostator or artificial pancreas. Subsequently, new generation sensors appeared, with mixed results.

Currently, there are 4 types of CGMS approved by the FDA available on the international market: CGMS® (Continuous Glucose Monitoring System) such as the Guardian®, the Guardian Real Time®, the Paradigm Real Time® (Medtronic MiniMed, Northridge, CA, USA); the GlucoDay® system (Menarini Diagnostics, Florence, Italy); the Seven® system (DexCom Inc., San Diego, CA, USA); and the Freestyle Navigator® monitor (Abbott Laboratories, Alameda, CA, USA) (Gross et al., 2000). Table 2 compares the main features of the currently available systems.

CGMS, approved by the FDA in 1999 was the first generation of sensors commercialised and, as such, the most widely used and, for which, there is the most clinical experience available. It is composed of a subcutaneous sensor and an external monitor. It needs to be

	Guardian, Guardian RT, Paradigm RT	Glucoday	Freestyle Navigator	Seven System
Range of glucose values (mg/dL)	40-400	40-400	20-500	40-400
Life-span of sensor (days)	3 in USA/ 6 in Europe	2	5	7
Warm-up period (hours)	2	2	10 (1 for latest system)	2
Calibration frequency	Every 12 h	One point	Post-insertion: -10, 12, 24, 72h -1, 2, 10, 24, 72h (latest system)	Every 72 hours
Sensor device	Amerometric sensor	Microdialysis glucose	Amperometric sensor	Amperometric sensor
Results timing	Retrospective	Retrospective and Real time	Real Time	Real Time
Sensor site	In situ	External	In situ	In situ
Frequency of blood glucose display (min)	5	3	1	5
Rate-of-change arrows	Yes	No	Yes	Yes
Integrate with pump	Yes (Paradigm RT)	No	No	No
Accuracy (error grid) (%)	61.7-76.3	64-88	76.3-81.7	70.4
Limitations	- Life span of 3 days (USA) - Update glycaemia data on the screen every 5 minutes - Calibrations are required every 2- 3 days	- Large system - Life span of 2 days - Skin irritation - No rate- of-change arrows	- Large sensor and transmitter - Warm- up period of 10 hours (first sensor)- - Calibration time programming required - Must use Freestyle strips for calibration - High cost	- Update glycaemia data on the screen every 5 minutes - Does not permit selecting specific points above

Table 2. Main features of the currently available CGMS devices (Torres et al, 2010)

calibrated a minimum of 4 times a day using measured capillary glucose levels, presenting an out-of-phase between the level of glycaemia and the sensor signal of about 4 minutes (Gross et al., 2000).

In the past few years, progressively improved new models have been developed. In 2004, the FDA approved the Guardian Monitor®, with improvements on the previous system that included an alarm not only to signal hyperglycaemia but also for hypoglycaemia. One year later the Guardian MiniMed Real Time® appeared on the market: It was the first continuous glucose monitor that provided the measurements of glucose in real time, every 5 minutes, and with direct connection to a CSII. The Paradigm Real Time® was approved in 2006 as the first sensor integrated with a CSII (Paradigm REAL-time 522/722) enabling it to create a closed circuit. More recently, MiniMed Paradigm Veo® system has been commercialised. It includes CSII with a CGMS with a mechanism that enables the infusion of insulin to be delayed when the levels of glucose are below the specified range. All these systems require at least 2 calibrations per day.

Another type of sensor known as the GlucoDay® system became available on the market in 2002. Its system is based on the technique of micro-dialysis applied to the interstitial fluid that, as has been commented-upon above, provides a reading of the glucose concentration in the subcutaneous cellular tissue that is very similar to the plasma value (Poscia et al.,2003; Varalli et al., 2003). The data collected can be visualised permanently in real time and to be used subsequently for different analyses regarding the behaviour of the glucose concentrations, such as its graphic representation. This system shows high precision and reliability, including at low glucose concentrations (Maran et al., 2002).

The Seven System® was approved by the FDA in 2007. It enables real time readings with measurements performed every 5 minutes and with a latency of 12 hours. It is the only one proven for use over a period of 7 days. The results can be stored for subsequent analyses. The system includes alarms that can be programmed not only for hyperglycaemia but also for hypoglycaemia. It needs to be calibrated every 12 hours with capillary glucose values. A new version is the Seven Plus System® which has improved not only the functionality but also has many additional functions included.

The latest system approved by the FDA in 2008 is the Freestyle Navigator® which has introduced important improvements to the CGM system (McGarraugh, 2009). It enables readings in real time following a latency period of 10 hours (1 hour in the more advanced versions). The concentration of glucose is measured every minute and enables analyses to be made every 10 minutes. The calibration requires capillary glucose measurement (only 4-5 in the first period). It has alarms not only for excessively elevated glucose levels but also for glucose decrease.

3.2.2.2 Clinical indications for continuous glucose monitoring (CGM)

The clinical applications for continuous glucose monitoring (CGM) have not, as yet, been well established. The system can be useful in determining patterns of glycaemia over a 24h period and to detect inadvertent hypoglycaemia. However, its role in improving control of diabetes is, as yet, unclear.

Currently, there are studies and preliminary data on the possible uses; the most extensive studies have focused on the detection of asymptomatic hypoglycaemia. Several studies show an elevated frequency of asymptomatic hypoglycaemia, especially during the nocturnal period and, above all, in patients with DM type 1, detected using CGMS, which have been underestimated with the conventional self-monitoring systems (DeVries et al., 2004). The CGMS also captures values of glucose which can change over a short period of time and, for which, it is not always practical to wait months to evaluate the reductions in the levels of HbA1c. CGM can show the time during which the patients remain in the glucose range that is normal, low or elevated. These values can be more useful than a single point when integrating the data such as the HbA1c levels. Prolonged exposure to intermediate levels of glucose may be preferred in some patients compared to the frequent peaks of hyperglycaemia and hypoglycaemia. This can obviate therapeutically targeting different HbA1c levels in response to oscillating levels of glucose. The CGMS can detect these oscillations as well as measure the mean amplitude and the index of variability of the glycaemia. As such, predictive information on trends during the different times of the day can be obtained (Manuel-y-Keenoy et al., 2004). The CGMS can also be used to evaluate the response of the glycaemia profile to specific treatment or therapeutic modalities such as, for example, the use of multiple doses of insulin vs. the CIIS (Weintrob et al., 2004). There are several studies that show the usefulness of CGMS in modifying treatment and achieving better metabolic control (Edelman et al., 2009; Hirsch et al., 2008; Leinung et al., 2010). Some authors consider this its most important use. In adolescents, apart from being a useful tool to improve glycaemia control, it also promotes communication and motivation of the patient (Schaepelynck-Bélicar et al., 2003) .

According to the data available, beneficial effects in metabolic control can be exercised in pregnant women with diabetes, but more studies are necessary to evaluate the reality of reducing perinatal complications (Festin, 2008).

As such, the possible indications of CGM comprise those situations that require detailed information on the fluctuations of glycaemia: diagnostic confirmation and management of hypoglycaemia (undetected hypoglycaemias or nocturnal hypoglycaemias); therapeutic adjustments in patients who do not achieve the control targets (discrepancy between HbA1c and capillary glycaemia, pregestational diabetes); diabetic educational tool (impact of intake on the glycaemia profile), physical exercise, intercurrent situations; diabetes and hospitalisation (unit for the treatment of the critically-ill patients and/or intensive coronary care), pancreatic tissue transplant and clinical investigation.

According to the recommendations of the American Diabetes Association (ADA, 2011), the CGM can be indicated in selected adult patients with DM type 1 on treatment with intensive insulin therapy to decrease the level of HbA1c (recommendation grade A). As well, CGM can be indicated in children, adolescents, and young adults in whom the adherence to treatment would be high (recommendation grade C). In patients with inadvertent hypoglycaemias, the CGM would be indicated as a complement to the SCCG.

3.2.2.3 Inconveniences

Currently, the CGMS is approved for the use in supplementing SCCG due to the inherent problems: limited level of precision for the isolated measurement of glucose, above all, at decreased levels (Klonoff, 2004); the need to calibrate the sensor several times a day using capillary measurements; short period of use (2-7 days) (Kovatchev et al., 2008).

Minimally invasive CGMS can present secondary effects related to the continuous measure of interstitial fluid. It can cause slight local distress at the site of catheter insertion which can occur on rare occasions. Further, because of its complicated technique, these systems require help from the health-care professional team (Tanenberg et al., 2004).

The major limitation of CGMS is, however, the current absence of scientific evidence of its usefulness. Methodologically appropriate studies are necessary to evaluate precisely the impact of these systems on improving the metabolic control in patients with diabetes, and their effect on hypoglycaemia decrease. The use can be extended in the future but CGMS needs to be improved with respect to the accuracy of glucose measurement, convenience for the patient, integration with other technologies such as CIIS.

4. Treatment of diabetes

As commented-upon earlier, intensive therapy of DM type 1 has been consolidated as the therapeutic strategy of choice since it has been demonstrated to delay the appearance and progression of the chronic complications (DCCT, 1993; Nathan et al., 2005). This strategy consists of multiple daily subcutaneous injections, or the use of CIIS with adjustment of insulin according to the intake of carbohydrates and the level of glycaemia (ADA, 2011).

4.1 Treatment with multiple doses of insulin

The objective of intensive insulin therapy is to arrive at levels of glycaemia close to that of normal, using a regimen of insulin similar to physiological conditions. To achieve this, basal insulin treatment (1 or 2 doses per day with intermediate or low insulin) is accompanied by pre-prandial bolus of quick-acting insulin which is adjusted according to the pre-prandial glycaemia and the intake of carbohydrates. To correctly fulfil this type of therapy, collaboration on the part of the patient is necessary and can be achieved with motivation and information using an appropriate program of diabetes education. As has been highlighted earlier, this type of treatment needs to be accompanied with frequent monitoring with capillary measurements.

Intensive therapy is associated with more frequent hypoglycaemias. Since the DCCT publication, analogues of fast- and slow-acting insulins have been developed which, currently, form the basis of intensive treatment with multiple doses of insulin. These insulin analogues have been associated with a lower risk of hypoglycaemias, and a comparable decrease in HbA1c. Among the analogues of slow-acting insulin are glargine and detemir. Glargine insulin is almost identical to human insulin, except for certain modifications in the molecular structure that enables delaying the absorption in subcutaneous tissue resulting in prolonged duration without peaks of activity. It can be administered at any time of the day without impairing its effectiveness. Detemir insulin is another slow-acting analogue that has a fatty acid in its structure that enables it to bind to albumin in the subcutaneous tissue and its slow release prolongs its action in the blood stream. Both insulins, glargine and detemir, have similar efficacy, similar to the NPH, and are especially indicated in patients with recurring hypoglycaemias (Sing et al., 2009).

The fast-acting insulin analogues have modifications in the molecular structure which facilitate more rapid absorption into the bloodstream. Currently, there are three fast-acting analogues (lispro, aspart and glulisine) whose duration of action and effects are similar. They commence action within 5-15 minutes of subcutaneous administration, with a maximum peak at 30-90 minutes and a duration of 2-4 hours. Compared to standard insulin that begins its effects at 30-45 minutes from injection and has a duration of 4-6 hours, the new fast-acting analogues decrease the post-prandial glucose peak more quickly, can be injected immediately before meals, and decrease hypoglycaemias (Plank et al., 2005; Porcellati et al., 2008). The election of one or other insulin for multiple dose therapy would depend on the characteristics of the patient. No one type of insulin has been elected as treatment-of-choice because a clear benefit on metabolic control has not as yet been demonstrated in a generic manner.

4.2 Continuous Insulin Infusion Systems (CIIS)

Pumps for CIIS are electro-mechanical, portable and small, with the administration of insulin from a reservoir at a programmable rate via a flexible catheter through a cannular inserted subcutaneously. This system delivers insulin continuously at a rhythm that is termed "basal rate" and which can be increased or decreased according to the requirements of the patient. In basal rate, the control of hepatic production of pre-prandial and overnight glucose is an objective. Further, the pump can provide specific amounts of extra "bolus" insulin which can administered before the intake allows the post-prandial glycaemia to become elevated. It can, as well, correct specific increases in glycaemia caused by other circumstances. Insulins used in the CIIS are exclusively fast-acting. Standard human, and preferably, the analogues lispro, aspart and glulisine, are used since these offer less variability in absorption, and show a pharmacokinetic profile closer to that of the physiologic state (Hirsch, 2005; Radermecker & Scheen, 2004).

Using CIIS in patients with DM type 1 began in the decade of the 1970s but, despite being effective in metabolic control, the initial devices had high risk of sepsis and thrombosis. At the start of the decade of the 1980s, evidence was communicated of an increase in mortality in patients having the CIIS; data that were not subsequently confirmed (Teutsch et al., 1984). The use of CIIS does not perform very well against the possibility of severe hypoglycaemia (Lock & Rigg, 1981) and frank ketoacidosis which was highlighted in some articles (Home & Marshall, 1984). The impact of the results of the DCCT became decisive for the widespread use of insulin pumps. The study highlighted a significant reduction in the levels of HbA1c in patients treated with CIIS compared with those who received multiple daily doses of insulin (DCCT, 1995). Since then, the use of CIIS has accelerated exponentially, and what was a research tool has become an established type of treatment for selected patients with DM type 1 (Cummins et al., 2010). On the other hand, the important technological development over the past few years has been to reduce the size of the pump considerably, to increase the benefits and to improve their safety. In the past decade, several studies have confirmed that therapy with CIIS has advantages in metabolic control while achieving greater decreases in the levels of HbA1c (Cummins et al., 2010; Pańkowska et al., 2009; Pickup & Sutton, 2008; Torres et al., 2009). Further, this improvement in glycaemia control is achieved with a lower quantity of insulin (Jeitler et al., 2008; Torres et al., 2009). Hence, CIIS has become established as the preferred modality of treatment, and an alternative to the multiple doses of insulin for those selected patients who do not achieve the target of glycaemia control with multiple injections of insulin (Bruttomesso et al., 2009).

The patients with DM type 1 treated with multiple injections of insulin frequently present with the "dawn phenomenon" which consists of a sharp increase in glucose in the small hours of the morning; increase due to the increase in the counter-regulatory hormones that occur during this period and which are not sufficiently counteracted by long-acting insulin administered at bedtime. The therapy with CIIS, enables basal infusion to be anticipated and programmed, which can be useful in controlling this phenomenon by increasing the basal rhythm to that suitable for the individual's needs (Bruttomesso et al., 2009; Cummins et al., 2010).

When CIIS therapy was used initially, there were cases of severe hypoglycaemia reported which brought the safety of the system into question (Lock & Rigg, 1981). In the subsequent years, the devices available were safer and used fast-acting analogues of insulin which resulted in reduction in the frequency of the severe hypoglycaemias. This form of treatment can achieve and maintain a grade of better metabolic control than can be achieved with multiple doses of insulin; the incidence of hypoglycaemia being significantly less, including at night (Pickup & Sutton, 2008; Torres et al., 2009). Brittle diabetes, with frequent and unannounced glycaemia oscillations, is improved with CIIS therapy.

Oscillations in glycaemia are reduced due to the use of fast-acting insulin analogues whose absorption variability is much lower than other insulins, and with which there is the possibility of programming different rhythms of infusion (Bruttomesso et al., 2008; Pickup et al., 2006).

The accumulated experience of CIIS use in children and adolescents is very promising. This modality of treatment reduces the incidence of acute complications, not only hypoglycaemias but also ketoacidosis, together with improved metabolic control, increased adherence to the treatment and promotion of family involvement. Treatment with CIIS in the paediatric population is safe and efficacious and represents a valid option in selected patients of whatever age provided that there is always appropriate family and health-care professional support (Boland et al., 1999; Danne et al., 2008; DiMeglio et al., 2004). The results of the use of CIIS in pregestational diabetes have not been quite conclusive. Although some trials had observed benefits in metabolic control (Lapolla et al., 2003), more studies are needed to confirm their advantages in achieving maternal and foetal objectives, and regards their safety during the gestation (Cummins et al., 2010; Mukhopadhyay et al., 2007; Volpe et al., 2010).
There are several studies that have found that the CIIS improves the quality-of-life of the patients because it allows better flexibility in relation to food intake and towards the conduct of various planned or unplanned activities. The considerable acceptance of this modality among users is due to the individual not being obliged to link food intake and social activities to insulin administration since several hours can elapse between the activities; as occurs when multiple dose insulin is used. The intake can be delayed or omitted and the content varied. Also, the intensity of the exercise can be modified as can the timing of the activity without compromising the glycaemia control target (EQuality1 Study Group, 2008; Radermecker & Scheen, 2004; Torres et al., 2009). The advantages of CIIS are summarised in Table 3.

Improvement in metabolic control
Correction of the dawn phenomenon
Decrease in hypoglycaemias
Improvement in brittle diabetes
Effective in adults, adolescents and children
Flexibility and improvement in quality-of-life

Table 3. Advantages of CIIS

Interruption of insulin delivery by mechanical failure in the system of infusion leads quickly to hypoglycaemia and ketoacidosis due to the absence of a subcutaneous deposit of insulin (Krzentowski et al., 1983). This and other similar circumstances are preventable by training the individual to identify a potential episode, to warn and to treat the elevated levels of glycaemia (Guilhem et al., 2006). At the site of insertion of the cannular there may appear atrophy, hypertrophy, pruritus, erythema and infection. In the majority of cases the clinical picture is slight and related to inadequate hygiene in the techniques used. Systematic rotation and changing the catheter a maximum of every 3 days would decrease, or pre-empt, these complications (Guilhem et al., 2006). The better strategy to prevent these complications is to instruct the patients using specific educative programs that highlight frequent monitoring of the glycaemia, objectives of glycaemia control, calculation of dietary carbohydrates and the adaptation of daily fluctuations in glycaemia induced by intake,

physical exercise and situations of stress or illness. Further, family help and social environment are important for outcomes (Jeandidier et al., 2008; Tamborlane et al., 2003).
The indications for CSII treatment are not universally established. Appropriate patient selection is fundamental in minimising the risks that these devices can involve. The best results are obtained in psychologically stable patients, with sufficient intellectual capacity, highly motivated and supervised by a multi-disciplinary team. CIIS therapy requires a specifically formed team of healthcare professionals with sufficient time dedication to their patients not only for the training but also for clinical follow-up. The circumstances for CIIS treatment apply to any age in achieving good metabolic outcomes (Bruttomesso et al., 2009; Cummins et al., 2010). The indications more widely accepted are collected in Table 4

HbA1c >7% despite good adherence to therapy with multi-injection systems
Severe hypoglycaemias, recurrent, nocturnal or inadvertent
Significant dawn phenomenon
Brittle diabetes. Wide glycaemia variation, independent of HbA1c
Planned pregnancy if no good control with multi-injection
Need for flexible life-style
Low insulin requirements (<20 UI/day)

Table 4. Indications for CIIS

4.3 CIIS monitoring

Frequent monitoring of glycaemia is a highly positive factor in obtaining good results with CIIS therapy (Shalitin et al., 2010). The information provided by CGMS enables better adaptation not only to the rhythm of basal infusion but also to the bolus. If it is accepted that if the patients treated with CIIS are more motivated, the outcomes resulting from the application of CGMS in this group could be greater (Leinung et al., 2010; Raccah et al., 2009). Currently, better practical advantages are to be gained in the *in situ* subcutaneous sensors with continuous reading in real time which integrate the CGMS in a continuous infusion of insulin using wireless communication; the technique termed continuous interactive monitoring. In this mode, the users of CIIS can adapt the insulin infusion and diet to the real metabolic status. This is possible because the information generated by CGMS allows for the detection of inadvertent hypoglycaemias, information on trends and speed-of-change of glucose, and provides help in planning the bolus to reduce the duration of the hyperglycaemic episode (Hirsch, 2009). A recent innovation has consisted of semi-automatic models that, apart from integrating the insulin infusion and the CGMS, automatically incorporates the delay in infusion over 2 hours in case of having produced an alarm for hypoglycaemia but had not obtained a response from the user (Hirsch et al., 2008a).
Real time information is an important advance in self-care by the patients but, as well, implies a challenge in applying this technology with safety and rigor. In the past 10 years the precision of these systems has improved and the durability of the sensor has increased up to 6-7 days. However, one important limitation is that none of the sensors currently available have the precision of the standard glucometers. This is because they do not measure the blood sugar directly but, rather, evaluate glucose in the subcutaneous interstitial fluid. The defects in precision are related to the low concentration of glucose in the interstitial fluid, the specific dynamics of the glucose in the capillary and interstitial fluids and the delays inherent in the measurement (Torres et al., 2010).

The patients with CIIS who are candidates for CGMS systems need to be very motivated and to have received verbal and written information in a program of therapeutic education. The effect is to avoid false expectations and to recognise the limitations of these systems. The educative program would be orientated towards training, management of the devices, and in the interpretation of the measurements of glucose in real time; all orientated towards achieving the euglycaemia state (Gilliam & Hirsch, 2009; Hirsch et al., 2008a; Juvenile Diabetes Research Foundation Continuous Glucose Monitoring Study Group, 2009a). In principle, the ideal candidate would be a patient with DM type 1, with excellent motivation and optimum therapeutic education, who has not been able to achieve HbA1c levels <7%.

Several studies have demonstrated that the use of CGMS in patients with CIIS has advantages in metabolic control, with significant decreases in the levels of HbA1c (Bergenstal et al., 2010; Deiss et al., 2006; Hirsch et al., 2008b; Juvenile Diabetes Research Foundation Continuous Glucose Monitoring Study Group, 2008) and less glycaemia variability (Garg et al., 2006; Kordonouri et al., 2010). Some studies have, as well, demonstrated improvement in the frequency of hypoglycaemia (Garg et al., 2006; Juvenile Diabetes Research Foundation Continuous Glucose Monitoring Study Group, 2009b; Leinung et al., 2010). The best results have been obtained in relation of adherence to the CGMS systems; continuous use being more efficient than intermittent use (Hirsch et al., 2008b; Juvenile Diabetes Research Foundation Continuous Glucose Monitoring Study Group, 2008, 2009a; Raccah et al., 2009) but, in practice, can be more difficult to fulfil (O'Connell et al., 2009).

A list of possible indication for the use of CGMS is summarised in Table 5 (American Diabetes Association, 2011; Fabiato et al., 2009).

Patients with DM type 1, excellent motivation and optimum therapeutic education, but who have not been able to achieve HbA1c <7%
Severe hypoglycaemias, inadvertent hypoglycaemias or fear of hypoglycaemias that impede achieving the targets of glycaemia control
Brittle diabetes
Planned pregnancy with difficulties achieving appropriate glycaemia control
Children and adolescents with significant glucose variability or frequent hypoglycaemias, severe or inadvertent despite adjustments of the therapies. It is indispensable that they and/or the family are motivated and have appropriate training.

Table 5. Indications for interactive CGMS

5. Future research

The challenge to achieve an optimum metabolic control in type 1 DM is being progressively better addressed. New insulins and technological devices have been designed to mimic beta cell function. However, to translate these findings into the clinical practice new research and clinical trials are needed. Technological advances have enabled the development of new CIIS devices with better performance in programming and for calculating optimal dose of insulin required. Systems security alerts are getting better, and the availability of sensors that promote CIIS devices has been a promising development. A closed-loop system should include an implantable continuous glucose sensor, an insulin pump and an algorithm control leading to insulin infusion adjusted to the glucose concentrations (Kumareswaran et al., 2009). In the

future, combined use of insulin pumps and glucose sensors could become an effective and safe strategy, with minimal constraints in optimising metabolic control in diabetic patients to achieve glycaemia very close to normal (Hirsch, 2009; Keenan et al., 2010; Kowalski, 2009).
Finally, we note that both CIIS therapy and the use of CGMS are expensive. The implementation of these technologies requires public health systems that have sufficient resources to initiate treatment and to ensure appropriate monitoring by the users. Further studies are needed on cost and effectiveness of these systems (Cummins et al., 2010; Fabiato et al., 2009; Huang et al., 2010).

6. Conclusions

Several prospective studies in Type 1 DM have demonstrated the tight association existing between glycaemia and the development of micro- and macro-angiopathy complications. The most significant study (the DCCT study) demonstrated that intensive treatment was accompanied by a reduction in the appearance and progression of the micro-vascular complications. Subsequent analyses of the DCCT study population demonstrated that the beneficial effects persisted even after the intervention and that they are extended to adverse cardiovascular events, as well. To achieve this objective, treatment of DM continues to be enriched by several novel therapeutic approaches. These have increased with the incorporation of insulin analogues and the introduction and optimisation of devices for the administration of insulin (continuous infusion system, CIIS) which achieves profiles of activity closer to the physiological equivalent. Several studies have demonstrated that the treatment with CIIS improves glycaemia variation with greater decrease in the HbA1c, less hypoglycaemias, and no increase in the frequency of ketoacidosis. Methods for evaluating response to treatment have been progressively improved. Recent clinical evidence has demonstrated that the glycaemia profile of the patients with DM, especially type 1 DM, is characterised by wide fluctuations related to physical activity, diet, and the specific treatment administered. The impact and the consequences of these variations are only partially known. Hence, the possibility of having continuous information available on glucose levels is an attractive option. Glucose sensors or CGMS provide maximum information on the changes in plasma glucose levels along the course of the day, and can be used in optimising treatment in patients with DM. However, the clinical applications of the CGMS have not, as yet, been well established.

7. Acknowledgments

This study was financed, in part, by grants from the Andalusia Department of Health (CTS-368). The authors declare that there is no conflict of interest that would prejudice the impartiality of this scientific work. Editorial assistance was by Peter R. Turner.

8. References

ADVANCE Collaborative Group; Patel, A., MacMahon, S., Chalmers, J., Neal, B., Billot, L., Woodward M., & Marre M. (2008). Intensive blood glucose control and vascular outcomes in patients with type 2 diabetes. *N Engl J Med*, Vol. 358, No. 24, (Jun. 2008), pp. 2560-2572, ISSN 0028-4793.

Alemzadeh, R., Lopnow, C., Parton, E., Kirby, & M. (2003). Glucose sensor evaluation of glycemic inestability in pediatric type 1 diabetes mellitus. *Diabetes Technol Ther*, Vol. 5, No. 2, (Jul. 2003), pp. 167-73. ISSN 1520-9156.

American Diabetes Association (2011). Standards of medical care in diabetes-2011. Diabetes Care, Vol. 34, Suppl. 1, (Jan. 2011), pp. S11-S61, ISSN 0149-5992.

Avignon, A., Radauceanu, A., & Monnier, L. (1997) Nonfasting plasma glucose is a better marker of diabetic control than fasting plasma glucose in type 2 diabetes. *Diabetes Care*, Vol. 20, (Dec. 1997) pp. 1822-1826, ISSN 0149-5992.

Baena, G., Carral, F., Roca, M., Cayón, M., Ortego, J., Escobar-Jiménez, L., Torres, I., Gavilán, I., Doménech, I., García, A., Coserria, C., López-Tinoco, C., & Aguilar-Diosdado, M. (2008). Can the metabolic control targets established for patients with type 1 diabetes be achieved in clinical practice? *Endocrino Nutr*, Vol. 55, No. 10, pp. 442-447, ISSN 1575-0922.

Bergenstal, R.M., & Gavin, J.R. (2005). The role of self-monitoring of blood glucose in the care of people with diabetes: report of a global consensus conference. *Am J Med*, Vol. 118, (Oct. 2005) pp. 1-6, ISSN 0002-9343.

Bergenstal, R.M., Tamborlane, W.V., Ahmann, A., Buse, J.B., Dailey, G., Davis, S.N., Joyce, C., Peoples, T., Perkins, B.A., Welsh, J.B., Willi, S.M., Wood, M.A. & STAR 3 Study Group (2010). Effectiveness of sensor-augmented insulin-pump therapy in type 1 diabetes. N Engl J Med, Vol. 363, No. 4, (Jul. 2010), pp. 311-320, ISSN 0028-4793.

Bode, B.W., Sabbad, H., & Davidson, P.C. (2001). What`s ahead in glucose monitoring? New techniques hold promise for improved ease and accuracy. *Postgrad Med*, Vol. 109, No. 4, (April 2001), pp. 41-9, ISSN 0032-5481.

Boland, E.A., Grey, M., Oesterle, A., Fredrickson, L. & Tamborlane, W.V. (1999). Continuous subcutaneous insulin infusion. A new way to lower risk of severe hypoglycaemia, improve metabolic control, and enhance coping in adolescents with type 1 diabetes. *Diabetes Care*, Vol. 22, No. 11, (Nov. 1999), pp. 1779-1784, ISSN 0149-5992.

Bruttomesso, D., Crazzolara, D., Maran, A., Costa, S., Dal Pos, M., Girelli, A., Lepore, G., Aragona, M., Iori, E., Valentini, U., Del Prato, S., Tiengo, A., Buhr, A., Trevisan, R., & Baritussio, A. (2008). In type 1 diabetic patients with good glycaemic control, blood glucose variability is lower during continuous subcutaneous insulin infusion than during multiple daily injections with insulin glargine. Diabet Med, Vol. 25, No. 3, (Mar. 2008), pp. 326-332, ISSN 0742-3071.

Bruttomesso, D., Costa, S. & Baritussio, A. (2009). Continuous subcutaneous insulin infusion (CSII) 30 years later: still the best option for insulin therapy. *Diabetes Metab Res Rev*, Vol. 25, No. 2, (Feb. 2009), pp. 99-111, ISSN 1520-7552.

Cavalot, F., Petrelli, A., Traversa, M., Bonomo, K., Fiora, E., Conti, M., Anfossi, G., Costa, G., & Trovati, M. (2006) Post-prandial blood glucose is a stronger predictor of cardiovascular events than fasting blood glucose in type 2 diabetes mellitus, particularly in women: lessons from the San Luigi Gonzaga Diabetes Study. *J Clin Endocrinol Metab*, Vol. 91, No. 3, (Dec. 2005) pp. 813-9, ISSN 0021-972X.

Ceriello, A., Taboga, C., Tonutti, L., Quagliaro, L., Piconi, L., Bais, B., Da Ros, R., & Motz, E. (2002). Evidence for an independent and cumulative effect of post-prandial hypertriglyceridemia and hyperglycemia on endothelial dysfunction and oxidative stress generation: effects of short- and long-term simvastatin treatment. *Circulation*, Vol. 106, No. 2, (Sept. 2002), pp. 1211– 1218, ISSN 0009-7322.

Ceriello, A. (2003). New insights on oxidative stress and diabetic complications may lead to a «causal» antioxidant therapy. *Diabetes Care,* Vol. 26, No. 5, pp. 1589-96, ISSN 0149-5992.

Ceriello, A. (2005). Post-prandial hyperglycemia and diabetes complications. Is it time to treat?. *Diabetes,* Vol. 54, No. 1, (Dec. 2004) pp. 1-7, ISSN 0012-1797.

Cooper, M., Glasziou, P., Grobbee, D., Hamet, P., Harrap, S., Heller, S., Liu, L., Mancia, G., Mogensen, CE., Pan, C., Poulter, N., Rodgers, A., Williams, B., Bompoint, S., de Galan, B.E., Joshi, R., & Travert, F. (2008). *Intensive Blood,* pp. 2560–2572, ISSN 1533-4406.

Cummins, E., Royle, P., Snaith, A., Greene, A., Robertson, L., McIntyre, L., & Waugh N. Clinical effectiveness and cost-effectiveness of continuous subcutaneous insulin infusion for diabetes: systematic review and economic evaluation. *Health Technol Assess,* Vol. 14, No. 11, (Feb. 2010), pp. 1-181, ISSN 1366-5278.

Danne, T., Battelino, T., Jarosz-Chobot, P., Kordonouri, O., Pánkowska, E., Ludvigsson, J., Schober, E., Kaprio, E., Saukkonen, T., Nicolino, M., Tubiana-Rufi, N., Klinkert, C., Haberland, H., Vazeou, A., Madacsy, L., Zangen, D., Cherubini, V., Rabbone, I., Toni, S., de Beaufort, C., Bakker-van Waarde, W., van den Berg, N., Volkov, I., Barrio, R., Hanas, R., Zumsteg, U., Kuhlmann, B., Aebi, C., Schumacher, U., Gschwend, S., Hindmarsh, P., Torres, M., Shehadeh, N., Phillip, M., & PedPump Study Group. (2008). Establishing glycaemic control with continuous subcutaneous insulin infusion in children and adolescents with type 1 diabetes: experience of the PedPump Study in 17 countries. *Diabetologia,* Vol. 51, No. 9, (Sept. 2008), pp. 1594-1601, ISSN 0012-186X

DCCT-EDIC. (2000). Retinopathy and nephropathy in patients with type 1 diabetes four years after a trial of intensive therapy. The Diabetes Control and Complications Trial/Epidemiology of Diabetes Interventions and Complications Research Group. *N Engl J Med,* Vol. 342, No. 6, (Feb. 2000), pp. 381–389, ISSN 0028-4793.

De Witt, D.E., & Hirsch, I.B. (2003). Outpatient insulin therapy in type 1 and type 2 diabetes mellitus: scientific review. *JAMA,* Vol. 289, No. 17, (May 2003), pp. 2254-2264, ISSN 0098-7484.

Deiss, D., Bolinder, J., Riveline, J.P., Battelino, T., Bosi, E., Tubiana-Rufi, N., Kerr, D. & Phillip, M. (2006). Improved glycemic control in poorly controlled patients with type 1 diabetes using real-time continuous glucose monitoring. Diabetes Care, Vol. 29, No. 12, (Dec. 2006), pp. 2730-2732, ISSN 0149-5992.

DeVries, J.H., Wentholt, I.M., Masurel, N., Mantel, I., Poscia, A., Maran, A., & Heine, R.J. (2004). Nocturnal hypoglycaemia in type 1 diabetes: consequences and assessment. *Diabetes Metab Res Rev,* Vol. 20, (Nov. 2004) pp. 43-6, ISSN 1520-7552.

Diabetes Control and Complications Trial Research Group. (1993). The effect of intensive treatment of diabetes on the development and progression of long-term complications in insulin-dependent diabetes mellitus. *N Engl J Med,* Vol. 329, No. 14 , (Sept. 1993), pp.977-986, ISSN 0028-4793.

Diabetes Control and Complications Trial Research Group. (1995). Implementation of treatment protocols in the Diabetes Control and Complications Trial. *Diabetes Care,* Vol. 18, No. 3, (Mar. 1995), pp. 361–376 ISSN 0149-5992

Diabetes Control and Complications Trial/Epidemiology of Diabetes Interventions and Complications (DCCT/EDIC) Research Group, Nathan, D.M., Zinman, B., Cleary, P.A., Backlund, J.Y., Genuth, S., Miller, R., & Orchard, T.J. (2009). Modern day clinical course of type 1 diabetes mellitus after 30 years' duration: the diabetes control and complications trial/epidemiology of diabetes interventions and complications and Pittsburgh epidemiology of diabetes complications experience (1983–2005). *Arch Intern Med*, Vol. 169, No. 14, (Jul. 2009), pp. 1307–1316, ISSN 0003-9926.

DiMeglio, L.A., Pottorff, T.M., Boyd, S.R., France, L., Fineberg, N., & Eugster E.A. (2004). A randomized, controlled study of insulin pump therapy in diabetic preschoolers. *J Pediatr*, Vol. 145, No. 3, (Sept. 2004), pp. 380-384, ISSN 0022-7476.

Duckworth, W., Abraira, C., Moritz, T., Reda, D., Emanuele, N., Reaven, P.D., Zieve, F.J., Marks, J., Davis, S.N., Hayward, R., Warren, S.R., Goldman, S., McCarren, M., Vitek, M.E., Henderson, W.G., Huang, G.D., & VADT Investigators. (2009). Glucose control and vascular complications in veterans with type 2 diabetes. *N Engl J Med*. Vol. 360, No. 2, (Jan. 2009), pp. 129–139, ISSN 0028-4793.

Edelman, S.V., & Bailey, T.S. (2009) Continuous glucose monitoring health outcomes. *Diabetes Technol Them*, Vol. 11, No. 1, (Jul. 2009), pp. 68-74, ISSN 1520-9156.

EQuality1 Study Group-Evaluation of quality of life and costs in diabetes type 1, Nicolucci, A., Maione, A., Franciosi, M., Amoretti, R., Busetto, E., Capani, F., Bruttomesso, D., Di Bartolo, P., Girelli, A., Leonetti, F., Morviducci, L., Ponzi, P., & Vitacolonna E. (2008). Quality of life and treatment satisfaction in adults with type 1 diabetes: a comparison between continuous subcutaneous insulin infusion and multiple daily injections. Diabet Med, Vol. 25, No. 2, (Feb. 2008), pp. 213-220, ISSN 0742-3071.

Ellison, J.M., Stegmann, J.M., Colner, S.L., Michael, R.H., Sharma, M.K., Ervin, K.R., & Horwithz, D.L. (2001). Rapid changes in post-prandial blood glucose produce concentration differences at finger, forearm, and thigh sampling sites. *Diabetes Care*, Vol. 25, No. 6, (May 2005) pp. 961-964, ISSN 0149-5992.

Esmatjes, E., Flores, L., Vidal, M., Rodriguez, L., Cortes, A., Almirall, L., Ricart, M.J., & Gomis, R. (2003). Hypoglycaemia after pancreas transplantation: usefulness of a continuous glucose monitoring system. *Clin Transplant*, Vol. 17, No. 6, (Feb. 2002) pp. 534-538, ISSN 0902-0063.

Fabiato, K., Buse, J., Duclos, M., Largay, J., Izlar, C., O'Connell, T., Stallings, J., & Dungan, K. (2009). Clinical experience with continuous glucose monitoring in adults. Diabetes Technol Ther, Vol. 11, Suppl. 1, (Jun. 2009), pp. S93-S103, ISSN 1520-9156.

Farmer, A., Wade, A., Goyder, E., Yudkin, P., French, D., Craven, A., Holman, R., Kinmonth, A.L., & Neil, A. (2007). Impact of self monitoring of blood glucose in the management of patients with non-insulin treated diabetes: open parallel group randomised trial. *BMJ*, Vol. 335, No. 7611, (Jun. 2007) pp. 1-8, ISSN 0959-535X.

Festin, M. (2008). Continuous glucose monitoring in women with diabetes during pregnancy. *BMJ*, Vol. 337, No. 1472, (Sept. 2008), pp. 1472, ISSN 0959-535X.

Fineberg, S.E., Bernstein, R.M., Laffel, L.M., & Schwartz, S.L. (2001). Use of an automated device for alternative site blood glucose monitoring. *Diabetes Care*, Vol. 24, No. 7, (Jul. 2001), pp. 1217-1220, ISSN 0149-5992.

Garg, S., Zisser, H., Schwartz, S., Bailey, T., Kaplan, R., Ellis, S., & Jovanovic, L. (2006). Improvement in glycemic excursions with a transcutaneous, real-time continuous glucose sensor: a randomized controlled trial. Diabetes Care, Vol. 29, No. 1, (Jan. 2006), pp. 44-50, ISSN 0149-5992

Garg, S.K. (2009). Role of continuous glucose monitoring in patients with diabetes using multiple daily insulin injections. *Infusystems International*. Vol. 8, No. 3, pp. 17-21.

Gerstl, E., Rabl, W., Rosenbauer, J., Grobe, H., Hofer, S., Krause, U., & Holl, R.W. (2008). Metabolic control as reflected by HbA1c in children, adolescents and young adults with type-1 diabetes mellitus: combined longitudinal analysis including 27035 patients from 207 centers in Germany and Austria during the last decade. *Eur J Pediatr*, Vol. 167, No. 4, (April 2008), pp. 447-453, ISSN 0340-6199.

Gilliam, L.K. & Hirsch, I.B. (2009). Practical aspects of real-time continuous glucose monitoring. Diabetes Technol Ther, Vol. 11, Suppl. 1, (Jun. 2009), pp. S75-S82, ISSN 1520-9156.

Goldstein, D.E., Lorenz, R.A., Malone, J.I., Nathan, D., & Peterson, C.M. (2004). Test of glycemia in diabetes. *Diabetes Care,* Vol. 27, Suppl. 1, (Jan. 2004), pp. 1761-1773, ISSN 0149-5992.

Gross, T.M., Einhorn, D., Kayne, D.M., Reed, J.H., White, N.H., & Mastrototaro, J.J. (2000). Performance evaluation of the MiniMed continuous glucose monitoring system during patient home use. *Diabetes Technol Ther,* Vol. 2, No. 1, (April 2001), pp. 49-56, ISSN 1520-9156.

Guerci, B., Tubiana-Rufi, N., Bauduceau, B., Bresson, R., Cuperlier, A., Delcroix,. C., Durain, D., Fermon, C., Le Floch, J.P., Le Devehat, C., Melki, V., Monnier, L., Mosnier-Pudar, H., Taboulet, P., & Hanaire-Broutin, H. (2005). Advantages to using capillary blood beta-hydroxybutyrate determination for the detection and treatment of diabetic ketosis. *Diabetes Metab,* Vol. 31, No. 4, Pt. 1, (Sept. 2005), pp. 401-406, ISSN 0742-3071.

Guilhem, I., Leguerrier, A.M., Lecordier, F., Poirier, J.Y., & Maugendre, D. (2006). Technical risks with subcutaneous insulin infusion. *Diabetes Metab,* Vol. 32, No. 3, (Jun. 2006), pp. 279-284, ISSN 0742-3071.

Diabetes Control and Complications Trial Research Group. (1999). Glucose tolerance and mortality: comparison of WHO and American DiabetesmAssociation diagnostic criteria. The DECODE study group. Collaborative analysis Of Diagnostic criteria in Europe. *Lancet,* Vol. 354, No. 9179, (Aug. 1999), pp. 617-21, ISSN 0140-6736.

Hanas, R. (2002). Selection for and initiation of continuous subcutaneous insulin infusion. Proceedings from a workshop. *Horm Res,* Vol. 57, Suppl. 1, (2002), pp. 101-104, ISSN 0301-0163.

Herman, W.H. (1999). Glycemic control in diabetes. *BMJ,* Vol. 319, No. 7202, (Jul. 1999), pp. 104-106, ISSN 0959-535X.

Hirsch, I.B. (2005). Insulin Analogues. *N Engl J Med,* Vol. 352, No. 2, (Jan. 2005), pp. 174-183, ISSN 0028-4793

Hirsch, I.B., Amstrong, D., Bergenstal, R.M., Buckingham, B., Childs, B.P., Clarke, W.L., Peters, A., & Wolpert H. (2008a). Clinical application of emerging sensor technologies in diabetes management: consensus guidelines for continuous glucose monitoring (CGM). *Diabetes Technol Ther,* Vol. 10, No. 4, (Aug. 2008), pp. 232-244, ISSN 1520-9156.

Hirsch, I.B., Abelseth, J., Bode, B.W., Fischer, J.S., Kaufman, F.R., Mastrototaro, J., Parkin, C.G., Wolpert, H.A., & Buckingham, B.A. (2008b). Sensor-augmented insulin pump therapy: results of the first randomized treat-to-target study. *Diabetes Technol Ther,* Vol. 10, No. 5, (Oct. 2008), pp. 377-383, ISSN 1520-9156.

Hirsch, I.B. (2009). Realistic expectations and practical use of continuous glucose monitoring for the endocrinologist. *J Clin Endocrinol Metab,* Vol. 94, No. 7, (Jul. 2009), pp. 2232-2238, ISSN 0021-972X.

Holman, R.R., Paul, S.K., Bethel, M.A., Matthews, D.R., & Neil, H.A. (2008). 10-year follow-up of intensive glucose control in type 2 diabetes. *N Engl J Med*, Vol. 359, No. 15, (Oct. 2008), pp. 1577- 1589, ISSN 0028-4793.

Home, P.D., & Marshall, S.M. (1984). Problems and safety of continuous subcutaneous insulin infusion. *Diabet Med*, Vol. 1, No. 1, (May 1984), pp. 41-44, ISSN 0742-3071.

Huang, E.S., O'Grady, M., Basu, A., Winn, A., John, P., Lee, J., Meltzer, D., Kollman, C., Laffel, L., Tamborlane, W., Weinzimer, S., Wysocki T., & Juvenile Diabetes Research Foundation Continuous Glucose Monitoring Study Group. (2010). The cost-effectiveness of continuous glucose monitoring in type 1 diabetes. Diabetes Care, Vol. 33, No. 6, (Jun. 2010), pp. 1269-1274, ISSN 0149-5992.

Ismail-Beigi, F., Craven, T., Banerji, M.A., Basile, J., Calles, J., Cohen, R.M., Cuddihy, R., Cushman, W.C., Genuth, S., Grimm, R.H. Jr., Hamilton, B.P., Hoogwerf, B., Karl, D., Katz, L., Krikorian, A., O'Connor, P., Pop-Busui, R., Schubart, U., Simmons, D., Taylor, H., Thomas, A., Weiss, D., Hramiak, I., & ACCORD trial group. (2010). Effect of intensive treatment of hyperglycaemia on micro-vascular outcomes in type 2 diabetes: an analysis of the ACCORD randomized trial. *Lancet*. Vol. 376, No. 9739, (Aug. 2010), pp. 419–430, ISSN 0140-6736.

Jeandidier, N., Riveline, J.P., Tubiana-Rufi, N., Vambergue, A., Catargi, B., Melki, V., Charpentier, G., & Guerci B. (2008). Treatment of diabetes mellitus using an external insulin pump in clinical practice. *Diabetes Metab*, Vol. 34, No. 4 ,Pt. 2, (Sept. 2008), pp. 425-438, ISSN 0742-3071.

Jeitler, K., Horvath, K., Berghold, A., Gratzer, T.W., Neeser, K., Pieber, T.R., & Siebenhofer, A. (2008). Continuous subcutaneous insulin infusion versus multiple daily insulin injections in patients with diabetes mellitus: systematic review and meta-analysis. *Diabetologia*, Vol. 51, No. 6, (Jun. 2008), pp. 941-951, ISSN 0012-186X

Juvenile Diabetes Research Foundation Continuous Glucose Monitoring Study Group, Tamborlane, W.V., Beck, R.W., Bode, B.W., Buckingham, B., Chase, H.P., Clemons, R., Fiallo-Scharer, R., Fox, L.A., Gilliam, L.K., Hirsch, I.B., Huang, E.S., Kollman, C., Kowalski, A.J., Laffel, L., Lawrence, J.M., Lee, J., Mauras, N., O'Grady, M., Ruedy, K.J., Tansey, M., Tsalikian, E., Weinzimer, S., Wilson, D.M., Wolpert, H., Wysocki, T., & Xing, D. (2008). Continuous glucose monitoring and intensive treatment of type 1 diabetes. *N Engl J Med*, Vol. 359, No. 14, (Oct. 2008), pp. 1464-1476, ISSN 0028-4793.

Juvenile Diabetes Research Foundation Continuous Glucose Monitoring Study Group, Beck, R.W., Buckingham, B., Miller, K., Wolpert, H., Xing, D., Block, J.M., Chase, H.P., Hirsch, I., Kollman, C., Laffel, L., Lawrence, J.M., Milaszewski, K., Ruedy, K.J., & Tamborlane, W.V. (2009a). Factors predictive of use and of benefit from continuous glucose monitoring in type 1 diabetes. *Diabetes Care*, Vol. 32, No. 11, (Nov. 2009), pp. 1947-1953, ISSN 0149-5992.

Juvenile Diabetes Research Foundation Continuous Glucose Monitoring Study Group, Bode, B., Beck, R.W., Xing, D., Gilliam, L., Hirsch, I., Kollman, C., Laffel, L., Ruedy, K.J., Tamborlane, W.V., Weinzimer, S., & Wolpert, H. (2009b). Sustained benefit of continuous glucose monitoring on A1C, glucose profiles, and hypoglycemia in adults with type 1 diabetes. Diabetes Care, Vol. 32, No. 11, (Nov. 2009), pp. 2047-2049, ISSN 0149-5992.

Katarina, E., Cederholm, J., Nilson, P., Gudbjornsdottir, S., & Eliasson, B. (2007). Glycemic and risk factor control in type 1 diabetes. Result from 13612 patients in a national diabetes register. *Diabetes Care*, Vol. 30, No. 3, (Mar. 2007), pp. 496-502, ISSN 0149-5992.

Keenan, D.B., Cartaya, R., & Mastrototaro, J.J. (2010). The pathway to the closed-loop artificial pancreas: research and commercial perspectives. *Pediatr Endocrinol Rev*, Vol. 7, Suppl. 3, (Aug. 2010), pp. 445-451, ISSN 1565-4753.

Klonoff, D.C. (2004). The need for separate performance goals for glucose sensors in the hypoglycemic, normomglycemic, and hyperglycaemic ranges. *Diabetes Care*, Vol. 27, No. 3, (Mar. 2004), pp. 834-836, ISSN 0149-5992.

Klonoff, D.C. (2005). Continuous glucose monitoring. Roadmap for 21st century diabetes therapy. *Diabetes Care*, Vol. 28, No. 5, (May 2008), pp. 1231-9, ISSN 0149-5992.

Kordonouri, O., Pankowska, E., Rami, B., Kapellen, T., Coutant, R., Hartmann, R., Lange, K., Knip, M., & Danne, T. (2010). Sensor-augmented pump therapy from the diagnosis of childhood type 1 diabetes: results of the Paediatric Onset Study (ONSET) after 12 months of treatment. Diabetologia, Vol. 53, No. 12, (Dec. 2010), pp. 2487-2495, ISSN 0012-186X.

Kowalski, A.J. (2009). Can we really close the loop and how soon? Accelerating the availability of an artificial pancreas: a roadmap to better diabetes outcomes. *Diabetes Technol Ther*, Vol. 11, Suppl. 1, (Jun. 2009), pp. S113-S119, ISSN 1520-9156.

Kovatchev, B., Anderson, S., Heinemann, L., & Clarke, W. (2008). Comparison of the numerical and clinical accuracy of four continuous glucose monitors. *Diabetes Care*, Vol. 31, No. 6, (Jun. 2008), pp. 1160-1164, ISSN 0149-5992.

Krzentowski, G., Scheen, A., Castillo, M., Luyckx, A.S., & Lefebvre, P.J. (1983). A 6-hour nocturnal interruption of a continuous subcutaneous insulin infusion. Metabolic and hormonal consequences and scheme for a prompt return to adequate control. *Diabetologia*, Vol. 24, No. 5, (May 1983), pp. 314-318, ISSN 0012-186X.

Kumareswaran, K., Evans, M.L., & Hovorka, R. (2009). Artificial pancreas: an emerging approach to treat type 1 diabetes. *Expert Rev Med Devices*, Vol. 6, No. 4, (Jul. 2009), pp. 401-410, ISSN 1743-4440.

Lapolla, A., Dalfrà, M.G., Masin, M., Bruttomesso, D., Piva, I., Crepaldi, C., Tortul, C., Dalla Barba, B., & Fedele, D. (2003). Analysis of outcome of pregnancy in type 1 diabetics treated with insulin pump or conventional insulin therapy. *Acta Diabetol*, Vol. 40, No. 3, (Sept. 2003), pp. 143-149, ISSN 0940-5429.

Leinung, M., Thompson, S., & Nardacci, E. (2010). Benefits of continuous glucose monitor use in clinical practice. *Endocr Pract*, Vol. 16, No. 3, (May-Jun. 2010), pp. 371-375, ISSN 1530-891X.

Lock, D.R., & Rigg, L.A. (1981). Hypoglycemic coma associated with subcutaneous insulin infusion by portable pump. *Diabetes Care*, Vol. 4, No. 3, (May-Jun. 1981), pp. 389-391, ISSN 0149-5992.

Malmberg, K., Ryden, L., Efendic, S., Herlitz, J., Nicol, P., Waldenstrom, A., Wedel, H., & Welin, L. (1995). Randomized trial of insulin-glucose infusion followed by subcutaneous insulin treatment in diabetic patients with acute myocardial infarction (DIGAMI study): effects of mortality at 1 year. *J Am Coll Cardiol*, Vol. 26, No. 1 (Jul. 1995), pp. 57-65, ISSN 0735-1097.

Manuel-y-Keenoy, B., Vertommen, J., Abrams, P., Van Gaal, L., De Leeuw, I., Messeri, D., & Poscia, A. (2004). Post-prandial glucose monitoring in type 1 diabetes mellitus: use of a continuous subcutaneous monitoring device. *Diabetes Metab Res Rev*, Vol. 20, Suppl. 2, (Dec. 2004), pp. S24-31, ISSN 1520-7552.

Maran, A., Crepaldi, C., Tiengo, A., Grassi, G., Vitali, E., Pagano, G., Bistoni, S., Calabrese, G., Santeusanio, F., Leonetti, F., Ribaudo, M., Di Mario, U., Annuzzi, G., Genovese, S., Riccardi, G., Previti, M., Cucinotta, D., Giorgino, F., Bellomo, A., Giorgino, R., Poscia, A., & Varalli, M. (2002). Continuous subcutaneous glucose monitoring in diabetic patients: a multicenter analysis. *Diabetes Care*, Vol. 25, No. 2, (Feb. 2002), pp. 347-52, ISSN 0149-5992.

Martin, C.L., Albers, J., Herman, W.H., Cleary, P., Waberski, B., Greene, D.A., Stevens, M.J., Feldman, E.L., & DCCT/EDIC Research Group. (2006). Neuropathy among the diabetes control and complications trial cohort 8 years after trial completion. *Diabetes Care*, Vol. 29, No. 2, (Feb. 2006), pp. 340–344, ISSN 0149-5992.

McGarraugh, G. (2009). The chemistry of commercial continuous glucose monitors. *Diabetes Technol Ther*, Vol. 11. Suppl. 1, (Jun. 2009), pp. 17-24, ISSN 1520-9156.

Mukhopadhyay, A., Farrell, T., Fraser, R.B., & Ola, B. (2007). Continuous subcutaneous insulin infusion vs intensive conventional insulin therapy in pregnant diabetic women: a systematic review and metaanalysis of randomized, controlled trials. *Am J Obstet Gynecol*, Vol. 197, No. 5, (Nov. 2007), pp. 447-456, ISSN 0002-9378.

Nathan, D.M., Cleary, P.A., Backlund, J.Y., Genuth, S.M., Lachin, J.M., Orchard, T.J., Raskin, P., Zinman, B., & Diabetes Control and Complications Trial/Epidemiology of Diabetes Interventions and Complications (DCCT/EDIC) Study Research Group. (2005). Intensive diabetes treatment and cardiovascular disease in patients with type 1 diabetes. N Engl J Med, Vol. 353, No. 25, (Dec. 2005), pp. 2643-2653, ISSN 0028-4793

O'Connell, M.A., Donath, S., O'Neal, D.N., Colman, P.G., Ambler, G.R., Jones, T.W., Davis, E.A., & Cameron, F.J. (2009). Glycaemic impact of patient-led use of sensor-guided pump therapy in type 1 diabetes: a randomised controlled trial. *Diabetologia*, Vol. 52, No. 7, (Jul. 2009), pp. 1250-1257, ISSN 0012-186X

Ohkubo, Y., Kishikawa, H., Araki, E., Miyata, T., Isami, S., Motoyoshi, S., Kojima, Y., Furuyoshi, N., & Shichiri, M. (1995). Intensive insulin therapy prevents the progression of diabetic micro-vascular complications in Japanese patients with non-insulin dependent diabetes mellitus: a randomized prospective 6-year study. *Diabetes Res Clin Pract*, Vol. 28, No. 2, (May 1995), pp. 103-17, ISSN 0168-8227.

Pańkowska, E., Błazik, M., Dziechciarz, P., Szypowska, A., & Szajewska, H. (2009). Continuous subcutaneous insulin infusion vs. multiple daily injections in children with type 1 diabetes: a systematic review and meta-analysis of randomized control trials. Pediatr Diabetes, Vol. 10, No. 1, (Feb. 2009), pp. 52-58, ISSN 1399-543X.

Pickup, J.C., Kidd, J., Burmiston, S., & Yemane, N. (2006). Determinants of glycaemic control in type 1 diabetes during intensified therapy with multiple daily insulin injections or continuous subcutaneous insulin infusion: importance of blood glucose variability. *Diabetes Metab Res Rev*, Vol. 22, No. 3, (May-Jun. 2006), pp. 232-237, ISSN 1520-7552.

Pickup, J.C., & Sutton, A.J. (2008). Severe hypoglycaemia and glycaemic control in type 1 diabetes: meta-analysis of multiple daily insulin injections compared with continuous subcutaneous insulin infusion. *Diabet Med*, Vol. 25, No. 7, (Jul. 2008), pp. 765-774, ISSN 0742-3071.

Plank, J., Siebenhofer, A., Berghold, A., Jeitler, K., Horvath, K., Mrak, P., & Pieber, T.R. (2005). Systematic review and meta-analysis of short-acting insulin analogues in patients with diabetes mellitus. *Arch Intern Med*, Vol. 165, No.12. (Jun. 2005), pp. 1337-1344, ISSN 0003-9926.

Porcellati, F., Rossetti, P., Busciantella, N.R., Marzotti, S., Lucidi, P., Luzio, S., Owens, D,R., Bolli, G.B., & Fanelli, C.G. (2007). Comparison of pharmacokinetics and dynamics of the long-acting insulin analogs glargine and detemir at steady state in type 1 diabetes: a double-blind, randomized, crossover study. *Diabetes Care*, Vol. 30, No.10 (Oct. 2007) pp. 2447-52. ISSN 0149-5992

Poscia, A., Mascini, M., Moscone, D., Luzzana, M., Caramenti, G., Cremonesi, P., Valgimigli, F., Bongiovanni, C., & Varalli, M. (2003). A microdialysis technique for continuous subcutaneous glucose monitoring in diabetic patients (part 1). *Biosens Bioelectron*, Vol. 18, No. 7, (Jul. 2003), pp. 891-898, ISSN 0956-5663.

Raccah, D., Sulmont, V., Reznik, Y., Guerci, B., Renard, E., Hanaire, H., Jeandidier, N., & Nicolino, M. (2009). Incremental value of continuous glucose monitoring when starting pump therapy in patients with poorly controlled type 1 diabetes: the RealTrend study. *Diabetes Care*, Vol. 32, No. 12, (Dec. 2009), pp. 2245-2250, ISSN 0149-5992.

Radermecker, R.P., & Scheen, A.J. (2004). Continuous subcutaneous insulin infusion with short-acting insulin analogues or human regular insulin: efficacy, safety, quality of life, and cost-effectiveness. *Diabetes Metab Res Rev*, Vol. 20, No. 3 , (May-Jun. 2004), pp. 178-188, ISSN 1520-7552.

Schaepelynck-Bélicar, P., Simonin, G., & Lassmann-Vague, V. (2003). Improved metabolic control in diabetic adolescents using the continuous glucose monitoring system. *Diabetes Metab*, Vol. 29, No. 6, (Dec. 2003), pp. 608-612, ISSN 0742-3071.

Selvin, E., Marinopoulos, S., Berkenblit, G., Rami, T., Brancati, F.L., Powe, N.R., & Golden, S.H. (2004). Meta-analysis: glycosylated hemoglobin and cardiovascular disease in diabetes mellitus. *Ann Intern Med*, Vol. 141, No. 6, (Sept. 2004), pp. 421–431, ISSN 0003-4819.

Shalitin, S., Gil, M., Nimri, R., de Vries, L., Gavan, M.Y., & Phillip, M. (2010). Predictors of glycaemic control in patients with Type 1 diabetes commencing continuous subcutaneous insulin infusion therapy. *Diabet Med*, Vol. 27, No. 3, (Mar. 2010), pp. 339-347, ISSN 0742-3071.

Shichiri, M., Kishikawa, H., Ohkubo, Y., & Wake, N. (2000). Long-terms results of de Kumamoto Study on Optimal Diabetes Control in Type 2 Diabetic Patients. *Diabetes Care*, Vol. 23, Suppl. 2, (April 2000), pp. B21-B29, ISSN 0149-5992

Simon, J., Gray, A., Clarke, P., Wade, A., Neil, A., Farmer, A., & Diabetes Glycaemic Education and Monitoring Trial Group. (2008). Cost effectiveness of self monitoring of blood glucose in patients with non-insulin treated type 2 diabetes: economic evaluation of data from the DiGEM trial. *BMJ*, Vol. 336, No. 7654, (May 2008), pp. 1177-1180, ISSN 0959-535X.

Singh, S.R., Ahmad, F., LaI, A., Yu, C., Bai, Z., & Bennett, H.C. (2009). Efficacy and safety of insulin analogues for the management of diabetes mellitus: a meta-analysis. CMAJ Vol. 17, No. 4, (Feb. 2009), pp. 385-97, ISSN 1488-2329.

Skyler, J.S. (2009). Continuous glucose monitoring: An overview of its development. *Diabetes Technol Ther*, Vol. 11, Suppl. 1, (Jun. 2009), pp. 5-10, ISSN 1557-8593.

Stettler, C., Allemann, S., Jüni, P., Cull, C.A., Holman, R.R., Egger, M., Krähenbühl. S., & Diem, P. (2006). Glycemic control and macrovascular disease in types 1 and 2 diabetes mellitus: Meta-analysis of randomized trials. *Am Heart J*, Vol. 152, No. 1, (Jul. 2006), pp. 27–38, ISSN 0002-8703.

Tamborlane, W.V., Fredrickson, L.P., & Ahern, J.H. (2003). Insulin pump therapy in childhood diabetes mellitus: guidelines for use. *Treat Endocrinol*, Vol. 2, No. 1, (Jan. 2003), pp. 11-21, ISSN 1175-6349.

Tanenberg, R., Bode, B., Lane, W., Levetan, C., Mestman, J., Harmel, A.P., Tobian, J., Gross, T., & Mastrototaro, J. (2004). Use of the continuous glucose monitoring system to guide therapy in patients with insulin-treated diabetes: a randomized controlled trial. *Mayo Clin Proc*, Vol. 79, No. 12, (Dec. 2004), pp. 1521-6, ISSN 0025-6196.

Teutsch, S.M., Herman, W.H., Dwyer, D.M., & Lane, J.M. (1984). Mortality among diabetic patients using continuous insulin-infusion pumps. *N Eng J Med*, Vol. 310, No. 6, (Feb. 1984), pp. 361-368, ISSN 0028-4793.

Torres, I., Ortego, J., Valencia, I., García-Palacios, M.V., & Aguilar-Diosdado, M. (2009). Benefits of continuous subcutaneous insulin infusion in type 1 diabetes previously treated with multiple daily injections with once-daily glargine and pre-meal analogues. *Exp Clin Endocrinol Diabetes*, Vol. 117, No. 8, (Sept. 2009), pp. 378-385, ISSN 0947-7349.

Torres, I., Baena, M.G., Cayon, M., Ortego-Rojo, J., & Aguilar-Diosdado, M. (2010). Use of sensors in the treatment and follow-up of patients with diabetes mellitus. *Sensors*, Vol. 10, No. 8, (Aug. 2010), pp. 7404-7420, ISSN 1424-8220.

U.K. Prospective Diabetes Study (UKPDS) Group. (1998). Intensive blood glucose control with sulphonylureas or insulin compared with conventional treatment and risk of complications in patients with type 2 diabetes. *Lancet*, Vol. 352, No. 9131, (Sept. 1998), pp. 837-853, ISSN 0140-6736.

Varalli, M., Marelli, G., Maran, A., Bistoni, S., Luzzana, M., Cremonesi, P., Caramenti, G., Valgimigli, F., & Poscia, A. (2003). A microdialysis technique for continuous subcutaneous glucose monitoring in diabetic patients (part 2). *Biosens Bioelectron*, Vol. 18, No. 7, (Jul. 2003), pp. 899-905, ISSN 0956-5663.

Valeri, C., Pozsilli, P., & Leslie, D. (2004). Glucose control in diabetes. *Diabetes Metab Res Rev*, Vol. 20, Suppl. 2 (Nov-Dec. 2004), pp. S1-8, ISSN 1520-7552.

Volpe, L., Pancani, F., Aragona, M., Lencioni, C., Battini, L., Ghio, A., Resi, V., Bertolotto, A., Del Prato, S., & Di Cianni, G. (2010). Continuous subcutaneous insulin infusion and multiple dose insulin injections in Type 1 diabetic pregnant women: a case-control study. *Gynecol Endocrinol*, Vol. 26, No. 3, (Mar. 2010), pp. 193-196, ISSN 0951-3590.

Weintrob, N., Schechter, A., Benzaquen, H., Shalitin, S., Lilos, P., Galatzer, A., & Phillip, M. (2004). Glycemic patterns detected by continuous subcutaneous glucose sensing in children and adolescents with type 1 diabetes mellitus treated by multiple daily injections vs continuous subcutaneous insulin infusion. *Arch Pediatr Adolesc Med*, Vol. 158, No. 7, (Jul. 2004), pp. 677-84, ISSN 1072-4710.

Welschen, L.M., Nijpels, G., Dekker, J.M., Heine, R.J., Stalman, W.A., & Bouter, L.M. (2005). Self-monitoring of blood glucose in patients with type 2 diabetes who are not using insulin: a systematic review. *Diabetes Care*, Vol. 28, No. 6, (Jun. 2005), pp. 1510-1517, ISSN 0149-5992.

9

Generation of Insulin Producing Cells for the Treatment of Diabetes

Guo Cai Huang and Min Zhao
Department of Diabetes and Endocrinology,
King's College London School of Medicine, London
Great Britain

1. Introduction

The are approx. 177 million people suffering from diabetes worldwide and this number will be doubled by 2030. Patients with type 1 diabetes require multiple injections of insulin daily with doses careful adjusted on carbohydrate intake, level of activity and stress. Often there is a mismatch between insulin requirements and the calculated dose, resulting in hyper or hypo-glycaemia. Between 20-30% of patients however suffer from recurrent hypoglycaemia, which may require third party help (Geddes et al. 2008). Islet transplantation has been a promising therapy since the "Edmonton protocol" was published in 2000 (Shapiro et al. 2000). However, numbers of transplants remain low for a variety of reasons (Shapiro et al. 2006). One major hurdle to more widespread provision of this treatment remains a shortage of supply of donor organs, with only 25-30% of isolations resulting in islets of sufficient quantity and quality to be used in clinical transplantation, indicating a huge waste of valuable resources (Nano et al. 2005). Studies using animal models have found the evidences of neogenisis of beta cells under non-physiological condition as well the limited proliferation capacity of beta cells. Unfortunately, human beings cannot be manipulated to generate insulin-producing cells. There are increasing evidence suggested that glucose response insulin-producing cells could be generated in large quantity for human use. The following are a few possible aspects that can be explored for this purpose.

1.1 Beta cell replication and regeneration

There are substantial evidences suggesting that the adult pancreas can generate new β-cells in response to pancreatic damage or increased demand for insulin (Wang et al., 1995; Bonner-Weir et al., 1993; Guz et al., 2001). The source of new β-cells is thought to be the replication of existing β-cells under normal growth condition (Dor et al., 2004). However, the capacity of mature β-cells to proliferation and then re-differentiate back into β-cells has not been demonstrated *in vitro* and it still remains a challenge. In addition to the replication, there are mounting evidences indicated that regeneration of beta cells also contribute significantly to the new beta cells when pancreas is under non-physiological conditions such as partial pancreas duct ligation (Wang et al., 1995) or partial pancreatectomy (Finegood et al., 1999). However, such mechanisms are believed to have little implication to diabetes patients, as it is not possible to mimic the situations in animals to humans. Furthermore, even though there is regeneration of beta cells; the patients need immunosuppressive drugs to control the self-destruction of beta cells by autoimmune mechanisms. In addition to the beta cell proliferation, whether there are other cell sources for the beta cell neogenesis is not clear. It has been shown that human adult pancreases contain cells expressing Oct4 and Sox2 proteins (Zhao et al., 2007). The expression of Oct4 and Sox2 is thought to be related to the stemness of stem cells in human pancreas. The location of these cells in the small ducts is interesting (Fig 1) as it reflects the development of pancreas. Whether these cells are a part of the undifferentiated stem cells retained in ducts during the formation of pancreas and are the sources of new beta cells in adulthood remains unknown to us. The question is whether these cells are truly functional adult stem cells? If they are, how these cells contribute to the balance of beta cell number warrants further investigations. Insulin positive cells were indeed observed in the pancreas ducts (Bonner-Weir et al., 1993; Dudek et al., 1991; Pour 1994; Bouwens and Pipeleers 1998; li et al., 2010) and the findings that cells derived from rodent and human islets were multiple potency (Smukler et al., 2011) have further confirmed the possibility of presence of stem cells in adult pancreas. For this reason, human pancreatic ducts have been the target material for insulin-producing cells (Gmyr et al., 2004). Unfortunately the experiment protocol seemed not be optimal enough and generating insulin-producing cells from these duct cells is remaining illusive. Further investigation is required to determine whether there would be possible means to increase beta cells from the stem cells to treat diabetes in newly diagnosed diabetes patients together with immune modulation drugs.

1.2 Immunosuppression approach

When the patient is newly diaganisd as type 1 diabetes, there is often associated with a "honey-noon" phenominon. It is thought that there are new beta cells generated during this transient phase of disease. Earlier clinical trial using immunosuppressive drugs to inhibit the T cells did show the improvement in insulin secretion but at the price of worsening renal functions (Mirouze et al., 1986; Mandrup-Poulsen et al., 1990). These are believed to be the side effects of the immunosuppressive drugs to the kidneys while modulating the autoimmunity to protect beta cells. In 1990s, the most widely used drugs is cyclosporine, which is known to be toxic to beta cells (Hahn et al., 1986), will also damage the beta cells overtime. The trials with less cell toxic drugs such as anti-CD3 or anti-CD4 antibodies also showed some benefits in altering the disease course (Chatenoud et al., 1993; Phillips et al., 2000; Herold et al., 2002) but the hope of increasing new beta cells suficient to cure the disease still meets difficulty (Keymeulen et al., 2005). It is believed that the time to initiate such treatment is crucial as the ability to increase new beta cells is limited. This treatment could be used to prevent type 1 diabetes in risk population when there is still a surficient number of beta cells and with potential renewing beta cells, if such a population is identified.

1.3 Pancreas organ transplantation vs. islet cell transplantation

Human pancreas transplantation has been the main option for replacing the lost beta cells in type 1 diabetes patients since 1960s (Kelly et al., 1967; Hermon-Taylor 1970). Even now it is still the best option to treat diabetes. The insulin independency following pancreas organ transplantation is around 70-90% when the surgical procedures are successful. However, it is a major surgical procedure and is normally reserved for kidney and pancreas

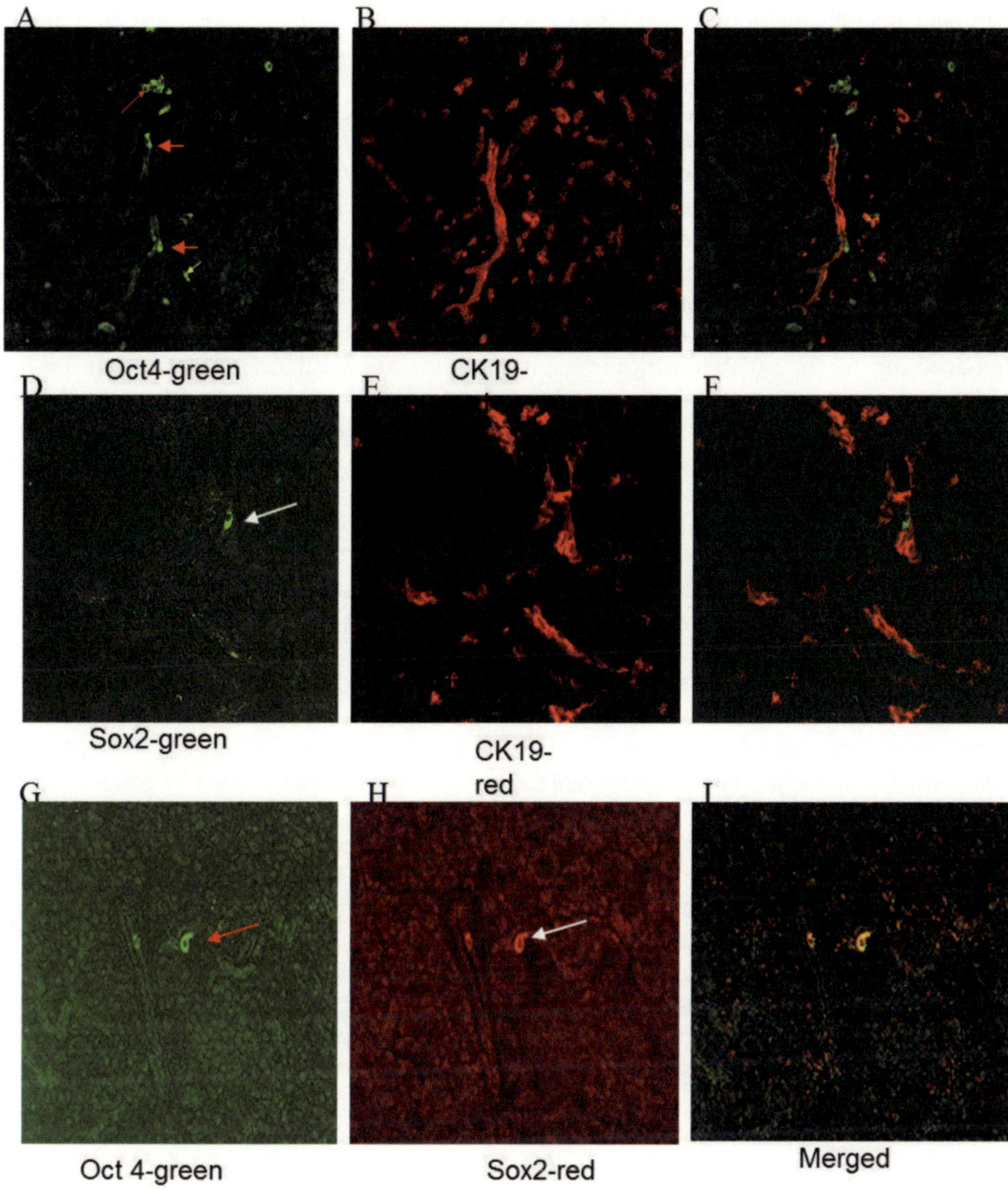

Typical immunohistochemical staining images of human pancreas sections for the Oct4, Sox2 expressing cells and their localization relevant to CK19^{+ve} cells. Panel A and G show Oct4^{+ve} cells (green) within the ductal structures and their surrounding area in a scattering pattern. Majority Oct4^{+ve} cells were shown cytopalsmic staining with only small number cells shown nuclei staining (arrowed). B and E show the CK19^{+ve} duct cells (red) and C is the merged of A and B. Panel D (green) and H (red) show Sox2 positive cells. F is the merge of D and E. Panel I is the merged of G (Oct4^{+ve}, Green) and H (Sox2^{+ve} Cells, Red), showing the colocalization of Oct4 and Sox2 positive cells.

Fig. 1. Immunohistochemical statining of the Oct-4 and Sox2 cells in human adult pancreas sections simultaneous transplantations just because it is a big operation procedure. Most old patients are not suitable for this approach as they are unable to tolerate the surgical procedures. The operation itself is associated with 10% mortality and mobility; often the patients need a second or third operation to correct the problem of exocrine enzyme leakage.

Human islet transplantation provides an alternative mean to restore the lost beta cells and it become a realistic option for a group of type 1 diabetes patients with bristle diabetes condition, especially for the group of patients with hypoglycaemia unawareness (Shapiro et al. 2000). The advantage for this approach is that it is a minor and less invasive procedure and a more safe approach for the replacement of lost beta cells. The disadvantages are that human pancreas is to be digested with a blend of collagenases and specialized proteases and human islets are purified from the exocrine tissues (Ricordi et al., 1989). Some islets are damaged during the isolation procedures. In addition, approximately 20-50% islets are lost under current density centrifugation purification techniques, which is based on the density differential between endocrine cells and exocrine cells. Therefore, it needs 2-3 pancreases to provide enough islet cell mass (~10,000 Islet IEQ/kg body weight) for one recipient. The human islets are then transplanted into the patient's liver via port vein, where the islets will set down in liver. The islets will function in the higher insulin concentration environment as comparison with those within pancreas. Therefore, this will require islets to work harder and lead to exhaustion of islets themselves. As the islets are digested away from the exocrine tissues, they are also cut away from the vascular system, which provides islets with essential nutrients, oxygen and neuron-regulating molecules and need to be revisualization following transplant. During the period of avascular state, the islets are very vulnerable to any attack, such as inflammatory factors and the cytotoxicity of the immunosuppressive drugs, as the cells take in nutrients and oxygen through passive perfusion, which is very inefficient. Since the body immune system destroys tissues it recognises as "foreign" and the nature of autoimmune disease in the patients, immunosuppressive drugs are given to the patients before, during and after transplant to protect the grafts from allo-rejection and the reoccurrence of autoimmunity. The immune regulation medication has several drawbacks currently. First, the immunosuppressive drugs have significant side effects and some patients cannot tolerate one or another immunosuppressive regimens. The patients have to take the drugs life long in order to protect the islet grafts and to prevent from getting sensitisation against donor tissues. There would be some implications for the risk of tumour generation, as the recipients may not have the full immune capacity to fight tumour cells although there is no such report yet. For the reason of toxicity of the immunosuppressive drugs, this approach is only suitable for a small group of patients. It is not yet suitable for young children simply it is not worthy taking immunosuppressive drugs. Secondly, the drugs also show some degrees of toxicity to beta cells and the drugs will reduce the islet cell mass overtime. The long-term prospect of islet transplantation currently is not yet satisfactory, with only ~13% of transplant patients remaining insulin independence for >5 years, although most patients still have endogenous C-peptide product and benefit from the better control of their blood glucose (Ryan et al., 2005). Thirdly, as to the drawback mentioned above, it requires 2-3 donor organs to generate enough islet cell mass to reach to >10,000 islet IEQ/kg body weight of the recipient. The large islet IEQ is needed because some islets will not survive during the avascular state, which deprive themselves of essential nutrients and oxygen, and the toxicity of immune modulation agents. This will obviously worsen the situation on the already limited supply of donor organs. Fourthly, the reoccurrence autoimmune attack on the grafts developed overtime, which seemed to be able to escape the current immunosuppressive regimens applied. The future work should concentrate on protecting islets during and post-transplantation and development of less toxic immune suppression drugs.

Despite the drawback mentioned above, for patients with bristle diabetic conditions and patients with pancreatectomy (due to prolonged pancreatitis), the beta cell replacement still remains the best option. To make this beta cell replacement as a wider applicable approach for the treatment of diabetes patients, the limitation of glucose responsive insulin-producing cells is the key obstacle and must be addressed. For patients with type 2 diabetes, current islet cell transplantation is insufficient as the demand for insulin-producing cells for these patients is far greater than type 1 diabetes patients. However, this approach could be applied to patients with type 2 diabetes, if the cell source of insulin surrogates is unlimited. For the later, there is only one need, that is, to prevent the allo-graft rejection.

2. Generation of glucose responsive insulin-producing cells

Many type of cells have been used to generate glucose responsive insulin-producing cells with limited success. These include the differentiation of embryonic and adult stem cells and transdifferentiation from other types of cells into insulin producing cells (Fujikawa et al., 2005; Zhao et al., 2005 and 2008; Kroon et al., 2008; Boyd et al., 2009; Tateishi et al., 2008; Zhou et al., 2008; Gabr et al., 2008; Zhang et al., 2009; Cai et al., 2010). However, the success has been limited to small animal models. The focus of this chapter is to briefly discuss the potentiality involved in our laboratories.

2.1 Islet cells replication *in vitro*

Islets of Langerhans are the endocrine mini-organs consisted of 4 major different endocrine cells: α-cells controlling the release of glucagon; β-cells for insulin, δ-cells for somatostatin and the pp cells-polypeptide. These 4 types of endocrine cells work together in a complex interplay in the maintaining of homeostasis of blood glucose level. Islet cells need to stay together as a cluster to function better as indicated by the finding that single Min 6 (mouse beta cell line) cells do not express and secret insulin as well as those when the Min 6 cells are forming as a cluster-called pseudoislets (Hauge-Evans et al., 1999). Human islets cultured in monolayer tend to lose the capacity gradually to express insulin within 5 weeks (Fig.2). Human islet cells cultured in 3-dimension seemed to be able to retain beta cell phenotype. However cells, particularly those at the centre of the clusters, will die due to necrosis if the cells cultured as 3-dimensional manner for too long. This is because that cells located in the centre of the 3-dimension will depend on the perfusion of nutrients and oxygen, which is very insufficient. We therefore developed a method to culture the cells in a rotation manner between monolayer culture (2-dimension) and cluster culture (3-dimension), the cells have acquired the survive signal through the 2-dimensional culture and can also maintain the capacity to express insulin through the 3-dimensional culture. The cells can maintain this capacity to express insulin and respond to glucose challenge for >4 months *in vitro*. When the cells were transplanted into SCID (an immune deficient mouse) mice, rendered diabetes by the injection of straptozotosin (STZ), they were able to correct the hyperglycaemia and maintaining the homeostasis of blood glucose (Fig. 3; Zhao et al., 2002). The beauty of this model is to provide a prototype model to analyse beta cell differentiation. The ability of beta cells to proliferate *in vitro* has been demonstrated in many studies (Beattie et al., 1999; 2000

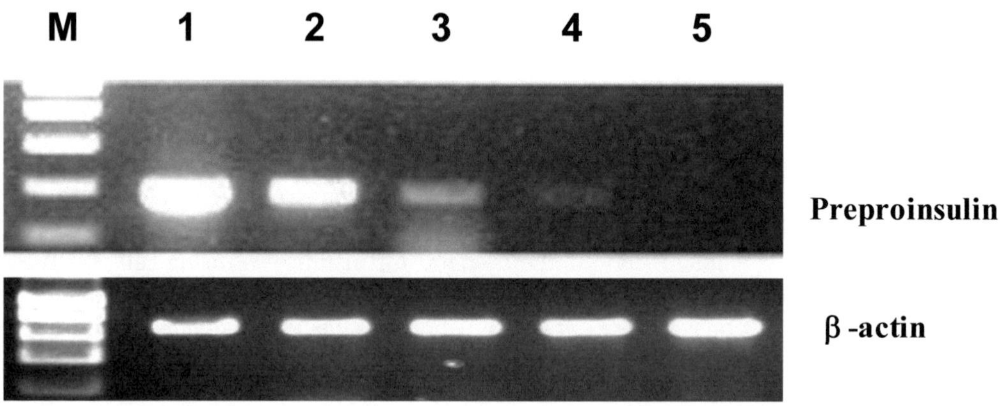

Semi-quantitative RT- PCR analysis. 5 weeks continuously monolayer cultured human islet cells were induced to express insulin. Total RNA were isolated from each different condition. cDNA derived from 4ng of total RNA were used to amplify preproinsulin and actin. 5 = 5weeks monolayer cultured human islet cells.

Fig. 2. Analyses the expression of insulin in continual monolayer culture

and 2002; Halvorsen et al., 2000; Gershengorn et al., 2004; Lechner et al., 2005; Ouziel-Yahalom et al., 2006;) and was directly confirmed in a study with GFP labelled beta cells using a lentinvirus system (Russ et al., 2008). However, the purpose of *ex vivo* expansion of human islets is to increase the glucose responsive insulin-producing cells for research and eventually for transplantation to treat diabetes. Unfortunately, making the proliferated insulin-producing cells to express insulin again in a glucose responsive manner is still a big challenge to us. Using a lentinvirus labelling system developed by Russ and colleagues, we were able to show that a small percentage of beta cells (GFP expressing cells) were found to be positive for insulin and Ki67--a proliferation marker *in vitro* (Fig. 4; Zhao et al., unpublished). This result illustrated that beta cells have the potential to be expanded *ex vivo*. The question is how to make this more efficient to achieve large number of cells for the treat of diabetes patients.

2.2 Human exocrine cells

From the development point of view, exocrine cells are the excellent candidate materials for insulin-producing cells as they share the same origin with the pancreatic endocrine cells (Slack 1995). Mouse exocrine cells have shown the flexibility to be converted into insulin-producing cells following chemical treatment (Lardon at al., 2004; Baeyens et al., 2005; Zhou et al., 2008). Therefore, there is good reason to believe that it is possible to convert human exocrine cells into endocrine cells. In terms of cell number, exocrine cells consist of 90% pancreatic cells with approximate 40-50 folds of their endocrine cell count apart, which consists of less than ~2% of total pancreatic cells. Secondly, it is already available. Following human islet isolation, the exocrine cells will be the waste material and are discarded at end. Thirdly, following dedifferentiation there is no obvious difference between the two types of cells. Both cells began to express CK19—a ductal cell marker. This is interesting because that both types of cells are derived from ductal cells during pancreas development (Slack 1995). Whether to differentiate into exocrine cells or into endocrine cells is under the complex interplays of complex genes at that stage. Gene Ptf1a may play a big role in the

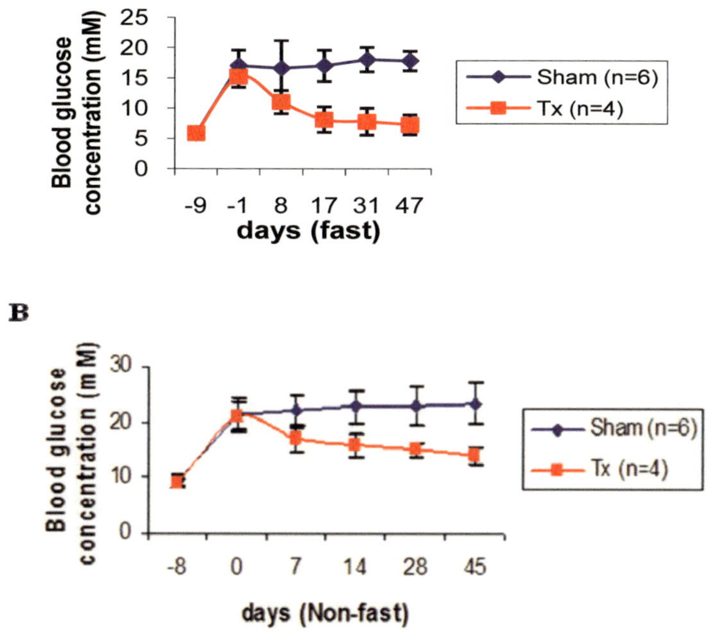

Blood glucose level (mM) of the STZ induced diabetic SCID mice before and after transplantation of long term cultured islets or sham control. Time of transplantation and sham was assigned as 0 day (d) and the time before surgery was indicated as –d. A shows the overnight fasting blood glucose level, solid square = islet cell transplanted (Tx), and the solid diamond shape = sham control. B shows the non-fasting blood glucose levels, solid square = islet cell transplanted (Tx), and solid diamond shape = sham control. The decrease in blood glucose levels was significant in both fasting and non-fasting with student t pair-test at $P<0.023$ and $P<0.002$ respectively. The difference in blood glucose levels between transplantation and sham groups was also significant ($P<0.02$and 0.023 respectively).

Fig. 3. Analyses of the blood glucose levels in mice transplanted with long term cultured human islet cells

determination of cells to exocrine cell fate (Dong et al., 2008). The mechanism of how exocrine cells being converted into endocrine cells is not clear and under our experimental conditions, it requires the gene products from beta cells and the right differentiation environments. Under the Pdx-1 gene influence, exocrine cells express some beta cell phenotype marker following differentiation induction with a cocktail of differentiation inducers (GLP-1, activin A, betacellulin, nicotinamide and glucose, Zhao et al., 2005) and expressed low level of insulin (Fig. 5) *in vitro*. The time to introduce Pdx-1 is seemed to be critical, although we did not have biomarkers to match this window exactly for the gene induction. We speculated that a short window existed during the dedifferentiation of exocrine cells. During which, exocrine cells would be more ready to be induced to express beta cell markers. The cells showed a glucose response *in vitro* when challenged with glucose. But the response was not typical as the background secretion is too high and the challenge secretion is too low in comparison with islet cells, suggesting the insulin-producing cells were immature. As predicted, these cells matured further following transplant in SCID mice, rendered diabetes with the injection of STZ solution. This approach is sufficient to work in small laboratory animals with ~40% mice recovered from the mild

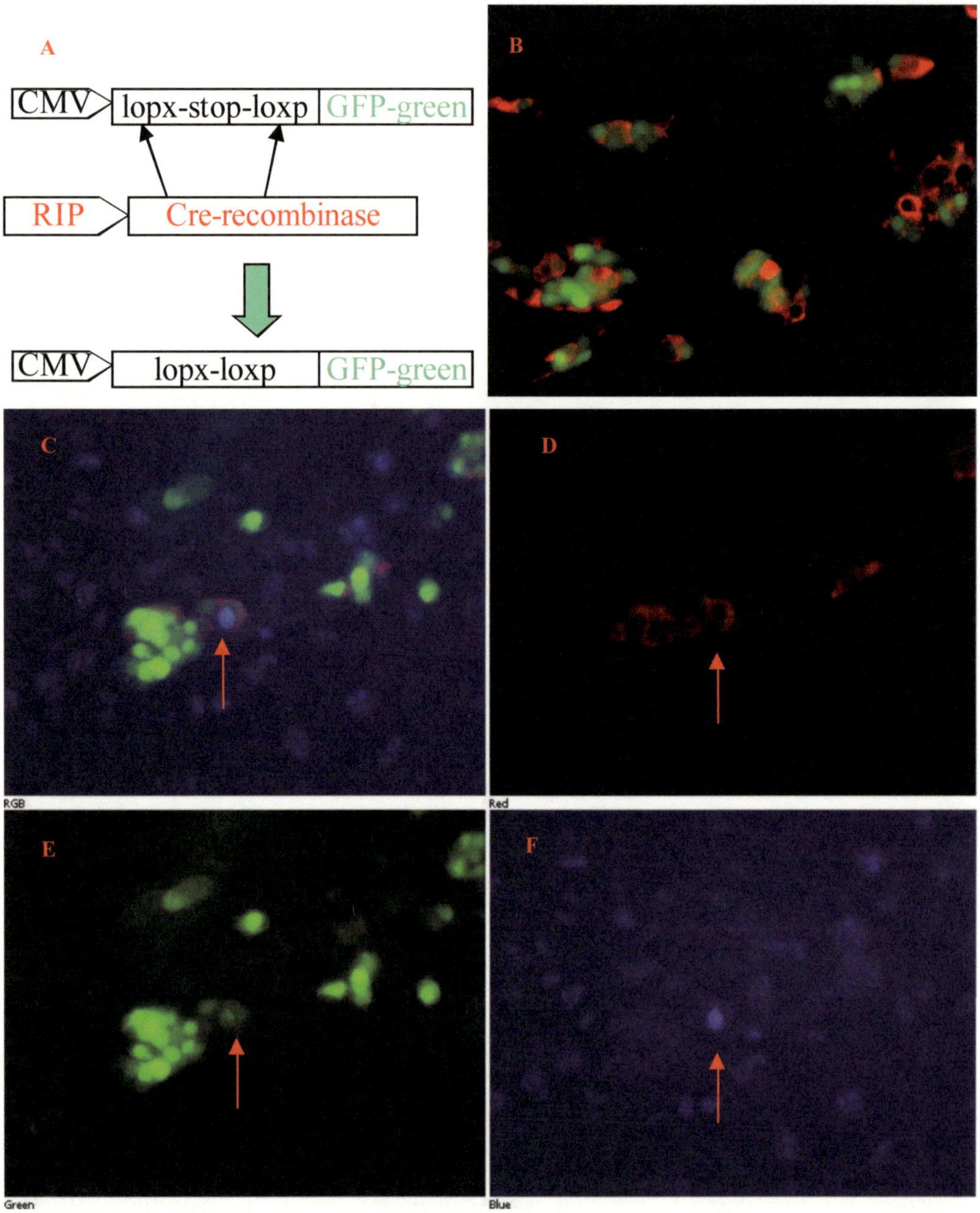

Genomic labelling of human beta cells and differentiation induction assessment. Panel A: the methed used in the labelling of human beta cells (Russ et al., 2008). Panel B: Control experiment of differentiation induction in the labelling beta cells. Beta cells were labelled as green and the cells were staining for insulin (Red). Panel D, E, F were images catched for red (insulin, D), green (beta cells, E) and blue (for Ki67 protein F). Panel C was the merged images of D, E, F. The proliferated beta cell was indicated by the arrow.

Fig. 4. Analyses the potential of proliferated adult human beta cells to reexpress insulin

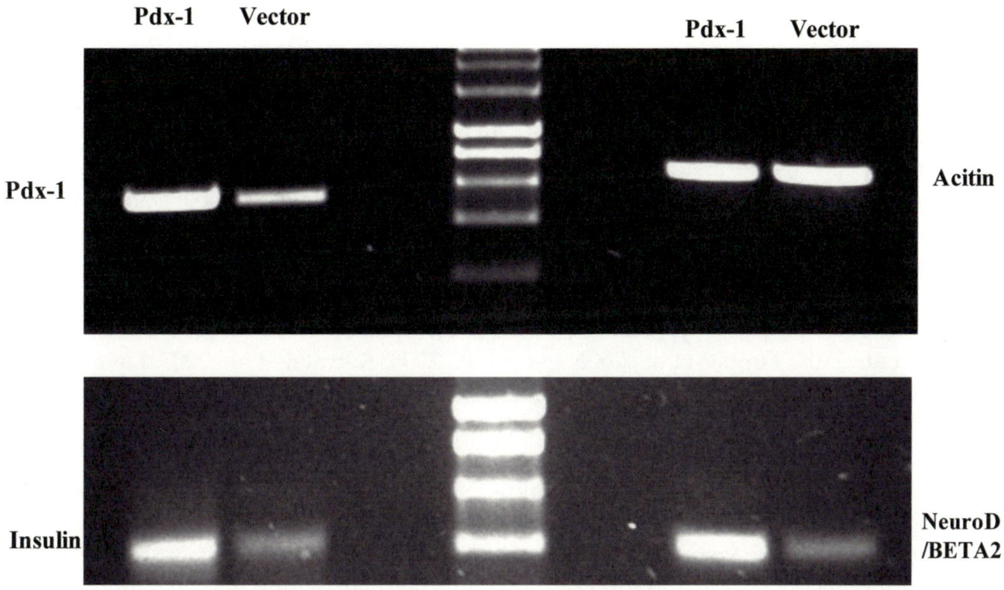

The dedifferentiated human pancreatic exocrine cells expressed insulin and NeuroD1/Beta 2 genes after transfection with Pdx-1 gene and differentiation induction, analysed by semi-quantitative RT-PCR.

Fig. 5. Expression of beta cell phenotype genes in manipulated human non-endocrine pancreatic cells in vitro

diabetes. The grafts showed that glucagon and somatostatin were also expressed in addition to the insulin (Fig.6), indicating that exocrine cells can be converted into whole pancreatic endocrine cells, not just insulin producing cells. Further works are required to explore the full potential of exocrine cells in order to create enough insulin producing materials for the treatment of diabetes.

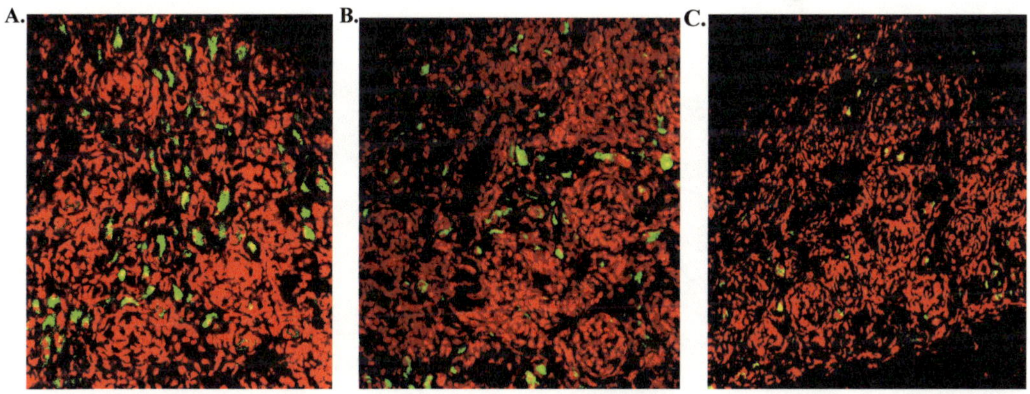

Immunohistochemical staining of the grafts (visulised by confocal microscope) for markers of the pancreatic endocrine cells. Insulin (A, 15±6.7%), Glucagon (B, 8±2.3%) and Somatostatin (C, 3±1.85%) positive cells are shown in green (FITC) and nuclei are stained with propidium iodide (red). Original amplification x40

Fig. 6. The expression of pancreatic endocrine cell hormones in the transdifferentiated cells.

2.3 Mesenchymal stem cell

Mesenchymal stem cells (MSCs) are the nonhematopoietic multipotent progenitor cells found in various adult tissues. Bone marrow derived MSC cells are those cells can adhere to plastic culture flask and proliferate *in vitro* (Kadiyala et al., 1997). The cells have the potential to be expanded *in vitro* in large quantity. MSC under specific differentiation environments can differentiate into cells with phenotypes of many specific tissues, such as bone, adipose and neurons (Pittenger et al., 1999; Deans and Moseley 2000; Deng et al., 2006; Gabr et al., 2008). MSC has the capacity to modulate host immune cells (see review papers in Bunnell et al., 2011) and express molecule help themselves evade the immune attack (El Haddad et al., 2011). The ability of MSC to become insulin-producing cells has been in debates and been controversy (Lechner et al., 2004; Taneera et al., 2006; Butle et al., 2007; Moriscot et al., 2005; Timper et al., 2006; Lee et al., 2006; Karnieli et al., 2007; Lavazais et al., 2007; Hasegawa et al., 2007; Denner et al., 2007). Human bone marrow MSC express low level of Oct4 and Sox2 as well Pdx-1—an important gene involve in the development of beta cells and the maintaining of beta cell phenotype in adult, indicative that these cells could be differentiated into glucose responsive insulin- producing cells. Under the influence of the gene products of Pdx-1, NeuroD1/BETA2 and Ngn3, the MSC express insulin gene *in vitro* following differentiation induction with a cocktail of differentiation inducers (GLP-1, activin A, betacellulin, nicotinamide and glucose). The cells seemed lacking insulin storage capacity and secreted insulin as it was synthesised. Therefore these cells were not glucose responsive *in vitro*. Following transplantation into SCID diabetes mice, the cells were able to mature further and expressed most beta cell phenotype gene markers, such as Glut-2 and Kir6.2 (Fig. 7A) and insulin processing enzymes, but the cells did not express Surl gene and therefore did not have a functional K-ATP channel. Interestingly the cells also expressed glucagon gene, indicating that some cells also differentiated into α-cells (Fig.7B) in addition to insulin producing cells. Nevertheless, the hyperglycaemia in the transplanted mice was corrected despite that the transplanted mice had some impairment in glucose tolerant in comparison with mice transplanted with human islets (Fig. 8 and Zhao et al., 2008). These

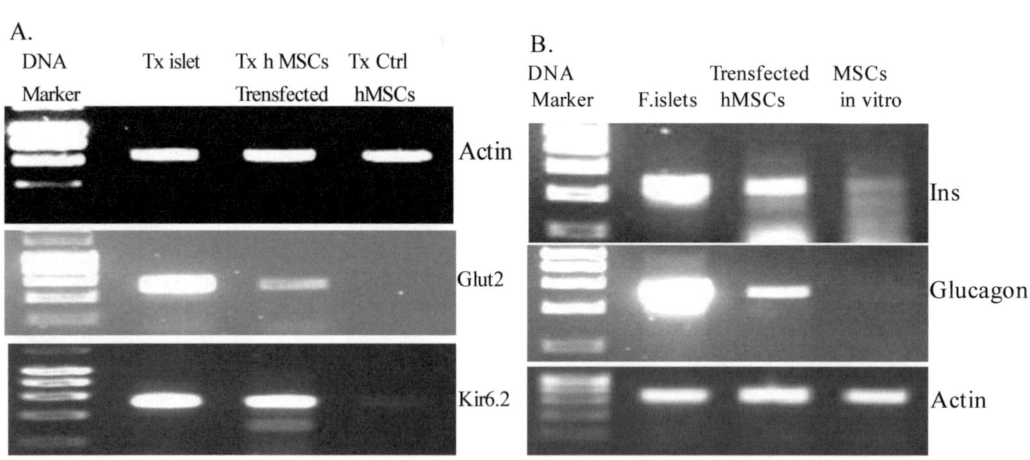

Analyses of the expression of β and α cell genes by semi-quatatative RT-PCR on kidneys transplanted with the cells.

Fig. 7. Gene expression analyses on the transplanted kidneys by semi-quatative RT-PCR data suggested that the MSC achieve partial glucose responsiveness through non-ATP K channel mechanism. The MSC did not form any teratoma structures *in vivo;* making it an idea candidate to be beta cell surrogates for the treatment of diabetes.

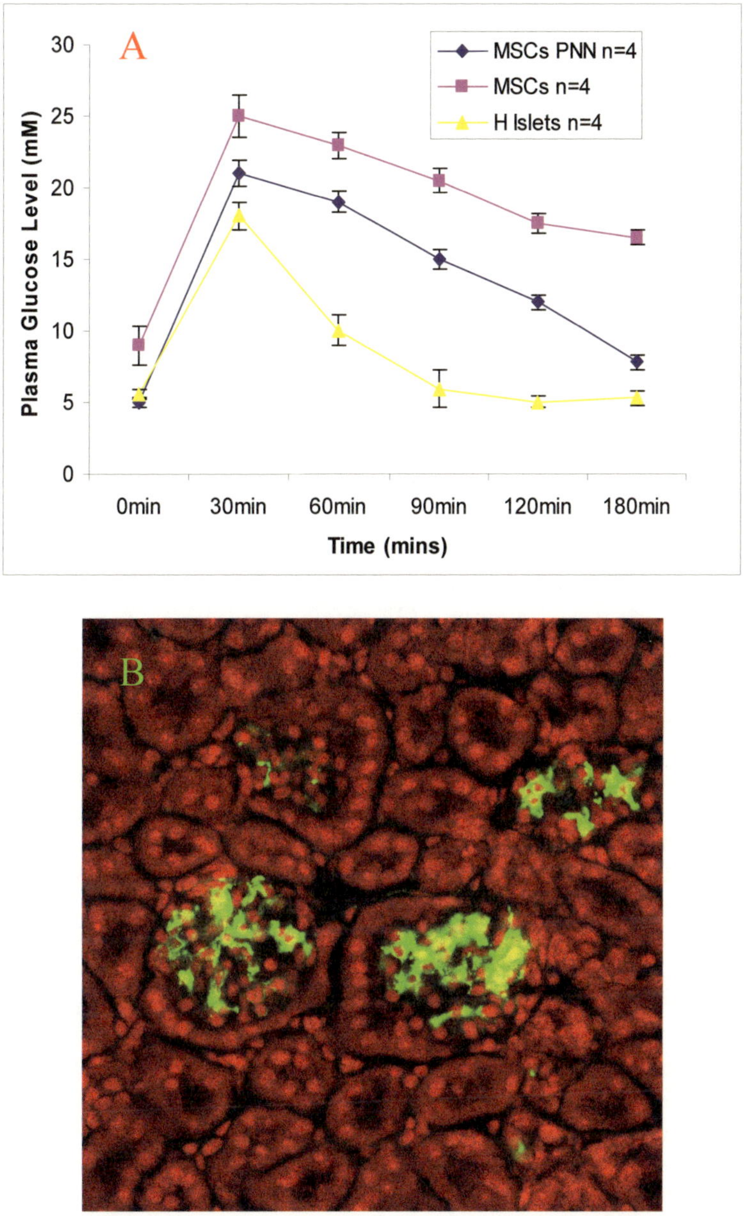

Panel A. Mice transplanted wtih the Pdx-1, Ngn3 and euroD1/Beta2 genes shows response to glucose challenge During a glucose tolerlant test. Panel B shows the manipulated human MSC expressing insulin (green fluorescence) in diabetic mice.

Fig. 8. Functional analyses in mice transplanted with human MSC cells

3. Conclusion and future direction of investigation

There are mounting evidences including our own data described above suggested that insulin-producing cells can be generated from many cells through the differentiation of stem cells (embryonic stem cells to adult stem cells) or via the transdifferentiation mechanisms. However, there are challenges ahead. The most urgent tasks are 1) to optimise the differentiation protocols to make them more efficiency by optimising the differentiation inducers and the extracellular environments; 2) to identify the molecular mechanisms associated with the differentiation to allow the translation of bench discovery to bedside treatments; 3) to enhance the efficacy to increase the cell mass for human usage.

4. References

Baeyens L. De Breuck S.. Lardon J... Mfopou J. K.Rooman I. Bouwens L. (2005) In vitro generation of insulin-producing cells from adult exocrine pancreatic cells. Diabetologia 48: 49–57

Beattie GM, Itkin-Ansari P, Cirulli V, Leibowitz G, Lopez AD, Bossie S, Mally MI, Levine F, Hayek A (1999): Sustained proliferation of PDX-1_ cells derived from human islets. *Diabetes* 48:1013–1019

Beattie GM, Leibowitz G, Lopez AD, Levine F, Hayek A (2000): Protection from cell death in cultured human fetal pancreatic cells. *Cell Transplant*9:431– 438,

Beattie GM, Montgomery AM, Lopez AD, Hao E, Perez B, Just ML, Lakey JR, Hart ME, Hayek A (2002): A novel approach to increase human islet cell mass while preserving _-cell function. *Diabetes* 51:3435–3439

Bonner-Weir S, Baxter LA, Schuppin GT, Smith FE (1993) A second pathway for regeneration of adult exocrine and endocrine pancreas. A possible recapitulation of embryonic development. Diabetes. 42:1715-20

Bouwens, L., and Pipeleers, D.G. (1998) Extra-insular beta-cells associated with ductules are frequent in adult human pancreas. Diabetologia, 41:629–633.

Boyd, A. S. & Wood, K. J (2009): Variation in MHC expression between undifferentiated mouse ES cells and ES cell-derived insulin-producing cell clusters. *Transplantation* 87, 1300–1304

Butler AE, Huang A, Rao PN, Bhushan A, Hogan WJ et al. (2007) Hematopoietic stem cells derived from adult donors are not a source of pancreatic beta-cells in adult nondiabetic humans. Diabetes. 56(7): 1810-6.

Bunnell BA, Betancourt AM, Sullivan DE. New concepts on the immune modulation mediated by mesenchymal stem cells. Stem Cell Res Ther. 2010 Nov 11;1(5):34.

Cai J, Yu C, Liu Y, Chen S, Guo Y, Yong J, Lu W, Ding M, Deng H (2009). Generation of homogeneous PDX1(+) pancreatic progenitors from human ES cell-derived endoderm cells. J Mol Cell Biol. 2010 Feb;2(1):50-60.

Chatenoud L, Thervet E, Primo J, Bach JF (1994): Anti-CD3 antibody induces long-term remission of overt autoimmunity in nonobese diabetic mice. *Proc Natl Acad Sci U S A* 91:123–127

Deans RJ, Moseley AB (2008). Mesenchymal stem cells: biology and potential clinical uses. Exp Hematol;28:875-884.

Deng J, Petersen BE, Steindler DA, Jorgensen ML, Laywell ED (2006). Mesenchymal stem cells spontaneously express neural proteins in culture and are neurogenic after transplantation. Stem Cells.24(4):1054-64.

Denner L, Bodenburg Y, Zhao JG, Howe M, Cappo J, Tilton RG, Copland JA, Forraz N, McGuckin C, Urban R. Stark (2007) Directed engineering of umbilical cord blood stem cells to produce C-peptide and insulin. Cell Prolif. 40(3):367-80.

Dong PD, Provost E, Leach SD, Stainier DY (2008). Graded levels of Ptf1a differentially regulate endocrine and exocrine fates in the developing pancreas. Genes Dev. 22(11):1445-50.

Dor Y, Brown J, Martinez OI, Melton DA (2004) Adult pancreatic beta-cells are formed by self-duplication rather than stem-cell differentiation. Nature. 429:41-6

Dudek, R.W., Lawrence, I.E., Hill, R.S., and Johnson, R.C. (1991) Induction of islet cytodifferentiation by fetal mesenchyme in adult pancreatic ductal epithelium. Diabetes, 40:1041–1048.

El Haddad N, Heathcote D, Moore R, Yang S, Azzi J, Mfarrej B, Atkinson M, Sayegh

MH, Lee JS, Ashton-Rickardt PG, Abdi R (2011). Mesenchymal stem cells express serine protease inhibitor to evade the host immune response. Blood.117(4):1176-83.

Finegood DT, Weir GC, Bonner-Weir S (1999). Prior streptozotocin treatment does not inhibit pancreas regeneration after 90% pancreatectomy in rats. Am J Physiol. 276(5 Pt 1):E822-7.

Fujikawa T, Oh SH, Pi L, Hatch HM, Shupe T, Petersen BE (2005) Teratoma formation leads to failure of treatment for type I diabetes using embryonic stem cell-derived insulin-producing cells. Am J Pathol.166(6):1781-91.

Gabr, M. M., Sobh, M. M., Zakaria, M. M., Refaie, A. F. & Ghoneim, M. A (2008). Transplantation of insulin-producing clusters derived from adult bone marrow stem cells to treat diabetes in rats. *Exp. Clin. Transplant.* 6, 236–243

Geddes J, Schopman JE, Zammitt NN, Frier BM. (2008). "Prevalence of impaired awareness of hypoglycaemia in adults with Type 1 diabetes." Diabet.Med. 25(4): 501-504.

Gershengorn MC, Hardikar AA, Wei C, Geras-Raaka E, Marcus-Samuels B, Raaka BM (2004): Epithelial-to-mesenchymal transition generates proliferative human islet precursor cells. *Science* 306:2261–2264

Guz Y, Nasir I, Teitelman G (2001) Regeneration of pancreatic beta cells from intra-islet precursor cells in an experimental model of diabetes. Endocrinology 142: 4956-68

Gmyr V, Belaich S, Muharram G, Lukowiak B, Vandewalle B, Pattou F, Kerr-Conte (2004). Rapid purification of human ductal cells from human pancreatic fractions with surface antibody CA19-9. Biochem Biophys Res Commun. 320(1):27-33.

Hahn HJ, Laube F, Lucke S, Klöting I, Kohnert KD, Warzock R (1986). Toxic effects of cyclosporine on the endocrine pancreas of Wistar rats. Transplantation. 41(1):44-7.

Halvorsen TL, Beattie GM, Lopez AD, Hayek A, Levine F (2000): Accelerated telomere shortening and senescence in human pancreatic islet cells stimulated to divide in vitro. *J Endocrinol* 166:103–109

Hasegawa Y, Ogihara T, Yamada T, Ishigaki Y, Imai J, Uno K, Gao J, Kaneko K, Ishihara H, Sasano H, Nakauchi H, Oka Y, Katagiri H (2007). Bone marrow (BM) transplantation promotes beta-cell regeneration after acute injury through BM cell mobilization. Endocrinology. 148(5):2006-15.

Hauge-Evans AC, Squires PE, Persaud SJ, Jones PM (1999). Pancreatic beta-cell-to-beta-cell interactions are required for integrated responses to nutrient stimuli: enhanced Ca2+ and insulin secretory responses of MIN6 pseudoislets. Diabetes. 48(7):1402-8.

Hermon-Taylor J (1970). [A review of pancreatic transplantation in man, and function of the pancreaticoduodenal graft]. Proc R Soc Med. 63(5):436.

Herold KC, Hagopian W, Auger JA, Poumian-Ruiz E, Taylor L, Donaldson D, Gitelman SE, Harlan DM, Xu D, Zivin RA, Bluestone JA (2002): Anti-CD3 monoclonal antibody in new-onset type 1 diabetes mellitus. *N Engl J Med* 346:1692–1698

Kadiyala S, Young RG, Thiede MA, Bruder SP (1997). Culture expanded canine mesenchymal stem cells possess osteochondrogenic potential in vivo and in vitro. Cell Transplant. 6(2):125-34.

Karnieli O, Izhar-Prato Y, Bulvik S, Efrat S (2007) Generation of Insulin-producing Cells From Human Bone Marrow Mesenchymal Stem Cells By Genetic Manipulation. Stem Cells. 25:2837-44.

Kelly W D, Lillehei R C, Merkel F K, Idezuki Y & Goetz F C (1967) Surgery 61, 827

Keymeulen B, Vandemeulebroucke E, Ziegler AG, Mathieu C, Kaufman L, Hale G, Gorus F, Goldman M, Walter M, Candon S, Schandene L, Crenier L, De Block C, Seigneurin JM, De Pauw P, Pierard D, Weets I, Rebello P, Bird P, Berrie E, Frewin M, Waldmann H, Bach JF, Pipeleers D, Chatenoud L (2005): Insulin needs after CD3-antibody therapy in new-onset type 1 diabetes. *N Engl J Med* 352:2598 –2608

Kroon E, Martinson LA, Kadoya K, Bang AG, Kelly OG, Eliazer S, Young H, Richardson M, Smart NG, Cunningham J, Agulnick AD, D'Amour KA, Carpenter MK, Baetge EE (2008). Pancreatic endoderm derived from human embryonic stem cells generates glucose-responsive insulin-secreting cells *in vivo*. *Nat. Biotechnol.* 26, 443–452

Lardon J, Huyens N, Rooman I, Bouwens L (2004) Exocrine cell transdifferentiation in dexamethasone-treated rat pancreas. Virchows Arch. 444:61-5

Lavazais E, Pogu S, SaÃ¯ P, Martignat L (2007). Cytokine mobilization of bone marrow cells and pancreatic lesion do not improve streptozotocin-induced diabetes in mice by transdifferentiation of bone marrow cells into insulin-producing cells. Diabetes Metab.33(1):68-78

Lechner A, Yang YG, Blacken RA, Wang L, Nolan AL, Habener JF. (2004) No evidence for significant transdifferentiation of bone marrow into pancreatic beta-cells in vivo. Diabetes. 53: 616-23.

Lechner A, Nolan AL, Blacken RA, Habener JF (2005): Redifferentiation of insulin-secreting cells after in vitro expansion of adult human pancreatic islet tissue. *Biochem Biophys Res Commun* 327:581–588

Lee RH, Seo MJ, Reger RL, Spees JL, Pulin AA, Olson SD, Prockop DJ. (2006) Multipotent stromal cells from human marrow home to and promote repair of pancreatic islets and renal glomeruli in diabetic NOD/scid mice. Proc. Natl. Acad. Sci. U.S.A. 103: 17438-43.

Li WC, Rukstalis JM, Nishimura W, Tchipashvili V, Habener JF, Sharma A, Bonner-Weir S (2010). Activation of pancreatic-duct-derived progenitor cells during pancreas regeneration in adult rats. J Cell Sci. 2010;123(Pt 16):2792-802.

Mandrup-Poulsen T, Mølvig J, Andersen HU, Helqvist S, Spinas GA, Munck M. Steno Memorial Hospital, Gentofte, Denmark (1990). Lack of predictive value of islet cell antibodies, insulin antibodies, and HLA-DR phenotype for remission in

cyclosporin-treated IDDM patients. The Canadian-European Randomized Control Trial Group. Diabetes. 39(2):204-10.
Mirouze J, Rodier M, Richard JL, Lachkar H, Monnier L (1986). Trial of mild immunosuppression by methisoprinol in acute onset diabetes mellitus: effects on rate and duration of remission. Diabetes Res. 3(7):359-62.
Moriscot C, de Fraipont F, Richard MJ, Marchand M, Savatier P, Bosco D, Favrot M, Benhamou PY. (2005) Human bone marrow mesenchymal stem cells can express insulin and key transcription factors of the endocrine pancreas developmental pathway upon genetic and/or microenvironmental manipulation in vitro. Stem Cells. 23: 594-603.
Nano R, Clissi B, Melzi R, Calori G, Maffi P, Antonioli B, Marzorati S, Aldrighetti L, Freschi M, Grochowiecki T, Socci C, Secchi A, Di Carlo V, Bonifacio E, Bertuzzi F. (2005). "Islet isolation for allotransplantation: variables associated with successful islet yield and graft function." Diabetologia 48(5): 906-12.
Ouziel-Yahalom L, Zalzman M, Anker-Kitai L, Knoller S, Bar Y, Glandt M, Herold K, Efrat S (2006): Expansion and redifferentiation of adult human pancreatic islet cells. *Biochem Biophys Res Commun* 341:291–298
Phillips JM, Harach SZ, Parish NM, Fehervari Z, Haskins K, Cooke A (2000): Nondepleting anti-CD4 has an immediate action on diabetogenic effector cells, halting their destruction of pancreatic beta cells. *J Immunol* 165:1949 –1955
Pittenger MF, Mackay AM, Beck SC, Jaiswal RK, Douglas R, Mosca JD, Moorman MA, Simonetti DW, Craig S, Marshak DR. (1999). Multilineage potential of adult human mesenchymal stem cells. Science 284:143-147.
Pour, P.M. (1994) Pancreatic centroacinar cells. The regulator of both exocrine and endocrine function. Int. J. Pancreatol., 15:51–64.
Ricordi C, Lacy PE, Scharp DW (1989). Automated islet isolation from human pancreas. Diabetes. 38 Suppl 1:140-2.
Russ HA, Bar Y, Ravassard P, Efrat S (2008).In vitro proliferation of cells derived from adult human beta-cells revealed by cell-lineage tracing. Diabetes 57(6):1575-83
Ryan EA, Paty BW, Senior PA, Bigam D, Alfadhli E, Kneteman NM, Lakey JR, Shapiro AM. (2005). Five-year follow-up after clinical islet transplantation. *Diabetes* 54: 2060-9.
Shapiro AM, Lakey JR, Ryan EA, Korbutt GS, Toth E, Warnock GL, Kneteman NM, Rajotte RV. (2000). Islet transplantation in seven patients with type 1 diabetes mellitus using a glucocorticoid-free immunosuppressive regimen." N Engl J Med 343(4): 230-8.
Shapiro AM, Ricordi C, Hering BJ, Auchincloss H, Lindblad R, Robertson RP, Secchi A, Brendel MD, Berney T, Brennan DC, Cagliero E, Alejandro R, Ryan EA, DiMercurio B, Morel P, Polonsky KS, Reems JA, Bretzel RG, Bertuzzi F, Froud T, Kandaswamy R, Sutherland DE, Eisenbarth G, Segal M, Preiksaitis J, Korbutt GS, Barton FB, Viviano L, Seyfert-Margolis V, Bluestone J, Lakey JR. (2006). International trial of the Edmonton protocol for islet transplantation. N Engl J Med 355(13): 1318-30.
Slack JM (1995) Developmental biology of the pancreas. Development. 121: 1569-80
Smukler SR, Arntfield ME, Razavi R, Bikopoulos G, Karpowicz P, Seaberg R, Dai F, Lee S, Ahrens R, Fraser PE, Wheeler MB, van der Kooy D (2011). The adult mouse and human pancreas contain rare multipotent stem cells that express insulin. Cell Stem Cell. 8(3):281-93.

Taneera J, Rosengren A, Renstrom E, Nygren JM, Serup P, Rorsman P, Jacobsen SE. (2006) Failure of transplanted bone marrow cells to adopt a pancreatic beta-cell fate. Diabetes. 55: 290-6.

Tateishi K, He J, Taranova O, Liang G, D'Alessio AC, Zhang Y (2008). Generation of insulin secreting islet-like clusters from human skin fibroblasts. *J. Biol. Chem.* 283, 31601–31607

Timper K, Seboek D, Eberhardt M, Linscheid P, Christ-Crain M, Keller U, Müller B, Zulewski H. (2006) Human adipose tissue-derived mesenchymal stem cells differentiate into insulin, somatostatin, and glucagon expressing cells. Biochem. Biophys. Res. Commun. 341: 1135-40.

Wang RN, Kloppel G, Bouwens L (1995). Duct- to islet-cell differentiation and islet growth in the pancreas of duct-ligated adult rats. Diabetologia. 38:1405-11

Zhang D, Jiang W, Liu M, Sui X, Yin X, Chen S, Shi Y, Deng H (2009). Highly efficient differentiation of human ES cells and iPS cells into mature pancreatic insulin-producing cells. *Cell Res.* 19, 429–438

Zhao M, Christie MR, Heaton N, George S, Amiel S, Cai Huang G (2002).Amelioration of streptozotocin-induced diabetes in mice using human islet cells derived from long-term culture in vitro. Transplantation. 73(9):1454-60.

Zhao M, Amiel SA, Christie MR, Rela M, Heaton N, Huang GC (2005). Insulin-producing cells derived from human pancreatic non-endocrine cell cultures reverse streptozotocin-induced hyperglycaemia in mice. Diabetologia. 48(10):2051-61.

Zhao M, Amiel SA, Christie MR, Muiesan P, Srinivasan P, Littlejohn W, Rela M, Arno M, Heaton N, Huang GC (2007). Evidence for the presence of stem cell-like progenitor cells in human adult pancreas. J Endocrinol.195(3):407-14.

Zhao M, Amiel SA, Ajami S, Jiang J, Rela M, Heaton N, Huang GC (2008). Amelioration of streptozotocin-induced diabetes in mice with cells derived from human marrow stromal cells. PLoS One. 3(7):e2666.

Zhou, Q., Brown, J., Kanarek, A., Rajagopal, J. & Melton, D. A (2008). *In vivo* reprogramming of adult pancreatic exocrine cells to beta-cells. *Nature* 455, 627–632

Part 2

Growth and Reproduction

10

GH-IGF-IGFBP Axis and Metabolic Profile in Short Children Born Small for Gestational Age

Daniëlle C.M. van der Kaay and Anita C.S. Hokken-Koelega
Erasmus Medical Center – Sophia Children's Hospital,
The Netherlands

1. Introduction

Small for gestational age (SGA) is defined as a birth weight and/or birth length below -2 standard deviation scores (SDS), adjusted for gestational age (Clayton et al., 2007). To determine whether a child is born SGA, accurate knowledge of gestational age, accurate measurements of weight and length at birth, and an appropriate reference population to calculate the standard deviation scores are required. The child can be further subclassified as SGA for weight, SGA for height or SGA for height and weight.

SGA only refers to size at birth and does not take fetal growth into account. The term intrauterine growth retardation (IUGR) is used when the fetus suffers from reduced fetal growth, based on at least 2 subsequent ultrasound measurements. A child born SGA has not necessarily suffered from IUGR, whereas a child with IUGR late in gestation can have a normal size at birth. These different fetal growth patterns are shown in Figure 1.

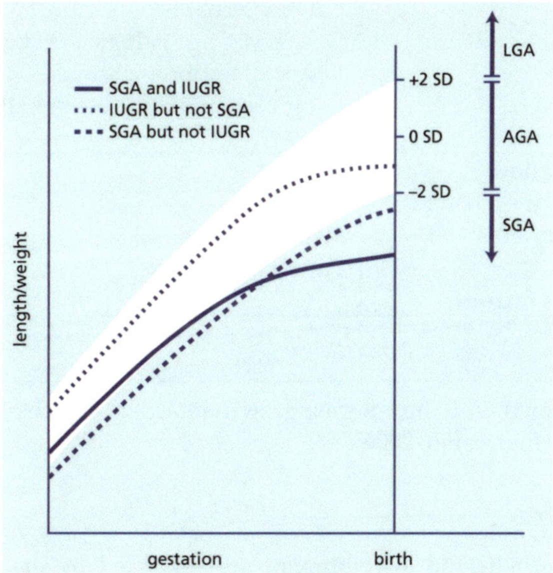

Fig. 1. Fetal growth chart demonstrating various growth curves in SGA and IUGR newborns. LGA=large for gestational age, AGA=appropriate for gestational age, SGA=small for gestational age, IUGR=intrauterine growth retardation.

1.1 Prevalence and etiology of SGA

By definition, 2.3% of all live-born neonates are born SGA when SGA is defined as a birth weight and/or length below -2 SDS. Intrauterine growth retardation might be caused by numerous fetal, maternal, placental and environmental factors which are outlined in Table 1. The cause of IUGR remains, however, unidentified in 40% of the children.

Fetal factors	
Multiple births	
Congenital malformations	
Chromosomal anomalies	Turner syndrome Down syndrome
Inborn errors of metabolism	
Intrauterine infections	Toxoplasmosis, Other infections, Rubella, Cytomegalovirus, Herpes simplex (TORCH)
Maternal factors	
Medical conditions	Pre-eclampsia Acute or chronic hypertension Severe chronic disease Severe chronic infections Systemic lupus erythematosus Antiphospholipid syndrome Anemia Malignancy Abnormalities of the uterus
Social conditions	Malnutrition Low prepregnancy body mass index Low maternal weight gain Delivery at age < 16 or > 35 years Low socioeconomic status Drug use (smoking, alcohol, illicit drugs)
Placental factors	
Reduced blood flow	
Reduced area for exchange of oxygen and nutrients	Infarcts Hematomas Partial abruption
Environmental factors	
Toxic substances	
High altitude	

Table 1. Factors associated with intrauterine growth retardation. Adapted from Bryan and Hindmarsh (Bryan & Hindmarsh, 2006).

2. GH-IGF-IGFBP axis

Fetal and postnatal growth and development are regulated by metabolic and endocrine processes, which are influenced by genetic and environmental factors. The Growth Hormone – Insulin-like Growth Factor – Insulin-like Growth Factor Binding Protein (GH-IGF-IGFBP) axis plays a major role in this system (Figure 2).

Growth hormone is secreted by the pituitary gland under the control of the hypothalamic hormones growth hormone releasing hormone (GHRH), somatostatin and ghrelin. The major effects of growth hormone on growth are mediated via Insulin-like Growth Factor I (IGF-I) expression. The physiological actions of growth hormone involve longitudinal bone growth and bone remodeling, skeletal muscle growth and immunomodulation (Holt, 2002).

The IGF-family consists of insulin, IGF-I and IGF-II. The metabolic actions of insulin are mediated through binding to the insulin receptor. The growth-promoting effects of IGF-I and IGF-II are primarily mediated through binding to the IGF-I receptor. Interactions between IGFs and the insulin receptor exist, because of strong homology between IGFs and insulin, and between the insulin receptor and IGF-I receptor (Steele-Perkins et al., 1988). Between 0.4% and 2% of IGF-I circulates as free or very easily dissociable IGF-I, the main biological active fraction. The physiological actions of IGFs involve growth, development and function of the central nervous system, skeletal muscle and reproductive organs.

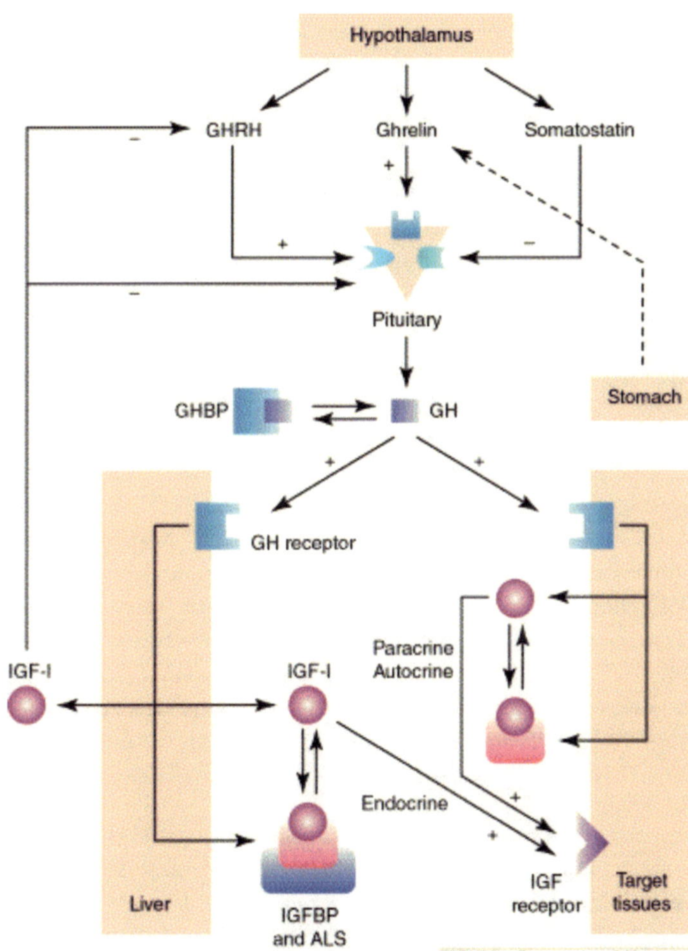

Fig. 2. Physiology of the GH-IGF-IGFPB axis (Holt, 2002).

Six IGF binding proteins (IGFBPs) form complexes with IGF-I and IGF-II, ensuring that more than 95% of IGF-I is bound. The majority of IGF-I and IGF-II (75%) is bound in a ternary complex with IGFBP-3 and an acid-labile subunit (ALS). IGFBP-3 is mainly produced in the liver. The concentration of IGFBP-3 in serum exceeds that of other IGFBPs and the affinity of IGFBP-3 for IGFs is higher than those of most other IGFBPs, reflecting its most important function as a carrier protein for IGFs. *In vitro* and *in vivo* studies have demonstrated that IGFBP-3 has IGF-mediated as well as IGF-independent effects on growth promotion and inhibition (Collet-Solberg & Cohen, 2000; Conover et al., 1996).

2.1 Genes involved in the GH-IGF-IGFBP axis

2.1.1 Growth hormone and growth hormone receptor gene

Common polymorphisms have small effects on a phenotype, but can provide important contributions to understanding complex diseases. Single nucleotide polymorphisms in the growth hormone gene have been associated with variability in normal adult height (Esteban et al., 2007). A common polymorphism in the growth hormone receptor gene (growth hormone receptor d3 polymorphism) was associated with size at birth and response to growth hormone treatment in some cohorts, although these findings were not reproduced by others (Carrascosa et al., 2006; de Graaff et al., 2008; Tauber et al., 2007).

Laron syndrome is caused by inactivating mutations affecting the expression or function of the growth hormone receptor. Clinical characteristics include severe postnatal growth failure, facial dysmorphism, truncal obesity, delayed puberty, hypoglycemia, elevated growth hormone levels, low IGF-I levels, absent/low or dysfunctional growth hormone binding protein (GHBP) and resistance to growth hormone (Laron et al., 1966).

2.1.2 IGF and IGF receptor genes

Animal knockout studies have demonstrated that IGF-I, IGF-II and their receptors are important regulators of fetoplacental growth. IGF-I gene knockout mice are 40% smaller than their littermates, without an alteration in placental size, whereas IGF-II gene knockout mice are also 40% smaller and have reduced placental growth. IGF-I gene receptor knockout mice are the most severely growth retarded (45% of normal birth weight) because of the loss of both IGF-I and IGF-II action (Baker et al., 1993). Liver IGF-I deficient mice, a mouse model where the IGF-I gene is specifically knocked out in the liver, have a normal birth weight and postnatal growth despite reduced circulating IGF-I and IGFBP3 levels. These data show that, at least in mice, liver-derived IGF-I is not essential for postnatal growth and development (Yakar et al., 1999).

Case reports in humans with defects in the IGF-I gene or IGF-I receptor gene demonstrated variable pre- and postnatal growth retardation as well as mental retardation in some cases (de Lacerda et al., 1999; Ester et al., 2009a; Veenma et al., 2010, Walenkamp et al., 2005).

Twin studies have shown that 40-65% of interindividual variability in IGF-I, IGF-II and IGFBP-3 levels is genetically determined (Harrela et al., 1996). Single nucleotide polymorphisms in the IGF-I gene are correlated with IGF-I levels, head circumference in short SGA children, birth weight and increased risk of type 2 diabetes and ischemic heart disease, although not all studies found similar associations (Ester et al., 2009b; Frayling et al., 2002; Johnston et al., 2003; Vaessen et al., 2001).

2.1.3 IGFBP genes

Knockout studies of genes encoding for IGFBPs or the acid-labile subunit demonstrated little effect on fetal growth. Knockout of the ALS gene resulted in a 60% reduction in IGF-I and IGFBP-3 levels, without an effect on fetal growth, only minor effects on postnatal growth and no effects on glucose metabolism, questioning the role of circulating IGF-I levels versus local autocrine-paracrine production of IGF-I (Ueki et al., 2000). Polymorphic variation in the IGFBP-3 gene promoter region is associated with IGFBP-3 levels, spontaneous growth and response to growth hormone treatment in short children born SGA (van der Kaay et al., 2009a).

3. The GH-IGF-IGFBP axis in fetal and postnatal growth

3.1 Fetal growth

Infants with congenital absence of the pituitary often have birth weights and birth lengths below the mean, although within the normal range, demonstrating that pituitary growth hormone has limited impact on late third trimester growth (Gluckman et al., 1992).

Fetal growth is determined by adequate delivery of oxygen and nutrients, in particular glucose, amino acids and lactate or ketone bodies across the placenta. Insulin, IGF-I and IGF-II and their receptors are the most important regulators of fetoplacental growth. IGF-II is the main growth factor in early embryonic growth, whereas IGF-I is more important during later stages of gestation. IGF-I and IGF-II levels are significantly influenced by the availability of adequate glucose levels. Glucose increases IGF-I levels through an increase in insulin secretion. In fetuses with intrauterine growth retardation, IGF-I levels are decreased during the second half of gestation. Cord blood IGF-I levels are significantly lower in infants born small for gestational age, compared to infants born appropriate for gestational age (Giudice et al., 1995; Gluckman et al., 1987).

All 6 IGFBPs have been found in fetal plasma and tissues. IGFBP-1 is the major IGF binding protein found in amniotic fluid. It binds IGF in fetal plasma, increases 20-fold from week 9 to week 12 and is the most important regulator of IGF-I bioavailability during pregnancy (Murphy et al., 2006). IGFBP-1 production is suppressed by insulin. IGFBP-1 levels are increased in infants born SGA, possibly reflecting the low insulin levels found in fetuses with intrauterine growth retardation (Holt, 2002). IGFBP-3 levels are significantly lower in infants born small for gestational age, compared to those born appropriate for gestational age (Giudice et al., 1995).

3.2 Postnatal growth

Growth hormone receptor expression is gradually upregulated after birth. Around 6 months of life, growth becomes dependent on pulsatile growth hormone secretion and growth hormone induced IGF-I and IGFBP-3 production. Serum IGF-I and IGFBP-3 levels are influenced by various factors such as sex steroids, nutritional status and liver function.

Catch-up growth is defined as a growth velocity greater than the median for chronological age and gender and is associated with a rise in IGF-I and IGFBP-3 levels (Cance-Rouzaud et al., 1998). In infants born SGA, catch-up growth occurs during the first 6 months of life in more than 80% of children. Prematurely born infants may take longer to catch-up (Hokken-Koelega et al., 1995). Catch-up growth is completed by the age of 2 years in most children born SGA (Figure 3).

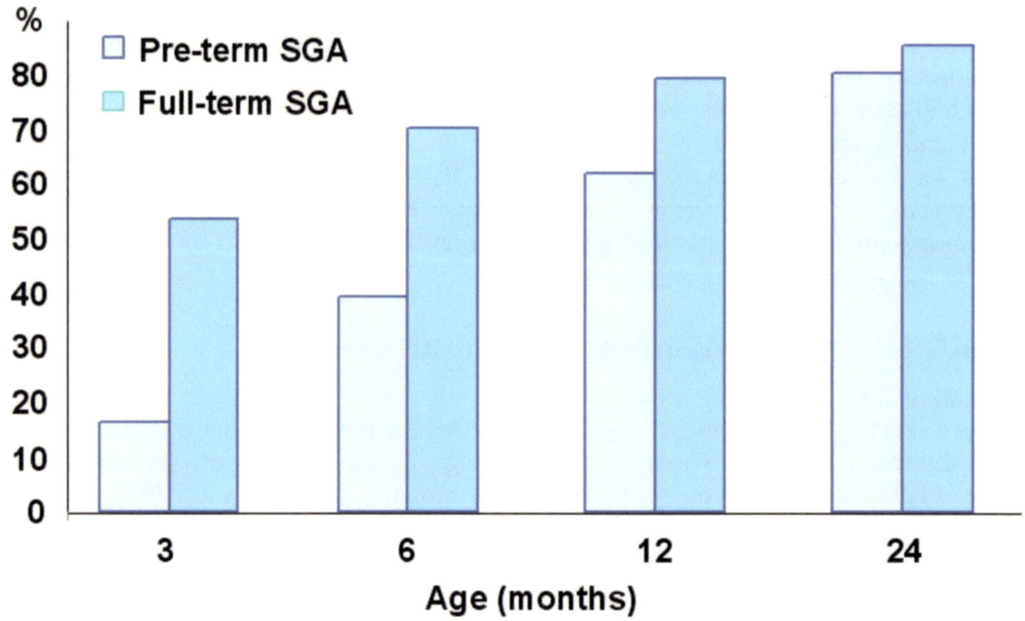

Fig. 3. Percentage of pre-term and full-term SGA infants with postnatal catch-up growth (Hokken-Koelega et al., 1995).

It is recommended that a child born SGA has measurements of height, weight, and head circumference every 3 months for the first year of life and every 6 months thereafter. Children without significant catch-up growth in the first 6 months of life and those who remain short by 2 years of age may have other conditions that are associated with short stature. These children require referral to a pediatrician because such conditions need to be identified and managed (Clayton et al., 2007).

Although catch-up growth occurs in most children born SGA, around 10% of infants remain short throughout childhood and adulthood (Leger et al., 1997). Alterations in the GH-IGF-IGFBP axis might underlie this failure in catch-up growth in short SGA children. Subnormal to low growth hormone levels during overnight growth hormone profiles have been found in prepubertal short SGA children in some cohorts, although others found normal growth hormone levels (Boguszewski et al., 1995; de Waal et al., 1994; Volkl et al., 2004). The wide variability in - and overlap between - growth hormone secretion in SGA cohorts and control populations are consistent phenomena. Within the heterogeneous SGA population, this probably reflects a continuum in growth hormone secretion, ranging from partial growth hormone deficiency to normal growth hormone secretion.

IGF-I and IGFBP-3 levels are significantly lower in short prepubertal and pubertal children, and young adults who were born SGA, compared to their age-matched peers with normal stature (de Waal et al., 1994; Carel et al., 2003; Verkauskiene et al., 2005).

4. Short children born small for gestational age

4.1 Metabolic status of short children born SGA

Body composition is greatly influenced by gender and height. It is important to adjust for these variables when comparing body composition in short SGA children and controls.

Prepubertal short SGA children have a significantly decreased fat mass. Lean body mass is comparable to controls in young prepubertal short SGA children. During a 3-year follow-up, however, it tended to decrease over time resulting in significantly lower levels in older prepubertal short SGA children compared to controls (Willemsen et al., 2007).

Epidemiological studies have demonstrated that development of type 2 diabetes mellitus and associated disorders such as hypertension, dyslipidemia and cardiovascular disease in adults is associated with low birth weight (Barker, 2004; Barker et al., 2005). Reduced insulin sensitivity plays a central role in the pathogenesis of these disorders. Short children born SGA are more insulin resistant, compared to controls born appropriate for gestational age. The disposition index - reflecting the capability of beta cells to compensate for the reduction in insulin sensitivity by increasing their insulin secretion - was comparable between short SGA subjects and controls (Leunissen et al., 2008). Young adults born SGA have a higher incidence of metabolic risk factors than those born appropriate for gestational age (2.3% versus 0.4%). More recent data indicate that insulin resistance and metabolic risk factors are mainly related to the accumulation of fat mass during early childhood. Rapid weight gain during the first 3 months of life results in a higher percentage of body fat, more central adiposity, reduced insulin sensitivity, lower high-density lipoprotein cholesterol levels and higher triglyceride levels in early adulthood (Arends et al., 2005; Jaquet et al., 2005; Leunissen et al., 2009). High blood pressure in childhood has been associated with an increased risk of developing hypertension in adulthood (Bao et al., 1995; Primatesta et al., 2005).

4.2 Intellectual consequences and health-related quality of life of short children born SGA

In large observational studies, cognitive impairment is independently associated with low birth weight, short birth length, and small head circumference. SGA children have poorer school performance and have more emotional, conduct, and attention deficit hyperactivity disorders, although the differences are mostly subtle (de Bie et al., 2010; van Pareren et al., 2004).

Adults who were born SGA show no difference in frequency of employment, marital status, or satisfaction with life. However, lower academic achievement and professional attainment with lower income have been found (Strauss, 2010).

Short children have reported to experience juvenilization and more teasing. Reports on health-related quality of life, the subjective perception of health, have been inconclusive (Sandberg & Colsman, 2005). More recently, a large British population study found that adult short stature may be associated with a reduction in health-related quality of life on five dimensions (mobility, self-care, usual activities, pain/discomfort and anxiety/depression) (Christensen et al., 2007).

5. Growth hormone treatment in prepubertal short children born SGA

5.1 Effects on linear growth

Growth hormone treatment in short children born SGA has been explored for over 40 years. Several studies have demonstrated that growth hormone treatment effectively induces catch-up growth in prepubertal short SGA children (Dahlgren & Wikland, 2005; de Zegher et al., 2006; Sas et al., 1999). Adult height data from a Dutch multicenter study demonstrated that 85% of children reached a height above -2 SDS and 98% reached a height within the target height range (Van Pareren et al., 2003) (Figure 4).

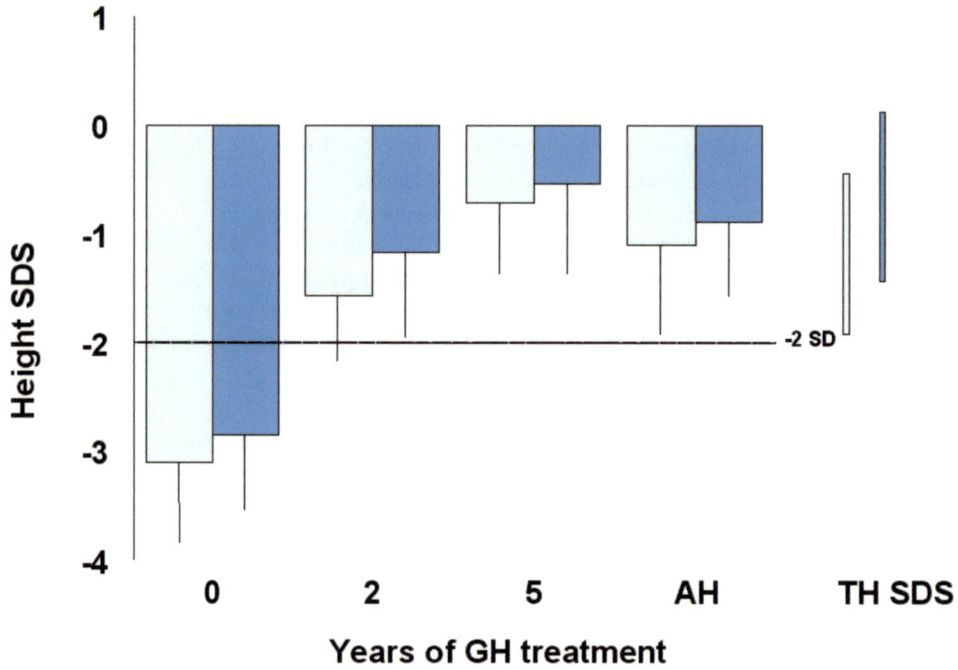

Fig. 4. Height SDS (± SD) during growth hormone treatment and at adult height (AH), in relation to target height (TH) SDS. Light blue boxes: 1 mg GH/m²/day, dark blue boxes: 2 mg GH/m²/day (Van Pareren et al., 2003).

This has led to the official registration of GH treatment for short children born SGA by the US Food and Drug Administration (FDA) in 2001 and by the European Agency for the Evaluation of Medicinal Products (EMEA) in 2003 (Table 2).

Discrepancies, for example in height at start of treatment and dose, between the 2 approved indications are recognized (Chernausek, 2005). A dose-dependent effect on growth is found during the first 4-5 years of growth hormone treatment, although growth hormone dose is less important for long-term growth (de Zegher & Hokken-Koelega, 2005; Van Pareren et al., 2003). Furthermore, there is no evidence for excluding children from growth hormone treatment when the distance to target height is less than 1 SDS (Lem et al., 2010).

There is considerable variation in the growth response to growth hormone treatment. This variation remains after adjustment for factors such as age, target height and duration of treatment. Short children born SGA form a heterogeneous group of patients and genetic variability in growth-related genes probably accounts for part of the variation in growth response.

A positive response to GH treatment could arbitrarily be defined as a height velocity SDS of more than 0.5 in the first year of treatment. In case of an inadequate response, reevaluation is necessary, including consideration of compliance, GH dose, diagnosis, and the decision to discontinue treatment. Discontinuation of GH treatment in adolescence is recommended when the growth rate is less than 2 cm/yr (Clayton et al., 2007).

5.2 Effects on the GH-IGF-IGFBP axis

Serum growth hormone, IGF-I and IGFBP-3 levels significantly increase in a dose-dependent manner during growth hormone treatment (Boguszewski et al., 1996; Sas et al., 1999; Van Dijk et al., 2006). During 1 year of treatment, IGF-I and IGFBP3 levels had increased to respectively +1.2 SDS and +0.2 SDS in children treated with 1 mg GH/m²/day and to respectively +1.9 SDS and +0.5 SDS in children treated with 2 mg GH/m²/day (Sas et al., 1999).

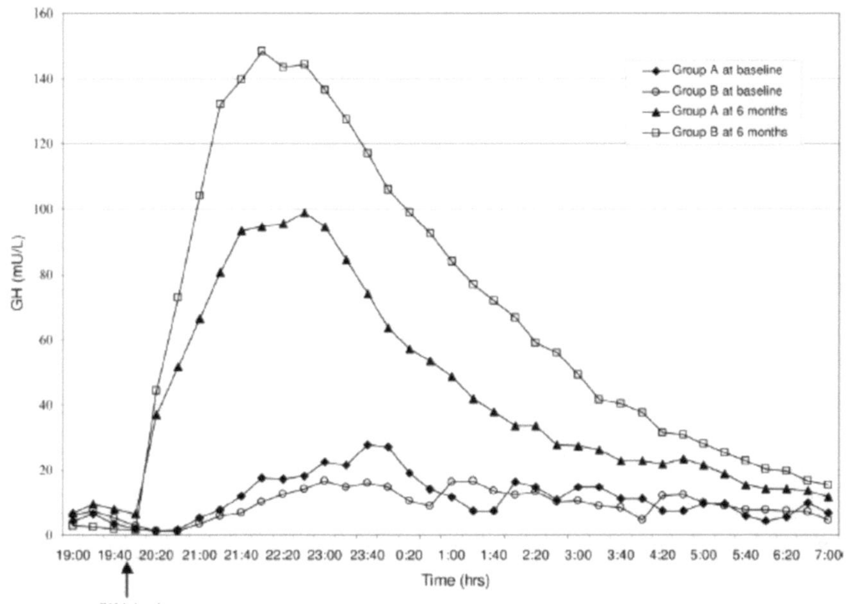

Fig. 5. Mean GH levels for each time point during an overnight GH profile before and after 6 months of growth hormone treatment. Closed figures: 1 mg GH/m²/day, open figures: 2 mg GH/m²/day (Van Dijk et al., 2006).

At 6.5 years after discontinuation of growth hormone treatment, IGF-I and IGFBP-3 levels had returned to levels comparable with those found in untreated short subjects born SGA and thus significantly lower than levels found in controls (Van Dijk et al., 2007).

5.3 Effects on insulin sensitivity, lipid profile and body composition

Large surveillance databases have demonstrated that growth hormone treatment is well-tolerated and adverse events are not more common in short SGA children than in other conditions that require growth hormone treatment (Cutfield et al., 2006).

Monitoring of glucose and insulin levels during growth hormone treatment is necessary, because growth hormone has insulin-antagonistic effects. Prepubertal short SGA children develop a relative insulin resistance during growth hormone treatment, which is largely reversible when treatment is terminated. Six years after discontinuation, insulin sensitivity in short SGA children who were treated with growth hormone was similar compared to untreated short individuals born SGA (de Zegher et al., 2002; van Dijk et al., 2007). Growth hormone treatment has positive effects on lipid metabolism and blood pressure in prepubertal short SGA children and these effects persisted after discontinuation (Sas et al., 2000; van Dijk et al., 2007). Growth hormone has well-documented anabolic effects on muscle mass and lipolytic effects on adipose tissue (Mukherjee et al., 2004). During treatment in prepubertal short SGA children, the increase in lean mass SDS adjusted for gender and height reflected the normal increase as a result of the increase in height, without an additional anabolic effect. Fat mass SDS adjusted for gender and height declined in prepubertal SGA children, especially during the first treatment year (Willemsen et al., 2007).

5.4 Effects on intellectual outcome and health-related quality of life

During 9 yr of GH treatment, IQ and psychosocial functioning had improved from scores significantly below average to scores comparable to Dutch peers (Figure 6) (van Pareren et al., 2004).

Health-related quality of life improves in growth hormone treated adolescents born SGA, according to the disorder-specific questionnaire which is designed to assess the impact of short stature on quality of life for children aged 5-15 years (The TNO AZL Children's Quality of Life-short stature (TACQOL-S)). This improvement continued until adult height. Health-related quality of life was not different between individuals treated with 1 or 2 mg $GH/m^2/day$ (Bannink et al., 2010). Other studies did not find a significant improvement (Stephen et al., 2011).

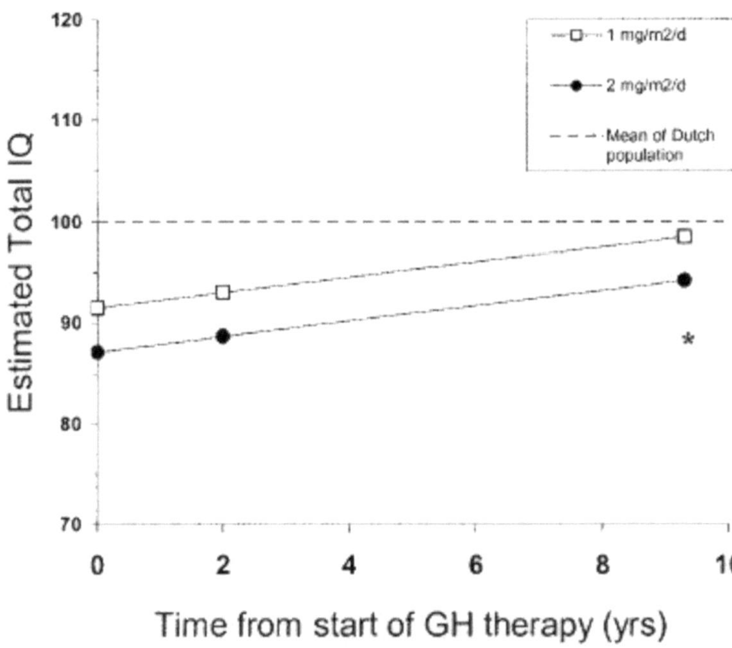

Fig. 6. Estimated total IQ score for both GH groups during growth hormone treatment, corrected for gender and age at start. Significant increase from start: *, $P < 0.001$ (van Pareren et al., 2004).

6. Puberty in short children born small for gestational age

Controversies exist about the relationship between being born SGA and reproductive function. In men born SGA, lower testosterone levels and smaller testicular size have been described (Cicognani et al., 2002). In women born SGA, smaller ovaries and uterus and lower anti-Mullerian hormone levels - a marker of follicle pool size - have been described

(Ibanez et al., 2003). These findings could not be replicated by others (Hernandez et al., 2006; Jensen et al., 2007). In a large cohort, it was recently shown that being born SGA does not have a negative effect on gonadal function in adult men. Factors that affect gonadal function are socio-economic status, fat mass, and maternal smoking during gestation, although all values of gonadal parameters remained within the normal range (Kerkhof et al., 2009). In women, being born SGA does not result in lower anti-Mullerian hormone levels. Catch-up growth after being born SGA might, however, be associated with increased anti-Mullerian hormone levels. Testosterone and androstenedione levels were comparable to levels in a control population. Other factors associated with serum anti-Mullerian hormone levels are oral contraceptive use, age at menarche, maternal smoking during gestation and socio-economic status (Kerkhof et al., 2010).

Growth hormone treatment has no detrimental effect on gonadal function in prepubertal short children born SGA (Boonstra et al., 2008; Lem et al., 2011).

7. Postponement of puberty in pubertal short children born small for gestational age

It has been indicated that a better growth response and greater adult height is achieved when children start growth hormone treatment at an early age (Carel et al., 2003). Although the age of onset and progression of puberty in short SGA children is comparable to healthy peers, some of these children only come under medical attention at onset of puberty.

Postponement of puberty with gonadotropin releasing hormone analogue (GnRH analogue) is the treatment of choice in children with central precocious puberty or early puberty. Most of these children reach an adult height within their target height range (Mul et al., 2002; Palmert et al., 1999; Pasquino et al., 2008). It is yet unknown whether the same applies to short children bon SGA who come under medical attention at onset of puberty.

7.1 Effects of GnRH analogue treatment on growth and the GH-IGF-IGFBP axis

During GnRH analogue treatment, a decline in growth velocity - even to levels below the age-appropriate normal range in some patients - is a well-known phenomenon (Carel et al., 1996; Saggese et al., 1993). Some studies in children with central precocious puberty found lower stimulated and spontaneous growth hormone levels during GnRH analogue treatment, others could not replicate these findings (DiMartino-Nardi et al., 1991; Sklar et al., 1991; Stanhope et al., 1988). Poor growth might also be directly related to reduced sex steroid levels or growth plate senescence by prior estrogen exposure (Savendahl, 2005; Weise et al., 2004).

In girls with normal stature, growth hormone secretion increases during puberty with the highest levels found at Tanner stage 3 and stage 4 (Rose et al., 1991). In contrast, pubertal short SGA girls have similar growth hormone levels compared to prepubertal short SGA girls (van der Kaay et al., 2009b). The lack of a rise in growth hormone levels during puberty in short SGA girls might play a role in the less intense pubertal growth spurt found in short SGA children who do not receive growth hormone treatment (Luo et al., 2003).

Treatment with subcutaneous leuprorelide acetate depots of 3.75mg every 4 weeks results in adequate pubertal suppression in pubertal short SGA children (van der Kaay et al., 2009c; van der Kaay et al., 2009d).

GnRH analogue treatment in pubertal short SGA girls results in a reduction of serum growth hormone levels, to levels lower than those found in prepubertal short SGA girls. The interindividual variability in growth hormone secretion in response to a GnRH analogue is significant (Figure 7). One third of short SGA girls had a reduction in growth hormone levels of more than 40%. These girls also demonstrated a greater decrease in IGF-I and IGFBP-3 levels, compared to girls who showed a reduction in growth hormone levels between 0 and 40%. There is no association between growth hormone levels and estrogen levels, or between growth hormone levels and luteinizing hormone levels. This implies that girls with the same degree of pubertal suppression have different growth hormone responses during GnRH analogue treatment (van der Kaay et al., 2009b).

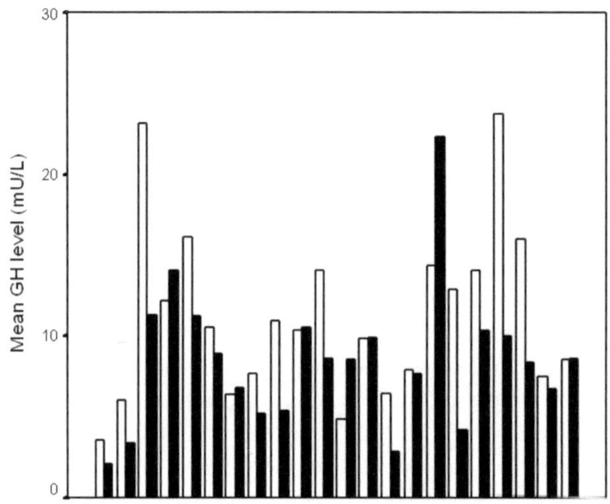

Fig. 7. Mean growth hormone levels for each individual girl during an overnight growth hormone profile before (white bars) and after 3 months of GnRHa treatment (black bars) (van der Kaay et al., 2009b).

7.2 Effects of GnRH analogue treatment on the metabolic profile

Most of the studies performed in children with central precocious puberty have focused on adult height, bone mineral density and restoration of the reproductive system after long-term treatment with GnRH analogues. Much less attention has been paid to changes in body composition. Some studies report an increase in fat mass or BMI during GnRH analogue treatment, with a return to values comparable to those at baseline after discontinuation (Pasquino et al., 2008; van der Sluis et al., 2002), whereas others report no changes (Palmert et al., 1999) or even a decreased BMI during GnRH analogue treatment (Arrigo et al., 2004). Lean body mass SDS decreases during GnRH analogue treatment (van der Sluis et al., 2002).

There is a physiological decrease in insulin sensitivity with pubertal progression (Hannon et al., 2006). Since both growth hormone and IGF-I levels significantly increase during puberty, the higher GH levels during puberty are thought to contribute to the pubertal insulin resistance (Moran et al., 2002). A brief period of GnRH analogue treatment in young, healthy women did not result in changes in insulin secretion (Toth et al., 2008). The effect of GnRH analogue treatment on insulin sensitivity in children with central precocious puberty is, however, unknown.

8. Combined treatment with a GnRH analogue and growth hormone in pubertal short children born small for gestational age

Studies in patients with idiopathic growth hormone deficiency demonstrated a beneficial effect on adult height in favor of combined treatment with a GnRH analogue and growth hormone, compared to growth hormone treatment alone (Mericq et al., 2000; Saggese et al., 2001). In children with idiopathic short stature contradictory results have been found (Lanes et al., 1998; Pasquino et al., 2000).

8.1 Effects on the GH-IGF-IGFBP axis

Similar to prepubertal short SGA children treated with either 1 or 2 mg GH/m^2/day, pubertal short SGA children treated with a GnRH analogue and either 1 or 2 mg GH/m^2/day show a dose-dependent increase in growth hormone levels (Figure 8). Growth hormone levels in pubertal short SGA children were, however, lower than levels in prepubertal short SGA children treated with a similar dose of growth hormone. Moreover, growth hormone levels in pubertal short SGA children treated with a GnRH analogue and 2 mg GH/m^2/day were similar to growth hormone levels in prepubertal short SGA children treated with 1 mg GH/m^2/day. Since growth hormone levels decrease during GnRH analogue treatment, these lower growth hormone levels might be the result of simultaneous treatment with a GnRH analogue, next to growth hormone (van der Kaay et al., 2010). Nevertheless, growth hormone levels in pubertal short SGA children treated with a GnRH analogue and 2 mg GH/m^2/day remain elevated for a great part of the day. Similar to prepubertal short SGA children, there is a wide interindividual variation in growth hormone levels in response to either 1 or 2 mg

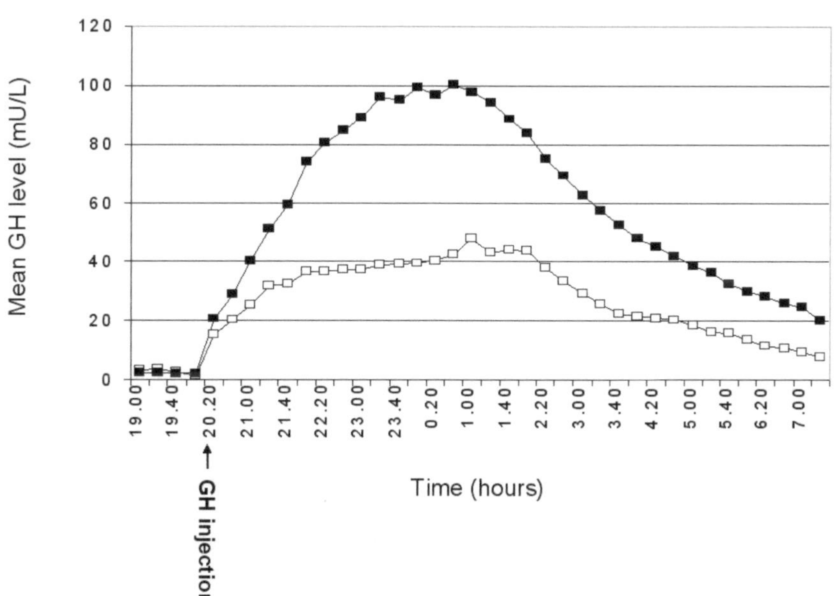

Fig. 8. Mean growth hormone levels for each time point during an overnight growth hormone profile after 1 year of combined treatment with a GnRH analogue and growth hormone. Open squares: 1 mg GH/m^2/day, solid squares: 2 mg GH/m^2/day (van der Kaay et al., 2010).

GH/m²/day. Genetic variability in growth-related genes probably accounts for part of this variation, next to variations in physiological mechanisms involved in degradation of growth hormone at the site of injection and in the systemic circulation.

Pubertal short SGA children treated with a GnRH analogue and either 1 or 2 mg GH/m²/day show a dose-dependent increase in IGF-I levels. Compared to the population mean, IGF-I levels are significantly lower at start of growth hormone treatment and significantly higher after 1 year of combined treatment. IGFBP-3 levels increase as well, but to a lesser extent than IGF-I levels. This results in an increase in levels of free, biologically active IGF-I which stimulates growth. Similar to prepubertal short SGA children treated with 2 mg GH/m²/day, a greater percentage of pubertal short SGA children treated with a GnRH analogue and 2 mg GH/m²/day have IGF-I SD scores in the highest quintile (> 0.84 SDS), compared to children treated with a GnRH analogue and 1 mg GH/m²/day. Reassuringly, the percentage of children with IGF-I SD scores above +2 SDS was not different between both growth hormone dosage groups (van der Kaay et al., 2010). Concern has been expressed about the association between high IGF-I levels during several years and long-term cancer risk (Renehan et al., 2004). Although pubertal short SGA children will be treated with growth hormone for a relatively short period of time, it is important to monitor IGF-I levels during growth hormone treatment in order to titrate the growth hormone dose to IGF-I levels within the age-appropriate normal range.

8.2 Effects on insulin sensitivity

In pubertal short SGA children, insulin sensitivity (Si) - measured by frequently sampled intravenous glucose tolerance tests - is lower and insulin secretion (acute insulin response (AIR)) is higher, compared to prepubertal short SGA children. This was expected since pubertal children have a physiological decrease in insulin sensitivity.

During combined treatment with a GnRH analogue and either 1 or 2 mg GH/m²/day, insulin sensitivity decreases and insulin secretion increases. The disposition index remained comparable to baseline, reflecting that β-cells are able to compensate for the reduction in insulin sensitivity by increasing their insulin secretion. Insulin sensitivity and secretion was comparable between children treated with either 1 or 2 mg GH/m²/day (Table 3) (van der Kaay et al., 2010).

8.3 Effect on lipid profile and blood pressure

In pubertal short SGA children, mean total cholesterol (TC), low density lipoprotein-cholesterol (LDL-c), high density lipoprotein-cholesterol (HDL-c), triglycerides (TG), non-esterified fatty acids (FFAs), apolipoprotein A1 (Apo-A1), apolipoprotein B (Apo B) and lipoprotein (a) (lp(a)) are within the normal range. Lipoprotein (a) levels are, however, above the normal range in 27% of pubertal short SGA children. High lipoprotein (a) levels have been associated with an increased risk of developing cardiovascular disease (Danesh et al., 2000).

During combined treatment with a GnRH analogue and either 1 or 2 mg GH/m²/day, very small increases and/or decreases of lipid levels are found. The clinical significance of these small changes is considered negligible. Lipid levels are comparable between children treated with either 1 or 2 mg GH/m²/day (Table 3) (van der Kaay et al., 2010).

Systolic blood pressure (BP) is higher in pubertal short SGA children than in controls and 27% of pubertal short SGA children have a systolic blood pressure above + 2 SDS adjusted for gender and height. Higher blood pressure in childhood has been associated with an increased risk of developing hypertension in adulthood. Systolic blood pressure does not change during 2 years of combined treatment with a GnRH analogue and either 1 or 2 mg GH/m^2/day (Table 3). This is in line with previous findings, where a decrease in blood pressure was found only after 3 years of growth hormone treatment (Willemsen et al., 2008).

	Start of GnRHa treatment (n=41)	One year of combined treatment (n=41)	Three months after the stop of GnRHa treatment (n=41)
Systolic BP SDS	1.59 (1.24–1.94)*	1.26 (0.87–1.65)*	1.39 (1.04–1.74)*
Diastolic BP SDS	0.22 (0.00–0.45)	0.52 (0.27–0.78)†	0.57 (0.36–0.79)‡
Si$\times 10^{-4}$/min (μU/ml)	7.38 (6.00–8.76)	4.61 (3.71–5.50)†	ND
Sg$\times 10^{-2}$/min	3.47 (2.98–3.96)	3.42 (2.94–3.89)	ND
AIR (mU/l)	421 (326–543)	790 (643–971)†	ND
DI (AIR$\times$Si)	2569 (2012–3279)	3105 (2514–3838)	ND
Insulin (pmol/l)	48.1 (41.7–55.5)	75.0 (63.8–88.1)†	79.2 (66.7–94.0)‡
HOMA-IR	0.91 (0.79–1.06)	1.39 (1.19–1.63)†	1.43 (1.20–1.70)‡
TC (mmol/l) (3.0–5.5)	4.16 (3.99–4.33)	4.20 (4.00–4.40)	4.33 (4.13–4.53)‡
LDL-c (mmol/l) (1.3–3.4)	2.28 (2.11–2.46)	2.44 (2.25–2.64)†	2.36 (2.19–2.52)
HDL-c (mmol/l) (0.9–1.9)	1.41 (1.31–1.52)	1.63 (1.51–1.76)†	1.55 (1.44–1.66)‡,§
TG (mmol/l) (0.4–1.6)	0.76 (0.66–0.86)	0.79 (0.67–0.94)	0.92 (0.75–1.13)‡
FFA (mmol/l) (0.2–1.0)	0.52 (0.45–0.59)	0.69 (0.59–0.79)†	0.51 (0.42–0.60)§
Apo-A1 (g/l) (0.9–1.6)	1.39 (1.32–1.46)	1.56 (1.47–1.65)†	1.45 (1.38–1.53)§
Apo-B (g/l) (0.5–1.3)	0.71 (0.66–0.75)	0.73 (0.68–0.77)	0.72 (0.67–0.77)
Lp(a) (g/l) ($\leq$0.3)	0.09 (0.06–0.13)	0.14 (0.09–0.21)†	0.14 (0.09–0.22)‡

ND = not determined; *P<0.0001 compared with the population mean (0 SDS); †P<0.03: 1 year of combined treatment, compared with the start of GnRH analogue treatment; ‡P<0.03: 3 months after the stop of GnRH analogue treatment, compared with the start of GnRH analogue treatment; §P<0.02: 3 months after the stop of GnRH analogue treatment, compared with 1 year of combined treatment (van der Kaay et al., 2010).

Table 3. Blood pressure, insulin sensitivity, and lipids at the start of GnRH analogue treatment, after 1 year of combined treatment and 3 months after the stop of GnRH analogue treatment in short SGA children with continuation of growth hormone treatment. Data are expressed as model estimate (95% CI), after adjustment for gender and Tanner stage at baseline. The values between brackets represent reference ranges for healthy children.

8.4 Effects on body composition

Fat mass adjusted for height and gender (SDS_{height}) in pubertal short SGA children is significantly lower than the population mean, consistent with findings in prepubertal short SGA children (Willemsen et al., 2007). During treatment with a GnRH analogue and 1 mg GH/m^2/day, fat mass SDS_{height} significantly increases to values comparable to the population mean. In contrast, during 1 year of treatment with a GnRH analogue and 2 mg GH/m^2/day, fat mass SDS_{height} decreases. During 2 years of combined treatment, fat mass SDS_{height} values return to those comparable before start of treatment - remaining significantly lower than the population mean in children treated with a GnRH analogue and 2 mg GH/m^2/day (Figure 9). Although the percentage of trunk fat increases in pubertal short SGA children treated with GnRHa and either 1 or 2 mg GH/m^2/day, values are lower in children treated with GnRHa and 2 mg GH/m^2/day (Figure 9). This indicates that pubertal short SGA children develop relatively more fat mass around the waist, but that the increase is less when GnRH analogue treatment is combined with 2 mg GH/m^2/day. In prepubertal short SGA children treated with 2 mg GH/m^2/day, percentage trunk fat remains comparable to untreated children. Thus, the increase in percentage trunk fat in pubertal short SGA children is most likely due to treatment with a GnRH analogue, next to growth hormone (van der Kaay et al., 2010).

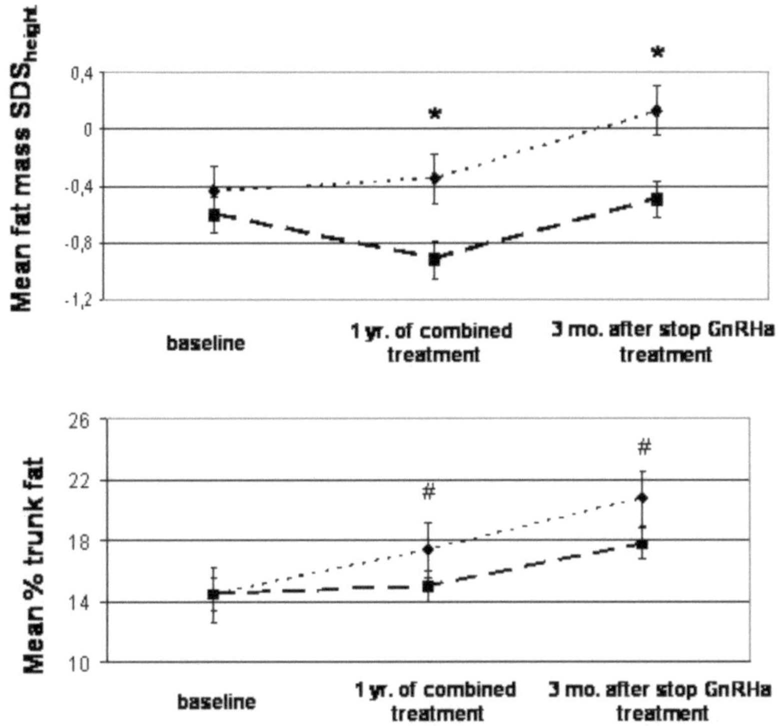

Fig. 9. Changes in fat mass SDS_{height} and percentage trunk fat during 27 months of GnRH analogue and growth hormone treatment. Data are expressed as mean (± standard error of the mean (SEM)). Diamonds represent values during treatment with a GnRH analogue and 1 mg GH/m²/day. Squares represent values during treatment with a GnRH analogue and 2 mg GH/m²/day. Mean percentage trunk fat=(trunk fat/total trunk mass)x100. * P<0.01, # P<0.05 (van der Kaay et al., 2010).

Several studies reported an increase in fat mass or BMI during GnRH analogue treatment in children with central precocious puberty. This might be explained by the lower growth hormone levels found during GnRH analogue treatment, as reported in children with growth hormone deficiency (Boot et al., 1997). Growth hormone has well-documented lipolytic effects and growth hormone treatment in prepubertal short SGA children results in a significant decrease in fat mass SDS_{height}, especially in the first treatment year. In pubertal short SGA children, treatment with 2 mg GH/m²/day counteracts the fat-accumulating effect of simultaneous treatment with a GnRH analogue, whereas treatment with 1 mg GH/m²/day is insufficient to prevent children from gaining fat mass during GnRH analogue treatment.

Epidemiological studies have shown that low birth weight followed by catch-up in fat mass during childhood and adolescence is associated with a higher risk of developing type 2 diabetes and cardiovascular disease, even when fat mass remains within the normal range. Follow-up until adult height is required to investigate the long-term effects of changes in body composition and metabolic profile in short SGA children treated with a combination of GnRH analogue and growth hormone.

Lean body mass SDS_{height} in pubertal short SGA children is significantly lower than the population mean. It was previously shown that older prepubertal short SGA children have a

lower lean body mass SDS_{height} compared with younger prepubertal short children born SGA (Willemsen et al., 2007).
During combined treatment with a GnRH analogue and either 1 or 2 mg GH/m²/day, lean body mass SDS_{height} increases only in pubertal short SGA children treated with a GnRH analogue and 2 mg GH/m²/day, although values remain significantly lower than the population mean. It is known that in children with central precocious puberty, lean body mass decreases during GnRH analogue treatment. Only combining 2 mg GH/m²/day with a GnRH analogue results in an increase in lean body mass SDS_{height} in older short SGA children (Figure 10) (van der Kaay et al., 2010).

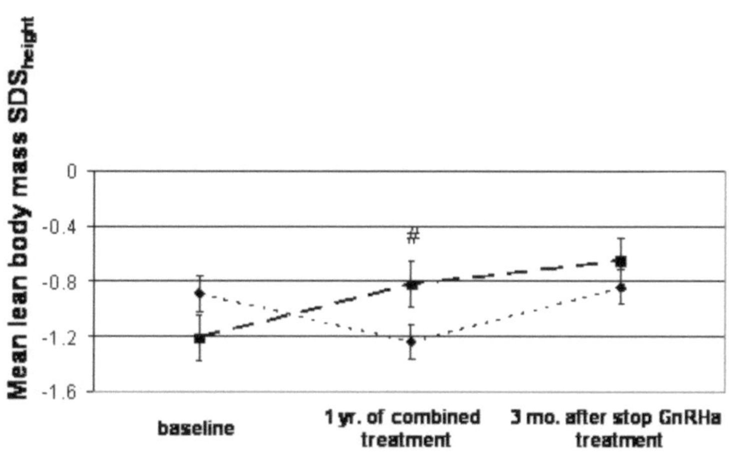

Fig. 10. Changes in lean body mass SDS_{height} during 27 months of GnRH analogue and growth hormone treatment. Data are expressed as mean (± standard error of the mean (SEM)). Diamonds represent values during treatment with a GnRH analogue and 1 mg GH/m²/day. Squares represent values during treatment with a GnRH analogue and 2 mg GH/m²/day. # $P<0.05$ (van der Kaay et al., 2010).

9. General conclusions and practical implications

Since growth hormone treatment was approved by the US Food and Drug Administration (FDA) in 2001 and by the European Agency for Evaluation of Medicinal Products (EMEA) in 2003, short children born small for gestational age comprise a large group of growth hormone treated children.
Various studies demonstrated that growth hormone treatment in prepubertal short SGA children effectively and safely induces catch-up growth. Better growth responses and greater adult height are achieved when children start growth hormone treatment at an early age. Some short SGA children, however, come under medical attention at onset of puberty.
Pubertal short SGA girls lack the usual increase in growth hormone levels that accompanies the pubertal growth spurt, as found in pubertal girls with normal stature. Furthermore, GnRH analogue treatment results in a decrease in growth hormone levels to levels lower than those found in prepubertal short SGA girls. The lack of a rise in growth hormone levels during puberty in short SGA girls might play a role in the less intense pubertal growth spurt found in short SGA children who do not receive growth hormone treatment.

During combined treatment with a GnRH analogue and either 1 or 2 mg GH/m²/day, growth hormone and IGF-I levels show a dose-dependent increase, although growth hormone levels are lower compared to levels in prepubertal short SGA children treated with the same GH dose. Moreover, growth hormone levels in pubertal short SGA children treated with a GnRH analogue and 2 mg GH/m²/day are similar to growth hormone levels in prepubertal short SGA children treated with 1 mg GH/m²/day. During 2 years of combined treatment, the higher dose of 2 mg GH/m²/day has a favorable effect on fat mass SDS, percentage trunk fat and lean body mass SDS. Blood pressure, insulin sensitivity and lipid profile are similar between children treated with a GnRH analogue and 1 or 2 mg GH/m²/day. Combined treatment has no adverse effect on these metabolic parameters.

Thus, combined treatment with a GnRH analogue and either 1 or 2 mg GH/m²/day - possibly in favor of treatment with a GnRH analogue and 2 mg GH/m²/day - can be considered as a safe treatment strategy in the short run for short children born small for gestational age who come under medical attention at onset of puberty. Adult height data need to be awaited before definitive conclusions can be drawn concerning the long-term efficacy and safety of this combined treatment.

10. References

Arends, N.J., Boonstra, V.H., Duivenvoorden, H.J., Hofman, P.L., Cutfield,W.S. & Hokken-Koelega,A.C. (2005). Clin Endocrinol (Oxf). *Reduced insulin sensitivity and the presence of cardiovascular risk factors in short prepubertal children born small for gestational age (SGA)*, 62, 44-50.

Arrigo, T., De Luca F., Antoniazzi, F., Galluzzi, F., Segni, M., Rosano, M., Messina, M.F. & Lombardo, F. (2004). Eur J Endocrinol. *Reduction of baseline body mass index under gonadotropin-suppressive therapy in girls with idiopathic precocious puberty*, 150, 533-537.

Baker, J., Liu J.P., Robertson, E.J. & Efstratiadis, A. (1993). Cell. *Role of insulin-like growth factors in embryonic and postnatal growth*, 75, 73-82.

Bannink, E., Djurhuus, C.B., Christensen, T., Jons, K. & Hokken-Koelega, A. (2010). J Med Econ. *Adult height and health-related quality of life after growth hormone therapy in small for gestational age subjects*, 13, 221-227.

Bao, W., Threefoot, S.A., Srinivasan, S.R. & Berenson, G.S. (1995). Am J Hypertens. *Essential hypertension predicted by tracking of elevated blood pressure from childhood to adulthood: the Bogalusa Heart Study*, 8, 657-665.

Barker, D.J. (2004). J Am Coll Nutr. *The developmental origins of adult disease*, 23, 588S-595S.

Barker, D.J., Osmond, C., Forsen, T.J., Kajantie, E. & Eriksson, J.G. (2005). N Engl J Med. *Trajectories of growth among children who have coronary events as adults*, 353, 1802-1809.

Boguszewski, M., Jansson, C., Rosberg, S. & Albertsson-Wikland, K. (1996). J Clin Endocrinol Metab. *Changes in serum insulin-like growth factor I (IGF-I) and IGF-binding protein-3 levels during growth hormone treatment in prepubertal short children born small for gestational age*, 81, 3902-3908.

Boguszewski, M., Rosberg, S. & Albertsson-Wikland, K. (1995). J Clin Endocrinol Metab. *Spontaneous 24-hour growth hormone profiles in prepubertal small for gestational age children*, 80, 2599-2606.

Boonstra, V. H., Weber R.F., Mulder, P. & Hokken-Koelega, A. (2008). Horm Res. *Testis function in prepubertal boys and young men born small for gestational age*, 70, 357-363.

Boot, A.M., Engels, M.A., Boerma, G.J., Krenning, E.P. & De Muinck Keizer-Schrama, S.M. (1997). J Clin Endocrinol Metab. *Changes in bone mineral density, body composition, and lipid metabolism during growth hormone (GH) treatment in children with GH deficiency*, 82, 2423-2428.

Bryan, S.M. & Hindmarsh P.C. (2006). Horm Res. *Normal and abnormal fetal growth*, 65, 19-27.

Cance-Rouzaud, A., Laborie, S., Bieth, E., Tricoire, J., Rolland, M., Grandjean, H., Rochiccioli, P. & Tauber, M. (1998). Biol Neonate. *Growth hormone, insulin-like growth factor-I and insulin-like growth factor binding protein-3 are regulated differently in small-for-gestational-age and appropriate-for-gestational-age neonates*, 73, 347-355.

Carel, J.C., Hay F., Coutant, R., Rodrigue, D. &Chaussain, J. L. (1996). J Clin Endocrinol Metab. *Gonadotropin-releasing hormone agonist treatment of girls with constitutional short stature and normal pubertal development*, 81, 3318-3322.

Carel, J. C., Chatelain P., Rochiccioli, P. &Chaussain, J.L. (2003). J Clin Endocrinol Metab. *Improvement in adult height after growth hormone treatment in adolescents with short stature born small for gestational age: results of a randomized controlled study*, 88, 1587-1593.

Carrascosa, A., Esteban, C., Espadero, R., Fernandez-Cancio, M., Andaluz, P., Clemente, M., Audi, L., Wollmann, H., Fryklund, L. &Parodi, L. (2006). J Clin Endocrinol Metab. *The d3/fl-growth hormone (GH) receptor polymorphism does not influence the effect of GH treatment (66 microg/kg per day) or the spontaneous growth in short non-GH-deficient small-for-gestational-age children: results from a two-year controlled prospective study in 170 Spanish patients*, 91, 3281-3286.

Chernausek, S.D. (2005). Horm Res. *Treatment of short children born small for gestational age: US perspective*, 2005, 64, 63-66.

Christensen, T.L., Djurhuus, C.B., Bentley, A., Djurhuus, C. & Baker-Searle, R. (2007). Clin Endocrinol (Oxf). *An evaluation of the relationship between adult height and health-related quality of life in the general UK population*, 67, 407-412.

Cicognani, A., Alessandroni, R., Pasini, A., Pirazzoli, P., Cassio, A., Barbieri, E. & Cacciari, E. (2002). J Pediatr. *Low birth weight for gestational age and subsequent male gonadal function*, 141, 376-379.

Clayton, P. E., Cianfarani, S., Czernichow, P., Johannsson, G., Rapaport, R. &Rogol, A. (2007). J Clin Endocrinol Metab. *Management of the child born small for gestational age through to adulthood: a consensus statement of the International Societies of Pediatric Endocrinology and the Growth Hormone Research Society*, 92, 804-810.

Collett-Solberg, P.F. & Cohen, P. (2000). Endocrine. *Genetics, chemistry, and function of the IGF/IGFBP system*, 12, 121-136.

Conover, C.A., Clarkson, J.T. & Bale, L.K. (1996). Endocrinology. *Factors regulating insulin-like growth factor-binding protein-3 binding, processing, and potentiation of insulin-like growth factor action*, 137, 2286-2292.

Cutfield, W.S., Lindberg, A., Rapaport, R., Wajnrajch, M.P. & Saenger, P. (2006). Horm Res. *Safety of growth hormone treatment in children born small for gestational age: the US trial and KIGS analysis*, 65, 153-159.

Dahlgren, J. & Wikland K.A. (2005). Pediatr Res. *Final height in short children born small for gestational age treated with growth hormone*, 57, 216-222.

Danesh, J., Collins, R. & Peto, R. (2000). Circulation. *Lipoprotein(a) and coronary heart disease. Meta-analysis of prospective studies*, 102, 1082-1085.

de Bie, H.M., Oostrom, K.J. & Delemarre-van de Waal, H.A. (2010). Horm Res Paediatr. *Brain development, intelligence and cognitive outcome in children born small for gestational age*, 73, 6-14.

de Graaff, L. C., Meyer, S., Els, C. & Hokken-Koelega, A.C. (2008). Clin Endocrinol (Oxf). *GH receptor d3 polymorphism in Dutch patients with MPHD and IGHD born small or appropriate for gestational age*, 68, 930-934.

de Lacerda, L., Carvalho, J.A., Stannard, B., Werner, H., Boguszewski, M.C., Sandrini, R., Malozowski, S.N., Leroith, D. & Underwood, L.E. (1999). Clin Endocrinol (Oxf). *In vitro and in vivo responses to short-term recombinant human insulin-like growth factor-1 (IGF-I) in a severely growth-retarded girl with ring chromosome 15 and deletion of a single allele for the type 1 IGF receptor gene*, 51, 541-550.

de Waal, W. J., Hokken-Koelega, A.C., Stijnen, T., de Muinck Keizer-Schrama, S. M. & Drop, S.L. (1994). Clin Endocrinol (Oxf). *Endogenous and stimulated GH secretion, urinary GH excretion, and plasma IGF-I and IGF-II levels in prepubertal children with short stature after intrauterine growth retardation. The Dutch Working Group on Growth Hormone*, 41, 621-630.

de Zegher, F., Ong, K., van Helvoirt, M., Mohn, A., Woods, K. & Dunger, D. (2002). J Clin Endocrinol Metab. *High-dose growth hormone (GH) treatment in non-GH-deficient children born small for gestational age induces growth responses related to pretreatment GH secretion and associated with a reversible decrease in insulin sensitivity*, 87, 148-151.

de Zegher, F. & Hokken-Koelega, A. (2005). Pediatrics. *Growth hormone therapy for children born small for gestational age: height gain is less dose dependent over the long term than over the short term*, 115, e458-e462.

de Zegher, F., Ong, K.K., Ibanez, L. & Dunger, D.B. (2006). Horm Res. *Growth hormone therapy in short children born small for gestational age*, 65, 145-152.

DiMartino-Nardi, J., Wu, R., Fishman, K. & Saenger, P. (1991). J Clin Endocrinol Metab. *The effect of long-acting analog of luteinizing hormone-releasing hormone on growth hormone secretory dynamics in children with precocious puberty*, 73, 902-906.

Esteban, C., Audi, L., Carrascosa, A., Fernandez-Cancio, M., Perez-Arroyo, A., Ulied, A., Andaluz, P., Arjona, R., Albisu, M., Clemente, M., Gussinye, M. & Yeste, D. (2007). Clin Endocrinol (Oxf). *Human growth hormone (GH1) gene polymorphism map in a normal-statured adult population*, 66, 258-268.

Ester, W.A., van Duyvenvoorde, H.A., de Wit, C.C., Broekman, A.J., Ruivenkamp, C.A., Govaerts, L.C., Wit, J.M., Hokken-Koelega, A.C. & Losekoot, M. (2009a). J Clin Endocrinol Metab. *Two short children born small for gestational age with insulin-like growth factor 1 receptor haploinsufficiency illustrate the heterogeneity of its phenotype*, 94, 4717-4727.

Ester, W.A., van Meurs, J.B., Arends, N.J., Uitterlinden, A.G., de Ridder, M.A. & Hokken-Koelega, A.C. (2009b). Horm Res. *Birth size, postnatal growth and growth during growth hormone treatment in small-for-gestational-age children: associations with IGF1 gene polymorphisms and haplotypes?* 72, 15-24.

Frayling, T.M., Hattersley, A.T., McCarthy, A., Holly, J., Mitchell, S.M., Gloyn, A.L., Owen, K., Davies, D., Smith, G.D. & Ben-Shlomo, Y. (2002). Diabetes. *A putative functional polymorphism in the IGF-I gene: association studies with type 2 diabetes, adult height, glucose tolerance, and fetal growth in U.K. populations*, 51, 2313-2316.

Giudice, L.C., de Zegher, F., Gargosky, S.E., Dsupin, B.A., de las Fuentes, L., Crystal, R.A., Hintz, R.L. &

Rosenfeld, R.G. (1995). J Clin Endocrinol Metab. *Insulin-like growth factors and their binding proteins in the term and preterm human fetus and neonate with normal and extremes of intrauterine growth*, 80, 1548-1555.

Gluckman, P.D., Butler, J.H., Comline, R. & Fowden, A. (1987). J Dev Physiol. *The effects of pancreatectomy on the plasma concentrations of insulin-like growth factors 1 and 2 in the sheep fetus*, 9, 79-88.

Gluckman, P.D., Gunn, A.J., Wray, A., Cutfield, W.S., Chatelain, P.G., Guilbaud, O., Ambler, G.R., Wilton, P. & Albertsson-Wikland, K. (1992). J Pediatr. *Congenital idiopathic growth hormone deficiency associated with prenatal and early postnatal growth failure. The International Board of the Kabi Pharmacia International Growth Study*, 121, 920-923.

Hannon, T.S., Janosky, J. & Arslanian, S.A. (2006). Pediatr Res. *Longitudinal study of physiologic insulin resistance and metabolic changes of puberty*, 60, 759-763.

Harrela, M., Koistinen, H., Kaprio, J., Lehtovirta, M., Tuomilehto, J., Eriksson, J., Toivanen, L., Koskenvuo, M., Leinonen, P., Koistinen, R. & Seppala, M. (1996). J Clin Invest. *Genetic and environmental components of interindividual variation in circulating levels of IGF-I, IGF-II, IGFBP-1, and IGFBP-3*, 98, 2612-2615.

Hernandez, M.I., Martinez, A., Capurro, T., Pena, V., Trejo, L., Avila, A., Salazar, T., Asenjo, S., Iniguez, G. & Mericq, V. (2006). J Clin Endocrinol Metab. *Comparison of clinical, ultrasonographic, and biochemical differences at the beginning of puberty in healthy girls born either small for gestational age or appropriate for gestational age: preliminary results*, 91, 3377-3381.

Hokken-Koelega, A.C., de Ridder, M.A., Lemmen, R.J., den Hartog, H., de Muinck Keizer-Schrama, S.M. & Drop, S.L. (1995). Pediatr Res. *Children born small for gestational age: do they catch up?* 38, 267-271.

Holt, R.I. (2002). Trends Endocrinol Metab. *Fetal programming of the growth hormone-insulin-like growth factor axis*, 13, 392-397.

Ibanez, L., Potau, N., Enriquez, G., Marcos, M.V. & de Zegher, F. (2003). Hum Reprod. *Hypergonadotrophinaemia with reduced uterine and ovarian size in women born small-for-gestational-age*, 18, 1565-1569.

Jaquet, D., Deghmoun, S., Chevenne, D., Collin, D., Czernichow, P. & Levy-Marchal, C. (2005). Diabetologia. *Dynamic change in adiposity from fetal to postnatal life is involved in the metabolic syndrome associated with reduced fetal growth*, 48, 849-855.

Jensen, R.B., Vielwerth, S., Larsen, T., Greisen, G., Veldhuis, J. & Juul, A. (2007). J Clin Endocrinol Metab. *Pituitary-gonadal function in adolescent males born appropriate or small for gestational age with or without intrauterine growth restriction*, 92, 1353-1357.

Johnston, L.B., Dahlgren, J., Leger, J., Gelander, L., Savage, M.O., Czernichow, P., Wikland, K. A. & Clark, A. J. (2003). J Clin Endocrinol Metab. *Association between insulin-like growth factor I (IGF-I) polymorphisms, circulating IGF-I, and pre- and postnatal growth in two European small for gestational age populations*, 88, 4805-4810.

Kerkhof, G.F., Leunissen R.W., Willemsen, R.H., de Jong, F.H., Stijnen, T. & Hokken-Koelega, A. C. (2009). J Clin Endocrinol Metab. *Influence of preterm birth and birth size on gonadal function in young men*, 94, 4243-4250.

Kerkhof, G.F., Leunissen, R.W., Willemsen, R.H., de Jong, F.H., Visser, J.A., Laven, J.S. & Hokken-Koelega, A. C. (2010). Eur J Endocrinol. *Influence of preterm birth and small birth size on serum anti-Mullerian hormone levels in young adult women*, 163, 937-944.

Lanes, R. & Gunczler, P. (1998). Clin Endocrinol (Oxf). *Final height after combined growth hormone and gonadotrophin-releasing hormone analogue therapy in short healthy children entering into normally timed puberty*, 49, 197-202.

Laron, Z., Pertzelan, A., Mannheimer, S. (1966). Isr J Med Sci. *Genetic pituitary dwarfism with high serum concentation of growth hormone--a new inborn error of metabolism?* 2, 152-155.

Leger, J., Levy-Marchal, C., Bloch, J., Pinet, A., Chevenne, D., Porquet, D., Collin, D. & Czernichow, P. (1997). BMJ. *Reduced final height and indications for insulin resistance in 20 year olds born small for gestational age: regional cohort study*, 315, 341-347.

Lem, A.J., de Kort, S.W., de Ridder, M.A. & Hokken-Koelega, A.C. (2010). Clin Endocrinol (Oxf). *Should short children born small for gestational age with a distance to target height <1 standard deviation score be excluded from growth hormone treatment?* 73, 355-360.

Lem, A.J., Boonstra, V.H., Renes, J.S., Breukhoven, P.E., de Jong, F.H., Laven, J.S. & Hokken-Koelega, A.C. (2011). Hum Reprod. *Anti-Mullerian hormone in short girls born small for gestational age and the effect of growth hormone treatment*, 26, 898-903.

Leunissen, R.W., Oosterbeek, P., Hol, L.K., Hellingman, A.A., Stijnen, T. & Hokken-Koelega, A.C. (2008). J Clin Endocrinol Metab. *Fat mass accumulation during childhood determines insulin sensitivity in early adulthood*, 93, 445-451.

Leunissen, R.W., Kerkhof, G.F., Stijnen, T. & Hokken-Koelega, A. (2009). JAMA. *Timing and tempo of first-year rapid growth in relation to cardiovascular and metabolic risk profile in early adulthood*, 301, 2234-2242.

Luo, Z.C., Cheung, Y.B., He, Q., Albertsson-Wikland, K. & Karlberg, J. (2003). Epidemiology. *Growth in early life and its relation to pubertal growth*, 14, 65-73.

Mericq, M.V., Eggers, M., Avila, A., Cutler, G.B. Jr. & Cassorla, F. (2000). J Clin Endocrinol Metab. *Near final height in pubertal growth hormone (GH)-deficient patients treated with GH alone or in combination with luteinizing hormone-releasing hormone analog: results of a prospective, randomized trial*, 85, 569-573.

Moran, A., Jacobs, D.R. Jr., Steinberger, J., Cohen, P., Hong, C.P., Prineas, R. & Sinaiko, A.R. (2002). J Clin Endocrinol Metab. Association between the insulin resistance of puberty and the insulin-like growth factor-I/growth hormone axis, 87, 4817-4820.

Mukherjee, A., Murray, R.D. & Shalet, S.M. (2004). Horm Res. *Impact of growth hormone status on body composition and the skeleton*, 62, 35-41.

Mul, D., Bertelloni, S., Carel, J.C., Saggese, G., Chaussain, J.L. & Oostdijk, W. (2002). Horm Res. *Effect of gonadotropin-releasing hormone agonist treatment in boys with central precocious puberty: final height results*, 58, 1-7.

Murphy, V.E., Smith, R., Giles, W.B. & Clifton, V.L. (2006). Endocr Rev. *Endocrine regulation of human fetal growth: the role of the mother, placenta, and fetus*, 27, 141-169.

Palmert, M.R., Mansfield, M.J., Crowley, W.F. Jr., Crigler, J.F. Jr., Crawford, J.D. & Boepple, P.A. (1999). J Clin Endocrinol Metab. *Is obesity an outcome of gonadotropin-releasing hormone agonist administration? Analysis of growth and body composition in 110 patients with central precocious puberty*, 84, 4480-4488.

Pasquino, A.M., Pucarelli, I., Accardo, F., Demiraj, V., Segni, M. & Di Nardo, R. (2008). J Clin Endocrinol Metab. *Long-term observation of 87 girls with idiopathic central precocious puberty treated with gonadotropin-releasing hormone analogs: impact on adult height, body mass index, bone mineral content, and reproductive function*, 93, 190-195.

Pasquino, A.M., Pucarelli, I., Roggini, M. & Segni, M. (2000). J Clin Endocrinol Metab. *Adult height in short normal girls treated with gonadotropin-releasing hormone analogs and growth hormone*, 85, 619-622.

Primatesta, P., Falaschetti, E. & Poulter, N.R. (2005). Hypertension. *Birth weight and blood pressure in childhood: results from the Health Survey for England*, 45, 75-79.

Renehan, A.G., Zwahlen, M., Minder, C., O'Dwyer, S.T., Shalet, S.M. & Egger, M. (2004). Lancet. *Insulin-like growth factor (IGF)-I, IGF binding protein-3, and cancer risk: systematic review and meta-regression analysis*, 363, 1346-1353.

Rose, S. R., Municchi, G., Barnes, K.M., Kamp, G.A., Uriarte, M.M., Ross, J.L., Cassorla, F. & Cutler, G.B. Jr. (1991). J Clin Endocrinol Metab. *Spontaneous growth hormone secretion increases during puberty in normal girls and boys*, 73, 428-435.

Saggese, G., Bertelloni, S., Baroncelli, G.I., Di Nero, G. & Battini, R. (1993). Acta Paediatr. *Growth velocity and serum aminoterminal propeptide of type III procollagen in precocious puberty during gonadotropin-releasing hormone analogue treatment*, 82, 261-266.

Saggese, G., Federico, G., Barsanti, S. & Fiore, L. (2001). J Clin Endocrinol Metab. *The effect of administering gonadotropin-releasing hormone agonist with recombinant-human growth hormone (GH) on the final height of girls with isolated GH deficiency: results from a controlled study*, 86, 1900-1904.

Sandberg, D.E. & Colsman, M. (2005). Horm Res. *Growth hormone treatment of short stature: status of the quality of life rationale*, 63, 275-283.

Sas, T., de Waal, W., Mulder, P., Houdijk, M., Jansen, M., Reeser, M. & Hokken-Koelega, A. (1999). J Clin Endocrinol Metab. *Growth hormone treatment in children with short stature born small for gestational age: 5-year results of a randomized, double-blind, dose-response trial*, 84, 3064-3070.

Sas, T., Mulder, P. & Hokken-Koelega, A. (2000). J Clin Endocrinol Metab. *Body composition, blood pressure, and lipid metabolism before and during long-term growth hormone (GH) treatment in children with short stature born small for gestational age either with or without GH deficiency*, 85, 3786-3792.

Savendahl, L. (2005). Horm Res. *Hormonal regulation of growth plate cartilage*, 64, 94-97.

Sklar, C.A., Rothenberg, S., Blumberg, D., Oberfield, S.E., Levine, L.S. & David, R. (1991). J Clin Endocrinol Metab. *Suppression of the pituitary-gonadal axis in children with central precocious puberty: effects on growth, growth hormone, insulin-like growth factor-I, and prolactin secretion*, 73, 734-738.

Stanhope, R., Pringle, P.J. & Brook, C.G. (1988). Acta Paediatr Scand. *Growth, growth hormone and sex steroid secretion in girls with central precocious puberty treated with a gonadotrophin releasing hormone (GnRH) analogue*, 77, 525-530.

Steele-Perkins, G., Turner, J., Edman, J.C., Hari, J., Pierce, S.B., Stover, C., Rutter, W.J. & Roth, R.A. (1988). J Biol Chem. *Expression and characterization of a functional human insulin-like growth factor I receptor*, 63, 1486-1492.

Stephen, M.D., Varni, J.W. Limbers, C.A., Yafi, M., Heptulla, R.A., Renukuntla, V.S., Bell, C.S. & Brosnan, P.G. (2011). Eur J Pediatr. *Health-related quality of life and cognitive functioning in pediatric short stature: comparison of growth-hormone-naive, growth-hormone-treated, and healthy samples*, 170, 351-358.

Strauss, R. S. (2000). JAMA. *Adult functional outcome of those born small for gestational age: twenty-six-year follow-up of the 1970 British Birth Cohort*, 283, 625-632.

Tauber, M., Ester, W., Auriol, F., Molinas, C., Fauvel, J., Caliebe, J., Nugent, T., Fryklund, L., Ranke, M.B., Savage, M.O., Clark, A.J., Johnston, L.B. & Hokken-Koelega, A.C. (2007). Clin Endocrinol (Oxf). *GH responsiveness in a large multinational cohort of SGA children with short stature (NESTEGG) is related to the exon 3 GHR polymorphism*, 67, 457-461.

Toth, M.J., Cooper, B.C., Pratley, R.E., Mari, A., Matthews, D.E. & Casson, P.R. (2008). Am J Physiol Endocrinol Metab. *Effect of ovarian suppression with gonadotropin-releasing hormone agonist on glucose disposal and insulin secretion*, 294, E1035-E1045.

Ueki, I., Ooi, G.T., Tremblay, M.L., Hurst, K.R., Bach, L.A. & Boisclair, Y.R. (2000). Proc Natl Acad Sci U S A. *Inactivation of the acid labile subunit gene in mice results in mild retardation of postnatal growth despite profound disruptions in the circulating insulin-like growth factor system*, 97, 6868-6873.

Vaessen, N., Heutink, P., Janssen, J.A., Witteman, J.C., Testers, L., Hofman, A., Lamberts, S.W., Oostra, B.A., Pols, H.A. & van Duijn, C.M. (2001). Diabetes. *A polymorphism in the gene for IGF-I: functional properties and risk for type 2 diabetes and myocardial infarction*, 50, 637-642.

van der Kaay, D.C., Hendriks, A.E., Ester, W.A., Leunissen, R.W., Willemsen, R.H., de Kort, S.W., Paquette, J.R., Hokken-Koelega, A.C. & Deal, C.L. (2009a). Growth Horm IGF Res. *Genetic and epigenetic variability in the gene for IGFBP-3 (IGFBP3): correlation with serum IGFBP-3 levels and growth in short children born small for gestational age*, 19, 198-205.

van der Kaay, D.C., Rose, S.R., van Dijk, M., Noordam, C., van Rheenen, E. & Hokken-Koelega, A.C. (2009b). Clin Endocrinol (Oxf). *Reduced levels of GH during GnRH analogue treatment in pubertal short girls born small for gestational age (SGA)*, 70, 914-919.

van der Kaay, D.C., de Jong, F.H., Laven, J.S. & Hokken-Koelega, A.C. (2009c). J Pediatr Endocrinol Metab. *Overnight luteinizing and follicle stimulating hormone profiles during GnRHa treatment in short girls born small for gestational age*, 22, 161-169.

van der Kaay, D.C., de Jong, F.H., Rose, S.R., Odink, R.J., Bakker-van Waarde, W.M., Sulkers, E.J. & Hokken-Koelega, A.C. (2009d). Horm Res. *Overnight levels of luteinizing hormone, follicle-stimulating hormone and growth hormone before and during gonadotropin-releasing hormone analogue treatment in short boys born small for gestational age*, 71, 260-267.

van der Kaay, D., Bakker, B., van der Hulst, F., Mul, D., Mulder, J., Schroor, E., van Elswijk, D., Rowaan, I., Willeboer, M., de Ridder, M. & Hokken-Koelega, A. (2010). Eur J Endocrinol. *Randomized GH trial with two different dosages in combination with a GnRH analogue in short small for gestational age children: effects on metabolic profile and serum GH, IGF1, and IGFBP3 levels*, 162, 887-895.

van der Sluis, I.M., Boot, A.M., Krenning, E.P., Drop, S.L. & de Muinck Keizer-Schrama, S.M. (2002). J Clin Endocrinol Metab. *Longitudinal follow-up of bone density and body composition in children with precocious or early puberty before, during and after cessation of GnRH agonist therapy*, 87, 506-512.

van Dijk, M., Mulder, P., Houdijk, M., Mulder, J., Noordam, K., Odink, R.J., Rongen-Westerlaken, C., Voorhoeve, P., Waelkens, J., Stokvis-Brantsma, J. & Hokken-Koelega, A. (2006). J Clin Endocrinol Metab. *High serum levels of growth hormone (GH) and insulin-like growth factor-I (IGF-I) during high-dose GH treatment in short children born small for gestational age*, 91, 1390-1396.

van Dijk, M., Bannink, E.M., van Pareren, Y.K., Mulder, P.G. & Hokken-Koelega, A.C. (2007). J Clin Endocrinol Metab. *Risk factors for diabetes mellitus type 2 and metabolic syndrome are comparable for previously growth hormone-treated young adults born small for gestational age (SGA) and untreated short SGA controls*, 92, 160-165.

Van Pareren, Y., Mulder, P., Houdijk, M., Jansen, M., Reeser, M. & Hokken-Koelega, A. (2003). J Clin Endocrinol Metab. *Adult height after long-term, continuous growth hormone (GH) treatment in short children born small for gestational age: results of a randomized, double-blind, dose-response GH trial*, 88, 3584-3590.

van Pareren, Y. K., Duivenvoorden, H.J., Slijper, F.S., Koot, H.M. & Hokken-Koelega, A. C. (2004). J Clin Endocrinol Metab. *Intelligence and psychosocial functioning during long-term growth hormone therapy in children born small for gestational age*, 89, 5295-5302.

Veenma, D. C., Eussen, H.J., Govaerts, L.C., de Kort, S.W., Odink, R.J., Wouters, C.H., Hokken-Koelega, A.C. & de Klein, A. (2010). J Med Genet. *Phenotype-genotype correlation in a familial IGF1R microdeletion case*, 47, 492-498.

Verkauskiene, R., Jaquet, D., Deghmoun, S., Chevenne, D., Czernichow, P. & Levy-Marchal, C. (2005). J Clin Endocrinol Metab. *Smallness for gestational age is associated with persistent change in insulin-like growth factor I (IGF-I) and the ratio of IGF-I/IGF-binding protein-3 in adulthood*, 90, 5672-5676.

Volkl, T.M., Schwobel, K., Simm, D., Beier, C., Rohrer, T.R., Dorr, H.G. (2004). *Growth Horm IGF Res. Spontaneous growth hormone secretion and IGF1:IGFBP3 molar ratios in children born small for gestational age (SGA)*, 14, 455-461.

Walenkamp, M.J., Karperien, M., Pereira, A.M., Hilhorst-Hofstee, Y., van Doorn, J., Chen, J.W., Mohan, S., Denley, A., Forbes, B., van Duyvenvoorde, H.A., van Thiel, S.W., Sluimers, C.A., Bax, J.J., de Laat, J.A., Breuning, M.B., Romijn, J.A. & Wit, J. M. (2005). J Clin Endocrinol Metab. *Homozygous and heterozygous expression of a novel insulin-like growth factor-I mutation*, 90, 2855-2564.

Weise, M., Flor, A., Barnes, K.M., Cutler, G.B. Jr. & Baron, J. (2004). J Clin Endocrinol Metab. *Determinants of growth during gonadotropin-releasing hormone analog therapy for precocious puberty*, 89, 103-107.

Willemsen, R.H., Arends, N.J., Bakker-van Waarde, W.M., Jansen, M., van Mil, E.G., Mulder, J., Odink, R.J., Reeser, M., Rongen-Westerlaken, C., Stokvis-Brantsma, W.H., Waelkens, J.J. & Hokken-Koelega, A.C. (2007). Clin Endocrinol (Oxf). *Long-term effects of growth hormone (GH) treatment on body composition and bone mineral density in short children born small-for-gestational-age: six-year follow-up of a randomized controlled GH trial*, 67, 485-492.

Willemsen, R.H., van Dijk, M., de Kort, S.W., van Toorenenbergen, A.W. & Hokken-Koelega, A.C. (2008). Clin Endocrinol (Oxf). *Plasma matrix metalloproteinase-9 levels and blood pressure in short children born small for gestational age and effects of growth hormone treatment*, 69, 264-268.

Yakar, S., Liu, J.L., Stannard, B., Butler, A., Accili, D., Sauer, B. & LeRoith, D. (1999). Proc Natl Acad Sci U S A. *Normal growth and development in the absence of hepatic insulin-like growth factor I*, 96, 7324-7329.

11

Failure to Thrive: Overview of Diagnosis and Management

Ayse Pinar Cemeroglu, Lora Kleis and Beth Robinson-Wolfe
Pediatric Endocrinology and Diabetes Division,
Spectrum Health Medical Group,
Helen DeVos Children's Hospital,
Grand Rapids, MI,
USA

1. Introduction

Failure to thrive (FTT) is a common and potentially serious growth problem identified in the first three years of life, affecting 5% to 10% of children seen in the primary care setting (Schwartz, 2000). It accounts for 5% to 10% of referrals to (Daniel et al., 2008) and 1% of hospital admissions in tertiary care centers (Berwick et al., 1982).

Although FTT is relatively common, there seems to be no consensus regarding its definition (Raynor & Rudolf, 2000). The term is most often used to describe persistently inadequate linear growth and/or weight gain within the first three years of life (Schwartz, 2000). FTT is a sign or finding rather than a diagnosis since it simply represents an abnormal growth pattern in young children. The underlying condition causing FTT might be difficult to determine, requiring a thorough history and physical examination with special attention to dietary and psychosocial factors. It requires close monitoring by the primary physician.

Poor growth or poor weight gain in children may be due to a variety of medical or psychosocial problems. Therefore, monitoring growth is an invaluable tool for primary care physicians and should be done vigilantly at every well-child visit. Growth charts are useful in comparing a child to appropriate standards for age, sex and ethnic background. If any abnormality in the growth pattern is detected, necessary measures should be undertaken to ensure appropriate evaluation for and treatment of any underlying condition.

Long-term FTT without significant underlying organic etiology has been shown to negatively impact neurodevelopmental outcome (Hufton et al., 1977). Studies have shown that five to eight years after a FTT diagnosis these children show disorders of personality trait, have decreased educational attainment and demonstrate lower IQ's despite having average anthropometric parameters at the time of evaluation (Hufton, et al., 1977). Therefore, early diagnosis and intervention are believed to be key factors in improving outcome in children with FTT (Casey et al., 1994). In the absence of effective treatment, children with FTT may develop irreversible cognitive and behavioral disorders that seem to correlate with the severity and duration of the FTT. However, other studies have reached the opposite conclusion. In a review and analysis of thirteen studies, there seemed to be no significant difference in the IQ of patients with failure to thrive compared to the general population (Wright et al., 1998). This discrepancy in outcome is probably due to the lack of large, randomized, controlled studies in children with FTT.

2. Normal growth in children less than three years of age

Evaluation of growth in children at well-child visits is an invaluable tool. Regular measurements of length/height and weight are vital, especially during the first three years of life, to facilitate early detection and treatment of any physical, nutritional or psychosocial factors that might negatively impact a child's growth and overall health.

Normal growth patterns may vary in different groups of children. Ethnicity, gestational age (premature infants should be corrected for their gestational age until age two years), birth weight and length, familial growth pattern (i.e. constitutional growth delay) and breast fed versus formula fed are some of the factors that should be considered to avoid unnecessary testing or referrals to pediatric subspecialists.

Effective growth monitoring requires accurate, consistent anthropometric measurements and meticulous plotting on the appropriate growth chart. Growth charts exist for age (length for ages 0-36 months; height for ages 2-20 years) and gender, as well as syndrome-specific charts. In the first three years of life, a length chart should be used for infants/toddlers measured in a recumbent position. For children between the ages of two and three who are able to cooperate with a standing measurement as well as children over the age of three, a 2-20 year height chart should be used.

Effective growth monitoring requires precise and consistent measurements by properly trained health care providers. The most common reason for an unexpected deviation in a child's height is an error in measuring technique (Pinyerd-Zipf & Amer, 2004). Use of the wrong growth chart or incorrect plotting of data can lead to an unnecessary evaluation of incorrectly perceived poor growth or failure to recognize a significant change in a child's growth pattern.

All children under the age of two and those from two to three years who are unable or unwilling to cooperate with a standing height should have a recumbent length measured. The preferred method is to utilize an infantometer (Figure 1) which has a fixed headplate and a moveable footplate. Measuring between two marks on exam table paper is often inaccurate and should be avoided. In general, children are transitioned from measuring a recumbent length to a standing height somewhere between the age of two and three years,

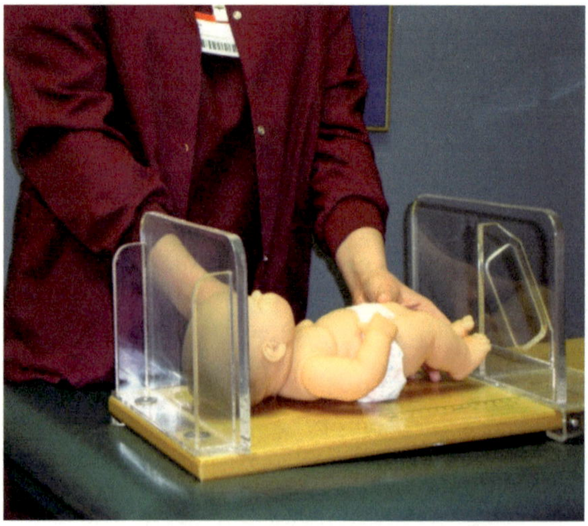

Fig. 1. Infantometer

once the child is able to cooperate with a standing measurement. Ideally both a recumbent length and a standing height should be performed at the time of this transition for comparison, as a standing height is usually slightly less than a recumbent length.

A stadiometer for measuring height requires a vertical board with a metric rule, preferably affixed to the wall (Figure 2). A horizontal headpiece can be brought down into contact with the superior part of the child's head. A flexible or "floppy" arm attached to a vertical rule can be unreliable for serial height measurements, as is standing a child against a tape measure or yardstick attached to the wall and using a ruler or piece of cardboard or plastic against the top of the head.

In the recumbent position, the head is held against the fixed headplate. The infant/toddler is gently stretched, legs together, toes pointing upward, as the footplate is moved against the bottom of the feet. The heels, back of the knees, buttocks and shoulders should be against the bottom platform. Ideally two people are needed to ensure an accurate measurement. The parent/care provider can assist in positioning the child.

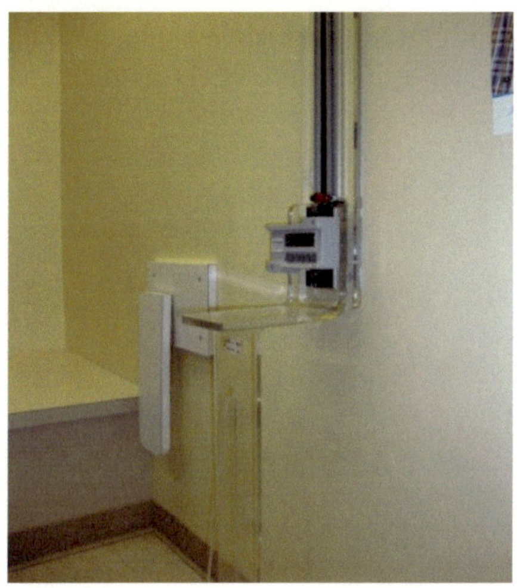

Fig. 2. Stadiometer

Shoes, bulky clothing, hats and hair accessories should be removed. The child should stand erect, weight evenly distributed, feet flat on the floor, heels together against the baseboard or wall. If possible the head, shoulders and buttocks should touch the vertical surface. The child's eyes should be in a straight horizontal line with the middle of the ear. Slight upward traction can be applied under the child's chin to avoid "turtling" of the neck when the fixed headpiece of the stadiometer comes in contact with the top of the child's head.

The weight measurement is usually less biased then a height or length measurement, however, infants and toddlers should be weighed naked for accuracy and continuity. If a toddler or child is uncooperative with a weight measurement, the parent or caregiver can be weighed alone and then holding the child, with the difference calculated as the child's weight.

Published in 2000, the CDC growth charts are used for monitoring the growth of infants and children (Figures 3-6). Primary care providers should ensure that recumbent measurements of children are plotted on the boy or girl birth to 36 months length- for- age chart (Figure 3), while a standing height should be plotted on a boy or girl 2-20 years stature for age (Figure 4).

Plotting anthropometric measurements on the incorrect growth chart (for example: height on the length chart or plotting height and weight on a chart for the incorrect gender) or not recording and plotting measurements accurately can cause the physician to believe that the child's growth is impaired, potentially leading to unnecessary testing and /or referral to a pediatric subspecialist.

Growth is a process. In evaluating growth in children, growth velocity or weight gain over a period of time is more important than attained length, height or weight percentiles. A single measurement of length, height or weight is of limited use.

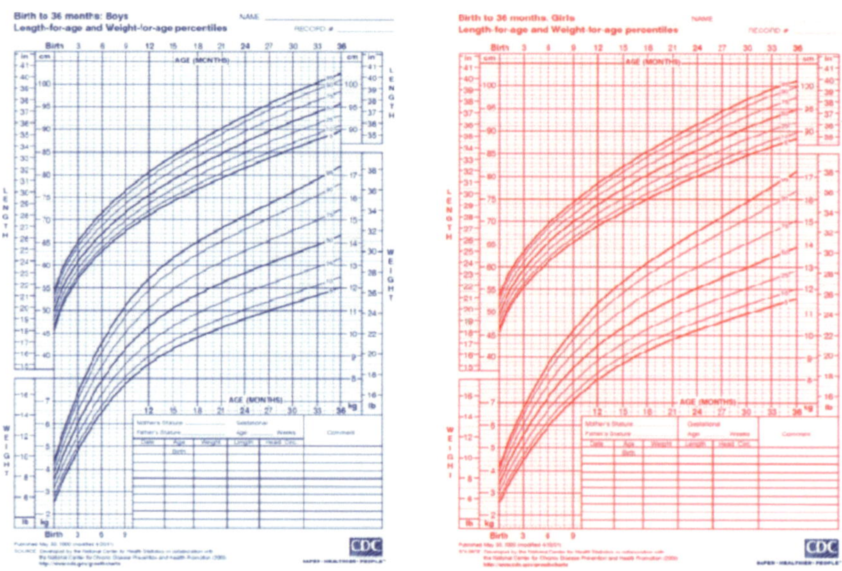

Fig. 3. Boy and girl length-for-age and weight-for-age charts for birth to 36 months

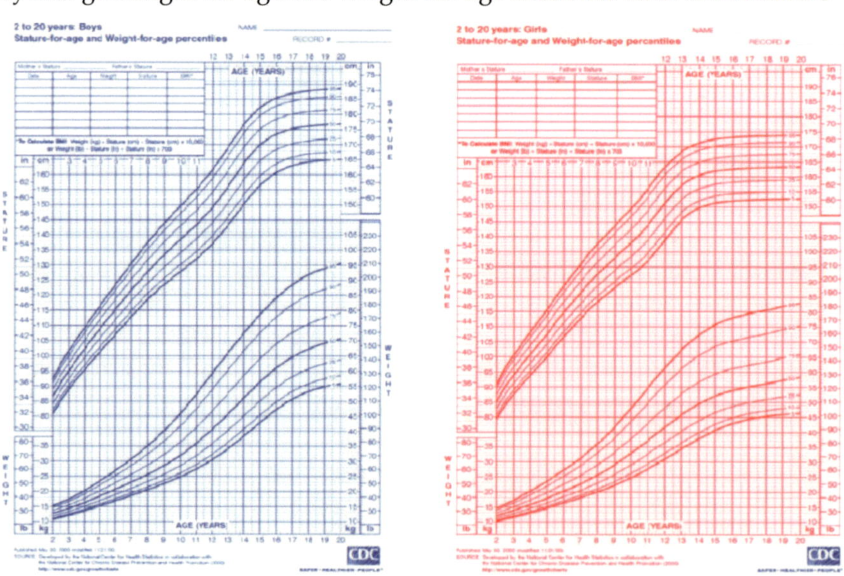

Fig. 4. Boy and girl stature-for-age and weight-for-age charts for 2-20 years

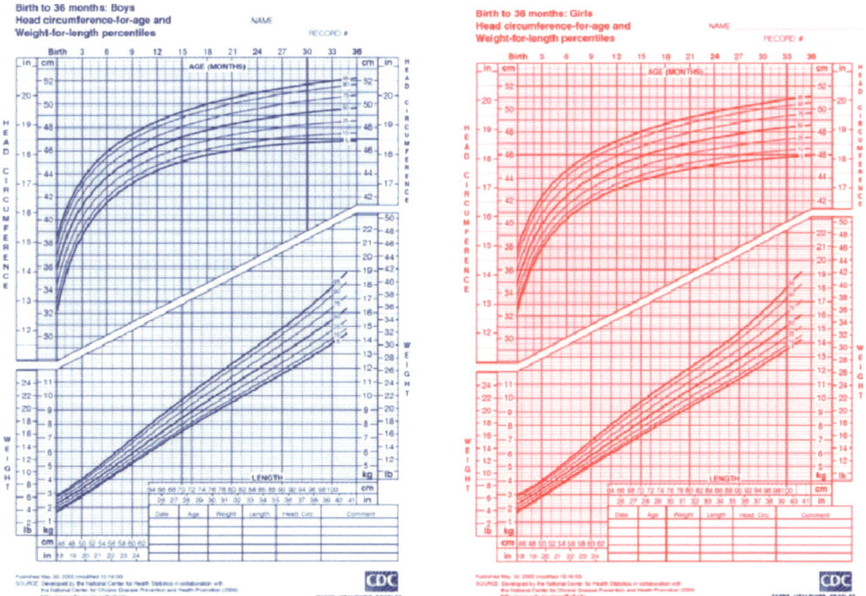

Fig. 5. Boy and girl head circumference/weight-for-length percentiles birth to 36 months

Weight for length is also a useful piece of information for children 36 months and younger, assisting with assessment of nutritional status (Figure 5). If a standing height is obtained, then a BMI chart with percentiles for age can be used for children two years of age and older (Figure 6).

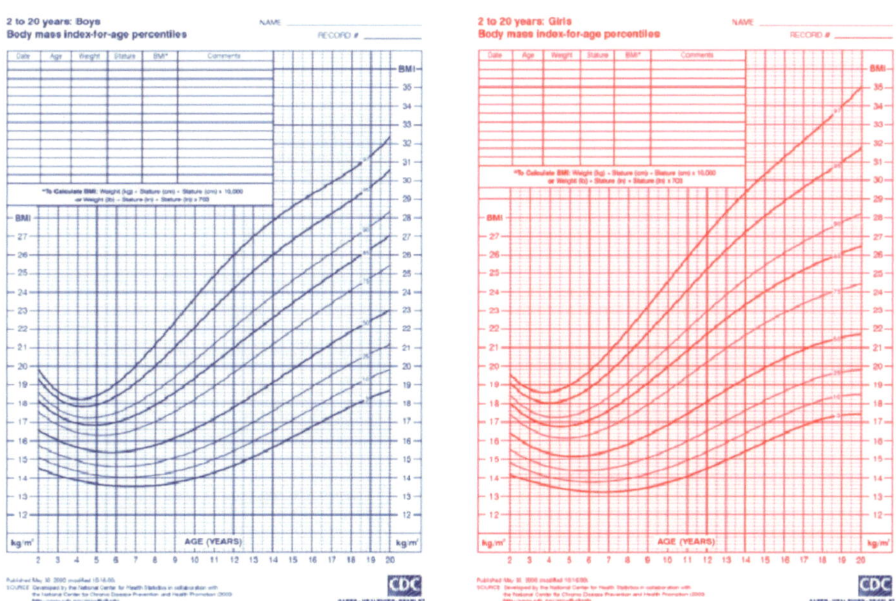

Fig. 6. Boy and girl body mass index-for-age (BMI) charts for 2-20 years (CDC)

In 2006, the World Health Organization (WHO) released new international growth charts for children ages birth to 59 months. The CDC now recommends using the WHO growth charts for children ≤ 24 months of age (Figures 7 and 8) and to continue using CDC charts for children older than 24 months of age (Grummer-Strawnet al., 2010).

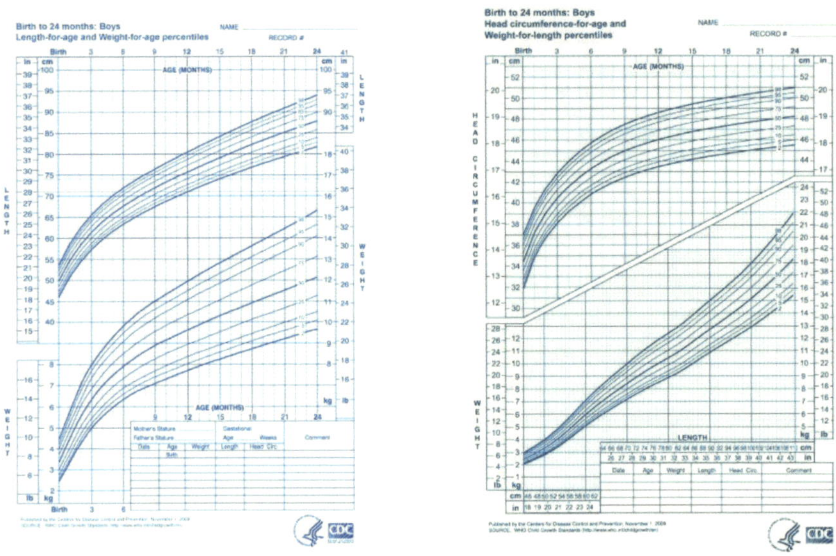

Fig. 7. WHO charts for boys birth to 24 months: length-for-age and weight-for age percentiles and head circumference-for-age and weight-for length percentiles

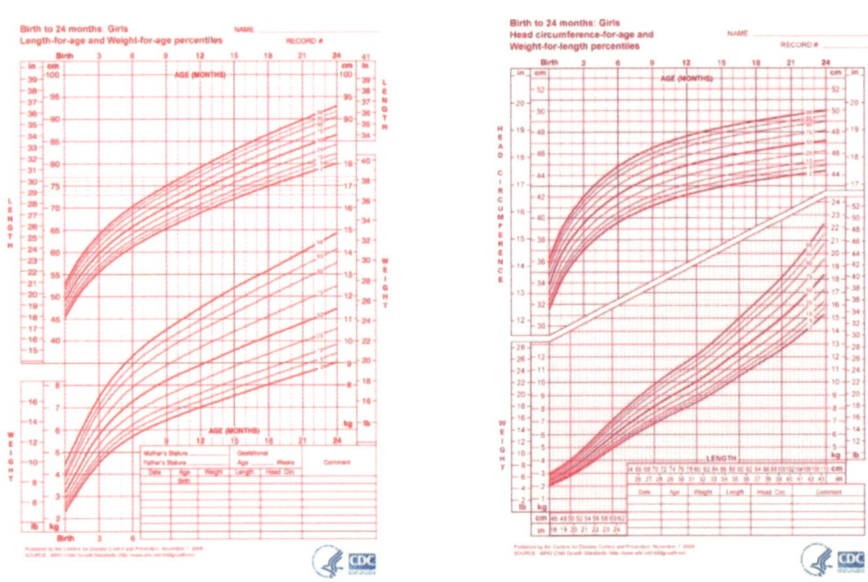

Fig. 8. WHO charts for girls birth to 24 months: length-for-age and weight-for age percentiles and head circumference-for-age and weight-for length percentiles

Fewer children will be diagnosed as having FTT if the WHO charts are used for exclusively breast fed infants. Slower growth among breast fed infants between the ages of three and eighteen months represents a normal growth variant. This slower growth rate should not be used to discourage mothers from exclusively breastfeeding their infants. There are numerous advantages to breastfeeding including increased protection from infectious disease.

On the other hand, the rapid, upward crossing of weight percentiles on the WHO charts might be an early indication of obesity (Grummer-Strawnet et al., 2010).

3. Definition of FTT

FTT has been a recognized condition for centuries. However, its precise definition remains unclear and often controversial. In order to verify the presence of FTT many physicians use weight gain over a period of time as the only anthropometric measurement, but others utilize two or more parameters.

In a cross-sectional review of studies published between 2002 and 2004, weight-for- age of less than the 10th percentile, height-for-age of less than the 5th percentile or weight-for-height of less than the 10th percentile were the most commonly used anthropometric measurements to define FTT (Olsen, 2006). Although using weight only to define FTT may be adequate in most cases, utilizing additional anthropometric measurements (such as weight-for-length, especially before the age of two years) is also helpful in determining the underlying problem. A study of 6090 Danish infants used seven different anthropometric measurements to define nutritional FTT and concluded that one single anthropometric parameter was inadequate to identify the condition and therefore more than one measurement should be used (Olsen et al., 2007).

4. Etiological classification of FTT

FTT is a sign or finding rather than a diagnosis and can be caused by several different conditions. Steps to identify the underlying cause should be undertaken when a child presents with FTT.

There are different definitions for the etiologies of FTT. The most commonly used etiologic classifications are nonorganic (inadequate nutrition in the absence of underlying organic disorders) or organic (underlying disease process such as endocrine, gastrointestinal, cardiac, genetic, metabolic, pulmonary, renal, hematologic or infectious). (Table 1)

Although organic FTT may have multiple etiologies, the majority of children have a nonorganic cause of their poor growth and/or weight gain (Mitchell et al., 1980).

4.1 Nonorganic FTT and psychosocial dwarfism (emotional deprivation syndrome)

The majority of cases of FTT presenting in a primary care setting are nonorganic with no underlying disease (Mitchell et al., 1980). Parental/caregiver nurturing is as important as nutrition for adequate growth and development in children. Neglected infants and toddlers have been known to stop growing, gaining weight and achieving normal developmental milestones. This was described in the 1940's (Talbot et al., 1946) and later in more detail as a form of hypopituitarism, commonly known as emotional deprivation or psychosocial dwarfism (Powell et al., 1967). This type of hypopituitarism is reversible as the home environment of the child improves (Albanese et al., 1994).

Nonorganic FTT **Neglect/abuse** (psychosocial dwarfism) **Hyper vigilance** (extreme parental attention) **Poor nutrition** (inexperienced or poorly educated parents/caregivers, poverty)
Organic FTT
Gastrointestinal: Gastroesophageal reflux, pyloric stenosis, malabsorptive conditions such as celiac disease, lactose intolerance, chronic liver disease, protein- losing enteropathy or food allergies
Pulmonary: Cystic fibrosis, bronchopulmonary dysplasia, chronic hypoxia
Endocrine: hyperthyroidism, adrenal failure, diabetes mellitus, diabetes insipidus, hypopituitarism
Neurologic: degenerative brain disease, cerebral palsy, mitochondrial disorders
Metabolic and genetic: inborn errors of metabolism, genetic syndromes, chromosomal defects including Prader-Willi Syndrome **Infectious**: parasites, tuberculosis, acquired immunodeficiency, congenital immune deficiency **Renal**: chronic renal failure, renal tubular acidosis, nephrogenic diabetes insipidus, recurrent urinary tract infections **Hematologic:** Fanconi's anemia

Table 1. Etiologic classifications of failure to thrive

Although the terms nonorganic FTT and psychosocial dwarfism are sometimes used interchangeably and the psychosocial family dynamics are similar in both conditions, the clinical features differ. The majority of children with nonorganic FTT are less than three years of age and often as young as eighteen months. They are often withdrawn and apathetic and weight loss or very poor weight gain is the most marked feature. Children with psychosocial dwarfism range between two and fifteen years of age and short stature is the most prominent feature. These children may steal and hoard food and display bizarre eating habits. In some cases a reversible hypopituitarism has been documented. Therefore, psychosocial dwarfism constitutes a subgroup of nonorganic FTT (Oates, 1984).

Behaviors that may be present in nonorganic FTT include inactivity, irritability, posturing, flat affect, rumination, excessive thumb sucking, disproportionate use of hands and fingers rather than arms, legs, and trunk, clenched fists, gross motor delay, crying when approached, wide-eyed expression, gaze aversion, lack of or decreased vocalization, lack of cuddling, poor eye contact, lack of response to a human stimulus and indifference to separation. Identification of these target behaviors may be valuable in diagnosing nonorganic FTT and providing early psychosocial assessment and intervention (Powell & Low, 1983).

A recent study of the neuroendocrine system in children with FTT included three groups: (1) a control group; (2) children suffering from attachment disorder (AD); and (3) children with non-organic FTT (NOFT) (Muñoz-Hoyos et al., 2010). In this study, the serum levels of melatonin, serotonin, β-endorphins, adrenocorticotropic hormone (ACTH) and tryptophan metabolites were measured both during the day and at night. There was a significant reduction in the levels of each of these markers in the group with AD and a more significant reduction in the group with NOFT. These findings suggest that AD and NOFT comprise a single process with a different evolutionary continuum of psychosocial dwarfism.

4.2 Organic FTT

Children suspected of having an organic FTT will require further evaluation and referral to the appropriate pediatric subspecialist for management once the underlying etiology has been identified. Primary care physicians are sometimes overly cautious, referring children with nonorganic FTT to pediatric subspecialties such as gastroenterology or endocrinology when these children could be managed by nutritional counseling and close follow-up alone. In a chart analysis of 97 patients referred for FTT by primary care physicians to a pediatric endocrinology clinic, the most common (52%) etiology was found to be nutritional deficiency or nonorganic FTT (Daniel et al., 2008). As these children were referred to a subspecialty clinic by their primary care physician for further evaluation, 52% having a nonorganic FTT is a surprisingly high number. These children could have been managed in the primary care setting with nutritional counseling and close monitoring. In the remaining 48% who had an organic FTT, endocrinologic etiologies included short stature due to low birth weight/small for gestational age (SGA), familial short stature and constitutional short stature. Gastrointestinal diseases included gastroesophageal reflux disease (GERD), multiple food allergies, celiac disease, selective immunoglobulin A deficiency and pyloric stenosis and were the third most common etiology (15.5%) for FTT in this study.

In order to reduce health care costs, pediatric subspecialty referral of children for FTT should be reserved for those with a proven underlying organic etiology. Differential diagnosis between nonorganic and organic FTT should be made by the primary care provider before referral to a subspecialty is considered.

5. Diagnostic evaluation of FTT

5.1 Initial evaluation and differential diagnosis of FTT

A child with FTT may present to the primary care physician crossing percentiles for weight and length as seen in Figure 9.

This growth chart may represent a child with an organic FTT such as celiac disease, a nonorganic FTT (psychosocial dwarfism) or a normal variant of growth such as constitutional delay (crossing percentiles and then following that channel until he/she enters puberty later than average). A growth chart alone cannot always provide enough data to determine whether the growth pattern is normal or abnormal. Further evaluation may be warranted to avoid unnecessary testing and increased parental anxiety for a child with a normal growth variant.

Assessing the length or height and weight of infants and toddlers during well-child visits is the standard of care. A comprehensive evaluation should include reviewing the past medical history, family history, feeding history, caloric intake, formula preparation, episodes of vomiting, family dynamics, number of caregivers; observing the interaction between the caregiver and the child and conducting a thorough physical examination. Each of these is crucial for an accurate appraisal of the child's growth pattern.

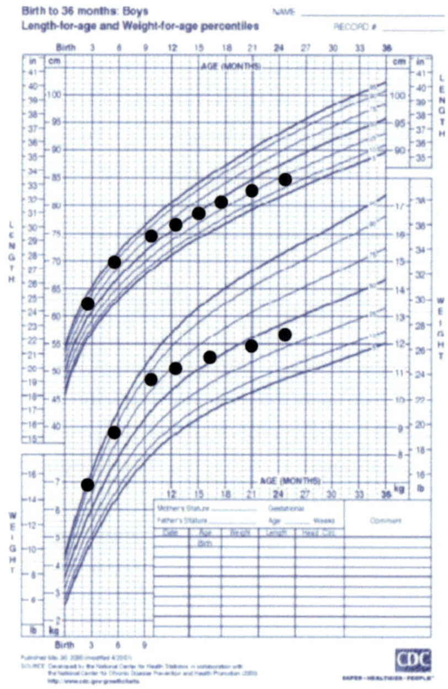

Fig. 9. A case of FTT

When a child is noted to have FTT, the health care provider should evaluate the child thoroughly, making certain to include the following:

- Prenatal and postnatal history
  - was the pregnancy unplanned?
  - gestational age
  - Apgar scores
  - birth weight and length
  - presence of feeding issues or any other neonatal problems (Table 2) (Ficicioglu et al., 2009, Tolia, 1995).
- Family history
  - history of neonatal or infant deaths
  - history of FTT, family members' growth patterns
  - parental heights/weights
- Past medical history (Table 2)
  - presence/absence of these findings may help differentiate between organic and nonorganic FTT (Ficicioglu et al 2009, Tolia 1995).
  - comprehensive dietary history (see Section 6.1, Nutritional counseling)
- Family dynamics and psychosocial factors
  - stressors in the family
  - is the parent/primary caregiver depressed?
  - is the parent/primary caregiver receiving adequate support from family/friends or does he/she feel overwhelmed?
  - socioeconomic status
  - level of education and parental/caregiver knowledge of infant feeding
  - family dietary patterns

  - observation of the child's behavior and parent/caregiver's interaction (for the possibility of psychosocial dwarfism or deprivation syndrome).
- Physical examination
  - anthropometric measurements including head circumference
  - facial features, presence of dysmorphology
  - cardiac murmur
  - organomegaly
  - muscle tone and other neurologic findings
  - developmental milestones

Neonatal	Infancy
• low birth weight/length • low apgar scores • respiratory distress in term baby • prolonged jaundice • cholestasis • hypoglycemia • poor feeding • hypotonia • sepsis • seizures • atypical face	• hypoglycemia • poor feeding • hypotonia • recurrent sepsis-like presentations • seizures • atypical face • micro or macrocephaly • recurrent infections • chronic diarrhea • recurrent vomiting • poor muscle tone • developmental delay • organomegaly • polyuria, polydipsia

Table 2. Significant findings suggesting an underlying organic etiology for FTT

5.2 Evaluation of suspected organic FTT

Children with findings suggesting an organic cause of FTT (Table 2) should be evaluated for an underlying condition. Since the organic reasons for FTT are relatively uncommon, the battery of tests depends on the primary care physician's index of suspicion. In some cases basic screening tests may be required for a differential diagnosis prior to ordering more specific studies. Referral to a pediatric subspecialty without a working diagnosis is not cost effective and should be avoided.

Basic screening tests usually include a complete blood count, comprehensive metabolic panel and urinalysis. In most cases a thorough history and physical examination will direct a skilled physician toward the possibility of one or two underlying organic etiologies and the appropriate diagnostic testing for the suspected condition(s) can be ordered (Sills, 1978). No specific battery of tests is recommended for FTT but rather the working diagnosis should direct the physician to order the appropriate diagnostic tests. The primary care physician is best suited to sort out the possible reasons for the child's FTT.

In a study of 122 infants less than two years of age admitted to a tertiary care pediatric hospital for FTT, an average of 40 tests and imaging studies were ordered per infant and only 0.8% of all tests led to a diagnosis of the underlying cause of the FTT. In most cases, a careful history and physical examination was sufficient for a differential diagnosis of the etiology of FTT (Berwick et al., 1982). An extensive work-up should be limited to cases of suspected organic FTT.

6. Management of FTT

Early identification of children with poor growth and weight gain and intervention with appropriate measures are important in determining the outcome of these children. Undiagnosed and untreated FTT may cause serious morbidity and mortality. Cognitive impairment and decreased IQ are potential serious consequences of long-standing, untreated FTT. Therefore, the role of the primary care physician in detecting and managing FTT is vital, especially since most (> 90%) of the FTT diagnosed in a primary care setting is nonorganic. Close follow-up of height/length and weight, either in a primary care physician's office or during home nursing visits, in conjunction with nutritional counseling will improve the majority of cases of FTT.

A randomized controlled study showed that, in FTT, a visiting nurse can significantly improve growth parameters compared to a control group who received no home nursing visits (Wright et al., 1998). Observation of the home environment and the child's behavior during daily routine by a trained health care professional will provide a more realistic picture of the family dynamics, psychosocial stressors and physical surroundings which may be affecting the child's growth and weight gain. Stress in the family, parental depression or abuse and neglect of the child requires prompt evaluation and effective intervention. Foster care placement should be considered in cases of suspected abuse and neglect.

In some cases of organic FTT where the underlying condition prevents the child from getting adequate oral intake and in rare occasions of nonorganic FTT, tube feeding may be indicated. Weaning from tube feeding may be a long process even after the underlying etiology of the FTT resolves. The child may require prolonged feeding therapy, preferably managed by a specialized feeding clinic.

6.1 Nutritional counseling

Nonorganic FTT is the most common and therefore nutritional counseling is the most important component in the management of FTT. Both nonorganic FTT and organic FTT with additional nutritional deficits should be evaluated by a dietitian. Close monitoring of the child's weight gain and growth rate by the primary care physician is an important component of management.

Nutritional assessment of a child with FTT is not simply an evaluation of food intake but also family feeding practices. Food allergies may affect macro and micronutrient intake. Social and environmental factors such as family budget, caregiver ability to prepare meals and family beliefs about the makeup of a nutritious diet may prevent the child from receiving an adequate diet.

A nutritional analysis of the current diet is needed. A 24-hour food recall combined with a food frequency questionnaire can be used to collect information. The best tool to analyze intake is a 3 to 5 day diet diary with a record of all foods and beverages consumed. An interview of the person recording the food intake should be done to fill in the missing information. Often, fluids taken between meals are not recorded. Meals eaten at daycare or away from home need to include the amounts eaten, not just the foods provided. If there are whole food groups missing from the food record, substitution for the food group should be questioned. Analysis of nutritional intake should provide average intake of calories, protein, and fat in the diet. When possible, a software program can be used that will give a comparison of all nutrients with Recommended Daily Allowance (RDA) for age. There are programs that will print the average intake using the Food Guide Pyramid servings eaten compared to recommended servings, or the percents of carbohydrate, protein and fat in the diet. These print outs can be used in the intervention and education for the parents.

Evaluating family feeding practices will show if there are changes that can be made to help enhance food intake.

- Is the child allowed to carry a sippy cup or bottle all day?
- What is in the sippy-cup/bottle?
- Is there one meal a day that is eaten at a table with the whole family?
- Is there a table in the house where the family can have a meal?
- Do the adults in the family eat fruits and vegetables?
- What are the beverages in the house?
- Is it difficult for the parents to get the child to sit down for a meal?
- Is the toddler fed or allowed to feed himself?
- Do the children have to eat everything put on their plates?
- If the child does not eat at mealtime do they get sweets between meals? Some families are so concerned with a family history of obesity, heart disease or other medical condition that they restrict their child's diet to try to prevent these conditions.
- What is used to measure the formula and water? Check how the formula is prepared.

Food avoidances due to food allergies need to be evaluated to make sure the nutrients in the offending foods are being provided by other foods or supplements. If the child is allergic to milk, he/she must receive the protein, calories, calcium and vitamins A and D from another food source. Children may avoid foods because the food makes them "feel bad" but are unable to explain this to their parents. Food avoidance might also be a sign of a metabolic disorder. For example, children with hyperammonemia tend to avoid a high protein diet.

All of the gathered information can be used to formulate a nutrition plan. Adequate calories and appropriate foods for age should be discussed with the family or care giver (Table 3).

Age (Month)	REE (kcals/kg/day) WHO	EER (kcal/day)	DRI (kcals/kg/day)	Protein (g/day)	Protein (g/kg/day)
0-3	52	610	102	9.1*	1.52
4-6	52	490	82	9.1*	1.52
7-12	55	720	80	11.0**	1.20
13-35	56	990	82	13.0**	1.05
36-48	64	1000	85	13.0**	1.05

Table 3. The estimated energy and protein requirements for birth to 48 months
(Bunting, et al., 2008.) * Adequate Intake, ** Recommended daily allowance (RDA),
REE: Resting energy expenditure; EER: Estimated energy requirements; DRI: Dietary reference intakes

For catch up growth a child may need 20-30% more calories. Increasing calories should be done slowly for the severely malnourished child to prevent re-feeding syndrome. Re-feeding syndrome is characterized by several life-threatening presentations including biochemical changes, clinical manifestations and complications that can occur as a consequence of feeding a malnourished baby in a catabolic state too rapidly (Khan et al., 2010).

Formulas for catch up growth:

$$\frac{\text{kcal/kg/day} = \text{IBW in kg}\left(50^{\text{th}}\text{percentile weight/height}\right) \text{ x kcal/kg/day }\left(\text{DRI for age}\right)}{\text{actual weight }\left(\text{kg}\right)}$$

IBW: Ideal body weight. (Bunting et al., 2008)

$$\frac{\text{kcal / kg / day } = \text{ 120 kcal / kg x median weight for height }\left(\text{kg}\right)}{\text{actual weight }\left(\text{kg}\right)}$$

(Orrales & Utter, 1999)

Nutritional intervention should begin by discussing proper nutrition with the caregiver(s). This should include diet for age and appropriate feeding techniques for catch-up growth. It is necessary to add calories and protein to the diet. This may mean concentrating the formula or breast milk to 24-27 calories per ounce.

Nutritional supplements may be an acceptable way to add calories and protein to a toddler's diet. Milk can be fortified with dry skim milk powder or commercially available instant breakfast powders. Adding calories without increasing serving sizes can be done with the use of oil, margarine or butter.

6.2 Inpatient management

In the past, inpatient evaluation and management was the standard of care for FTT. However, it is now necessary only in the small number of children for whom outpatient management fails.

An inpatient evaluation of FTT may be necessary in suspected neglect or abuse or in psychosocial dwarfism. The child can be observed for caloric intake, daily weight change, interaction with the parent/caregiver and behaviors during feeding. Valuable information can be gathered during the period of hospitalization and a final decision can be made regarding possible foster care placement, especially if the child shows adequate weight gain and catch-up growth as an inpatient after failing outpatient management. Changing the home environment with foster care placement often resolves the FTT in these children.

Occasionally a case of FTT with a complex underlying etiology may require admission for an extensive evaluation. This constitutes a very small portion of cases, however (Berwick et al., 1982).

6.3 Referral to subspecialty clinics

Referral to a pediatric subspecialist should be reserved for FTT with an underlying organic etiology. Nonorganic (nutritional) FTT should be managed by a primary care physician to avoid the unnecessary expenditure of health care dollars, as well as the cost to families for travel, insurance co-pays and time away from their employment. Parents or caregivers often experience anxiety or feelings of guilt related to a child's poor growth or weight gain. This may be exacerbated by an unnecessary, extensive and often expensive work-up when, in most situations, the FTT may resolve simply with nutritional counseling and a period of close monitoring of weight gain and linear growth. When organic FTT is suspected by history and/or physical examination, evaluation based on the suspected etiology should be performed and then the corresponding pediatric subspecialty (gastroenterology, allergy and immunology, pulmonary, cardiology, endocrinology, nephrology, hematology, neurology, infectious disease or genetic/metabolic disorders) should be considered based on the findings.

7. Conclusions

Failure to thrive is a common but potentially serious growth problem requiring early recognition, thorough evaluation and vigilant management to avoid possible long-term morbidity, especially in regard to a child's neurodevelopment. Although there seems to be no consensus regarding definition, the term FTT is most commonly used to describe persistently inadequate linear growth and/or weight gain within the first three years of life.

Health care providers should be familiar with anthropometric measurements and normal growth patterns of children to avoid either misdiagnosis or unnecessary work-up of children with FTT. Unnecessary testing not only increases health care costs, but also can delay dietary or psychosocial intervention and contribute to parental/caregiver anxiety and guilt which may potentially exacerbate the problem.

FTT is a sign or finding rather than a diagnosis and may either have a nonorganic or organic etiology. Steps to identify the underlying cause should be undertaken when a child presents with FTT. The most common cause is inadequate caloric intake (nonorganic). In most cases of organic FTT, a thorough history and physical examination will direct a skilled physician to one or more possible etiologies and then the appropriate diagnostic testing for the suspected underlying condition(s) can be ordered.

Majority of children with FTT have a nonorganic etiology and should be managed by a primary care physician with nutritional counseling and close monitoring of linear growth and weight gain. Extensive evaluation and referral to a pediatric subspecialist for children with FTT should be reserved for the limited number of children suspected of having an underlying organic disease.

8. References

Albanese, A., Hamill, G., Jones, J., Skuse,D., Matthews,D.R. & Stanhope, R. (1994). Reversibility of physiological growth hormone secretion in children with psychosocial dwarfism. *Clin Endocrinol (Oxf)*, Vol. 40, No.5, pp. 687-692, ISSN 0300-0664

Berwick, D.M., Levy, J.C. & Kleinerman, R. (1982). Failure to thrive: diagnostic yield of hospitalisation. *Arch Dis Child*, Vol. 57, No. 5, pp. 347-351, ISSN 0003-9888

Bunting, D., D'Souza, S., Nguyen, J., Phillips, S., Rich, S. & Trout, S. (2008). *Pediatric Nutrition Reference Guide*, Texas Children's Hospital, Houston, Texas.

Casey, P.H., Kelleher, K.J., Bradley, R.H., Kellogg, K.W., Kirby, R.S. & Whiteside, L. (1994). A multifaceted intervention for infants with failure to thrive, A prospective study. *Arch Pediatr Adoles Med*, Vol. 148, No. 10, pp. 1071-1077, ISSN 1072-4710

Daniel, M., Kleis, L. & Cemeroglu, A.P. (2008). Etiology of failure to thrive in infants and toddlers referred to a pediatric endocrinology outpatient clinic. *Clin Pediatr (Phila)*, Vol. 47, No. 8, pp. 762-5, ISSN 0009-9228

Ficicioglu, C. & Haack, K. (2009) Failure to Thrive: When to Suspect Inborn Errors of Metabolism. *Pediatrics*, Vol. 124, pp. 972–979 ISSN 0031-4005

Grummer-Strawn, L.M., Reinold, C. & Krebs, N.F. (2010). Centers for Disease Control and Prevention (CDC). Use of World Health Organization and CDC growth charts for children aged 0-59 months in the United States. *MMWR Recomm Rep,* vol. 10, No.59, pp. 1-15, ISSN: 1057-5987

Hufton, I.W. & Oates, R.K. (1977). Nonorganic failure to thrive: a long-term follow-up. *Pediatrics,* Vol. 59, No. 1, pp. 73-77, ISSN 0031-4005

Khan, L.U., Ahmed, J., Khan, S. & Macfie, J. (2010). Refeeding syndrome: a literature review. *Gastroenterol Res Pract,* [Epub]. Aug 25, ISSN 1687-630X (Electronic), ISSN 1687-6121 (Print)

Mitchell, W.G., Gorrell ,R.W. & Greenberg, R.A. (1980). Failure to thrive: A study in a primary care setting epidemiology and follow-up. *Pediatrics,* Vol. 65, pp. 971-977, ISSN 0031-4005

Muñoz-Hoyos, A., Molina-Carball, A., Augustin-Morales, M., Contreras-Choya, F., Naranjo-Gómez, A., Justicia-Martínez, F. & Uberos, J. (2010). Psychosocial dwarfism: Psychopathological aspects and putative neuroendocrine markers. *Psychiatry Res,* Nov 9. [Epub], ISSB 0165-1781 (Print), ISSN 1872-7123 (Electronic)

Oates, R.K. (1984). Similarities and differences between nonorganic failure to thrive and deprivation dwarfism. *Child Abuse Negl,* Vol. 8, No. 4, pp. 439-45, ISSN 0145-2134

Olsen, E.M. (2006). Failure to thrive: still a problem of definition. *Clin Pediatr,* Vol. 45, pp. 1-6, ISSN 0009-9228

Olsen, E.M., Petersen, J., Skovgaard, A. M., Weile, B., Jørgensen, T. & Wright, C. M. (2007). Failure to thrive: the prevalence and concurrence of anthropometric criteria in a general infant population. *Arch Dis Child,* Vol. 92, pp. 109–114. ISSN 0003-9888

Orrales, K. & Utter, S. (1999). Failure to Thrive. *Handbook of Pediatric Nutrition,* Samour, P., Helm, K. & Lang, C. pp. 395-407, Aspen Publishers, Inc., Gaitherburg, Maryland. ISBN 0-8342-1199-8

Pinyerd-Zipf, B. & Amer, K. (2004). Clinical Perspectives on Growth Monitoring. *Partners in Education,* Pediatric Endocrinology Nursing Society

Powell, G.F., Brasel, J.A. & Blizzard, R.M. (1967). Emotional Deprivation and Growth Retardation Simulating Idiopathic Hypopituitarism—Clinical Evaluation of the Syndrome. *N Engl J Med,* Vol. 276, pp.1271-1278, ISSN 0028-4793

Powell, G. F. & Low, J. (1983). Behavior in nonorganic failure to thrive. *J Dev Behav Pediatr,* Vol. 4, No. 1, pp. 26-33, ISSN 0196-206X

Raynor, P. & Rudolf, M.C.J. (2000) Anthropometric indices of failure to thrive. *Arch Dis Child,* Vol. 82, pp. 364–365, ISSN 0003-9888

Reinhart, J.B. & Drash, A.L. (1969). Psychosocial dwarfism: environmentally induced recovery. *Psychosom Med,* Vol. 31, No.2, pp.165-72, ISSN 0033-3174

Ruldolf, M.C. & Logan, S. (2005). What is the long-term outcome for children who fail to thrive? A systemic review. *Arch Dis Child,* Vol.90, pp. 925-931, ISSN 0003-9888

Schwartz, D. (2000). Failure to thrive: an old nemesis in the new millennium. *Pediatr Rev,* Vol. 21, pp. 257-264, ISSN 0191-9601

Sills, R.H. (1978). Failure to Thrive: The role of clinical and laboratory evaluation. *Am J Dis Child,* Vol. 132, No.10, pp. 967-969, ISSN 0096-8994

Talbot, N.B., Sobel, E.H., Burke, B.S., Lindemann, E. & Kaufman, S.B. (1946). Dwarfism in healthy children; its possible relation to emotional nutritional and endocrine disturbances. *Am J Dis Child,* Vol. 72, No. 4, pp. 450-454, ISSN 0002-922X

Tolia, V. (1995). Very early onset nonorganic failure to thrive in infants. *J Pediatr Gastroenterol Nutr,* Vol. 20, pp. 73-80, ISSN 0277-2116

Wright, C.M., Callum, J., Birks, E. & Jarvis, S. (1998). Effect of community based management in failure to thrive: a randomized controlled trial. *BMJ,* Vol.317, No. 7158, pp. 571-574, ISSN 0959-8138

12

Hormonal Regulation of Circadian Pacemaker in Ovary and Uterus

Masa-aki Hattori
Kyushu University, Fukuoka
Japan

1. Introduction

Ovarian folliculogenesis is characterized by drastic proliferation and differentiation of granulosa cells and theca cells. Although it is well accepted that gonadotropins and ovarian steroids play the central roles in follicular development by controlling follicular microenvironments, intrafollicular substances including growth factors and cytokines are known to function as modulators of ovarian follicular growth and development. Differentiation of granulosa cells involves follicle-stimulating hormone (FSH)-induced maturation of immature cells into mature cells. The expressions of related genes are rigidly controlled until ovulation, and then granulosa and theca cells are finally differentiated into luteal cells, which produce progesterone. On the other hand, the uterus is closely synchronized to the ovary: increasing ovarian steroids regulate the uterus as one of the principal targets to prepare for embryo implantation following fertilization. In the uterus—composed of heterogeneous cell types including luminal and glandular epithelial cells, stroma cells, and muscle layers—estradiol stimulates the proliferation of epithelial cells, whereas progesterone inhibits estradiol-induced hyperplasia of the epithelial compartments (Carson et al., 2000). In rodents, the endometrial stroma cells undergo proliferation and decidualization in response to ovarian steroids and embryo implantation at the early stage of pregnancy (Clarke & Sutherland, 1990; Dey et al., 2004). Thus, cellular functions in the ovary and uterus are accompanied by cyclic changes of cell proliferation, differentiation and apoptosis. The circadian clock system may contribute to the progress of follicular development, luteinization and luteolysis, and steroid hormone-induced proliferation and differentiation of uterine cells through fluctuating hormones. Recently, there is a growing body of evidence that circadian clock genes are expressed in reproductive tissues including the ovary and uterus (Johnson et al., 2005; Nakamura et al., 2005; Fahrenkrug et al., 2006; Dolatshad et al., 2006; Karman & Tischkau, 2006; He et al., 2007a, 2007b, 2007c; Nakao et al., 2007; Hirata et al., 2009; Sellix & Menaker, 2010; Uchikawa et al., 2011). Many regulatory elements are located at the upstream of clock genes, such as steroid hormone response element half-sites and the adenosine 3′,5′-cyclic monophosphate (cAMP) response element site as well as E-box and D-box elements. The mammalian circadian system is composed of three components: input pathways, central pacemaker, and output pathways. The input pathways transmit environmental signals to the central pacemaker, which coordinates the external signals with the central endogenous rhythm of the body by neural, hormonal and behavioural cues (Reppert & Weaver, 2001; Schibler & Sassone-Corsi, 2002; Yamamoto et al.,

2004; Duguay & Cermakian, 2009). At the molecular level, the circadian systems through expression of clock genes generate circadian changes in cell functions via identified transcriptional and posttranscriptional regulatory processes. The CLOCK-BMAL1 heterodimers formed by the bHLH-PAS-activating clock-controlled genes, including *Per*, *CKIε*, *Clock*, *Bmal1*, and *Cry*, bind to the canonical E-box element of these promoters and initiate the transcription activities of these genes. The PER and CRY proteins, in turn, form multimeric complexes and feed back to repress the transactivation by CLOCK/BMAL1 in the nucleus (Ueda et al., 2005). The peripheral oscillators, synchronized by the central clock, control the expression of downstream clock-controlled genes in tissue-specific relationships. Here, the hormonal regulation of the circadian clock system in ovarian and uterine cells is reviewed and studied in rats. The study indicated that the circadian pacemaker is altered in ovarian and uterine cells during cellular differentiation, which is induced by hormonal stimulation.

2. Real-time monitoring of circadian oscillation in primary cultured cells

Cell lines such as fibroblasts also display several oscillations of the clock gene expression when treated with dexamethasone, serum shock or other stimuli (Balsalobre et al., 2000a, 2000b). To precisely analyze the circadian clock system, a real-time system for monitoring gene expression has been employed using transgenic rats constructed with mouse *Per2*

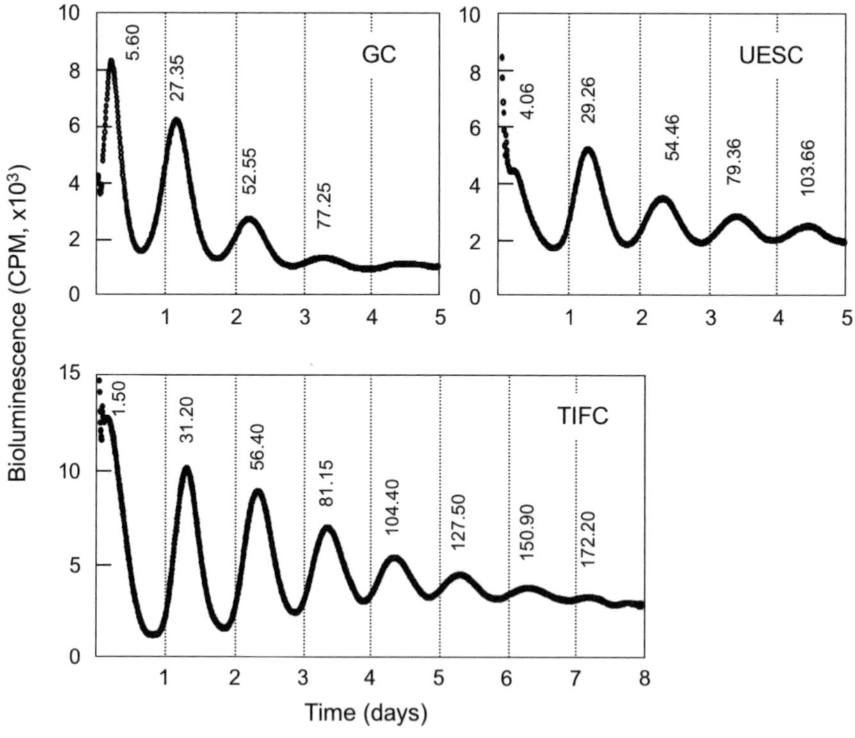

Fig. 1. Profiles of circadian *Per2-dLuc* oscillations in ovarian granulosa cells (GC), uterine endometrial stroma cells (UESC) and testicular interstitial fibroblast-like cells (TIFC) treated with dexamethasone. The values are the peak times (hours) in each oscillation.

promoter-destabilized luciferase (*Per2-dLuc*) reporter gene (Ueda et al., 2002). Transgenic rats were maintained under 12-h L and 12-h D (zeitgeber time, ZT0; 08:00 h light on; ZT12: 20:00 h light off). Three cell types were prepared from the ovary, uterus and testis: i.e., ovarian granulosa cells, uterine endometrial stroma cells and testicular interstitial fibroblast-like cells. These cell types exhibited several oscillations after exposure to dexamethasone, but the number of oscillations for each cell type was distinct (Fig. 1). The times of the second oscillation were 27.35 h in the granulosa cells, 29.26 h in the stroma cells, and 31.20 h in the testicular interstitial fibroblast-like cells, but the cycle times were similar (~24 h).

3. Circadian rhythm in ovarian cells under hormonal stimulation

Several laboratories have reported the expression of clock genes in the ovarian follicles and corpora lutea *in vivo*, but their conclusions are mostly conflicting. Studies on the circadian clock in the *Drosophila* ovary suggested that *period* and *timeless* were constantly expressed in the follicular cells (Beaver et al., 2003). The diurnal rhythms of *Per1* and *Per2* expression were reported in the corpora lutea of rat ovaries (Fahrenkrug et al., 2006). In contrast, *Bmal1* and *Per2* were rhythmically expressed in the rat ovarian follicles but not in the corpora lutea (Karman & Tischka, 2006). In the current study, preantral and antral ovarian follicles of immature transgenic rats were primed with diethylstilbestrol and equine chorionic gonadotropin (eCG), respectively (Fig. 2, A), to obtain granulosa cells. In both cell types, an oscillation of *Per2* promoter activity was observed at approximately 4 h after exposure to dexamethasone. While oscillation was induced in both, the oscillatory patterns of two cell types were different. In the granulosa cells from preantral follicles only one weak oscillation was induced, subsequent to the initial oscillation, which occurred at approximately 24 h (Fig. 2, B & C). Conversely, a few robust oscillations were detected in the granulosa cells from antral follicles, albeit with a continuous decreasing of amplitude (He et al., 2007a). FSH was also effective at inducing the oscillation seen at approximately 24 h (Fig. 2, C). This distinctness may be related to each cellular physiology. Granulosa cells spontaneously undergo cellular apoptosis *in vitro* (Tilly et al., 1992). However, it is unlikely that the cell death caused the cessation of oscillation in the granulosa cells after only one cycle, as 90% of the cells were still viable, and additional oscillation could be evoked by replacement with fresh medium or stimulation with forskolin (Fig. 2, B). This finding suggests that, *in vivo*, the circadian clockwork is somewhat influenced in follicular granulosa cells during the process of cell differentiation or maturation. The clock system was also analyzed in the luteal cells that were prepared from ovaries of immature rats primed by eCG and human chorionic gonadotropin (hCG). The luteal cells exhibited several circadian oscillations with high amplitude after exposure to forskolin or dexamethasone (Fig. 2, D). However, the oscillation shifted forward approximately 3 h when the cells were treated with forskolin. The profiles of oscillation for dexamethasone and forskolin treatments were distinct, although the cycle times were the same, approximately 24 h. The first oscillation was found at 3-5 h after the initiation of monitoring, although the time was dependent upon the stimulant. LH was also effective at inducing circadian oscillation in luteal cells (Fig. 2, D).

4. Circadian rhythm in uterine cells under hormonal stimulation

Ovarian steroids regulate the proliferation and differentiation of uterine endometrial stroma cells (Carson et al., 2000). In addition, in the rat *Per2* gene, many estrogen response element (ERE) half-sites and progesterone response element (PRE) half-sites are located at the

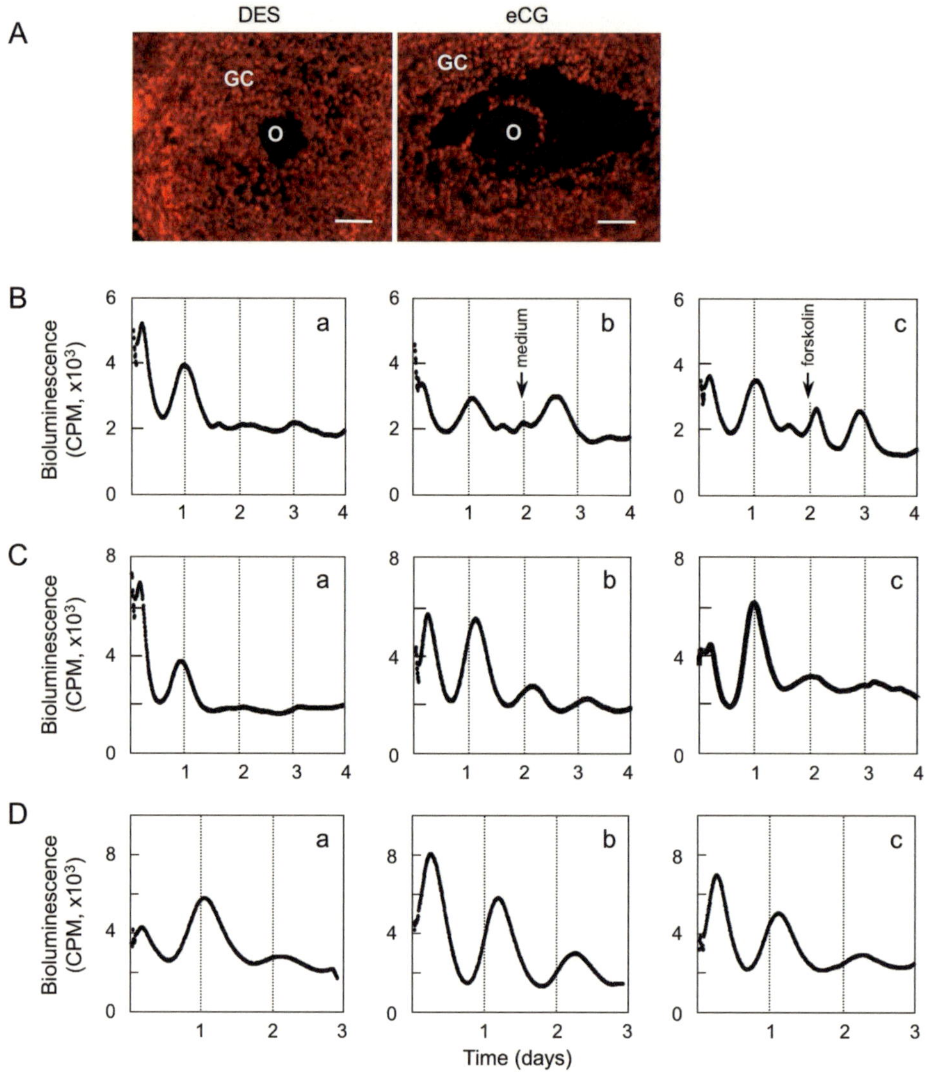

Fig. 2. Circadian oscillation of *Per2-dLuc* in granulosa cells and luteal cells. A, Observation of the PER2 protein in preantral (DES injection for 3 days) and antral (eCG injection) follicles of ovaries by fluorescent immunohistochemistry. GC, granulosa cells; O, oocytes. *Scale bar*, 50 μm. B, The granulosa cells isolated from preantral follicles were cultured for 48 h with medium containing 5% FBS. The oscillation of *Per2-dLuc* was induced after exposure to dexamethasone (a). Culture medium containing with (c) or without (b) 10 μM forskolin was replaced at 48 h after the initiation of bioluminescent monitoring. C, Granulosa cells from preantral (a) and antral follicles (b, c) were cultured as described above and treated with dexamethasone (a, b) for 2 h, and then subjected to real-time monitoring of bioluminescence. FSH was contained in the culture medium during monitoring (c). D, Luteal cells prepared from luteinized ovaries of rats primed by eCG and hCG were cultured as described above and treated with forskolin (a) or dexamethasone (b) for 2 h, and then subjected to real-time monitoring of bioluminescence. LH was contained in the culture medium during monitoring (c).

upstream of the transcription start site. These sites may contribute to the expression of the *Per2* gene by ovarian steroid hormones. It is well known that eCG injection causes the formation of antral follicles in ovaries that produce estradiol, and hCG injection thereafter results in luteinization of ovarian follicles that produce large amounts of progesterone. The large amounts of estradiol and progesterone promote proliferation and differentiation in the uterus. The stroma cells proliferate in the eCG-primed rat uterus, compared to those in the hCG-primed rat uterus. The stroma cells were treated with dexamethasone or forskolin. In the stroma cells prepared from intact immature rats, cyclic *Per2* oscillation was observed after exposure to dexamethasone or forskolin (Fig 3, a & e) (Hirata et al., 2009). This suggests that the glucocorticoid response element (GRE) and cAMP response element (CRE) sites in the rat *Per2* promoter are operative and transactivate the transcription of the *Per2* gene (Travnickova-Bendova et al., 2002; Yamamoto et al., 2004). Although the second oscillation in the stroma cells was delayed compared to that in the ovarian cells (He et al., 2007c), the circadian oscillator was operative with approximately 24 h per cycle. In contrast, the stroma cells from eCG-primed rats exhibited an irregular rhythm of *Per2* oscillation with a smaller trough (Fig. 3, b & f). Disrupted oscillation was also observed in the cells 2 days after hCG priming subsequent to eCG priming (Fig. 3, c & g). However, in the cells of rats 4 days after hCG priming subsequent to eCG priming, the disrupted oscillation recovered to a rhythmic

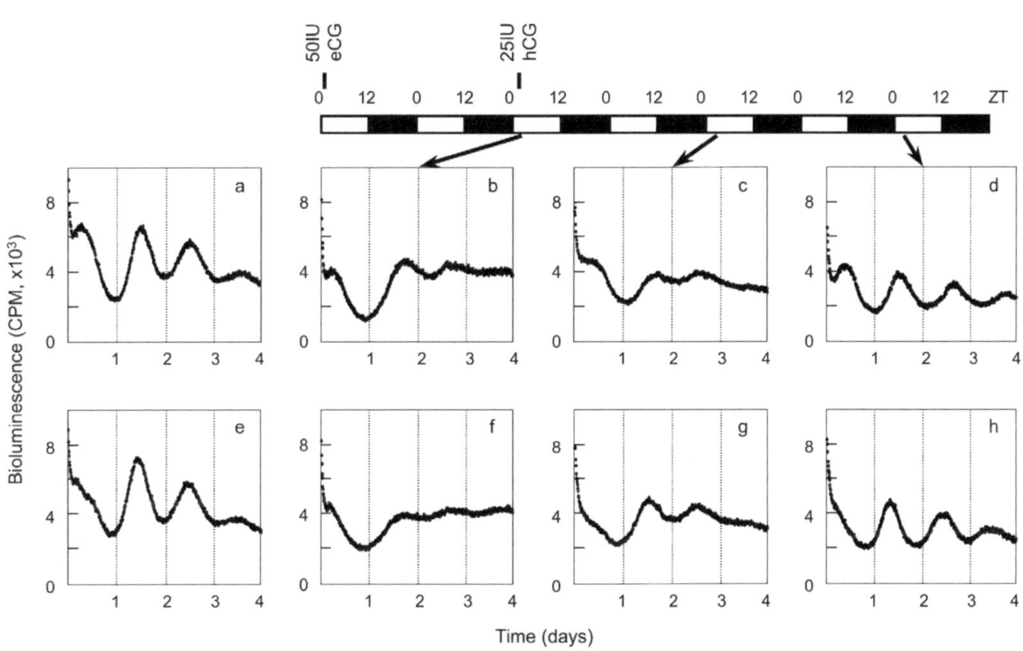

Fig. 3. Circadian oscillation of *Per2-dLuc* in uterine endometrial stroma cells prepared from intact or gonadotropin-primed rats. Immature rats were primed with or without 25IU hCG following 50IU eCG, and the stroma cells isolated were cultured for 48 h with medium containing 10% FBS. The cells were treated with dexamethasone (a-d) or forskolin (e-h), and then subjected to real-time monitoring of bioluminescence. a, e: stroma cells from intact rats; b, f: cells from rats 2 days after priming with eCG; c, g: cells from rats 2 days after priming with hCG subsequent to eCG priming; d, h: cells from rats 4 days priming with hCG subsequent to eCG priming.

pattern with a 24-h cycle, similar to those observed in intact immature rats (Fig. 3, d & h). Chronic treatment with estradiol is known to disrupt the circadian rhythms of *Per1* and *Per2* expression in the liver, kidney and uterus (Nakamura et al., 2005). Furthermore, the phase of the estrous cycle has a profound effect on the oscillation of the PER2 protein within the brain (Perrin et al., 2006). The circadian oscillator may be operative in the stroma cells after progesterone administration, through the transcriptional and feedback loops of the clock system. Consequently, it is possible that estradiol does not induce rhythmic *Per2* oscillation, whereas progesterone promotes the rhythmic pattern.

5. Expression of *Per1* gene in uterine cells by ovarian steroids

The uterus undergoes profound remodelling, implicating cyclic proliferation, differentiation and differential gene expression dependent on the levels of circulating ovarian steroids. Recent studies have demonstrated that circadian clock genes are rhythmically expressed in the uterus (Nakamura et al., 2005; Dolatshad et al., 2006). Expression of *Per1* mRNA was analyzed by *in situ* hybridization in different compartments of the uterus at ZT 0 and ZT 8 (He et al., 2007c). The expression could be readily detected in both the endometrium and myometrium at ZT 0 and ZT 8 (Fig. 4). Strong signals were observed in the luminal epithelium and glandular epithelium, as compared to that in the stromal cell layer. The staining intensity of *Per1* mRNA was approximately two-fold higher at ZT 8 than at ZT 0 in the stroma, luminal epithelium and myometrium compartments. It is noted that the staining signal did not apparently change at ZT 0 and ZT 8 in the glandular epithelium compartment. This suggests the lack of rhythmical clockwork in the control of uterine glandular physiology. The effects of estradiol and progesterone on the expression of *Per1*

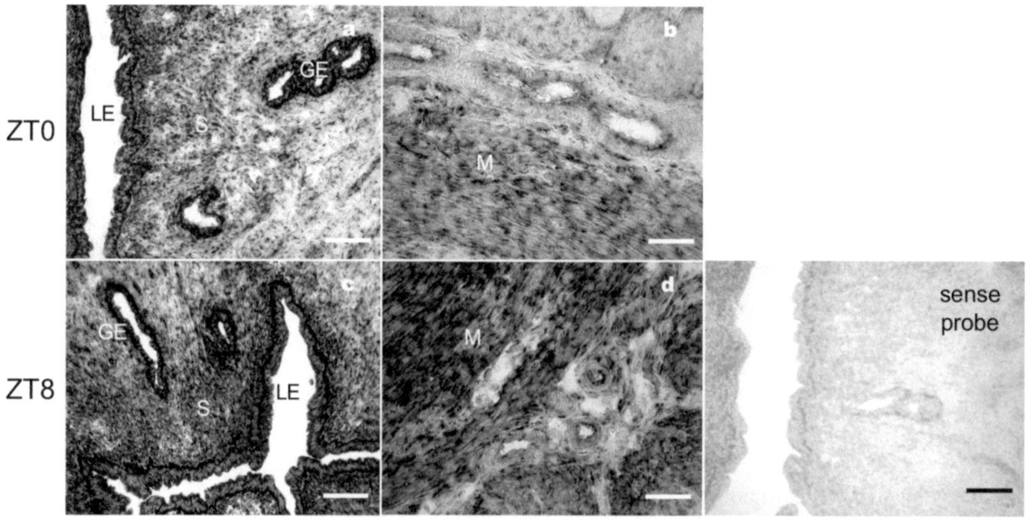

Fig. 4. Representative photomicrographs of *in situ* hybridization analyses for *Per1* mRNA in diestrous uteri. The uterine samples were obtained at ZT0 (a, b) and ZT8 (c, d). Dark shades show the staining of *Per1* mRNA. No signal was obtained in the uteri stained with a sense probe. S, stroma; LE, luminal epithelium; GE, glandular epithelium; M, myometrium. *Scale bars*, 100 μm.

mRNA were evaluated in the uteri of ovariectomied rats. All the uteri were collected at ZT 0 after a single injection of ovarian steroids. *In situ* hybridization analysis revealed that the estradiol-primed uteri exhibited much stronger staining in the luminal epithelium, glandular epithelium and myometrium compartments (Fig. 5). However, the staining signal was weak in the stroma compartment. In addition, treatment with an ER antagonist (ICI182,780) caused a decrease of the staining intensity of *Per1* mRNA in all examined compartments (Fig. 6). This indicates that the *Per1* expression is at least partly through the

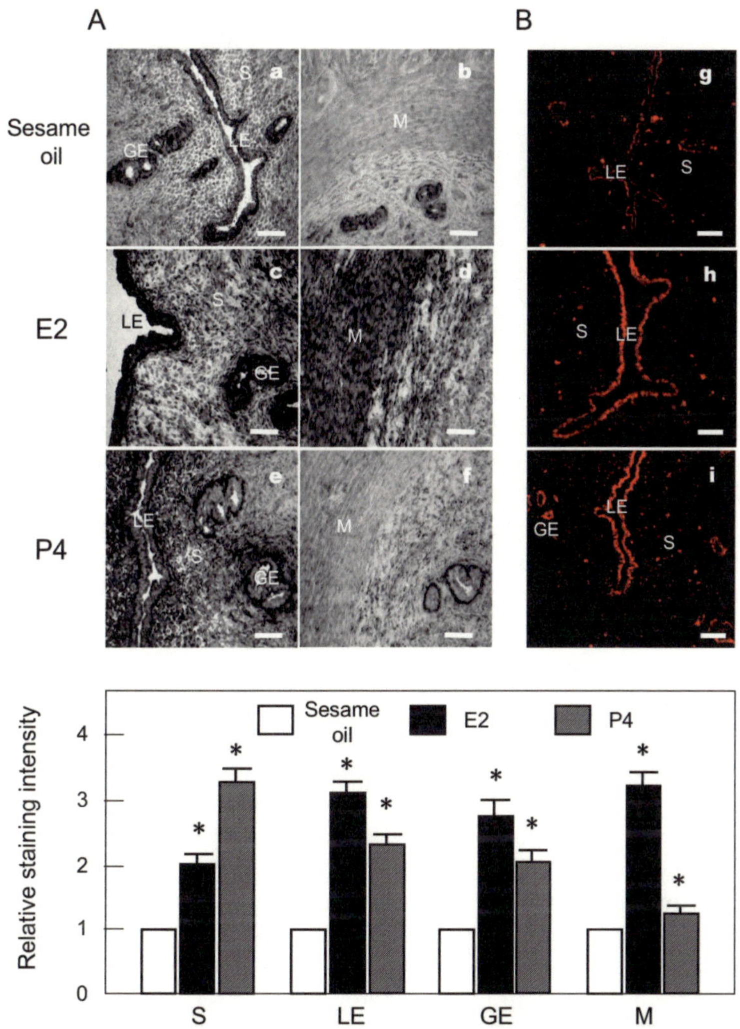

Fig. 5. Representative photomicrographs of *in situ* hybridization analyses for *Per1* mRNA (A) and immunofluorescent analyses for PER1 protein (B) in the uteri treated with estradiol (E2) or progesterone (P4). At ZT0, the OVX rats were injected subcutaneously with 100 μl sesame oil-containing vehicle (a, b, g), 50 μg/kg E2 (c, d, h), or 10 mg/kg P4 (e, f, i), and uteri were removed after 24 h. The relative changes of *Per1* mRNA staining are presented as means ± SEM of three independent sections. S, stroma; LE, luminal epithelium; GE, glandular epithelium; M, myometrium. *Scale bars*, 100 μm.

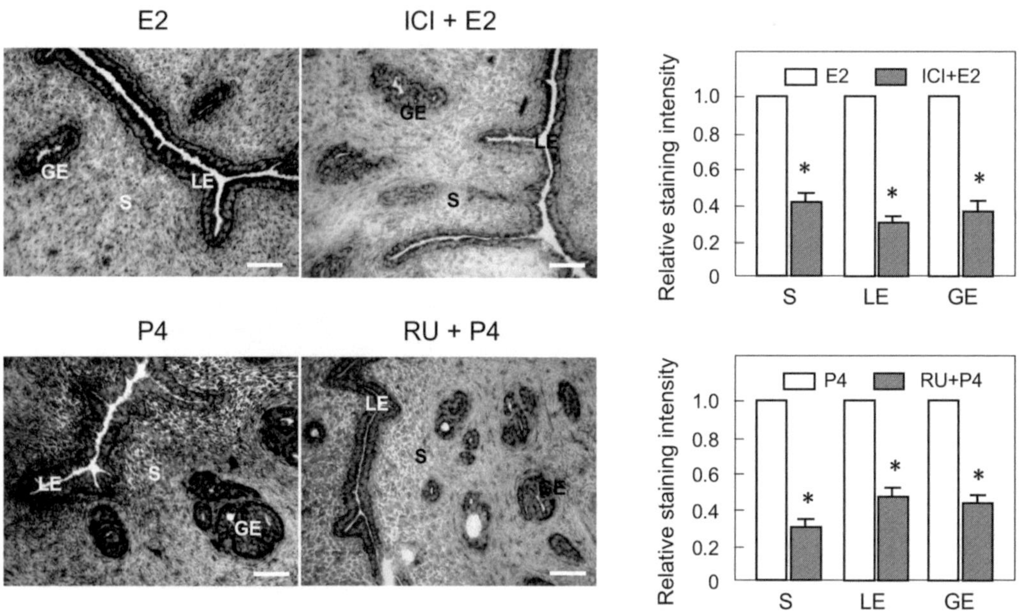

Fig. 6. Representative photomicrographs of *in situ* hybridization analyses for *Per1* mRNA in the uteri treated with estradiol (E2), E2 + ICI182780, progesterone (P4), or P4 + RU486. At ZT0, the OVX rats were injected subcutaneously with 100 μl sesame oil-containing vehicle, 3 mg/kg ICI182780, or 30 mg/kg RU486, after 2 h, followed by injection with 50 μg/kg E2 or 10 mg/kg P4. The uteri were collected at ZT0 the following day. The relative changes of *Per1* mRNA staining are presented as means ± SEM of three independent sections. S, stroma; LE, luminal epithelium; GE, glandular epithelium; M, myometrium. *Scale bars*, 100 μm. *Statistical significance vs. the control ($p<0.05$).

ER-mediated pathway. The differences in *Per1* mRNA expression among the compartments might result from differential expression of ER. Actually, the ER mRNA or protein is expressed at higher levels in the luminal epithelium, glandular epithelium and myometrium compartments than in the stroma at 24 h after estradiol administration (Nephew et al., 2000). This pattern of ER distribution, to some extent supports the current *Per1* mRNA expression profile in the uterus in response to estradiol. On the other hand, progesterone administration resulted in intense staining in the stroma, luminal epithelium and glandular epithelium compartments, but not in the myometrium compartment (Fig. 5). Treatment with a PR antagonist (RU486) remarkably inhibited *Per1* mRNA expression in the stroma and glandular epithelium compartments (Fig. 6). These observations indicate that ER and PR might mediate estradiol- and progesterone-regulated *Per1* expression in the uterus, respectively. Immunofluorescent staining for the PER1 protein was performed in estradiol- and progesterone-administered uteri. In the control uteri, relatively stronger staining was observed in the luminal epithelium and glandular epithelium compartments, with weak staining in the stroma. With estradiol treatment, the PER1 protein was more intensively expressed in the stroma, luminal epithelium and glandular epithelium compartments. Treatment with progesterone also resulted in stronger immunostaining of PER1 in the stroma, luminal epithelium and glandular epithelium compartments. Immunohistochemical observations of PER1 expression in response to ovarian steroids were similar to the results revealed by *in situ* hybridization. The activated expression of *Per1* by ovarian steroids might result from the direct binding of receptors for estrogen and progesterone to some potential elements (ERE, PRE) in the *Per1* promoter. There is no consensus ERE (5′-GGTCANNNTGACC-3′) site, but some ERE half-sites are located in the 5′ flanking region of the *Per1* promoter (Nakamura et al. 2005).

6. Expression and distribution of the PER2 protein in the uterus during gestation

In studies on the expression pattern of the *Per2* mRNA in the uterus of estrous mice, a robust daily variation was reported with a peak around early dark periods (Dolatshad et al., 2006). However, little is known about whether the circadian clockwork is modulated during gestation. In rodents and humans, uterine endometrial stroma cells undergo proliferation and differentiation into decidual cells, ultimately leading to the formation of the placenta. We previously described that the rhythmic *Per2-dLuc* oscillation is not observed in the stroma cells undergoing decidualization induced by medroxyprogesterone acetate plus N6, 2-O-dibutyryl adenosine 3′:5′-cyclic monophosphate (He et al., 2007b). Stroma cells isolated from pregnant rats on day 4.50 of gestation are proliferative in culture. Cells isolated from the transgenic rats were employed to analyze circadian oscillation on day 4.50 (ZT 4) and day 6.50 (ZT 4). On day 4.50, treatment of the stroma cells with dexamethasone caused the generation of circadian *Per2-dLuc* oscillation. This indicates that GREs in the rat *Per2* promoter are functional and transactivate the transcription of the *Per2* gene (Travnickova-Bendova et al., 2002; Yamamoto et al., 2004; He et al., 2007b). Although the second oscillation in the stroma cells is delayed compared with that of ovarian cells (He et al., 2007b), the circadian oscillation was obvious, with approximately 24 h per cycle at least during the stage of implantation. In contrast, the circadian oscillation was attenuated in the decidualizing cells only 2 days after implantation. However, the times of each oscillation in the stroma cells on day 4.50 and day 6.50 of gestation were mostly identical. The expression and distribution of the PER2 protein were investigated by fluorescent immunohistochemistry in different compartments of the uteri (day 4.5) at ZT 4 and ZT12 (Uchikawa et al., 2011). A strong immunostaining signal was detected in the luminal epithelium, as compared to that in the stroma cell layer (Fig. 7), which was similar to the distribution of the PER1 protein. The cytoplasm of the luminal epithelium especially exhibited a strong signal at both ZT4 and ZT12. This suggests a continuous expression of the PER2 protein. On the other hand, in the stromal cell layer, immunostaining signals were observed in both the nuclei and cytoplasms at ZT4, whereas signals were observed predominantly in the nuclei at ZT12. Fluorescent immunohistochemical studies may support the circadian rhythm of the PER2 protein at least in the stroma cell layer. In contrast to the implantation stage, no significant rhythm of the PER2 protein was found during the decidualization stage (day 6.5 to day 6.8). Fluorescent immunohistochemistry revealed a strong signal in the cytoplasm of the luminal epithelium at both ZT4 and ZT12 (Fig. 7). As compared to the implantation stage, immunostaining signals were observed predominantly in the nuclei of stroma cell layers at both ZT4 and ZT12.

7. Circadian rhythm in uterine endometrial stroma cells during gestation

The uterine endometrial stroma cells prepared from several stages of gestation (pregnancy days 2.5, 4.5 and 6.5; P2.5, P4.5, P6.5, respectively) exhibited different responses to

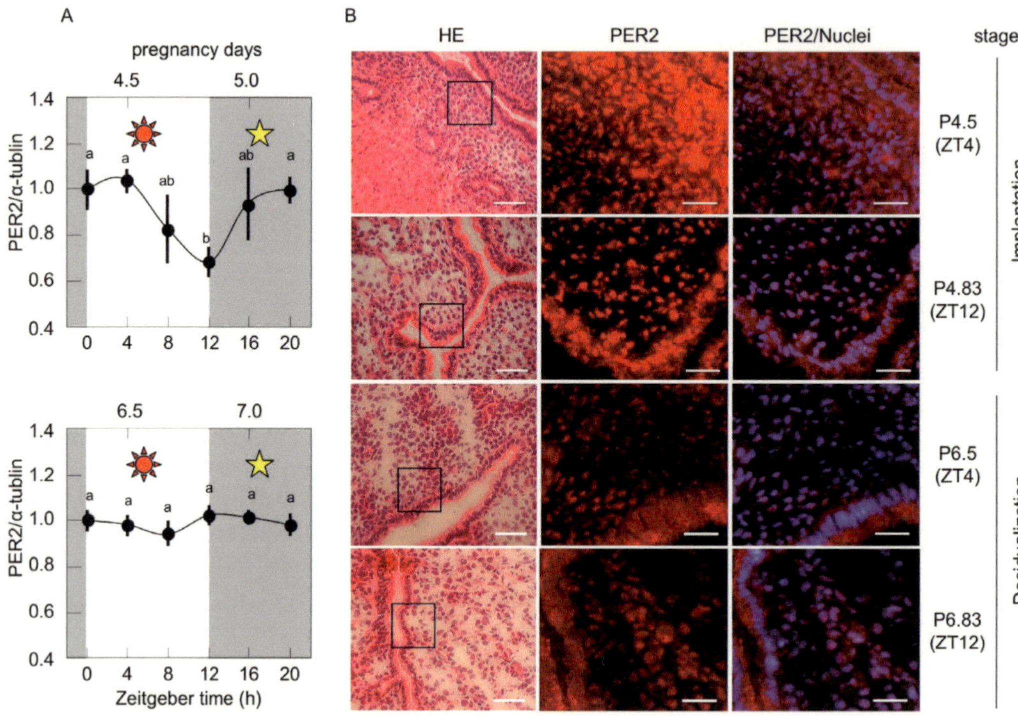

Fig. 7. Circadian rhythm of the PER2 protein and representative photomicrographs of immunofluorescent analyses for PER2 protein in the uteri of pregnant rats during the stages of implantation and decidualization. A, Pregnant rats were killed at 4-h intervals over a daily cycle (ZT0, 0800h). Proteins (30 μg) prepared from a part of the uterine horns were separated on SDS-PAGE, and analyzed by immunodetection using anti-mPER2 antibody. Data are means ± SEM from three independent experiments normalized to the values given by α-tubulin. Values with different letters are significantly different ($p<0.05$). *Shaded areas*, during the night. B, Parts of uterine horns at ZT4 and ZT12 were subjected to fluorescent immunohistochemistry. The square regions shown in HE were magnified from a serial section subjected to immunofluorescent studies of the PER2 protein (*red*) and Hoechst staining (*blue*). *Scale bars*: 150 μm (HE), 50 μm (PER2, PER2/Nuclei).

dexamethasone and forskolin. Circadian oscillation was generated in these cells, albeit with a continuous decrease of amplitude (Fig. 8). However, the response to forskolin showed a greater decrease from P2.5 to P6.5 than the response to dexamethasone. This suggests that the effect of cAMP signalling on the circadian rhythm of clock genes is weak. Of interest, the oscillatory intensity was low in the stroma cells at day 7, at which these cells undergo decidualization. This suggests that the circadian oscillator is impaired in the stroma cells during decidualization. During the stage of implantation, dramatic changes are observed in the expression of hypoxia-inducible factor 1α (HIF1α) and vascular endothelial growth factor (VEGF), angiogenesis, down-regulation of anti-adhesion proteins, and up-regulation of adhesion proteins. Several of these genes are known to interact with the clock gene transcription factors. BMAL1 can dimerize with HIF1α and may bind to the hypoxia response elements in the promoters and drive the transcription of target genes (Hogenesch et al., 1998). On the other hand, during the stage of decidualization, the decidual cells

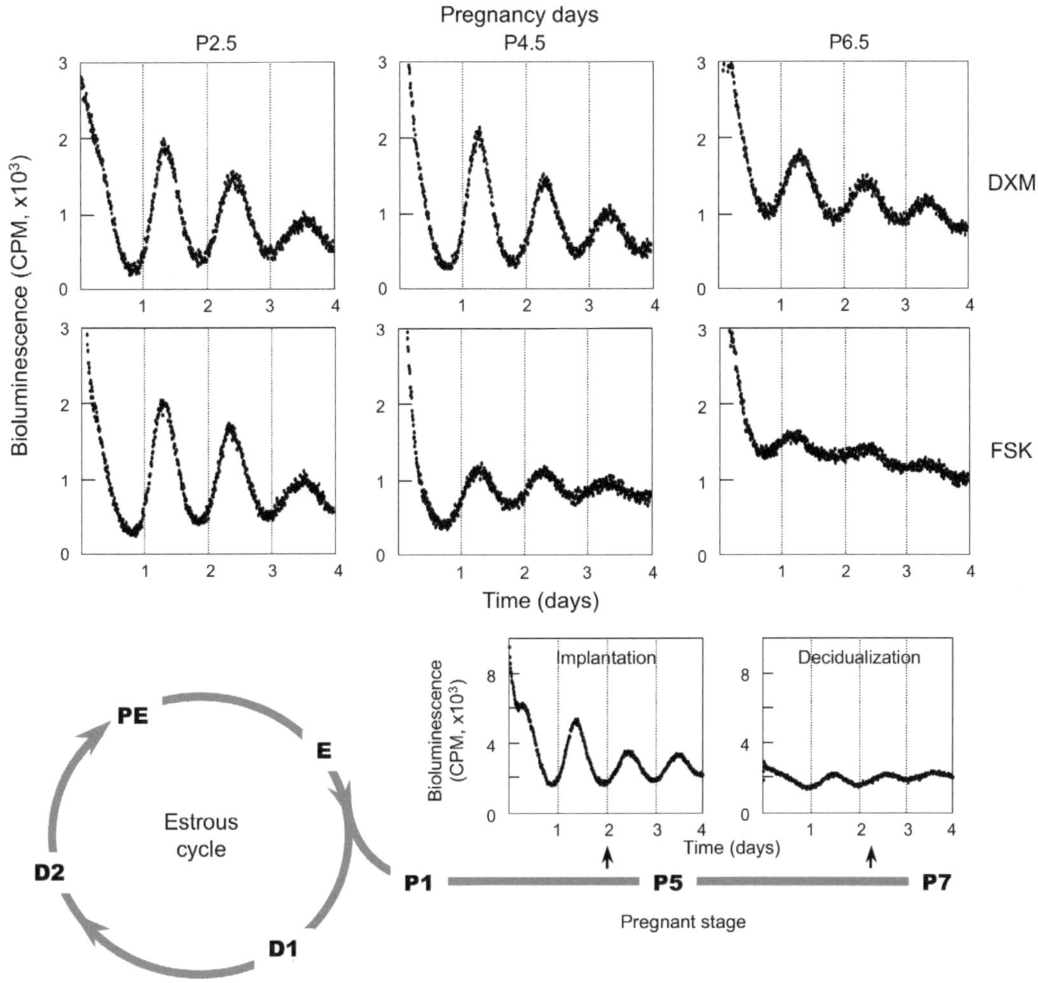

Fig. 8. Profiles of *Per2-dLuc* oscillation in uterine endometrial stroma cells prepared from pregnant rats at day 2.5 (P2.5), day 4.5 (P4.5) and day 6.5 (P6.5) of gestation. After the stroma cells were cultured for 48 h, they were treated with dexamethasone (DXM) or forskolin (FSK) for 2 h, and then subjected to real-time monitoring of bioluminescence.

express many peptides including desmin, IGF-binding proteins, tumor necrosis factor, and decidual prolactin-related protein. Some of these factors may be controlled under the circadian clockwork. For example, the *Vegf* gene has at least 7 E-box and E-box-like sites within the -5000 upstream of the transcription start site (NC_005108). Circadian oscillation of *Vegf* mRNA was observed during the stage of implantation, whereas it was not seen during the stage of decidualization (Fig. 9). In addition, the circadian rhythm of the *Vegf* mRNA was consistent with that of the *Per2* mRNA (Uchikawa et al., 2011). This suggests a clock regulation of the *Vegf* gene. Clearly, the circadian oscillator is down-regulated in the uterine endometrial stroma cells during decidualization. This strongly suggested that cellular differentiation in the stroma cells interferes with the circadian clockwork.

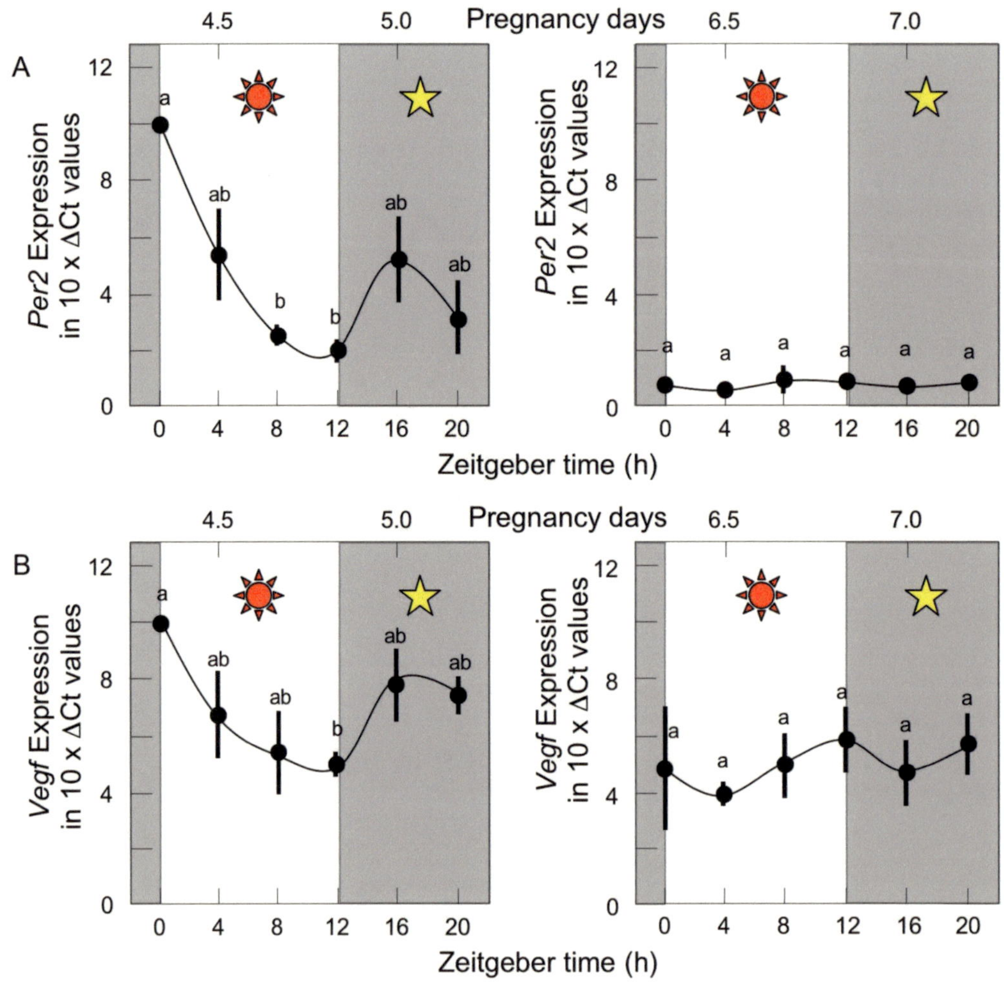

Fig. 9. Circadian rhythms of *Per2* and *Vegf* transcripts in the uterine tissues of pregnant rats during the implantation and decidualization stages. RNA was extracted from a part of uterine horns and reverse transcribed. The resulting cDNA was used for real-time qPCR for *Per2* and *Vegf* mRNAs. (A) *Left*, *Per2* mRNA expression was significantly altered in the uterine tissues of pregnant rats during implantation (day 4.33–5.16 of gestation). *Right*, *Per2* mRNA expression did not change significantly in the uterine tissues of pregnant rats during decidualization (day 6.33–7.16 of gestation). (B) *Left*, *Vegf* mRNA expression was significantly altered in the uterine tissues of pregnant rats during implantation. *Right*, *Vegf* mRNA expression did not significantly change in the uterine tissues of pregnant rats during decidualization. Data are means ± SEM from three independent experiments normalized to the values given by *Gapdh*. Values with different letters are significantly different (p<0.05).

8. Conclusions

The circadian pacemaker undergoes changes in ovarian and uterine cells during cellular differentiation as follows. Firstly, the circadian pacemaker in ovarian cells is modulated during follicular development. Secondly, ovarian steroids promote expression of *Per1* and *Per2* in uterine endometrial stroma cells. Especially, progesterone may recover the deregulation of the circadian oscillator induced by eCG-produced estradiol. Thirdly, the circadian oscillator is down-regulated in the uterine endometrial stroma cells during decidualization. The alteration of the circadian pacemaker in the ovarian and uterine cells results largely from hormonal inputs such as gonadotropins and ovarian steroids, possibly via the regulatory elements such as the cAMP response element and steroid hormone response element half-sites (Fig. 10). However, cell differentiation may also disrupt the circadian pacemaker.

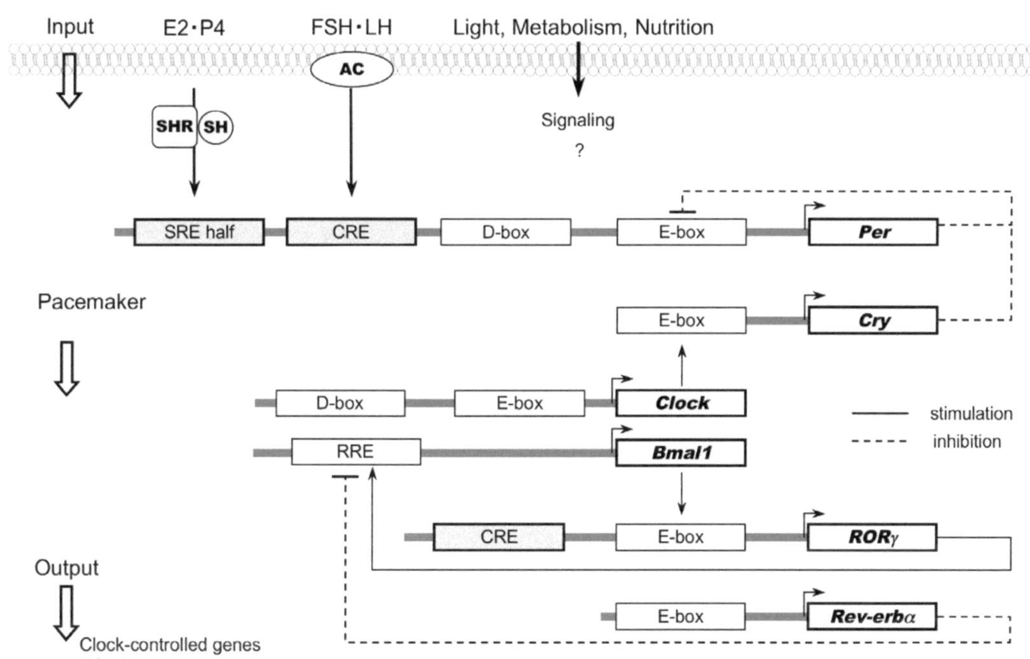

Fig. 10. Hormonal regulation of circadian clock system in cell functions via identified transcriptional and posttranscriptional regulatory processes. The CLOCK-BMAL1 heterodimers bind to the canonical E-box element of clock genes and initiate the transcription activities of these genes. In addition to the E-box and D-box elements, many SHE half and CRE sites are located at the upstream of clock genes. As the input pathway, hormonal and environmental signals are transmitted to the pacemaker. The clock system may contribute to the progress of follicular development, luteinization and luteolysis, and steroid hormone-induced proliferation and differentiation of uterine cells through fluctuating hormones. SH: steroid hormones, AC: adenylate cyclase.

9. Acknowledgments

This research was collaborated with Dr. P-J. He (Emory University, GA, USA), Dr. N. Yamauchi (Kyushu University, Fukuoka, Japan), Dr. Y. Xi (Zhejiang University, Hangzhou, China), Dr. S. Hashimoto (The University of Tokyo, Tokyo, Japan) and Dr. Y. Shigeyoshi (Kinki University School of Medicine, Osaka, Japan). This work was funded by a Grant-in-Aid for Scientific Research from the Japan Society for the Promotion of Sciences (JSPS; 19658099, 22380152).

10. References

Balsalobre, A., Brown, S.A., Marcacci, L., Tronchen, F., Kellendonk, C., Reichardt, H.M., Schutz, G. & Schibler, U. (2000a). Resetting of circadian time in peripheral tissues by glucocorticoid signalling. *Science* 289:2344-2347.

Balsalobre, A., Marcacci, L. & Schibler, U. (2000b). Multiple signaling pathways elicit circadian gene expression in cultured Rat-1 fibroblasts. *Curr. Biol.* 10:1291-1294.

Beaver, L.M., Rush, B.L., Gvakharia, B.O. & Giebultowicz, J.M. (2003). Noncircadian regulation and function of clock genes period and timeless in oogenesis of Drosophila melanogaster. *J. Biol. Rhythms* 18:463-472.

Carson, D.D., Bagchi, I., Dey, S.K., Enders, A.C., Fazleabas, A.T., Lessey, B.A. & Yoshinaga, K. (2000). Embryo implantation. *Dev. Biol.* 223:217-237.

Clarke, C.L. & Sutherland, R.L. (1990). Progestin regulation of cellular proliferation. *Endocr. Rev.* 11:266-301.

Dey, S.K., Lim, H., Das, S.K., Reese, J., Paria B.C., Daikoku, T. & Wang, H. (2004). Moecular cues to implantation. *Endocr. Rev.* 25:341-373.

Dolatshad, H., Campbell, E.A., O'hara, L., Maywood, E.S., Hastings, M.H. & Johnson, M.H. (2006). Developmental and reproductive performance in circadian mutant mice. *Hum. Reprod.* 21:68-79.

Duguay, D. & Cermakian, N. (2009). The crosstalk between physiology and circadian clock proteins. *Chronobiol. Int.* 26:1479-1513.

Fahrenkrug, J., Georg, B., Hannibal, J., Hindersson, P. & Gras, S. (2006). Diurnal rhythmicity of the clock genes Per1 and Per2 in the rat ovary. *Endocrinology* 147:3769-3776.

He, P-J., Hirata, M., Yamauchi, N., Hashimoto, S. & Hattori, M-A. (2007a). Gonadotropic regulation of circadian clockwork in rat granulosa cells. *Mol. Cell. Biochem.* 302:111-118.

He, P-J., Hirata, M., Yamauchi, N., Hashimoto, S. & Hattori, M-A. (2007b). The disruption of circadian clockwork in differentiating cells from rat reproductive tissues as identified by in vitro real-time monitoring system. *J. Endocrinol.* 193:413-420.

He, P-J., Hirata, M., Yamauchi, N. & Hattori, M-A. (2007c). Up-regulation of Per1 expression by estradiol and progesterone in the rat uterus. *J. Endocrinol.* 194:511-519.

Hirata, M., He, P-J., Shibuya, N., Uchikawa, M., Yamauchi, N., Hashimoto, S. & Hattori, M-A. (2009). Progesterone, but not estradiol, synchronizes circadian oscillator in the uterus endometrial stroma cells. *Mol. Cell. Biochem.* 324:31-38.

Hogenesch, J.B., Gu, Y.Z., Jain, S. & Bradfield, C.A. (1998). The basic-helix-loop-helix-PAS orphan MOP3 forms transcriptionally active complexes with circadian and hypoxia factors. *Proc. Natl. Acad. Sci. USA* 95:5474-5479.

Horard, B., Rayet, B., Triqueneaux, G., Laudet, V., Delaunay, F. & Vanacker, J.M. (2004). Expression of the orphan nuclear receptor ERRα is under circadian regulation in estrogen-responsive tissues. *J. Mol. Endocrinol.* 33:87-97.

Johnson, M.H., Lim, A., Fernando, D. & Day, M.L. (2002). Circadian clockwork genes are expressed in the reproductive tract and conceptus of the early pregnant mouse. *Reprod. Biomed. Online* 4:140-145.

Karman, B.N. & Tischkau, S.A. (2006). Circadian clock gene expression in the ovary: effects of luteinizing hormone. *Biol. Reprod.* 75:624-632.

Nakamura, T.J., Moriya, T., Inoue, S., Shimazoe, T., Watanabe, S., Ebihara, S. & Shinohara, T. (2005). Estrogen differentially regulates expression of Per1 and Per2 genes between central and peripheral clocks and between reproductive and nonreproductive tissues in female rats. *J. Neurosci. Res.* 82:622-630.

Nakao, N., Yasuo, S., Nishimura, A., Yamamura, T., Watanabe, T., Anraku, T., Okano, T., Fukada, Y., Sharp. P.J., Ebihara, S. & Yoshimura, T. (2007). Circadian clock gene regulation of steroidogenic acute regulatory protein gene expression in preovulatory ovarian follicles. *Endocrinology* 148:3031-3038.

Nephew, K.P., Long, X., Osborne, E., Burke, K.A., Ahluwalia, A. & Bigsby, R.M. (2000). Effect of estradiol on estrogen receptor expression in rat uterine cell types. *Biol. Reprod.* 62:168-177.

Perrin, J.S., Segall, L.A., Harbour, V.L., Woodside, B. & Amir, S. (2006). The expression of the clock protein PER2 in the limbic forebrain is modulated by the estrous cycle. *Proc. Natl. Acad. Sci. USA* 103:5591-5596.

Reppert, S.M. & Weaver, D.R. (2001). Molecular analysis of mammalian circadian rhythms. *Annu. Rev. Physiol.* 63:647-676.

Schibler, U. & Sassone-Corsi, P. (2002). A web of circadian pacemakers. *Cell* 111:919-922.

Sellix, M.T. & Menaker, M. (2010), Circadian clocks in the ovary. *Trends Endocrinol. Metab.* 21:628-636.

Tilly, J.L., Billig, H., Kowalski, K.I. & Hsueh, A.J. (1992). Epidermal growth factor and basic fibroblast growth factor suppress the spontaneous onset of apoptosis in cultured rat ovarian granulosa cells and follicles by a tyrosine kinase-dependent mechanism. *Mol. Endocrinol.* 6:1942-1950.

Travnickova-Bendova, Z., Cermakian, N., Reppert, S.M. & Sassone-Corsi, P. (2002). Biomodal regulation of mPeriod promoters by CREB-dependent signaling and CLOCK/BMAL1 activity. *Proc. Natl. Acad. Sci. USA* 99:7728-7733.

Uchikawa, M., Kawamura, M., Yamauchi, N. & Hattori, M-A. (2011). Down regulation of circadian clock gene Period 2 in uterine endometrial stromal cells of pregnant rats during decidualization. *Chronobiol. Int.* 28:1-9.

Ueda, H.R., Chen, W., Adachi, A., Wakamatsu, H., Hayashi, S., Takasugi, T., Nagano, M., Nakahara, K., Suzuki, Y., Sugano, S., Iino, M., Shigeyoshi, Y., Iino, M. & Hashimoto, S. (2002). A transcription factor response element for gene expression during circadian night. *Nature* 418:534-539.

Ueda, H.R., Hayashi, S., Chen, W., Sano, M., Machida, M., Shigeyoshi, Y., Iino, M. & Hashimoto, S. (2005). System-level identification of transcriptional circuits underlying mammalian circadian clocks. *Nat. Genet.* 37:187-192.

Yamamoto, T., Nakahata, Y., Soma, H., Akashi, M., Mamine, T. & Takumi, T. (2004). Transcriptional oscillation of canonical clock genes in mouse peripheral tissues. *BMC Mol. Biol.* 5:18.

13

Role of Leptin in the Reproduction and Metabolism: Focus on Regulation by Seasonality in Animals

Malgorzata Szczesna and Dorota A. Zieba
University of Agriculture in Krakow
Poland

1. Introduction

The hypothesis of the existence of a peripheral factor that provides the brain with information on energy status was first proposed in the 1950s (Kennedy, 1953). This hypothesis formed the basis for further investigations that eventually led to the characterization of the obese (*ob/ob*) mouse, a homozygous mutant that lacks a critical factor for the regulation of body weight (Friedman & Halaas, 1998).

This key element of the system regulating food intake has proven to be leptin, a protein hormone produced in adipose tissue. The concentration of this hormone in the blood provides an organism with information about its nutritional status and energy reserves. Leptin acts on hunger and satiety centers in the hypothalamus that affect the regulation of appetite (Halaas et al., 1995). This hormone's activity has primarily been observed in the central nervous system, especially within various parts of the hypothalamus and hypothalamic nuclei. Leptin activity was confirmed in the arcuate nucleus (ARC), ventro-medial hypothalamus (VMH), dorso-medial hypothalamus (DMH), mammillary nuclei, lateral hypothalamic area (LHA) and preoptic area (POA) by Elmquist and colleagues (1998), Williams and colleagues (1999) and Morgan & Mercer (2001). In peripheral tissues, leptin directly stimulates lipolysis and inhibits lipogenesis. Direct effects of leptin were also observed in pancreatic β cells, indicating effects on the regulation of glucose homeostasis independent of the central nervous system (Kieffer et al., 1997; Zieba et al., 2003) and suggesting that leptin may affect energy balance in various ways.

The metabolic status of an organism, which is defined in part by the availability of energy and nutrients to tissues, influences almost all biological functions. Among these functions, reproductive capacity is one of the most important. In linking energy homeostasis to feeding behavior and procreative functions, leptin plays a crucial role in the regulation of reproductive processes, acting at all levels of the gonadotropic axis. Additionally, apart from the mechanisms of energy homeostasis and regulation of reproduction, where leptin plays relatively well-known roles, this protein is also an important regulator of neuroendocrine functions (Wauters et al., 2000). Its impact has been observed on different levels of hormonal axes, ranging from releasing hormone secretion from the hypothalamus and influencing pituitary hormone secretion to a direct influence on the secretory activity of peripheral tissues.

2. Leptin is a potent regulator of energy homeostasis

Leptin receptor expression occurs at the highest levels in the ARC, which is known to affect appetite regulation (Elmquist et al., 1999). There are two main types of neurons with opposite effects. Activation of the orexigenic neurons, which produce neurotransmitters such as neuropeptide Y (NPY) and agouti-related peptide (AgRP), stimulates the appetite and decreases metabolism, while activation of anorectic neurons leads to the release of such factors as proopiomelanocortin (POMC) and cocaine- and amphetamine-regulated transcript (CART), which reduce the consumption of food (Morgan & Mercer, 2001). When an organism's energy reserves that are stored in adipose tissue decrease and serum leptin concentration is reduced, NPY/AgRP neurons are activated, and POMC neurons are inhibited, stimulating the organism to acquire and store energy. These neurons have also been implicated in transducing the action of leptin on GnRH neuronal activity and are sensitive to negative energy balances (Lin et al., 2000).

2.1 Leptin and the leptin receptor

Leptin is a non-glycosylated polypeptide with a molecular mass of approximately 16 kDa encoded by the *ob* gene (*Obese Gene*; Zhang et al., 1994). The leptin gene is highly conserved across species, and it is located on chromosome 7q31.3 in humans (Green et al., 1995) and on chromosome 4q32 in cattle (Stone et al., 1996). This gene's DNA sequence includes more than 15,000 base pairs and contains 3 exons, which are separated by 2 introns (Green et al., 1995). The mouse protein exhibits 83% homology with human leptin (Zhang et al., 1994), and both share many structural similarities with other members of the helical cytokine family, including interleukin-6 (IL-6), prolactin (PRL) and growth hormone (GH) (Zhang et al., 1997). Leptin is synthesized as a pro-hormone (167 amino acids) and released into the bloodstream following the cleavage of a signaling segment (21 amino acids) in the form of a hormone 146 amino acids in length (Prolo et al., 1998; Zhang et al., 1994).

Although adipose tissue is the primary source of leptin, the production of leptin has been observed in a variety of other tissues, including the stomach (Sobhani et al., 2000), skeletal muscle (J. Wang, 1998), fetal cartilage (Hoggard et al., 1998), pituitary tissue (Jin et al., 1999), mammary tissue (Smith-Kirwin et al., 1998), and placenta (Masuzaki et al., 1997). Leptin may be found in the bloodstream in its free form or complexed with leptin-binding proteins, and this characteristic appears to be species-specific (Garcia et al., 2002; Houseknecht et al., 1996). In humans, the half-life of free leptin is approximately 30 min (Trayhurn et al., 1999), with the kidneys being responsible for approximately 80% of leptin clearance from the peripheral circulation (Meyer et al., 1997). Additionally, leptin secretion follows a circadian rhythm (Licinio et al., 1998b), with a nadir early in the morning (0800–0900 h), an increase during the day, and a peak between 2400 and 0200 h.

The multitude of organs in which the presence of leptin receptors has been identified confirms the pleiotropic character of leptin's action. Expression of the *db* gene (*Diabetes Gene*), which encodes a leptin receptor (Tartaglia et al., 1995) has been confirmed within pituitary (Iqbal et al., 2000), adipose tissue in sheep (Dyer et al., 1997), on the granulosa, theca and interstitial cells of the ovary (Karlsson et al., 1997), in testis (Caprio et al., 1999), and in heart, liver, lung, kidney, adrenal gland (Hoggard et al., 1997), small intestine and lymph nodes.

The leptin receptor has a single membrane-spanning domain and exists in different isoforms (Ob-Ra, Ob-Rb, OB-Rc, Ob-Rd, Ob-Re and Ob-Rf) derived from alternative splicing of its mRNA (Bjorbaek et al., 1997). All isoforms have similar ligand-binding domains but differ at the C-terminus in the intracellular domain. The Ob-Rb isoform, which contains a long intracellular domain, is the only one with both of the protein motifs necessary for activation of the Janus kinase 2 and signal transducers and activators of transcription (JAK-STAT) pathway (Uotani et al., 1999). The leptin receptor lacks intrinsic enzymatic activity and mediates signals through the activation of receptor-associated intracellular JAKs. The leptin receptor homodimerizes upon ligand binding and activates JAK/STAT pathways. Phosphorylated STATs dimerize and then translocate to the nucleus, where they bind to DNA and affect target gene transcription (Banks et al., 2000). This system can be modulated by a large variety of cellular factors. Although the JAK2/STAT3 pathway has been considered the major signaling mechanism activated by the leptin receptor, mitogen-activated protein kinase (MAPK) (Niswender et al., 2001) and phosphatidylinositol-3 kinase (PI-3 K) (Niswender et al., 2001) have also been implicated in leptin receptor signaling.

2.2 Factors influencing the synthesis and secretion of leptin

The concentration of leptin circulating in the bloodstream depends primarily on the amount of the protein stored in body fat deposits, and this relationship presents a positive correlation (Maffei et al., 1995). The levels of leptin mRNA are variable in different adipose tissue depots, suggesting that there are site-specific variations in the expression of the leptin gene (Maffei et al., 1995). In humans, leptin expression in subcutaneous fat is higher than in other kinds of adipose tissue (Montague et al., 1997), while in rats, the highest level of leptin mRNA is observed in internal fat depots, especially in perirenal and epididymal adipose tissue (Maffei et al., 1995; Trayhurn et al., 1995).

The expression level of leptin is also dependent on age (Rayner et al., 1997) and sex (Montague et al., 1997). Sexual dimorphism involves not only the level of leptin mRNA expression but also the correlation between the mass of adipose tissue and the concentration of the hormone. The concentration of leptin circulating in the blood is 2 to 3 times higher in women than in men. Additionally, female synthesis of leptin in relation to body weight is not only approximately 75% higher, but leptin is also much more easily released from adipose tissue in females (Licinio et al., 1998a). It has been suggested that these observed differences may be partly due to the impact of sex hormones.

Changes in leptin concentrations are dependent on age and physiological state. In pre-menopausal women, the plasma concentrations of leptin are higher than in post-menopausal individuals (Rosenbaum et al., 1996). Higher levels of this protein are also noted in women of procreative age, and the concentration of leptin increases with the maturation of ovarian follicles in the menstrual cycle. Moreover, its concentration is higher in the luteal phase compared with the follicular phase of the ovarian cycle (Popovic & Casanueva, 2002). In cattle, however, the concentration of leptin decreases in the luteal phase and early follicular phase (G.L. Williams et al., 2002).

Pregnancy and lactation are important factors that determine the amount of leptin in the bloodstream. Interestingly, hyperleptinemia occurring during pregnancy is not associated with a reduction in food intake, which suggests that this state induces a kind of leptin resistance. In sheep, the concentration of leptin in the bloodstream increases during the first half of pregnancy (Ehrhardt et al., 2001) and depends on the number of fetuses, presenting higher values in the case of a multiple pregnancy (Kulcsar et al., 2006). The concentration of leptin is reduced in the second half of pregnancy, and a low concentration of this hormone is maintained during the first weeks of lactation (Ehrhardt et al., 2001). Lactation significantly

reduces the expression of leptin mRNA in adipose tissue, and the concentration of this protein in the bloodstream is approximately five times lower in lactating compared with non-lactating ewes (Sorensen et al., 2002).
Nutritional status also has an impact on the concentration of leptin in the blood. Undernutrition, or even short-term restriction of access to food, results in a significant reduction in leptin concentrations in ruminants (Amstalden et al., 2000), rodents (Trayhurn et al., 1995) and humans (Boden et al., 1996).
Photoperiod can also affect leptin expression in numerous species, including sheep. Exposure of ovariectomized adult ewes to a long day length for 4-6 weeks stimulated leptin release and expression in perirenal adipose tissue, and this effect was independent of any change in the number of adipocytes or feed intake (Bocquier et al., 1998). A similar effect of long days on leptin expression was previously reported in Syberian hamster (*Phodopus sungorus*) (Klingenspor et al., 1996). In lactating dairy cows, exposure to different photoperiodic conditions significantly affects the gene expression of leptin and its receptors in adipose tissue. Cows exposed to long-day conditions (18:6) exhibited higher expression of leptin compared with cows housed under neutral (12:12) or short day-length (6:18) conditions. Additionally, expression of the long form of the leptin receptor (*Ob-Rb*) was found to be downregulated by short-day conditions (Bernabucci et al., 2006). Bertolucci and co-workers (2005) demonstrated the circadian rhythms of leptin release from adipose tissue in sheep, with a minimum concentration of the hormone occurring during the light phase and peak secretion being observed during the dark phase. Moreover, the amplitude of these changes was higher during the short days (Marie et al., 2001). Diurnal variations in circulating leptin concentrations have also been reported in humans (Licinio et al., 1998b). The mechanisms involved in photoperiod-induced differences in adipose tissue leptin expression remain unknown. Direct effects of the sympathetic nervous system and interactions between melatonin and PRL have been suggested to play a role in this process.
In the membranes of adipocytes, there are many receptors mediating the sensitivity of adipose tissue to various hormonal factors. For example, on mammalian adipocytes, it has been observed that receptors for leptin (Dyer et al., 1997), insulin (Jarett et al., 1980), melatonin (Alonso-Vale et al., 2005; Zalatan et al., 2001), PRL (Ling et al., 2000) and GH (Carter-Su et al., 1984) are present, suggesting that these hormones may directly regulate the activity of adipocytes, including their secretory activity.

2.3 State of leptin resistance

Although it was originally referred to as an *anti-obesity* hormone in humans, leptin's effects are counteracted in some individuals by a natural resistance associated with hyperleptinemia, which is related to changes in hypothalamic sensitivity to leptin associated with, for example, pregnancy and lactation, malnutrition or obesity. In sheep, it was observed that the hypothalamus is resistant to leptin in some periods, and this phenomenon is related to the adaptation of these animals to annual changes in energy supply and demand (Marie et al., 2001). During the long-day season, the concentration of leptin in blood plasma increases by 180% compared with during the short-day season (Marie et al., 2001), but this is not associated with the anorectic action of leptin. During this period, when there is an abundance of food and it is readily accessible, sheep exhibit increased appetite and appear to be insensitive to high concentrations of leptin (resulting from increased adiposity). Seasonal leptin resistance allows these animals to live in a changing climate and store energy that they will be able to use in periods of reduced food availability. In autumn and winter, sheep exhibit sensitivity to leptin at the physiological level, and their appetite adjusts approximately to their nutritional status. This paradox can be explained by the state of leptin resistance or leptin insensitivity occurring during long days, but the neuroendocrinal basis of this phenomenon remains unknown. Suggestions that hypothalamic sensitivity to the anorexic effects of leptin in sheep changes in a seasonally dependent manner were confirmed in studies using exogenous leptin (Miller et al., 2002). The amount of food intake was found to be affected by exogenous leptin only during a period of days of decreasing length, while in the spring, this response was not observed (Miller et al., 2002).

Changes during the year related to leptin sensitivity have been observed in other seasonal animal species. In Siberian hamsters, the potency of exogenous leptin in reducing food intake is significantly more marked in periods of short days than during long days (Atcha et al., 2000; Klingenspor et al., 2000). These observations provide insight into the phenomenon of seasonal changes in sensitivity to leptin, not only in relation to the regulation of food intake, but also related to the modifying effects of season on other leptin-induced responses.

It appears that an intracellular protein induced by leptin receptor activation, suppressor of cytokine signaling-3 (SOCS-3), may mediate leptin resistance at the molecular level, mainly within the region of the arcuate nucleus, as it effectively blocks leptin signaling (Bjorbaek et al., 2000). Uotani and colleagues (1999) suggest the desensitization of leptin receptors as the cause of reduced sensitivity, and El-Haschimi & Lehnert (2003) suggest disturbances in the transport of the hormone across the blood-brain barrier. Leptin resistance is probably not caused by a single mechanism but, rather, results from a combination of the above-mentioned factors. However, the critical mechanism(s) underlying this process remain unclear.

3. Seasonality of leptin action

In the last decade, many factors affecting the appetite and energy expenditure have been described. It has been shown that the effects of many of these factors are dependent on photoperiod. Melatonin, which is a biochemical indicator of changes in light conditions, is functionally and anatomically involved in the modulation of numerous interactions linked with adaption to changes in food intake according to circadian and annual changes in the environment. Moreover, many other hormones involved in maintaining energy homeostasis are characterized by daily and annual fluctuations of their concentrations in the bloodstream. In temperate latitudes, sheep are seasonal breeders for which reproductive activity is controlled mainly by photoperiod. Nocturnal secretion of pineal-derived melatonin provides information about day length, but neither the target sites for its action in the brain nor the neuropeptide circuits engaged by the melatonin signal are well defined (Adam & Mercer, 2004). Recently, attention has been focused on the role of leptin, in this process, which is strongly implicated as one of the major peripheral signals controlling body fat reserves and appetite in mammals.

In numerous animal species, food intake and the amount of fat stored change over the annual cycle. Melatonin can affect adipose tissue through sympathetic innervation. The presence of neurons projecting directly into fat tissue from suprachiasmatic nuclei (SCN), which are structures in the brain that are particularly rich in melatonin receptors, has been observed (Bartness et al., 2001), which was confirmed by experiments carried out on the Siberian hamster. Infusion of melatonin to the SCN caused a reduction in fat mass analogous to the reduction observed during short days (Bartness et al., 1993).

Furthermore, receptors for melatonin have been found in the DMH and anterior hypothalamic area, but not in the ARC, in seasonal species (Morgan & Mercer, 1994). The ARC theoretically rule out the possibility of direct effects of melatonin on leptin signaling within the ARC, which is the primary site of leptin receptors in brain. Colocalization of these receptors elsewhere has not yet been demonstrated; however, both melatonin and leptin receptors have been independently localized to the DMN. Morgan et Mercer (2001) reported that neurons from the DMH, SCN, and ARC project to the paraventricular nucleus (PVN). Adam & Mercer (2004) proposed that melatonin could contribute to hypothalamic sensitivity to leptin through acting on the PVN region (the center of appetite regulation), with the PVN thus representing a site at which melatonin and leptin feedback may be coordinated. Relative leptin insensitivity during long days (LD) may be necessary to prevent the observed increase in leptin concentrations, which would cause appetite reduction and thereby counteract photoperiod-driven increases in voluntary food intake and body weight (Tups et al., 2004). Collectively, these observations imply that there is a distinct system of regulation in which normal responses to leptin and energy deficits are overridden by photoperiod (Tups et al., 2004).

In addition to the indirect effects of melatonin, which occur through the nervous system, melatonin may directly modulate the activity of adipose tissue via the endocrine system by acting on specific receptors on membranes of adipocytes. In isolated rat adipocytes, melatonin inhibits basal and insulin-induced lipogenesis (Ng & Wong, 1986). These observations were confirmed in studies by Zalatan and colleagues (2001), in which melatonin inhibited isoproterenol-induced lipolysis, and this effect was blocked by pertussis toxin and a melatonin receptor agonist. Moreover, effects of melatonin were demonstrated only in the case of adipocytes derived from adipose tissue taken from the groin area, but not the epididymal region, suggesting a site-specific nature of these interactions (Zalatan et al., 2001). Melatonin was observed to enhance leptin expression in primary cultures of rat adipocytes in the presence of insulin; this effect was blocked by pertussis toxins and forskolin, which are known to be selective antagonists of the melatonin receptor (Alonso-Vale et al., 2005). This type of stimulation was promoted when melatonin was added in a circadian-like manner (12 h +/ 12 h -; Alonso-Vale et al., 2006).

The role of melatonin in leptin secretion is still poorly understood. Several authors have reported that melatonin reduces the leptin concentration in the blood, while authors have reported an opposite tendency. The removal of the pineal gland in rats was associated with an elevated concentration of leptin circulating in the bloodstream, and the application of exogenous melatonin reversed this effect (Canpolat et al., 2001). Other studies indicate that intraperitoneal injection of exogenous melatonin (1 mg) did not affect the secretion of leptin in rats when it was administered during the day; however, it slightly reduced the leptin concentration at night (Mastronardi et al., 2000). Exogenous melatonin reduced the levels of leptin in Siberian hamsters (*Mesocricetus auratus*) (Korhonen et al., 2008). In Syrian hamsters, high levels of melatonin in the blood were associated with a decrease in leptin concentrations, and the removal of the pineal gland resulted in increases in the leptin level (Gunduz, 2002). In contrast, in seasonally breeding mink (*Mustela vision*), melatonin implantation in the fall was linked to a stimulating effect on leptin in the bloodstream (Mustonen et al., 2000). Similarly, these hormones exhibited positive relationships with circadian rhythms in sheep (Bertolucci et al., 2005). However, regarding seasonal rhythms, the pattern observed for leptin concentrations is the opposite of that found for the release of melatonin.

Interestingly, there are also several reports indicating that leptin can affect melatonin secretion. It has been shown that recombinant ovine leptin is able to modulate melatonin release in ovine pineal gland explants *in vitro*, and this effect is seasonally dependent (Zieba et al., 2007). Exogenous leptin inhibits the secretion of melatonin from pineal gland explants during LD and stimulates this process during short days (SD) (Zieba et al., 2007). A seasonal switch in the sensitivity of the ovine pineal gland to leptin was also reported based on *in vivo* studies in sheep. Following intracerebroventricular (icv) infusion of leptin, stimulatory effects on melatonin secretion during SD and inhibitory effects during LD were observed (Zieba et al., 2008).

4. SOCS-3 as a negative regulator of leptin signaling

SOCS-3 is a potent inhibitor of the JAK/STAT signaling pathway, negatively regulating the signal transduction of a variety of factors, including leptin. Despite the fact that proteins currently classified as SOCS were identified and characterized as negative regulators of cytokine signaling in the late twentieth century (Endo et al., 1997; Naka et al., 1997; Starr et al., 1997), their role in the coordination of hormonal interactions is still poorly understood. In physiological conditions, the expression of SOCS mRNA in the majority of tissues, with the exception of the brain, is rather low. However, it is known that some specific factors (cytokines, growth factors, hormones) can rapidly alter the level of SOCS expression.

Leptin supplied through intraperitoneal or intravenous injection was found to result in a significant increase of SOCS-3 expression in numerous hypothalamic nuclei in male *ob/ob* mice (Bjorbaek et al., 1998). A lack of changes in SOCS-3 mRNA levels in mice without functional leptin receptors (*db/db*) confirms that this process is associated with the activation of leptin receptors (Bjorbaek et al., 1998). Additionally, *in vitro* studies on hamster ovary cell lines have confirmed that leptin induces SOCS-3 mRNA transcription and protein expression (Bjorbaek et al., 1999). Moreover, these investigators demonstrated that increases in the SOCS-3 level caused by preincubation in the presence of leptin were linked to leptin resistance during sequent incubation.

Localization of this protein in the hypothalamic nucleus and the wide variety of factors that are able to induce its expression suggest that SOCS-3 may play a pivotal role in the modulation of neuroendocrinal interactions. Additionally, there is evidence implying that SOCS-3 has an important function within the pituitary. Recent experiments indicate that the SOCS-3 expression level is also dependent on environmental factors, such as photoperiodic conditions and nutritional status.

4.1 The role of SOCS-3 in seasonal leptin resistance

If the major control of seasonal changes in leptin sensitivity takes place at the hypothalamic level, the question arises as to how this effect is mediated. Although several potential mechanisms to account for this process have been proposed (Levin et al., 2004; Münzberg et al., 2005), the one receiving the most attention has been the inhibition of intracellular leptin signaling by SOCS-3.

Studies in the Siberian hamster (Tups et al., 2004) have demonstrated that reduced SOCS-3 activity during short day period contributes to increased sensitivity to leptin and that, conversely, increased activity of SOCS-3 signaling contributes to the relative leptin insensitivity seen in LD. Moreover, leptin was able to induce SOCS-3 expression exclusively in short days and had no effect during long days, which indicates that this interaction is also seasonally dependent (Adam & Mercer, 2004; Tups et al., 2004). Changes in hypothalamic sensitivity to leptin at different times of the year have previously been reported in sheep (Adam et al., 2003; Miller et al., 2002). However, these studies mainly investigated the photoperiodic regulation of appetite and reproductive axes.

Studies conducted by the authors of the present paper indicated that intracerebroventricular leptin infusions were also able to alter hypothalamic SOCS-3 expression in sheep. However, this effect was observed only during long day', but not during short day', conditions (Zieba et al., 2008), while in the pituitary, leptin affects this expression only during short days (Szczesna et al., 2011). This explains the existence of leptin resistance in the hypothalamus with simultaneous maintenance of leptin sensitivity in the pituitary. Seasonally dependent changes in the responsiveness of the ovine hypothalamus to leptin have also been reported (Miller et al., 2002). This may be the result of increased levels of SOCS-3 expression and, to some extent, may explain the phenomenon of a lack of sensitivity of the hypothalamus with respect to the anorexic effects of leptin in the long day season.

One of the key reports presenting the results of experiments on changes in the expression of SOCS-3 factors in response to annual environmental rhythms was produced by Tups and colleagues (2004). Based on studies in the Siberian hamster, these investigators described the changes in SOCS-3 mRNA levels in response to short-term fasting and long-term dietary restrictions and the effects of exogenous leptin relative to short (8 h light: 16 h darkness)- and long (16 h light: 8 h dark)-day conditions. The authors showed that the expression of SOCS-3 in the ARC was significantly higher during long days than during short days in all of the experimental systems studied (Tups et al., 2004). It was found that leptin administered through intraperitoneal injections (2 mg/kg BW) significantly increased the expression of SOCS-3 factors in the ARC in animals kept in short-day conditions, without changing the expression in individuals remaining under the influence of a long day (Tups et al., 2004). The lack of an effect of leptin during LD observed in these experiments could result from a high endogenous photoperiod-induced SOCS-3 level, which, in turn, led to the occurrence of leptin resistance.

Based on the wide range of factors affecting SOCS-3 expression and the large number of potential interactions occurring in organisms, the impact of other hormones on the modulation of endocrine relationships (also relative to the season) should not be neglected. Presumably, during LD, at least in hamsters, the SOCS-3 gene is expressed constitutively at a high rate, regardless of the level of endogenous leptin (Tups et al., 2004), and it is very possible that maintaining a high level of SOCS-3 results from interactions other than with leptin.

The complexity of this issue may underlie the results of studies on the daily fluctuations in SOCS-3 expression. In rats, which are characterized by nocturnal increases of activity, including in relation to food intake and increased levels of leptin secretion during the dark phase, the mRNA expression of SOCS-3 is much lower at night than during the day (Denis et al., 2004). However, studies on daily changes in the expression of SOCS-3 in the hypothalamus of Siberian hamsters found no correlation between the time of day and the level of SOCS-3 mRNA, as its expression remained at comparable levels in the light and dark phases (Ellis et al., 2008). In relation to other genes involved in the regulation of energy balance, diurnal variations in expression level were observed only in the case of leptin receptor mRNA, for which the level increased in the dark phase, but only in a long day photoperiod (Ellis et al., 2008). This indicates that depending on the season, hypothalamic sensitivity to leptin may be regulated by several mechanisms simultaneously.

Taking into account that melatonin is the main cue of changes in day length, pineal hormone or other hormones for which the concentration in the bloodstream is highly dependent on the concentration of melatonin (for example, PRL) may be involved in the seasonally dependent modulation of the expression of SOCS-3. It is possible that the differences observed between seasons with respect to when exogenous leptin can influence the expression of SOCS-3 in the hypothalamus that were observed in hamsters (Tups et al., 2004) and sheep (Zieba et al., 2008) resulted from the action of other hormones (steroids) associated with differences in the timing of seasonal reproduction activity in these species.

4.2 SOCS-3 and obesity

It is believed that changes in the expression of SOCS-3 factors are also associated with pathological states of insensitivity to cytokines, as in the case of obesity. In rats with experimentally induced obesity (initiated by lesions in the VMH or the administration of a high-fat diet), the expression of these factors in adipose tissue was significantly increased (Z. Wang et al., 2000). Particularly interesting information regarding the role of SOCS-3 in the induction of leptin resistance has been provided by research on mice in which the SOCS-3 gene was specifically knocked-out (Mori et al., 2004). Total absence of the SOCS-3 gene is lethal in the early stages of fetal life because of the numerous disturbances that occur, for example, in the development of the placenta (Roberts et al., 2001) or in erythropoiesis (Marine et al., 1999). Based on these findings, Mori and colleagues (2004) carried out studies using two animal models in which deletions in the SOCS-3 gene occurred exclusively in nerve tissue. Leptin infusions were not associated with increased levels of SOCS-3 factors within the hypothalamus, a characteristic of individuals with a wild-type genotype, and the observed reduction in food consumption and body weight was significantly higher in both experimental models compared with control subjects with normal genes (Mori et al., 2004). Through analysis of the impact of obesity and high-fat diet-induced leptin resistance, it was also found that while wild animals are susceptible to the occurrence of both of these phenomena, individuals with the SOCS-3 deficient are more resistant to weight gain (Mori et al., 2004). Similar conclusions were drawn based on research conducted on mice with an SOCS-3 +/- genotype with haploinsufficiency of SOCS-3 (Howard et al., 2004). Other studies have found that the lethal yellow mouse (Ay/a), characterized by obesity, hyperleptinemia and leptin resistance, presents significantly elevated levels of SOCS-3 mRNA compared with wild-type individuals (Bjorbaek et al., 1998). However, experiments conducted by Emilsson and colleagues (1999) demonstrated that the basal expression of SOCS-3 mRNA in the hypothalamus is higher in obese animals lacking the genes encoding leptin (*ob/ob*) compared to wild-type individuals. This suggests that, at least in this case, expression of SOCS-3 mRNA was not caused by leptin but by other factors associated with obesity, once again indicating the role of those suppressors in integrating of the activities of various factors.

Because of the wide range of actions and strong biological activity of leptin, the effects of its action must be strictly controlled to prevent disadvantageous consequences of excessive stimulation of leptin receptors. Localization of SOCS-3 mRNA in neurons of the hypothalamus and a significant induction of their expression in response to numerous factors indicates that SOCS-3 plays a crucial role in cytokine-induced regulation of neuroendocrine interactions. The observations presented above suggest that SOCS-3 proteins are important regulators playing a key role in feeding-induced or genetic-origin obesity and leptin resistance, leading to the hypothesis that therapy consisting of a reduction in the levels of these proteins within the hypothalamus might be helpful in treating obesity associated with reduced sensitivity to leptin.

5. Leptin and reproduction

Leptin also plays a crucial role in the regulation of reproductive processes. It is generally accepted that there is a close relationship between reproductive processes and nutritional status. There is some evidence that leptin is one of the pivotal factors modulating these processes (Sahu, 2003). Exogenous leptin accelerates entry into a period of sexual maturity of female rodents, including mice (Ahima et al., 1997) and rats (Cheung et al., 1997). High levels of endogenous leptin, associated with excess body fat, are responsible for the earlier occurrence of first menstruation in girls who are overweight compared with lean girls at the same age (Jaruratanasirikul et al., 1997).

Malnutrition has a negative impact on reproductive processes, ranging from a reduction in libido to negative effects on pregnancy (implantation disorders, increased fetal resorption, abortion) and the inhibition of ovulation. Nutritional deprivation of females, whether as a result of an insufficient supply of energy in the diet or excessive demands for energy (e.g., lactation), inhibits GnRH release, leading to reduced secretion of LH and even to anovulation and anestrus (Scaramuzzi & Martin, 2008). Both chronic undernutrition and acute fasting with associated hypoglycemia quickly lead to suppression of the GnRH system and a cessation of LH pulsatility in monogastric species (Bronson, 1988). In contrast, stimulation by leptin of the hypothalamic–gonadotropic axis by ruminant species is observed predominantly in animals and tissues pre-exposed to an intense negative energy balance (Zieba et al., 2003).

The hypothalamic GnRH pulse generator in ruminant species (cattle, sheep and goats) is much less sensitive to nutritional deprivation due to the fact that ruminant species derive metabolizable energy primarily from volatile fatty acid production in the rumen. Therefore, both serious and chronic food restrictions are required to result in negative reproductive consequences in adults. Importantly, the central reproductive axis of pre-pubertal ruminants is much more sensitive to nutritional perturbations, such as acute fasting, than that of sexually mature individuals (Zieba et al., 2005). It was demonstrated that short-term fasting (48-72 h) is sufficient to suppress the frequency of LH pulses in peripubertal heifers (Amstalden et al., 2000). Moreover, treatment with exogenous leptin prevented these decreases, implying a direct action of leptin at the hypothalamic level (Maciel et al., 2004a). In contrast, mature cows subjected to similar feeding restrictions, resulting in analogous metabolic responses to those seen peripubertal heifers (e.g., decreased leptin mRNA expression in adipose tissue, decreased plasma concentrations of leptin, insulin and IGF-1), did not exhibit a decrease in the pulsatile secretion of LH (Maciel et al., 2004b). However, similar to the heifers, mature cows subjected to short-term fasting became intensely hypersensitive to exogenous leptin. Intravenous infusion of leptin in this animal model promptly increased baseline and overall mean concentrations of LH and markedly augmented the amplitude of individual pulses of LH (Amstalden et al., 2000). Studies conducted by Nonaka and co-workers (2005) have provided clear evidence demonstrating a direct effect of leptin on LH release from primary cultured anterior pituitary cells collected from fully fed steers.

Although leptin's action on GnRH neuronal activity was confirmed in several studies, the neuroendocrine mechanisms associated with this process remain unclear. Although few

GnRH neurons, if any, have been found to express the leptin receptors in the rat (Zamorano et al., 1997) and monkey (Finn et al., 1998), leptin has been found to stimulate the release of GnRH from rat and porcine hypothalamic explants and from hypothalamus of cattle during *in vivo* study (Zieba et al., 2005). Expression of leptin receptor mRNA has been demonstrated in both the anterior pituitary gland and hypothalamus (Amstalden et al., 2002), and the leptin receptors has been identified within regions rich in GnRH neurons, such as the ARC, the medial preoptic area, and the median eminence (Ahima et al., 2000; Sahu, 2003), and *in vitro* studies using explants collected from normally fed rodents indicate that leptin can act directly at both sites (Amstalden et al., 2002; Watanobe, 2002) to stimulate the release of GnRH and LH, respectively. Data from Watanobe (2002) strongly suggest that leptin could act at both the cell bodies and axon terminals of GnRH neurons to stimulate the release of the neurohormone *in vivo*, with greater sensitivity of the ARC to leptin observed in fasted than in fed rats. Based upon increases in both receptor mRNA and protein levels (Baskin et al., 1998, 1999), fasting may enhance the leptin receptor concentration in the ARC. Similarly, the expression of the full-length leptin receptor, both in the ventromedial hypothalamus and in the pituitary gland, was found to be much greater in feed-restricted ewes than in ewes that were well fed (Dyer et al., 1997), which in turn suggests that dietary restriction can increase the sensitivity of both of these tissues to the action of leptin. In castrated yearling rams subjected to 72 h of food deprivation, leptin restores pulsatile LH secretion, although direct leptin action is not sufficient to influence LH release in satiated animals (Nagatani et al., 2000). In properly nourished ovariectomized ewes, icv infusion of leptin did not affect LH secretion, although the dose of leptin used was sufficient to reduce food intake (Henry et al., 1999), while in long-term food-restricted animals, leptin partially restores LH release without affecting appetite (Henry et al., 2001). In prepubertal female lambs, central (Morrison et al., 2001) and intravenous (Morrison et al., 2002) infusion of leptin did not affect LH release in either well-fed or undernourished animals, despite the fact that LH pulse frequencies were lower in diet-restricted than fed animals (Morrison et al., 2001).

The discrepancies linked with the observations mentioned above may be connected with the influence of the different times of year in which the studies were carried out, as seasonally dependent changes in sensitivity to leptin have been reported in sheep. It was shown that in spring, icv infusions of leptin in castrated, adequately nourished rams cause a significant increase in LH secretion compared with the results obtained when the infusions were performed in the fall (Miller et al., 2002). In turn, Adam et al. (2003) observed that a single, pharmacological icv dose of leptin in sheep specifically stimulated the frequency of LH pulses and simultaneously decreased appetite in late autumn. In contrast, no effect was observed when leptin was applied to the same sheep in the spring. However, the latest results from this group (Adam et al., 2006) do not support the hypothesis that leptin stimulates the reproductive neuroendocrine axis under the influence of photoperiod, although photoperiod modulates intrahypothalamic leptin sensitivity related to appetite. These observations in sheep concerning voluntary feed intake and the lack of effects observed on the GnRH/LH system are consistent with similar studies in Siberian hamsters, which are resistant to leptin during the long days but become responsive to leptin treatment in terms of body weight and abdominal fat loss during the short days (Atcha et al., 2000).

An influence of leptin is also observed in the peripheral sites of the reproductive axis. Additionally, leptin exhibits direct action within the ovary, including inhibition of estradiol secretion from ovarian follicles (Spicer & Francisco, 1997), thus participating in the regulation of the growth and maturation of this organ. Placental leptin, acting by paracrine and autocrine mechanisms, appears to be involved in the modulation of maternal-fetal interactions, including angiogenesis and the processes of growth and metabolism within the fetus and the uterus (Ashworth et al., 2000).

6. *Pas de trois*: leptin, ghrelin and orexin interaction

In addition to the previously described effects of leptin, the growing interest in the regulation of both metabolic and reproductive function has led to increased interest in orexin A and B, produced in the hypothalamus (De Lecea et al., 1998; Sakurai et al., 1999), and ghrelin, produced mainly in the stomach (Kojima et al., 1999).

The LHA is one of the sites that mediates the orexigenic properties of ghrelin (Cowley et al., 2003). As an integrator of ghrelin-derived input, the lateral hypothalamus acts as part of a larger feeding-related network that includes the PVN, ARC, and DMH. Ghrelin receptors are present in hypothalamic NPY/AgRP neurons, and ghrelin activates those neurons to stimulate food intake. It was observed that the mRNA levels of ghrelin in the stomach, hypothalamus and pituitary gland increase significantly during starvation. Furthermore, it was found that changes in the level of ghrelin in plasma are correlated with the level of leptin (Cummings & Foster, 2003). During fasting, plasma ghrelin concentrations increase, with a simultaneous decrease in leptin concentrations, and during feeding, the situation is reversed. Moreover ghrelin, activates the neurons of the ARC in a dose-dependent manner, whereas leptin inhibits these neurons. To emphasize the close relationship that exists between leptin and ghrelin in the regulation of energy, appetite and body weight, Cummings and Foster (2003) used the term "ghrelin-leptin tango", which accurately describes the nature of the interaction between these hormones. Kim et al. (2004) demonstrated that long-term intracerebellar or intraventricular administration of leptin reduced the levels of glucose and insulin, decreased food intake by 39% and reduced body fat weight by 41%, while co-administration of ghrelin nullified these effects. Barazzoni et al. (2003) demonstrated that leptin functions as an adiposity signal to negatively regulate ghrelin concentrations in the rat.

Interestingly, there are several pieces of evidence indicating that some of ghrelin's actions are under the influence of photoperiod. Central infusions of ghrelin, depending on the season, stimulated food intake, modulated the secretion of GH and inhibited the release of GnRH/LH in castrated rams (Harrison et al., 2008). Injections of ghrelin into the third ventricle of the brain caused a temporary increase in food intake during long days, with no similar effect seen during short days. In turn, inhibition of the release of GnRH/LH was observed only when ghrelin was administrated in short days during the breeding season of sheep. Furthermore, it has been demonstrated that in the rat, exogenous melatonin decreases ghrelin concentration (Mustonen et al., 2001). In turn, Brunetti et al. (2002) showed that ghrelin inhibits the melatonin precursor serotonin in the rat hypothalamus. Studies conducted in sheep indicate a lack of any effect of day length on ghrelin-treated pineal gland explants in relation to melatonin concentration (Zieba et al., 2011). It is noteworthy that the length of day had no effect on circadian or annual concentrations of endogenous ghrelin in sheep. However, during both seasons - long and short days, ghrelin decreased melatonin concentrations when administered at either low or high doses (Harrison et al., 2008).

In analyzing the interactions between leptin and ghrelin, the finding of greatest interest is that opposite effects of their actions are found not only in relation to the regulation of food intake, but also to the season in which adjustments in food intake occur. During short days, injections of leptin inhibit appetite (Miller et al., 2002), while centrally administered ghrelin has no effect on food intake (Harrison et al., 2008). Intriguing results were obtained by Zieba and co-workers (2011) through *in vitro* studies on ovine pineal glands. They showed that the addition of leptin to ghrelin-treated cultures increased melatonin concentrations compared to cultures supplemented with ghrelin alone during both long and short photoperiods. Although leptin decreased melatonin secretion during long days (Zieba et al., 2007), leptin and ghrelin acted synergistically to increase melatonin concentration to higher levels than in either individually-treated or untreated cultures (Zieba et al., 2011). These findings contribute to the formation of hypotheses concerning the joint action of leptin and ghrelin in the regulation of energy homeostasis depending on photoperiod.

Among the orexygenic peptides, orexins (also known as hypocretins) have also attracted considerable attention in recent years. Studies in rats have shown that exogenous administration of orexins increases food intake (Sakurai et al., 1998). Subsequently, other functions of these proteins were confirmed in studies demonstrating their role in the regulation of sleep-wake rhythms (Chemelli et al., 1999). Despite the fact that orexin-containing neurons represent a relatively small group of cells, it has been proven that their projections are spread through many parts of the central nervous system. Experimental data indicate the involvement of these proteins in various regulatory processes. Recent studies suggest that orexins play important roles as neurotransmitters within the central nervous system, and the orexins involved in this system may represent a link between the hypothalamus and other parts of the brain. It was found incontrovertibly that the expression of orexin receptors (OxR1 and OxR2) is not confined to the area of the hypothalamus, though it is the strongest in this region. The largest quantity of OxR1 mRNA was detected in the VMH. Additionally, it OxR1 mRNA was located in the lateral and posterior hypothalamus, POA, hippocampus and in the pituitary and the pineal gland. In turn, the highest expression of hypothalamic OxR2 mRNA was found in the PVN. Studies conducted in 2000 by Date and co-workers confirmed that there is strong expression of OxR1 and OxR2 mRNA in the middle, anterior (glandular) and posterior (neural) lobes of the pituitary gland of the rat. It has been shown that in sheep, orexin gene expression varies depending on the length of day: levels are higher during short days compared to long days (Archer et al., 2002). Moreover, prepro-orexin mRNA and orexin immunoreactivity display diurnal variation in the hypothalamic area, supporting the involvement of this hypothalamic peptide in the daily rhythm of melatonin synthesis (Archer et al., 2002).

Furthermore, orexin neurons are anatomically linked to components of the circadian system and innervate the pineal gland directly via a central input, but they may also be a part of the multineuronal pathway culminating in noradrenergic input from the superior cervical ganglion (Mikkelsen et al., 2001). They demonstrated that through its receptors present in the pineal gland, orexin (mainly B) decreases melatonin releases and reduces the activation of N-acetyltransferase, which is a key enzyme involved in the synthesis of pineal hormone. Studies carried out on explants of ovine pineal glands (Zieba et al., 2011) demonstrated a dose-dependent orexin stimulatory effect on melatonin release, mainly during the long photoperiod, with a lower dose having a stronger effect. No such effect was observed during short photoperiod, whereas a decrease in melatonin release was noted, as described by Mikkelsen et al. (2001), in cultured rat pinealocytes treated with orexin B. Hakansson and co-workers (1999) confirmed the presence of leptin receptor immunoreactivities in orexin neurons of the lateral hypothalamus. Therefore, it is possible that leptin can modulate food intake and reproduction via an interaction with the activity of orexin neurons.

Interesting links are also found between ghrelin and orexins. Intraventricular injections of ghrelin demonstrated anatomical and functional synaptic connections between neurons secreting orexins and ghrelin in the region of the lateral hypothalamus (Toshinai et al., 2003). Injections of ghrelin induced an immediate expression of C-Fos protein, which is the marker of neuronal activity in the neurons synthesizing orexin (Toshinai et al., 2003).

Taking into account the role of ghrelin and orexins in the regulation of energy homeostasis, it is not surprising that, as in the case of leptin, both ghrelin and orexin affect processes associated with reproduction. Intraventricular injections of orexin in ovariectomized female rats were associated with a decrease in LH pulse frequency (Tamura et al., 1999). Orexin A was also found to be an inhibitor of LH release from the pituitaries of female rats by Russell et al. (2001). Kohsaka et al. (2001) indicate the involvement of this peptide in the regulation of the pre-ovulatory output of LH and PRL in rats. They showed that administration of orexin to fasted animals can lead to a return of the concentrations of these hormones to the state observed prior to food restriction. Additionally, anti-orexin sera completely abolish the flow of both hormones in normally fed rats (Kohsaka et al., 2001). Studies on mammals have demonstrated that ghrelin is able to suppress pulsatile LH secretion in a diffrent species. However, in castrated rams, the effect of exogenous ghrelin on the release of GnRH/LH has been shown only during the short day period (Harrison et al., 2008). Acetylated ghrelin inhibited spontaneous LH pulsatility and the LH response to naloxone (Lanfranco et al., 2008). It was also provided, that ghrelin decreased GnRH release by hypothalamic explants *in vitro*, so its action for inhibitory effects on the gonadotropic release take place also in a higher level of this axis (Fernandez-Fernandez et al., 2005a). Ogata et al. (2009) provided that suppresive efect of central injection of ghrelin on pulstalile LH secretion was mediated by β-endorphin which suppressed pulsatile GnRH secretion from hypothalamus. In turn, studies conducted on goldfish pituitary cells inicate that ghrelin may also stimulate LH release via mechanism linked with Ca^{2+} entry and voltage-sensitive Ca^{2+} channels (Grey et al., 2010). Expression of ghrelin gene and gene of ghrelin receptor was reported also on gonadal stage - in the testis (Barreiro et al., 2003) and in the ovary (Caminos et al., 2003). It was also suggested that elevated ghrelin levels may be a negative modifier for embryo implantation (Kawamura et al., 2003) and development (Fernandez-Fernandez et al., 2005b) during pregnancy.

Taken together, these findings indicate an abundance of functions performed by proteins engaged in the regulation of energy homeostasis, in which these proteins form a close web of interactions and interrelationships. Based on these results, we can compare this relationship not to a tango of two partners, as suggested by Cummings and Foster, but rather to a *Pas de trois* - a dance of three, where not only leptin and ghrelin, but also orexin play very important roles. In this dance, there is a place for individual variations in each of these players, but their joint actions play the primary role. Due to the complexity of these interactions, as in a *Pas de trois*, this dance is spectacular and technically difficult, and the dancers exhibit a masterly precision and grace.

7. Conclusion

Intense research has been carried out to provide explanations for the relationships between hormones engaged in the regulation of energy homeostasis, metabolism and reproduction resulting from the importance of these interactions and the processes controlled by them. These studies have been conducted not only in theoretical, but also in practical terms, for the treatment of pathological phenomena associated with endocrine dysfunction in humans and animals or related to the economic viability of farming. Because of their strictly regulated adaptation to environmental conditions related to the plasticity of their endocrine system, as well as the presence of physiological leptin resistance, sheep represent a particularly interesting model for such studies. The observations described above emphasize the close relationship that exists between photoperiod, which is a powerful factor that influences the course of many processes in sheep, its main biochemical indicator, melatonin, and peptides involved in the regulation of energy homeostasis.

8. Acknowledgment

This work was supported by a grant from the Polish National Research Council (MNiSW NN 311 318436)

9. References

Adam, CL., Archer, ZA. & Miller, DW. (2003). Leptin actions on the reproductive neuroendocrine axis in sheep. *Reproduction. Supplement*, Vol.61, pp. 283-297, ISSN 1477-0415

Adam, CL. & Mercer, JG. (2004). Appetite regulation and seasonality: implications for obesity. *The Proceedings of the Nutrition Society*, Vol.63, No.3, pp. 413-419, ISSN 0029-6651

Adam, CL., Findlay, PA. & Miller, DW. (2006). Blood-brain leptin transport and appetite and reproductive neuroendocrine responses to intracerebroventricular leptin injection in sheep: influence of photoperiod. *Endocrinology*, Vol.147, No.10, pp. 4589-4598, ISSN 0013-7227

Ahima, RS., Dushay, J., Flier, SN., Prabakaran, D. & Flier, JS. (1997). Leptin accelerates the onset of puberty in normal female mice. *Journal of Clinical Investigation*, Vol.99, No.3, pp. 391-395, ISSN 0021-9738

Ahima, RS., Saper, CB., Flier, JS. & Elmquist, JK. (2000). Leptin regulation of neuroendocrine systems. *Frontiers in Neuroendocrinology*, Vol.21, No.3, pp. 263-307, ISSN 0091-3022

Alonso-Vale, MIC., Andreotti, S., Peres, SB., Anhe, GF., Borges-Silva, CN., Cipolla-Neto, J. & Lima, FB. (2005). Melatonin enhances leptin expression by rat adipocytes in the presence of insulin. *American Journal of Physiology. Endocrinology and Metabolism*, Vol.288, No.4, pp. 805-812, ISSN 0193-1849

Alonso-Vale, MIC., Andreotti, S., Borges-Silva, CN., Mukai, PY., Cipolla-Neto, J. & Lima, FB. (2006). Intermittent and rhythmic exposure to melatonin in primary cultured adipocytes enhances the insulin and dexamethasone effects on leptin expression. *Journal of Pineal Research*, Vol.41, No.1, pp. 28-34, ISSN 0742-3098

Amstalden, M., Garcia, MR., Williams, SW., Stanko, RL., Nizielski, SE., Morrison, CD., Keisler, DH. & Williams, GL. (2000). Leptin gene expression, circulating leptin, and luteinizing hormone pulsatility are acutely responsive to short-term fasting in prepubertal heifers: relationships to circulating insulin and insulin-like growth factor I. *Biology of Reproduction*, Vol.63, No.1, pp. 127-133, ISSN 0006-3363

Amstalden, M., Garcia, MR., Stanko, RL., Nizielski, SE., Morrison, CD., Keisler, DH. & Williams, GL. (2002). Central infusion of recombinant ovine leptin normalizes plasma insulin and stimulates a novel hypersecretion of luteinizing hormone after short-term fasting in mature beef cows. *Biology of Reproduction*, Vol.66, No.5, pp. 1555-1561, ISSN 0006-3363

Archer, ZA., Findlay, PA., Rhind, SM., Mercer, JG. & Adam, CL. (2002). Orexin gene expression and regulation by photoperiod in the sheep hypothalamus. *Regulatory Peptides*, Vol.104, No.1-3, pp. 41-45, ISSN 0167-0115

Ashworth, CJ., Hoggard, N., Thomas, L., Mercer, JG., Wallace, JM. & Lea, RG. (2000). Placental leptin. *Reviews of Reproduction*, Vol.5, No.1, pp. 18-24, ISSN 1359-6004

Atcha, Z., Cagampang, FR., Stirland, JA., Morris, ID., Brooks, AN., Ebling, FJ., Klingenspor, M. & Loudon, AS. (2000). Leptin acts on metabolism in a photoperiod-dependent manner, but has no effect on reproductive function in the seasonally breeding Siberian hamster (*Phodopus sungorus*). *Endocrinology*, Vol.141, No.11, 4128-4135, ISSN 0013-7227

Banks, AS., Davis, SM., Bates, SH. & Myers Jr., MG. (2000). Acivation of downstream signals by the long form of the leptin receptor. *Journal of Biological Chemistry*, Vol.275, No.19, pp. 14563-14572, ISSN 0021-9258

Barazzoni, R., Zanetti, M., Stebel, M., Biolo, G., Cattin, L. & Guarnieri, G. (2003). Hyperleptinemia prevents increased plasma ghrelin concentration during short-term moderate caloric restriction in rats. *Gastroenterology*, Vol.124, No.5, pp. 1188-1192, ISSN 0016-5085

Barreiro, ML., Suominen, JS., Gaytan, F., Pinilla, L., Chopin, LK., Casaneuva, FF., Dieguez, C., Aguilar, C., Toppari, J. & Tena-Sempere, M. (2003). Developmental, stage-specific and hormonally regulated expression of growth hormone secretagogue receptor messenger RNA in rat testis. *Biology of Reproduction*, Vol.68, No.5, pp. 1631-1640, ISSN 0006-3363

Bartness, TJ., Powers, JB., Hastings, MH., Bittman, EL. & Goldman, BD. (1993). The timed infusion paradigm for melatonin delivery: What has it taught us about melatonin signal, its reception, and the photoperiodic control of seasonal responses? *Journal of Pineal Research*, Vol.15, No.4, pp. 161-190, ISSN 0742-3098

Bartness, TJ., Song, CK. & Demas, GE. (2001). SCN efferents to peripheral tissues: implications for biological rhythms. *Journal of Biological Rhythms*, Vol.16, No.3, pp. 196-204, ISSN 0748-7304

Baskin, DG., Seeley, RJ., Kuijper, JL., Lok, S., Weigle, DS., Erickson, JC., Palmiter, RD. & Schwartz, MW. (1998). Increased expression of mRNA for the long form of the leptin receptor in the hypothalamus is associated with leptin hypersensitivity and fasting. *Diabetes*,Vol.47, No.4, pp. 538-543, ISSN 0012-1797

Baskin, DG., Breininger, JF., Bonigut, S. & Miller, MA. (1999). Leptin binding in the arcuate nucleus is increased during fasting. *Brain Research*, Vol.828, No.1-2, pp. 154-158, ISSN 0006-8993

Bernabucci, U., Basirico, L., Lacetera, N., Morera, P., Ronchi, B., Accorsi, PA., Seren, E. & Nardone, A. (2006). Photoperiod affects gene expression of leptin and leptin receptors in adipose tissue from lactating dairy cows. *Journal of Dairy Science*, Vol.89, No.12, pp. 4678-4686, ISSN 0022-0302

Bertolucci, C., Caola, G., Foa, A. & Piccione, G. (2005). Daily rhythms of serum leptin in ewes: effects of feeding, pregnancy and lactation. *Chronobiology International*, Vol.22, No.5, pp. 817-827, ISSN 0742-0528

Bjorbaek, C., Uotani, S., Da Silva, B. & Flier, JS. (1997). Divergent signaling capcities of the long and the short isoforms of the leptin receptor. *Journal of Biological Chemistry*, Vol.272, No.51, pp. 32686-32695, ISSN 0021-9258

Bjorbaek, C., Elmquist, J., Frantz, J., Shoelson, S. & Flier, J. (1998). Identification of SOCS-3 as a potential mediator of central leptin resistance. *Molecular Cell*, Vol.1, No.4, pp. 619-625, ISSN 1097-2765

Bjorbaek, C., El-Haschimi, K., Frantz, JD. & Flier, JS. (1999). The role of SOCS-3 in leptin signaling and leptin resistance. *Journal of Biological Chemistry*, Vol.274, No.42, pp. 30059-30065, ISSN 0021-9258

Bjorbaek, C., Lavery, HJ. & Bates, SH. (2000). SOCS-3 mediates feedback inhibition of the leptin receptor via Tyr985. *Journal of Biological Chemistry*, Vol.275, No.51, pp. 40649-40657, ISSN 0021-9258

Bocquier, F., Bonnet, M., Faulconnier, Y., Guerre-Millo, M., Martin, P. & Chilliard, Y. (1998). Effects of photoperiod and feeding level on perirenal adipose tissue metabolic activity and leptin synthesis in the ovariectomized ewe. *Reproduction, Nutrition, Development*, Vol.38, No.5, pp. 489-498, ISSN 0926-5287

Boden, G., Chen, X., Mazzoli, M. & Ryan, I. (1996). Effect of fasting on serum leptin in normal human subjects. *Journal of Clinical Endocrinology and Metabolism*, Vol.81, No.9, pp. 2419-2423, ISSN 0021-972X

Bronson, FH. (1988). Effect of food manipulation on the GnRH-LH-estradiol axis of young female rats. *The American Journal of Physiology*, Vol.254, No.4 Pt 2, pp. R616-R621, ISSN 0002-9513

Brunetti, L., Recinella, G., Orlando, B., Michelotto, C., Di Nisio, C. & Vacca, M. (2002). Effects of ghrelin and amylin on dopamine, norepinephrine and serotonin release in the hypothalamus. *European Journal of Pharmacology*, Vol.454, no.2-3, pp. 189–192, ISSN 0014-2999

Caminos, JE., Tena-Sempere, M., Gaytan, F., Sanchez-Criado, JE., Barreiro, ML., Nogueiras, R., Casanueva, FF., Aguilar, E. & Dieguez, C. (2003). Expression of ghrelin in the cyclic and pregnant rat ovary. *Endocrinology*, Vol.144, No.4, pp. 1594-602, ISSN 0013-7227

Canpolat, S., Sandal, S., Yilmaz, B., Yasar, A., Kutlu, S., Baydas, G. & Kelestimur, H. (2001). Effects of pinealectomy and exogenous melatonin on serum leptin levels in male rat. *European Journal of Pharmacology*, Vol.428, No.1, pp. 145-148, ISSN 0014-2999

Caprio, M., Isidori, AM., Carta, AR., Moretti, C., Dufau, ML. & Fabbri A. (1999). Expression of leptin receptors in rodents Leydig cells. *Endocrinology*, Vol.140, No.11, pp. 4939-4947, ISSN 0013-7227

Carter-Su, C., Schwartz, J. & Kikuchi, G. (1984). Identification of a high-affinity growth hormone receptor in rat adipocytes. *Journal of Biological Chemistry*, Vol.259, No.2, pp.1099-1104, ISSN 0021-9258

Chemelli, RM., Willie, JT., Sinton, CM., Elmquist, JK., Scammell, T., Lee, C., Richardson, JA., Williams, SC, Xiong, Y., Kisanuki, Y., Fitach, TE., Nakazato, M, Hammer, RE., Saper, CB. & Yanagisawa, M. (1999). Narcolepsy in orexin knockout mice: molecular genetics of sleep regulation. *Cell*, Vol.98, No.4, pp. 437–451, ISSN 0092-8674

Cheung, CC., Thornton, JE., Kuijper, JL., Weigle, DS., Clifton, DK. & Steiner, RA. (1997). Leptin is metabolic gate for the onset of puberty in the female rat. *Endocrinology*, Vol.138, No.2, pp. 855-858, ISSN 0013-7227

Chilliard, Y., Delavaud, C. & Bonnet, M. (2005). Leptin expression in ruminants: nutritional and physiological regulations in relation with energy metabolism. *Domestic Animal Endocrinology*, Vol.29, No.1, pp. 3-22, ISSN 0739-7240

Cowley, MA., Smith, RG., Diano, S., Tschöp, M., Pronchuk, N., Grove, KL., Strasburger, CJ., Bidlingmaier, M., Esterman, M., Heiman, ML., Garcia-Segura, LM., Nillni, EA., Mendez, P., Low,MJ., Sotonyi, P., Friedman, JM., Liu, H., Pinto, S., Colmers, WF., Cone, RD. & Horvath, TL. (2003). The distribution and mechanism of action of ghrelin in the CNS demonstrates a novel hypothalamic circuit regulating energy homeostasis. *Neuron* , Vol.37, No.4, pp. 649-661, ISSN 0896-6273

Cummings, DE. & Foster, KE. (2003). Ghrelin-leptin tango in body-weight regulation. *Gastroenterology*, Vol.124, No.5, pp. 1532-1535, ISSN 0016-5085

Date, Y., Mondal, MS., Matsukura, S., Ueta, Y., Yamashita, H., Kaiya, H., Kangawa, K. & Nakazato, M. (2000). Distribution of orexin/hypocretin in the rat median eminence and pituitary. *Brain Research. Molecular Brain Research*, Vol.76, No.1, pp. 1-6, ISSN 0169-328X

De Lecea, L., Kilduff, TS., Peron, C., Gao, X-B., Foye, PE., Danielson, PE., Fukuhara, C., Battenberg, ELF., Gautvik, VT., Bartlett, FS., Frankel, WN., Van den Pol, AN., Bloom, FE., Gautvik, KM. & Sutcliffe, JG. (1998). The hypocretins: hypothalamus-specific peptides with neuroexcitatory activity. *Proceedings of the National Academy of Sciences of the United States of America*, Vol.95, No.1, pp. 322-327, ISSN 0027-8424

Denis, RPG., Bing, C., Brocklehurst, S., Harrold, JA., Vernon, RG. & Williams, G. (2004). Diurnal changes in hypothalamic neuropeptide and SOCS-3 expression: effects of lactation and relationship with serum leptin and food intake. *Journal of Endocrinology*, Vol.183, No.1, pp. 173-181, ISSN 0022-0795

Dyer, CJ., Simmons, JM., Matteri, RL. & Keisler, DH. (1997). Leptin receptor mRNA is expressed in ewe anterior pituitary and adipose tissues and is differentially expressed in hypothalamic regions of well-fed and feed-restricted ewes. *Domestic Animal Endocrinology*, Vol.14, No.2, pp. 119-128, ISSN 0739-7240

Ehrhardt, RA., Slepetis, RM., Bell, AW. & Boisclair, YR. (2001). Maternal leptin is elevated during pregnancy in sheep. *Domestic Animal Endocrinology*, Vol.21, No.2, pp. 85-96, ISSN 0739-7240

El-Haschimi, K. & Lehnert, H. (2003). Leptin resistance - or why leptin fails to work in obesity. *Experimental and Clinical Endocrinology & Diabetes*, Vol.111, No.1, pp. 2-7, ISSN 0947-7349

Ellis, C., Moar, KM, Logie, TJ., Ross, AW., Morgan, PJ. & Mercer, JG. (2008). Diurnal profiles of hypothalamic energy balance gene expression with photoperiod manipulation in the Siberian hamster, *Phodopus sungorus*. *American Journal of Physiology. Regulatory, Integrative and Comparative Physiology*, Vol.294, No.4, pp. R1148-R1153, ISSN 0363-6119

Elmquist, JK., Bjorbaek, C., Ahima, RS., Flier, JS. & Saper, CB. (1998). Distributions of leptin receptor mRNA isoforms in the rat brain. *Journal of Comparative Neurology*, Vol.395, No.4, pp. 535-547, ISSN 0021-9967

Elmquist, JK., Elias, CF. & Saper, CB. (1999). From lesions to leptin: hypothalamic control of food intake and body weight. *Neuron*, Vol.22, No.2, pp. 221-232, ISSN 0896-6273

Emilsson, V., Jonathan, ARS, de Groot, RD., Lister, CA. & Cawthorne, MA. (1999). Leptin treatment increases suppressors of cytokine signaling in central and peripheral tissues. *FEBS Letters*, Vol.455, No.1-2, pp. 170-174, ISSN 0014-5793

Endo, TA., Masuhara, M., Yokouchi, M., Suzuki, R., Sakamoto, H., Mitsui, K., Matsumoto, A., Tanimura, S., Ohtsubo, M., Misawa, H., Miyazaki, T., Leonor, N., Taniguchi, T., Fujita, T., Kanakura, Y., Komiya, S. & Yoshimura, A. (1997). A new protein containing an SH2 domain that inhibits JAK kinases. *Nature*, Vol.387, No.6636, pp. 921-924, ISSN 0028-0836

Fernandez-Fernandez, R., Tena-Sempere, M., Navarro., VM., Barreiro, ML., Castellano, JM., Aguilar, E. & Pinilla, L. (2005a). Efffects of ghrelin upon gonadotropin-releasing hormone and gonadotropin secretion in adult female rats: in vivo and in vitro studies. *Neuroendocrinology*, Vol.82, No.5-6, pp. 245-255, ISSN 0028-3835

Fernandez-Fernandez, R., Navarro, VM., Barreiro, ML., Vigo, EM., Tovar, S., Sirotkin, AV., Casanueva, FF., Aguilar, E., Dieguez, C., Pinilla, L. & Tena-Sempere, M. (2005b). Effects of chronic hyperghrelinemia on puberty onset and pregnancy outcome in the rat. *Endocrinology*, Vol.146, No.7, pp. 3018-3025, ISSN 0013-7227

Finn, PD., Cunningham, MJ., Pau, KY., Spies, HG., Clifton, DK. & Steiner, RA. (1998). The stimulatory effect of leptin on the neuroendocrine reproductive axis of the monkey. *Endocrinology*, Vol.139, No.11, pp. 4652-4662, ISSN 0013-7227

Friedman, JM. & Halaas, JL. (1998). Leptin and the regulation of the body weight in mammals. *Nature*, Vol.395, No.6704, pp. 763-770, ISSN 0028-0836

Garcia, MR., Amstalden, M., Williams, SW., Stanko, RL., Morrison, CD., Keisler, DH., Nizielski, SE. & Williams GL. (2002). Serum leptin and its adipose gene expression during pubertal development, the estrous cycle, and different seasons in cattle. *Journal of Animal Science*, Vol.80, No.8, pp. 2158-2167, ISSN 0021-8812

Green, ED., Maffei, M., Braden, VV., Porenca, R., De Silva, U., Zhang, Y., Chua, SC., Leibel, R., Weissanbach, J. & Friedman, JM. (1995). The human obese (OB) gene: RNA expression pattern and mapping on the physical, cytogenic and genetic maps of chromosome 7. *Genome Research*, Vol.5, No.1, pp. 5-12, ISSN 1088-9051

Grey, CL., Grayfer, L., Belosevic, M. & Chang, JP. (2010). Ghrelin stimulation of gonadotropin (LH) release from goldfish pituitary cells: presence of the growth hormone secretagogue receptor (GHS-R1a) and involvement of voltage-sensitive Ca2+ channels. *Molecular and Cellular Endocrinology*, Vol.317, No.1-2, pp. 64-77, ISSN 0303-7207

Gunduz B. (2002). Daily rhythm in serum melatonin and leptin levels in the Syrian hamster (*Mesocricetus auratus*). *Comparative Biochemistry and Physiology. Part A, Molecular & Integrative Physiology*, Vol.132, No.2, pp. 393-401, ISSN 1095-6433

Hakansson, ML., de Lecea, L., Sutcliffe, JG., Yanagisawa, M. & Meister, B. (1999). Leptin receptor-abd STAT-3- immunoreactivities in hypocreti/orexin neurons of the lateral hypothalamus. *Journal of Neuroendocrinology*, Vol.11, No.8, pp. 653-663, ISSN 0953-8194

Halaas, JL., Gajiwala, KS., Maffei, M., Cohen, SL., Chait, BT., Rabinowitz, D., Lallone, RL., Burley, SK. & Friedman, JM. (1995). Weight-reducing effects of the plasma protein encoded by the obese gene. *Science*, Vol.269, No.5223, pp. 543-546, ISSN 0193-4511

Harrison, JL., Miller, DW., Findlay, PA. & Adam, CL. (2008). Photoperiod influences the central effects of ghrelin on food intake, GH and LH secretion in sheep. *Neuroendocrinology*, Vol.87, No.3, pp. 182-192, ISSN 0028-3835

Henry, BA., Goding, JW., Alexander, WS., Tilbrook, AJ., Canny, BJ., Dunshea, F., Rao, A., Mansell, A. & Clarke, IJ. (1999). Central administration of leptin to ovariectomised ewes inhibits food intake without affecting the secretion of hormones from pituitary gland: evidence for a dissociation of effects on appetite and neuroendocrine function. *Endocrinology*, Vol.140, No.3, pp. 1175-1182, ISSN 0013-7227

Henry, BA., Goding, JW., Tilbrook, AJ., Dunshea, F. & Clarke, IJ. (2001). Intracerbroventicular infusion of leptin elevates the secretion of luteinizing hormone without affecting food intake in long-term food-restricted sheep, but increases growth hormone irrespective of body weight. *Journal of Endocrinology*, Vol.168, No.1, pp. 67-77, ISSN 0022-0795

Hoggard, N., Mercer, JG., Rayner, DV., Moar, K., Trayhurn, P. & Williams, LM. (1997). Localization of leptin receptor mRNA splice variants in murine peripheral tissues by RT-PCR and in situ hybridization. *Biochemical and Biophysical Research Communications*, Vol.232, No.2, pp. 383-387, ISSN 0006-291X

Hoggard, N., Hunter, L., Trayhurn, P., Williams, LM. & Mercer JG. (1998). Leptin and reproduction. *The Proceedings of the Nutrition Society*, Vol.57, No.3, pp. 421-427, ISSN 0029-6651

Houseknecht, KL., Mantzoros, CS., Kuliawat, R., Hadro, E., Flier, JS. & Kahn, BB. (1996). Evidence for leptin binding to proteins in serum of rodents and humans: modulation with obesity. *Diabetes*, Vol.45, No.11, pp. 1638-1643, ISSN 0012-1797

Howard, JK., Cave, BJ., Oksanen, LJ., Tzameli, I., Bjorbaek, C. & Flier, JS. (2004). Enhanced leptin sensitivity an attenuation of diet-induced obesity in mice with haploinsufficiency of Socs3. *Nature Medicine*, Vol.10, No.7, pp. 739-743, ISSN 1078-8956

Iqbal, J., Pompolo, S., Considine, RV. & Clarke, IJ. (2000). Localization of leptin receptor-like immunoreactivity in the corticotropes, somatotropes, and gonadotropes in the ovine anterior pituitary. *Endocrinology*, Vol.141, No.4, pp. 1515-1520, ISSN 0013-7227

Jarett, L., Schweitzer, JB. & Smith, RM. (1980). Insulin receptors: differences in structural organization on adipocyte and liver plasma membranes. *Science*, Vol.210, No.4474, pp. 1127-1128, ISSN 0193-4511

Jaruratanasirikul, S., Mo-Suwan, L. & Lebel, L. (1997). Growth pattern and age at menarche of obese girls in a transitional society. *Journal of Pediatric Endocrinology & Metabolism*, Vol.10, No.5, pp. 487-490, ISSN 0334-018X

Jin, L., Burguera, BG., Couce, ME., Scheithauer, BW., Lamsan, J., Eberhardt, NL., Kulig, E. & Lloyd, RV. (1999). Leptin and leptin receptor expression in normal and neoplastic human pituitary: evidence of a regulatory role for leptin on pituitary cell proliferation. *Journal of Clinical Endocrinology and Metabolism*, Vol.84, No.8, pp. 2903-2911, ISSN 0021-972X

Karlsson, C., Lindell, K., Svensson, E., Bergh, C., Lind, P., Billig, H., Carlsson, LM. & Carlsson, B. (1997). Expression of functional leptin receptors in human ovary. *Journal of Clinical Endocrinology & Metabolism*, Vol.82, No.12, pp. 4144-4148, ISSN 0021-972X

Kawamura, K., Sato, N., Fukuda, J., Kodama, H., Kumagai, J., Tanikawa, H., Nakamura, A., Honda, Y., Sato, T. & Tanaka, T. (2003). Ghrelin inhibits the development of mouse preimplantation embryos in vitro. *Endocrinology*, Vol.144, No.6, pp. 2623-2633, ISSN 0013-7227

Kennedy, GC. (1953). The role of depot fat in the hypothalamic control of food intake in the rat. *Proceedings of the Royal Society of London, Series B, Biological Sciences*, Vol.140, No.901, pp. 579-592, ISSN 0080-4649

Kieffer, TJ., Heller, RS., Lech, CA., Holz, GG. & Habaner, JF. (1997). Leptin supression of insulin secretion by activation of ATP-sensitive K channels in pancreatic beta-cells. *Diabetes*, Vol.46, No.6, pp. 1087-1093, ISSN 0012-1797

Kim, MS., Namkoong, C., Kim, HS., Jang, PG., Kim Pak, YM., Katakami, H., Park, JY. & Lee, KU. (2004). Chronic central administration of ghrelin reverses the effects of leptin. *International Journal of Obesity and Related Metabolic Disorders*, Vol.28, No.10, pp. 1264-1271, ISSN 0307-0565

Klingenspor, M., Dickopp, A., Heldmaier, G. & Klaus, S. (1996). Short photoperiod reduces leptin gene expression in white and brown adipose tissue of Djungarian hamsters. *FEBS Letters*, Vol.399, No.3, pp. 290-294, ISSN 0014-5793

Klingenspor, M., Niggemann, H. & Heldmaier, G. (2000). Modulation of leptin sensitivity by short photoperiod acclimation in the Djungarian hamster, *Phodopus sungorus*. *Journal of Comparative Physiology. Biochemical, Systemic, and Environmental Physiology*, Vol.170, No.1, pp. 37-43, ISSN 0174-1578

Kohsaka, A., Watanobe, H., Kakizaki, Y., Suda, T., Schiöth, HB. (2001). A significant participation of orexin-A, a potent orexigenic peptide, in the preovulatory luteinizing hormone and prolactin surges in the rat. *Brain Research*, Vol.898, No.1, pp.166-170, ISSN 0006-8993

Kojima, M., Hosoda, H., Date, Y., Nakazato, M., Matmo, H. & Kangawa, K. (1999). Ghrelin is a growth hormone-releasing acylated peptide from stomach. *Nature*, Vol.402, No. 6762, pp. 656-660, ISSN 0028-0836

Korhonen, T., Mustonen, AM., Nieminen, P. & Saarela, S. (2008). Effects of cold exposure, exogenous melatonin and short-day treatment on the weight-regulation and body temperature of the Siberian hamster (*Phodopus sungorus*). *Regulatory Peptides*, Vol.149, No.1-3, pp. 60-66, ISSN 0167-0115

Kulcsar, M., Danko, G., Magdy, HGI., Reiczigel, J., Forgach, T., Prohaczik, A., Delavaud, C., Magyar, K., Chilliard, Y., Solti, L. & Huszenicza, G. (2006). Pregnancy stage and number of fetuses may influence maternal plasma leptin in ewes. *Acta Veterinaria Hungarica*,Vol.54, No.2, pp. 221-234, ISSN 0236-6290

Lanfranco, F., Bonelli, L., Baldi, M., Me, E., Broglio, F. & Ghigo, E. (2008). Acylated ghrelin inhibits spontaneous luteinizing hormone pulsatility and responsiveness to naloxone but not that to gonadotropin-releasing hormone in young men: evidence for a central inhibitory action of ghrelin on the gonadal axis. *Journal of Clinical Endocrinology and Metabolism*, Vol.93, No.9, pp. 3633-3639, ISSN 0021-972X

Levin, B.E., Dunn-Meynell, AA. & Banks, WA. (2004). Obesity-prone rats have normal blood-brain barrier transport but defective central leptin signaling before obesity onset. *American Journal of Physiology. Regulatory, Integrative and Comparative Physiology*, Vol.286, No.1, pp. 143-150, ISSN 0363-6119

Licinio, J., Negrao, AB., Mantzoros, C., Kaklamani, V., Wong, M-L., Bongiorno, PB., Negro, P., Mulla, A., Veldhuis, J., Cearnal, L., Flier, J. & Gold, P. (1998a). Sex differences in circulating human leptin pulse amplitude: clinical implications. *Journal of Clinical Endocrinology and Metabolism*, Vol.83, No.11, pp. 4140-4147, ISSN 0021-972X

Licinio, J., Negrao, AB., Mantzoros, C., Kaklamani, V., Wong, M., Bongiorno, PB., Mull, A., Cearnal, L., Veldhuis, JD., Flier, JS., McCann, SM. & Gold, PW. (1998b).

Synchronicity of frequently sampled 24-h concentrations of circulating leptin, luteinizing hormone, and estradiol in healthy women. *Proceedings of the National Academy of Sciences of the United States of America*, Vol.95, No.5, pp. 2541-2546, ISSN 0027-8424

Lin, J., Barb, CR., Matteri, RL., Kraeling, RR., Chen, X., Meinersmann, RJ. & Rampacek, GB. (2000). Long form leptin receptor mRNA expression in the brain, pituitary, and other tissues in the pig. *Domestic Animal Endocrinology,* Vol.19, No.1, pp. 53-61, ISSN 0739-7240

Ling, C., Hellgren, G., Gebre-Medhin, M., Dillner, K., Wennbo, H., Carlsson, B. & Billig, H. (2000). Prolactin receptor gene expression in mouse adipose tissue: increases during lactation and in PRL-transgenic mice. *Endocrinology,* Vol.141, No.10, pp. 3564-3572, ISSN 0013-7227

Maciel, MN., Zieba, DA., Amstalden, M., Keisler, DH., Neves, JP. & Williams, GL. (2004a). Chronic administration of recombinant ovine leptin in growing beef heifers: effects on secretion of LH, metabolic hormones, and timing of puberty. *Journal of Animal Science,* Vol.82, No.10, pp. 2930-2936, ISSN 0021-8812

Maciel, MN., Zieba, DA., Amstalden, M., Keisler, DH., Neves, JP., Williams & GL. (2004b). Leptin prevents fasting-mediated reductions in pulsatile secretion of luteinizing hormone and enhances its gonadotropin-releasing hormone-mediated release in heifers. *Biology of Reproduction,* Vol.70, No.1, pp. 229-35, ISSN 0006-3363

Maffei, M., Halaas, J., Ravussin, E., Pratley, RE., Lee, GH., Zhang, Y., Fei, H., Kim, S., Lallone R., Ranganathan, S., Kern, PA. & Friedman, JM. (1995). Leptin levels in human and rodent: measurement of plasma leptin and *ob* RNA in obese and weight-reduced subjects. *Nature Medicine,* Vol.1, No.11, pp. 1155-1161, ISSN 1078-8956

Marie, M., Findlay, PA., Thomas, L. & Adam, CL. (2001). Daily patterns of plasma leptin in sheep: effect of photoperiod and food intake. *Journal of Endocrinology,* Vol.170, No.1, pp. 277-286, ISSN 0022-0795

Marine, JC., McKay, C., Wang, D., Topham, DJ., Parganas, E., Nakajima, H., Pendeville, H., Yasukawa, H., Sasaki, A., Yoshimura, A., Ihle, JN. (1999). SOCS3 is essential in the regulation of fetal liver erythropoiesis. *Cell,* Vol.98, No.5, pp. 617-627, ISSN 0092-8674

Mastronardi, CA., Walczewska, A., Yu, WH., Karanth, S., Parlow, A.F. & McCann, S.M. (2000). The possible role of prolactin in the circadian rhythm of leptin secretion in male rats. *Proceedings of The Society for Experimental Biology and Medicine,* Vol.224, No.3, pp. 152-158, ISSN 0037-9727

Masuzaki, H., Ogawa, Y., Ssie, N., Satoh, N., Okazaki, T., Shigemoto, M., Mori, K., Tamura, N., Hosoda, K., Yoshimasa, Y., Jingami, H., Kawada, T. & Nakao, K. (1995). Human obese gene expression: adipocyte-specific expression and regional differences in the adipose tissue. *Diabetes,* Vol.44, No.7, pp. 855-858, ISSN 0012-1797

Masuzaki, H., Ogawa, Y., Sagawa, N., Hosoda, K., Matsumoto, T., Mise, H., Nishimura, H., Yoshimasa, Y., Tanaka, I., Mori, T. & Nakao, K. (1997). Nonadipose tissue production of leptin: leptin as a novel placenta-derived hormone in humans, *Nature Medicine,* Vol.3, No.9, pp. 1029-1033, ISSN 1078-8956

Meyer, C., Robson, D., Rackovsky, N., Nadkarni, V. & Gerisch, J. (1997). Role of the kidney in human leptin metabolism. *The American Journal of Physiology,* Vol.273, No.5Pt1, pp. E903-E907, ISSN 0002-9513

Mikkelsen, JD., Hauser, F., deLecea, L., Sutcliffe, JG., Kilduff, TS., Calgari, C., Pévet, P. & Simonneaux, V. (2001). Hypocretin (orexin) in the rat pineal gland: a central transmitter with effects on noradrenaline-induced release of melatonin. *European Journal of Neuroscience*, Vol.14, No.3, pp. 419-25, ISSN 0953-816X

Miller, DW., Findlay, PA., Morrison, MA., Raver, N. & Adam, CL. (2002). Seasonal and dose-dependent effects of intracerebroventricular leptin on LH secretion and appetite in sheep. *Journal of Endocrinology*, Vol.175, No.2, pp. 395-404, ISSN 0022-0795

Montague, CT., Prins, JB., Sanders, L., Digby, JE. & O'Rahilly, S. (1997). Depot- and sex-specific differences in human leptin mRNA expression: implications for the control of regional fat distribution. *Diabetes*, Vol.46, No.3, pp. 342-347, ISSN 0012-1797

Morgan, PJ. & Mercer, JG. (1994). Control of seasonality by melatonin. *The Proceedings of the Nutrition Society*, Vol.53, No.3, pp. 483-93, ISSN 0029-6651

Morgan, PJ. & Mercer, JG. (2001). The regulation of body weigh: lessons from the seasonal animals. *The Proceedings of the Nutrition Society*,Vol.60, No.1, pp. 127-134, ISSN 0029-6651

Mori, H., Hanada, R., Hanada, T., Aki, D., Mashima, R., Nishinakamura, H., Torisu, T., Chien, KR., Yasukawa, H. & Yoshimura, A. (2004). Socs3 deficiency in the brain elevates leptin sensitivity and confers resistance to diet-induced obesity. *Nature Medicine*,Vol.10, No.7, pp. 739-743, ISSN 1078-8956

Morrison, CD., Daniel, JA., Holmberg, BJ., Djiane, J., Raver, N., Gertler, A. & Keisler, DH. (2001). Central infusion of leptin into well-fed and undernourished ewe lambs: effects on feed intake and serum concentrations of growth hormone and luteinizing hormone. *Journal of Endocrinology*, Vol.168, No.2, pp. 317-324, ISSN 0022-0795

Morrison, CD., Wood, R., McFadin, EL., Whitley, NC. & Keisler, DH. (2002). Effect of intravenous infusion of recombinant ovine leptin on feed intake and serum concentrations of GH, LH, insulin, IGF-I, cortisol and thyroxine in growing prepubertal ewe lambs. *Domestic Animal Endocrinology*, Vol.22, No.2, pp. 103-112, ISSN 0739-740

Münzberg, H., Bjonholm, M., Bates, SH. & Meyers Jr, MG. (2005). Leptin receptor action and mechanism of leptin resistance. *Cellular and Molecular Life Science*, Vol.62, No.6, pp. 642-652, ISSN 1420-682X

Mustonen, AM., Nieminen, P., Hyvarinen, H. & Asikainen, J. (2000). Exogenous melatonin elevates the plasma leptin and thyroxine concentrations of the mink (*Mustela vision*). *Zeitschrift für Naturforschung. C, Journal of Biosciences*, Vol.55, No.9-10, pp. 806-813, ISSN 0939-5075

Mustonen, AM., Nieminen, P. & Hyvarinen, H. (2001). Preliminary evidence that pharmacological melatonin treatment decreases rat ghrelin levels. *Endocrine*, Vol.16, No.1, pp. 43–46, ISSN 1355-008X

Nagatani, S., Zeng, Y., Keisler, DH., Foster, DL., Jaffe & CA. (2000). Leptin regulates pulsatile luteinizing hormone and growth hormone secretion in sheep. *Endocrinology*, Vol.141, No.11, pp. 3965-3975, ISSN 0013-7227

Naka, T., Narazaki, M., Hirata, M., Matsumoto, T., Minamoto, S., Aono, A., Nishimoto, N., Kajita, T., Taga, T., Yoshizaki, K., Akira, S. & Kishimoto T. (1997). Structure and function of a new STAT-induced STAT inhibitor. *Nature*, Vol.387, No.6636, pp. 924-929, ISSN 0028-0836

Ng, TB. & Wong, CM. (1986). Effects of pineal indoles and arginine vasotocin on lipolysis and lipogenesis in isolated adipocytes. *Journal of Pineal Research*, Vol.3, No.1, pp. 55-66, ISSN 0742-3098

Niswender, KD., Morton, GJ., Stearns, WH., Rhodes, CJ., Myers, Jr. MG. & Schwartz MW. (2001). Intracellular signaling. Key enzyme in leptin-induced anorexia. *Nature*, Vol.413, No.6858, pp. 794-795, ISSN 0028-0836

Nonaka, S., Hashizume, T. & Kasuya, E. (2005). Effects of leptin on the release of luteinizing hormone, growth hormone and prolactin from cultured bovine anterior pituitary cells. *Animal Science Journal*, Vol.76, pp. 435-440, ISSN 1344-3941

Ogata, R., Matsuzaki, T., Iwasa, T., Kiyokawa, M., Tanaka, N., Kuwahara, A., Yasui, T. & Irahara, M. (2009). Hypothalamic Ghrelin suppresses pulsatile secretion of luteinizing hormone via beta-endorphin in ovariectomized rats. *Neuroendocrinology*, Vol.90, No.4, pp. 364-370, ISSN 0028-3835

Popovic, VD. & Casanueva, FF. (2002). Leptin, nutrition and reproduction: new insights. *Hormones*, Vol.1, No.4, pp. 204-217, ISSN 1109-3099

Prolo, P., Wong, M-L. & Licinio, J. (1998). Leptin. *International Journal of Biochemistry and Cell Biology*, Vol.30, No.12, pp. 1285-1290, ISSN 1357-2725

Rayner, DV., Dalgliesh, GD., Duncan, JS., Hardie, LJ., Hoggard, N. & Trayhurn, P. (1997). Postnatal development of the *ob* gene system: elevated leptin levels in suckling *fa/fa* rats. *American Journal of Physiology. Regulatory, Integrative and Comparative Physiology*, Vol.273, No.1-2, pp. R446-R450, ISSN 0363-6119

Roberts, AW., Robb, L., Rakar, S., Hartley, L., Cluse, L., Nicola, NA., Metcalf, D., Hilton, DJ. & Alexander, W.S. (2001). Placental defects and embryonic lethality in mice lacking suppressor of cytokine signaling 3. *Proceedings of the National Academy of Sciences of the United States of America*, Vol.98, No.16, pp. 9324-9329, ISSN 0027-8424

Rosenbaum, D., Nicolson, M., Hirsch, J., Heymsfield, SB., Gallagher, D., Chu, F., Leibel, RL. (1996). Effects of gender, body composition, and menopause on plasma concentrations of leptin. *Journal of Clinical Endocrinology and Metabolism*, Vol.81, No.9, pp. 3424-3427, ISSN 0021-972X

Russell, SH., Small, CJ., Kennedy, AR., Stanley, SA., Seth, A., Murphy, KG., Teheri, S., Ghatei, MA. & Bloom, SR. (2001). Orexin A interactions in the hypothalamo-pituitary gonadal axis. *Endocrinology*, Vol.142, No.12, pp. 5294–5302, ISSN 0013-7227

Sahu, A. (2003). Leptin signaling in the hypothalamus: emphasis on energy homeostasis and leptin resistance. *Frontiers in Neuroendocrinology*, Vol.24, No.4, pp. 225-253, ISSN 0091-3022

Sakurai, T., Moriguchi, T., Furuya, K., Kajiwara, N., Nakamura, T., Yanagisawa, M. & Goto, K. (1999). Structure and function of human prepro-orexin gene. *Journal of Biological Chemistry*, Vol.274, No.25, pp. 17771-17776, ISSN 0021-9258

Scaramuzzi, RJ. & Martin, GB. (2008). The importance of interactions among nutrition, seasonality and socio-sexual factors in the development of hormone-free methods for controlling fertility. *Reproduction in Domestic Animals*, Vol.43, Suppl.2, pp. 129-136, ISSN 0936-6768

Smith-Kirwin, SM., O'Conor, DM., De Johston, J., Lancey, ED., Hassink, SG. & Funanage, VL. (1998). Leptin expression in human mammary epithelial cells and breast milk. *Journal of Clinical Endocrinology and Metabolism*, Vol.83, No.5, pp. 1810-1813, ISSN 0021-972X

Sobhani, I., Vissuzaine, C., Buyse, M., Kermorgant, S., Laigneau, JP., Attoub, S., Lahy, T., Henin, D., Mignon, M. & Lewin, MJ. (2000). Leptin secretion and leptin receptor in the human stomach. *Gut*, Vol.47, No.2, pp. 178-183, ISSN 0017-5749

Sorensen, A., Adam, CL., Findlay, PA., Marie, M., Thomas, L., Travers, MT. & Vernon, RG. (2002). Leptin secretion and hypothalamic neuropeptide and receptor gene expression in sheep. *American Journal of Physiology. Regulatory, Integrative and Comparative Physiology*, Vol.282, No.4, pp. R1227-R1235, ISSN ISSN 0363-6119

Spicer, LJ. & Francisco, CC. (1997). The adipose obese gene product, leptin: evidence of a direct inhibitory role in ovarian function. *Endocrinology*, Vol.138, No.8, pp. 3374-3379, ISSN 0013-7227

Starr, R., Willson, TA., Viney, EM., Murray, LJ., Rayner, JR., Jenkins, BJ., Gonda, TJ., Alexander, WS., Metcalf, D., Nicola, NA. & Hilton, DJ. (1997). A family of cytokine-inducible inhibitors of signalling. *Nature*, Vol.387, No.6636, pp. 917-921, ISSN 0028-0836

Stone, RT., Kappes, SM. & Beattie, CW. (1996). The bovine homolog of the obese gen maps to chromosome 4. *Mammalian Genome*, Vol.7, No.5, pp. 399-400, ISSN 0938-8990

Szczesna, M., Zieba, DA., Klocek-Gorka, B., Misztal, T. & Stepien, E. (2011). Seasonal effects of central leptin infusion and prolactin treatment on pituitary SOCS-3 gene expression in ewes. *Journal of Endocrinology*, Vol.208, No.1, pp. 81-88, ISSN 0804-4643

Tamura, T., Irahara, M., Tezuka, M., Kiyokawa, M. & Aono, T. (1999). Orexins, orexigenic hypothalamic neuropeptides, suppress the pulsatile secretion of luteinizing hormone in ovariectomized female rats. *Biochemical and Biophysical Research Communications*, Vol.264, No.3, pp. 759-762, ISSN 0006-291X

Tartaglia, LA., Dembski, M., Weng, X., Den, N., Culpepper, J., Devos, R., Richards, GJ., Campfield, LA., Clark, FT., Deeds, J., Muir, C., Skaner, S., Moriarty, A., Moore, KJ., Smutko, JS., Mays, GG., Woolf, EA., Monero, CA. & Tepper, RI. (1995). Identification and expression cloning of a leptin receptor, OB-R. *Cell*, Vol.83, No.7, pp. 1263-1271, ISSN 0092-8674

Toshinai, K., Date, Y., Murakami, N., Mitsushi, S., Muhtashan, S., Shimbara, T., Guan, J-L., Wang, Q-P. Funashashi, H., Sukurai, T., Shioda, S., Matsukura, S., Kangawa, K. & Nakazato, M. (2003). Ghrelin-induced food intake is mediated via the orexin pathway. *Endocrinology*, Vol.144, No.4, pp. 1506-1512, ISSN 0013-7227

Trayhurn, P., Thomas, MEA., Duncan, JS. & Rayner, DV. (1995). Effects of fasting and refeeding on *ob* gene expression in white adipose tissue of lean and obese (*ob/ob*) mice. *FEBS Letters*, Vol.368, No.3, pp. 488-490, ISSN 0014-5793

Trayhurn, P., Hoggard, N., Mercer, JG. & Rayner, DV. (1999). Leptin: fundamental aspects. *International Journal of Obesity*, Vol.23, Suppl.1, pp. 22-28, ISSN 0307-0565

Tups, A., Ellis, C., Moar, KM., Logie, TJ., Adam, CL., Mercer, JG. & Klingenspor, M. (2004). Photoperiodic regulation of leptin sensitivity in the Siberian hamster, Phodopus sungorus, is reflected in arcuate nucleus SOCS-3 (Suppressor of Cytokine Signaling) gene expression. *Endocrinology*, Vol.145, No.3, pp. 1185-1193, ISSN 0013-7227

Uotani, S., Bjorbaek, C., Tornoe, J. & Flier, JS. (1999). Functional properties of leptin receptor isoforms: Internalization and degradation of leptin and ligand-induced receptor downregulation. *Diabetes*, Vol.48, No.2, pp. 279-286, ISSN 0012-1797

Wang, J. (1998). A Nutrient sensing pathway regulates leptin gene expression in muscle and fat. *Nature*, Vol.393, No.6686, pp. 684-688, ISSN 0028-0836

Wang, Z., Zhou, Y-T., Kakuma, T., Lee, Y., Kalra, SP., Kalra, PS., Pan, W. & Unger, RH. (2000). Leptin resistance of adipocytes in obesity: role of suppressor of cytokine signaling. *Biochemical and Biophysical Research Communications*, Vol.277, No.1, pp. 20-26, ISSN 0006-291X

Watanobe, H. (2002). Leptin directly acts within the hypothalamus to stimulate gonadotropin-releasing hormone secretion in vivo in rats. *Journal of Physiology*, Vol.545, No.Pt 1, pp. 255-268, ISSN 0022-3751

Wauters, M., Considine, RV. & van Gaal, LF. (2000). Human leptin: from an adipocyte hormone to an endocrine mediator. *European Journal of Endocrinology*, Vol.143, No.3, pp. 293-311, ISSN 0804-4643

Williams, LM., Adam, CL., Mercer, JG., Moar, KM., Slater, D., Hunter, L., Findlay, PA. & Hoggard, N. (1999). Leptin receptor and neuropeptide Y gene expression in the sheep brain. *Journal of Neuroendocrinology*, Vol.11, No.3, pp. 165-169, ISSN 0953-8194

Williams, GL., Amstalden, M., Garcia, MR., Stanko, RL., Nizielski, SE., Morrison, CD. & Keisler, DH. (2002). Leptin and its role in the central regulation of reproduction in cattle. *Domestic Animal Endocrinology*, Vol.23, No.1-2, pp. 339-349, ISSN 0739-7240

Zalatan, F., Krause, JA. & Blask, DE. (2001). Inhibition of isoproterenol-induced lipolysis in rat inguinal adipocytes *in vitro* by physiological melatonin *via* a receptor-mediated mechanism. *Endocrinology*, Vol.142, No.9, pp. 3783-3790, ISSN 0013-7227

Zamorano, PL., Mahesh, VB., De Sevilla, LM., Chorich, LP., Bhat, GK. & Brann, DW. (1997). Expression and localization of the leptin receptor in endocrine and neuroendocrine tissues of the rat. *Neuroendocrinology* , Vol.65, No.3, pp. 223-228, ISSN 0028-3835

Zhang, Y., Proenca, R., Maffei, M., Barone, M., Leopold, L. & Friedman, JM. (1994). Positional cloning of the mouse obese gene and its human homologue. *Nature*, Vol.372, No.6505, pp. 425-432, ISSN 0028-0836

Zhang, Y., Basinski, MB., Beals, JM., Briggs, SL., Churgaj, LM., Clawson, DK., DiMarchi, RD., Furman, TC., Hale, JE., Hsiung, HM., Schoner BE, Smith, DP., Zhang, XY., Wery, JP. & Schevitz, RW. (1997). Crystal structure of the obese protein leptin-E100. *Nature*, Vol.387, No.6629, pp. 206-209, ISSN 0028-0836

Zieba, DA., Amstalden, M., Maciel, MN., Keisler, DH., Raver, N., Gertler, A. & Williams, GL. (2003). Divergent effects of leptin on luteinizing hormone and insulin secretion are dose dependent. *Experimental Biology and Medicine*, Vol.228, No.3, pp. 325-330, ISSN 1535-3702

Zieba, DA., Amstalden, M. & Williams, GL. (2005). Regulatory roles of leptin in reproduction and metabolism: a comparative review. *Domestic Animal Endocrinology*, Vol.29, No.1, pp. 166-185, ISSN 0739-7240

Zieba, DA., Klocek, B., Williams, GL., Romanowicz, K., Boliglowa, L. & Wozniak, M. (2007). *In vitro* evidence that leptin supresses melatonin secretion during long days and stimulates its secretion during short days in seasonal breeding ewes. *Domestic Animal Endocrinology*, Vol.33, No.3, pp. 358-365, ISSN 0739-7240

Zieba, DA., Szczesna, M., Klocek-Gorka, B., Molik, E., Misztal, T., Williams, GL., Romanowicz, K., Stepien, E., Keisler, DH. & Murawski, M. (2008). Seasonal effects of central leptin infusion on secretion of melatonin and prolactin and on SOCS-3 gene expression in ewes. *Journal of Endocrinology*, Vol.198, No.1, pp. 147-155, ISSN 0804-4643

Zieba, DA., Kirsz, K., Molik, E., Romanowicz, K. & Wojtowicz, AK. (2011). Effects of orexigenic peptides and leptin on melatonin secretion during different photoperiods in seasonal breeding ewes. An in vitro study. *Domestic Animal Endocrinology*, Vol.40, No.3, pp. 139-146, ISSN 0739-7240

14

Attenuin: What It Is, How It Works and What It Does

Ana Gordon, José C. Garrido-Gracia, Rafaela Aguilar, Carmina Bellido, Juana Martín de las Mulas and José E. Sánchez-Criado
University of Córdoba
Spain

1. Introduction

The reproductive function in female mammals, unlike that of males, is cyclical in nature. Whilst testosterone exerts a wholly negative control, regulation of the ovarian cycle is effected through a complex series of positive and negative feedback mechanisms involving the ovary, the pituitary and the hypothalamus. Although the role of these feedback mechanisms has been known for many years, our knowledge of the detailed workings involved continues to expand. Reproductive-axis hormones have proved to be similar in all the mammalian species studied to date. The female cycle can generally be divided into the follicular, periovulatory (preovulatory and ovulatory) and luteal phases. The pituitary hormones - the gonadotropins luteinizing hormone (LH) and follicle-stimulating hormone (FSH) - remain at basal levels throughout most of the reproductive cycle, due to negative regulation by ovarian hormones (mainly estradiol and progesterone; see fig. 1 for additional details). The physiological capacity of steroids to control gonadotropin secretion is evident in a marked increase in plasma LH and FSH levels after the menopause or following ovariectomy. During the preovulatory phase, the estradiol negative feedback switches to positive. Major positive actions by estrogens include: a 20- to 50-fold increase in pituitary sensitivity to gonadotropin-releasing hormone (GnRH) (Speight et al., 1981); an increase in pituitary GnRH receptors, in concert with GnRH (Clayton et al., 1980); an increase in progesterone receptors (PR) in both pituitary and hypothalamus (Conneely et al., 1989); stimulation of GnRH synthesis and release, resulting in preovulatory GnRH secretion (Sarkar et al., 1976); and a drop in GnRH metabolism by pituitary cells (Danforth et al., 1990). These positive actions of estradiol lead to the appearance of GnRH self-priming. GnRH self-priming is an event with a twofold effect: it prompts an exponential increase in pituitary responsiveness to GnRH, and it coordinates increased responsiveness with enhanced GnRH release, ensuring that both occur at the same time and thus guaranteeing preovulatory LH secretion (Fink, 1995). In rats, this self-priming effect has been found to be more effective when GnRH pulses occur at hourly intervals (Fink, 1995), a frequency also reported to be optimal in monkeys with hypothalamic lesions (Knobil, 1980) and in women with idiopathic hypogonadotropic hypogonadism (Crowley et al., 1985). How does GnRH come to possess this unique property? Probably because the preovulatory LH surge is indispensable for species reproduction, and the fact that a very small amount of GnRH induces a disproportionate release of LH makes the process both economic and efficient

(Fink, 1995). In conclusion, although the cyclical nature of reproduction has been recognized in both humans and animals for centuries, the sequence of events involved has only recently become clear, and a number of questions remain unanswered (Schwartz, 2000).

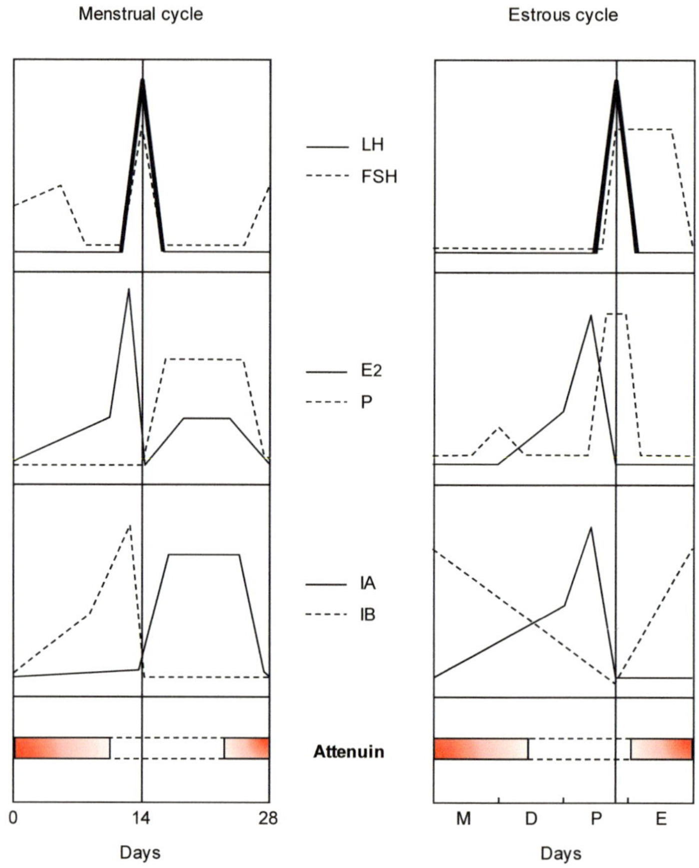

Fig. 1. **Diagram showing pituitary and ovarian hormone fluctuation during menstrual (woman) and estrous (rat) cycles.** LH: luteinizing hormone; FSH: follicle-stimulating hormone; E2: estradiol; P: progesterone; IA: inhibin A; IB: inhibin B; M: metestrus; D: diestrus; P: proestrus; E: estrus. Days of cycle are synchronized with the LH surge (day 14 in women and proestrous afternoon in rats). During the menstrual cycle, and shortly after functional luteolysis (drop in E2, P and IA) the secretion of FSH increased, stimulating the ovaries and inducing follicular recruitment. In the rat, secondary FSH secretion during early estrus stimulated the ovaries, similarly inducing follicular recruitment. In both cases, increased FSH secretion augmented attenuin bioactivity by stimulating the ovaries (lower panels). Attenuin bioactivity prevented premature occurrence of the LH surge (see text for additional details).

One crucial and still-unresolved question is how the negative feedback exerted by estradiol suddenly switches to positive, resulting in the preovulatory LH surge. Though this issue has been argued back and forth, no agreement has yet been reached. The positive effects of estradiol do not all occur at the same time, nor are they present only during preovulatory secretion. For example, the increased steroid-induced pituitary response to GnRH is directly linked to steroid levels during the follicular phase (Yen et al., 1972). Moreover, GnRH self-priming can be observed experimentally long before the LH surge is due (Waring & Turgeon, 1980). All this would suggest that steroids have to reach a critical threshold before generating any LH surge (de Koning, 1995), or alternatively that some factor is exerting a "braking" effect on the estradiol positive feedback (Whitehead, 1990). Studies of *in vitro* fertilization (IVF) methods argue against the idea of a critical level of estradiol (200 pg/ml during 36-48 h): reports indicate that in FSH-treated women with multiple follicles able to produce supraphysiological levels of estradiol from the beginning of the follicular phase, preovulatory LH secretion does not occur prematurely, and when it does appear it is diminished (Ferraretti et al., 1983; Glasier et al., 1988; Messinis et al., 1986). High levels of steroids are unlikely to inhibit the preovulatory LH surge, and high exogenous doses of estradiol are unable to suppress LH secretion in normal menstrual cycles (Messinis & Templeton, 1987). There is thus no evidence to support the hypothesis that abnormal estradiol levels inhibit preovulatory LH secretion in stimulated cycles; indeed, the evidence so far points to the existence of some non-steroidal factor, produced by stimulated ovaries and able to suppress steroidal positive feedback. Over recent decades, the search for putative new substances secreted by the ovaries has provided new insights into the role of the ovaries in gonadotropin secretion. This chapter focuses on the factor known as attenuin (Messinis & Templeton, 1989; Sopelak & Hodgen, 1984).

1.1 Evidence for the existence of attenuin

The development of IVF methods for addressing infertility in the 1970s and 1980s also shed new light on the role of FSH. In addition to its classic functions (stimulation of aromatase activity and estradiol secretion in granulosa cells, and participation in follicular selection mechanisms), FSH was found to stimulate the production of an ovarian factor with a special ability to reduce preovulatory LH secretion in women. The first evidence for an ovarian factor that attenuated GnRH-induced LH secretion appeared in the late 70s, when de Jong et al. (1979), using bovine follicular fluid (bFF), observed a drop in the responsiveness of rat pituitary cells to GnRH. Over the following decade, a number of studies pointed to the existence of a non-steroidal ovarian factor that reduced preovulatory LH release when FSH was administered during the follicular phase in women (Ferraretti et al., 1983; Messinis & Templeton, 1986), monkeys (Littman & Hodgen, 1984; Schenken et al., 1984) and rats (Busbridge et al., 1988; Geiger et al., 1980). This factor was called gonadotropin surge-attenuating factor (GnSAF), gonadotropin surge-inhibiting factor (GnSIF) or simply attenuin. In 1984, Schenken et al. demonstrated for the first time a direct effect of FSH on gonadotropin secretion, involving one or more ovarian factor(s). Ovarian venous serum (OVS) was collected from FSH-treated monkeys before and after aspiration of the right ovarian follicle; the left ovarian follicle remained intact. Serum from right ovaries before aspirated and from intact left ovaries inhibited GnRH responsiveness in rat pituitary cultures, suggesting that exogenous FSH increased OVS concentrations of a non-steroidal ovarian factor with gonadotropin-inhibiting activity. The ovarian origin of attenuin was confirmed when Fowler et al. (2002), culturing theca, stroma and granulosa cells from cyclic women, showed that attenuin bioactivity was present only in granulosa-cell-conditioned medium. Use of a superovulated protocol as a model for increased attenuin bioactivity posed a number of problems, including elevated peripheral estradiol and inhibin levels during gonadotropin administration (de Jong, 1988; Messinis & Templeton, 1988;

Muttukrishna et al., 1994), which raised doubts as to the origin of this bioactivity. With regard to estradiol, studies carried out in women have proved that effects on LH secretion are not due to negative feedback: Messinis et al. (1991, 1993) demonstrated that a single FSH injection had dose-dependent suppressive effects on pituitary responsiveness to exogenous GnRH pulses. This effect was seen as early as 8 h after FSH administration, although circulating estradiol did not increase significantly until at least 24 h after gonadotropin administration. Subsequently, this group also concluded that attenuin bioactivity in FSH-treated women could not be due to an increase in circulating total α-inhibin (Messinis et al., 1991, 1993, 1994, 1996).

Attenuin bioactivity has so far been found in serum, FF and ovarian extracts from superovulated (Fowler et al., 1994a) and cyclic women (Fowler et al., 1995a), in bFF (Van Dieten et al., 1999), in porcine FF (pFF; Danforth et al., 1987; Kita et al., 1994), in rat ovarian extracts (de Koning et al., 1989) and in rat testicular extracts (Tio et al., 1994). It should be stressed that attenuin bioactivity has been observed in human FF (hFF) from women during an untreated spontaneous cycle, suggesting that it plays a physiological role as a central regulator (Busbridge et al., 1990; Byrne et al., 1993).

1.2 Current status of attenuin characterization

In 1987 Danforth et al., using pFF, showed that attenuin bioactivity displayed certain characteristics: it was resistant to moderate heating (60 °C for 60 min), fully recoverable from an acetone precipitation, and not bound by a heparin/sepharose affinity matrix of the sort widely used to isolate inhibin. To date, attempts to characterize attenuin have proved relatively unsuccessful. Purification strategies have obtained very small amounts of bioactive material and an abundance of different proteins. The fact that the protein is present at very low concentrations makes it difficult to use Edman sequencing, leading to a whole range of different results. Tio et al. (1994) isolated inhibin and attenuin by high performance liquid chromatography from 32 liters of rat Sertoli cell-conditioned medium. Both peptides were separated on polyacrylamide gel; however the partial N-terminal sequence of the 37 kDa protein with attenuin bioactivity did not match gene and protein databases (Genbank and PIR). Subsequently, employing an elegant sequential series of purification techniques, Danforth & Cheng (1995) found a 69 kDa monomeric polypeptide in pFF that inhibited GnRH-stimulated LH secretion, but partial N-terminal analysis showed no homology with other reproductive hormones. Mroueh et al. (1996) also found a protein with attenuin bioactivity in hFF, similar to that reported in pFF (63 kDa). However, Pappa et al. (1999), starting from the same source (hFF) treated with multiple and complex purification techniques, described a protein with a molecular mass of 12.5 kDa. This protein was identified by mass spectrometry as a truncated part of the C-terminus of human serum albumin (HSA). The next published purification procedure side-stepped serum albumin contamination problems by using a serum- and BSA-free granulosa-luteal cell culture system (Fowler et al., 2002). The isolated attenuin-bioactivity protein had a molecular weight of 60-70 kDa and an isoelectric point (pI) of 5.7-5.8 pH. The internal and N-terminal amino acid sequences did not display significant homology with other accessions in the protein-sequence database. Attenuin is therefore thought to be a peptide, different from inhibin, with a postulated molecular weight which varies from less than 37 kDa (Tio et al., 1994) to 64-69 kDa (Danforth & Cheng, 1995; Fowler et al., 2002). These differences may reflect the presence either of small active subunits or of larger aggregates with or without carrier proteins, and may also reflect species differences. Ingeniously, using the expression-secretion system of a yeast (*Pichia Pastoris* GS115), it has proved feasible to produce recombinant polypeptides of HSA. Various polypeptides thus obtained were added to rat pituitary cultures and only those corresponding to subdomain IIIB (specifically residues 490-585) presented attenuin bioactivity, while the whole molecule and even the whole subdomain IIIB were inactive (Tavoulari et al., 2004). More recently, Karligiotou et al. (2006) used the retrotranscriptase-polymerase chain reaction (RT-PCR) technique and appropriate primers to amplify different transcripts from HSA gene in granulosa cells. Results showed that while all HSA fragments were expressed in the nucleus, only two fragments (the promoter and a C-terminal fragment) were expressed in granulosa cell cytoplasm, indicating a differential expression of the HSA gene, probably leading to attenuin synthesis. Finally, the current attenuin purification strategy involves the use of phage display techniques to produce antibodies against partially-purified human-granulosa-luteal cell-conditioned medium. Three of these antibodies were found to block human attenuin bioactivity on GnRH-induced LH secretion from rat pituitary cell cultures. Subsequently, these antibodies were used to immunopurify attenuin; the antigen-antibody complexes obtained were separated by electrophoresis. Candidate attenuin spots (around 66 kDa and pI 5.5-6.0) were excised for peptide mass mapping. The main molecules identified were HSA precursor and variants. All these data suggest that attenuin may be a post-translationally modified form of serum albumin, or else may be very tightly bound to, and transported by, serum albumin (Sorsa-Leslie et al., 2005).

1.3 Synthesis and secretion pattern of attenuin

In women, the production of attenuin in the ovarian follicle is clearly related to follicular size in both spontaneous and stimulated cycles. FF from follicles smaller than 11 mm (stimulated cycles, Fowler et al., 1994b) or 6-8 mm (spontaneous cycles, Fowler et al., 2001) has been found to contain the greatest amount of attenuin. In women receiving fertility treatment, there is an increase both in the number of follicles and in serum attenuin bioactivity with respect to spontaneous cycles (Byrne et al., 1993). Similarly, small follicles in pig ovaries contain the highest attenuin concentrations, while bioactivity falls sharply in preovulatory follicles (Kita et al., 1994). Thus, medium from granulosa cell cultures showed more attenuin bioactivity when these cells were obtained from aspiration of small follicles (Seo & Danforth, 1994). All these findings suggest that small and growing follicles are the major producers of attenuin. In summary, attenuin levels are highest during the early part of the menstrual cycle (days 1 to 8), falling thereafter as follicular size increases, and disappearing at the appropriate preovulatory time (Fowler et al., 2003). The corpus luteum does not appear to produce attenuin in women, but small developing follicles may produce attenuin during the luteal phase (Messinis et al., 1996; fig. 1 lower panel).

2. Methods of study

2.1 In vivo

In the absence of purified bioactive molecule, for the reasons indicated above, the effect of attenuin on the LH surge in rats is currently studied using both *in vivo* and *in vitro* procedures. The *in vivo* approach consists in administration of exogenous FSH during the diestrous phase in cycling rats as a tool to increase the biological activity of endogenous attenuin (Geiger et al., 1980; Gordon et al., 2008). In addition to attenuin, FSH also stimulates the synthesis and secretion by granulosa cells of a number of steroidal and non-steroidal factors (mainly estradiol and inhibin) that affect pituitary gonadotropin secretion (Arai et al., 1996; Watanabe et al., 1990). However, this treatment attenuates the magnitude of the proestrous afternoon LH surge despite the presence of high circulating levels of estradiol (Geiger et al., 1980; Gordon et al., 2008, de Koning et al., 1987; see fig. 2A for additional details).

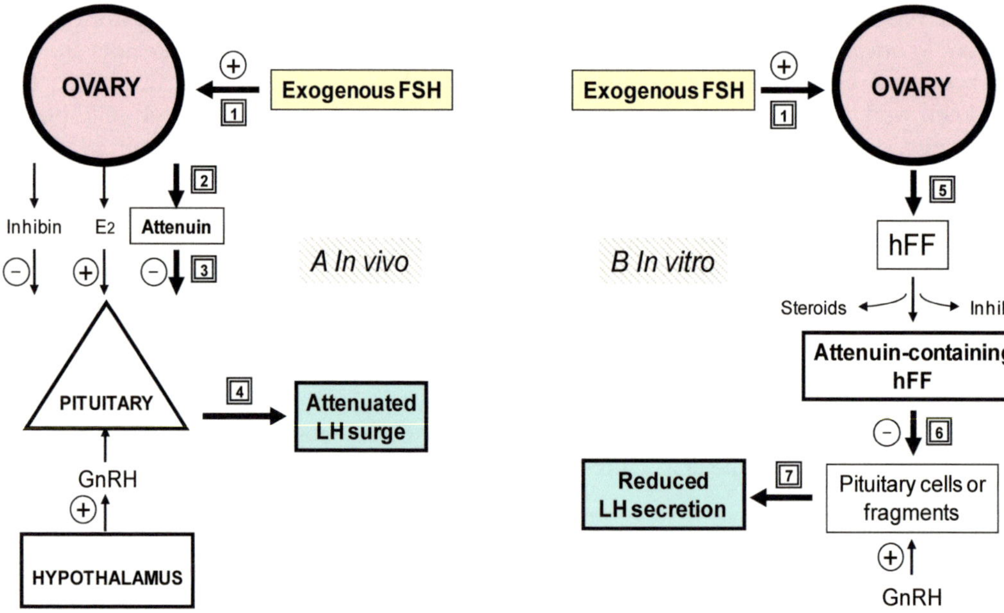

Fig. 2. **Schematic representation of current approaches to the study of attenuin effects on luteinizing hormone (LH) secretion.** GnRH: gonadotropin releasing hormone; E2: 17β-estradiol; FSH: follicle-stimulating hormone; hFF: human follicular fluid. A: *in vivo.* [1] Administration of FSH stimulates the synthesis/secretion of ovarian hormones (E2, inhibin and attenuin) [2]. Whereas in proestrus inhibin suppresses FSH secretion (Gordon et al., 2010a, 2010c) and E2 acts on LH secretion in its positive feedback mode [2], attenuin acting on gonadotrope membrane receptor [3] results in a reduction of the magnitude of the LH surge [4]. B: *in vitro.* Administration of FSH stimulates follicular growth and recruitment [1]. Pooled hFF from women undergoing IVF treatments [5] is submitted to steroid charcoal-extraction and inhibin immunoprecipitation (Gordon et al., 2010c). Attenuin-containing hFF is then added to cultured pituitary cells or fragments [6]. This results in a reduction of GnRH-stimulated LH secretion [7].

At the same time, the bioactivity of attenuin can be promoted and/or prolonged by removing endogenous inhibin and consequently increasing endogenous FSH. One option is the neutralization of inhibin's biological activity by injection of an anti-inhibin serum on metestrus that increases FSH serum levels during diestrus and proestrus, induces superovulation and again reduces the magnitude of the proestrous afternoon LH surge (Ishigame et al., 2004).

2.2 In vitro

However, it is difficult to delineate, *in vivo,* the precise bioactivity of attenuin in the rat pituitary using exogenous FSH. Alternatively, attenuin bioactivity can be studied by *in vitro* procedures, using cultured anterior pituitary cells or pituitary fragments treated with murine FF (Busbridge et al., 1990; Fowler & Spears, 2004), pFF (Danforth & Cheng, 1995) or hFF from women undergoing IVF treatments (Byrne et al., 1995a, 1996; Fowler & Templeton 1996) as a source of exogenous attenuin, following steroid and inhibin depletion (see fig. 2B for additional details).

3. Mechanism of attenuin action

3.1 Background

Despite considerable research and the availability of improved molecular techniques, little is known about how attenuin acts. This section outlines the key findings reported to date. *In vitro* experiments have highlighted the potentiating effects of increased intracellular calcium, stimulation of both intracellular GnRH signalling pathways (calcium- and cAMP-dependent protein kinases, PKC and PKA respectively), as well as progesterone treatment on GnRH-induced LH secretion (Kile & Nett, 1994; Sánchez-Criado et al., 2006). A further clue regarding the mechanism by which attenuin acts was discovered when, in rat pituitary monolayers, GnRH was co-incubated with either estradiol, progesterone, PMA (phorbol 12-myristate 13-acetate, a stimulator of PKC) or calcium ionophore. All treatments potentiated the effects of GnRH on LH synthesis and release, but administration of hFF counteracted the enhancing effects of all these compounds, with one exception: the augmentative effect of progesterone on GnRH-induced LH synthesis (Cowking et al., 1995). Shortly afterwards, the authors found that while progesterone augmented GnRH self-priming in rat pituitary monolayers, this secretion was blocked when hFF and the antiprogestagen RU486 were added to the medium (Byrne et al., 1995b). All these findings suggest that the mechanism of action of attenuin on preovulatory LH secretion might involve the pituitary PR. There is considerable evidence, both *in vivo* and *in vitro,* to suggest that attenuin has a suppressant effect on GnRH self-priming (Byrne et al., 1996; Koppenaal et al., 1992, 1993). This action has been shown to be linked to a blockade of GnRH second messenger pathways rather than to competition between attenuin and GnRH for GnRH receptors (Fowler et al., 1994c; Tijssen et al., 1997). A study by Helder et al. (1997) reported that the unknown attenuin receptor located in the gonadotrope membrane might act through the cAMP pathway. It might thus be hypothesized that the inhibiting effect of attenuin on LH secretion is exerted through this GnRH second pathway. Both hypotheses, i.e. attenuin acting through a GnRH second pathway or through the PR, are feasible, since it has been shown that GnRH can activate the PR in a ligand-independent manner through the PKA and/or PKC pathways (Garrido-Gracia et al., 2006; Turgeon & Waring, 1994).

3.2 The relationship between attenuin and LH release

A number of published studies report a reduction of the preovulatory LH surge *in vivo* in rats treated with FSH during metestrus and diestrus (Culler, 1992; Geiger et al., 1980; Gordon et al., 2008; de Koning et al., 1987; Shuiling et al., 1999). Additionally, this FSH treatment *in vivo* causes an *in vitro* suppression of GnRH-stimulated LH secretion, GnRH self-priming and progesterone-potentiating effect on GnRH-stimulated LH secretion, without affecting basal LH levels (Byrne et al., 1996; Gordon et al., 2008; Koppenaal et al., 1992, 1993). *Pace* Geiger et al. (1980), the possibility that these effects are produced by an increase in estradiol levels can be ruled out, since animals treated with estradiol benzoate display greater LH secretion both *in vivo* and *in vitro;* more important, FSH plus estradiol-injected ovariectomized rats do not display any suppressant effect on LH secretion (Gordon et al., 2008). All this proves conclusively that FSH treatment stimulates the production of some ovarian factor(s) other than estradiol, that reduces the preovulatory LH surge but not basal LH secretion. Subsequent *in vitro* research has shown that attenuin produces this inhibiting effect on pituitary sensitivity to GnRH in a dose-dependent manner: administration of different doses of FSH (0.1, 1 and 10 I.U.) caused variable inhibition of LH secretion, partially reversed by simultaneous administration of estradiol (Gordon et al., 2009a). Attenuin would thus appear to bind to its gonadotrope membrane receptor and activate a secondary pathway in order to inhibit preovulatory LH secretion (Fowler & Templeton, 1996). The potentiating effects of progesterone, 8-bromo cAMP and PMA on GnRH-stimulated LH secretion are antagonized in rat hemipituitaries incubated with steroid-free bFF (bFF) or with FF from women undergoing a superovulation protocol (Cowking et al., 1995; Tijssen et al., 1997). All this suggests that attenuin may exert a suppressant effect on the GnRH secondary pathway. Subsequent research has shown that neither progesterone, nor GnRH, nor activation of PKA and PKC has any effect on GnRH-stimulated LH secretion in FSH-treated cyclic rats (Gordon et al., 2008; 2009b), indicating that this effect is probably produced downstream of PKA, PKC and progesterone. Given these findings, and the fact that attenuin decreases all PR-dependent parameters of LH secretion, it may be postulated that this action is exerted through a modification of PR expression and/or action (Garrido-Gracia et al., 2007).

3.3 The relationship between attenuin, PR and LH release

With regard to the effect of FSH-treatment on PR gene expression in rats, RT-PCR analysis has revealed a partial decrease in PR mRNA (Gordon et al., 2008). Nevertheless, immunohistochemical examination revealed no difference in the number of PR-positive pituitary cells in FSH injected rats (Gordon et al., 2008, 2009b) or rats in which inhibin was immunoneutralized; the latter group, however, did not display a similar partial decrease in PR mRNA (Gordon et al., 2010a). These differences may be due to different FSH and/or attenuin levels between experimental groups. In most species and tissues, PR is expressed by a single gene but transcribed into separate mRNAs as two distinct molecular forms, PR-A and PR-B. The B (stimulatory) form contains an additional N-terminal sequence and is the main transcription factor, while the A form is modulatory of B in nature (Vegeto et al., 1993; Wen et al., 1994). For this reason, the present authors decided to analyze two inhibiting possibilities: an increase in PR-A and a decrease in PR-B protein levels. While passive immunization against inhibin with an anti-inhibin serum attenuated preovulatory LH secretion in cyclic rats, pituitary protein levels of both PR isoforms were unaffected by the absence of inhibin. This was the first time the two PR isoform protein levels had been demonstrated using the western blot technique in rat pituitaries (Gordon et al., 2010a). Although attenuin could exert its negative action on LH secretion by several mechanisms, the results pointed to a possible involvement of attenuin in post-translational modifications of PR, leading to its inactivation. Phosphorylation at serine residues is the most frequent post-translational processing event in PR modification (Beck et al., 1992; Takimoto & Horwitz, 1993) and is involved in PR-regulated gene transcription (Denner et al., 1990; Faus & Haendler, 2006). To explore this question, two studies were carried out: the first sought to measure PR phosphorylation levels, while the second aimed to determine the effect of phosphatases on pituitary sensitivity to GnRH.

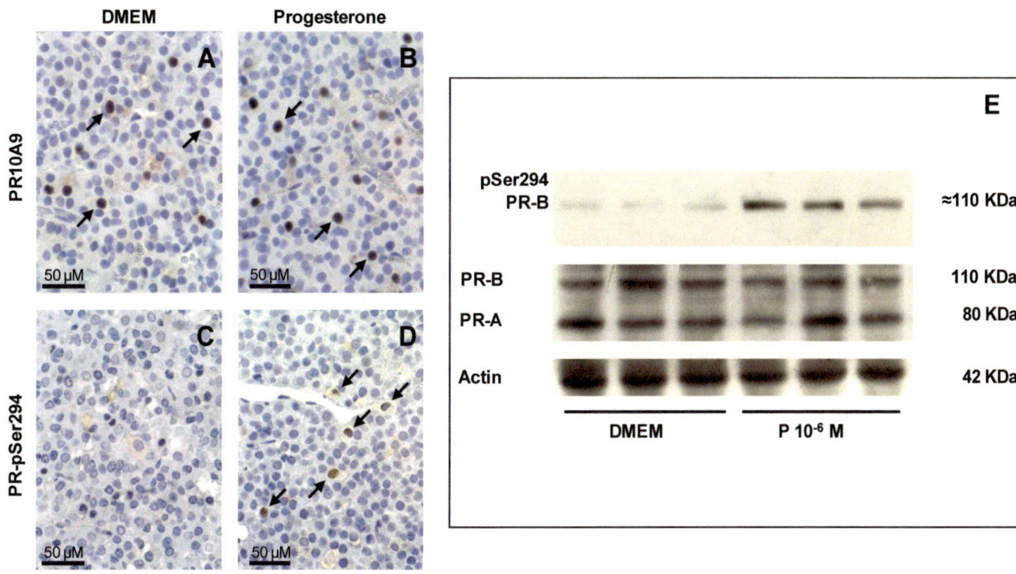

Fig. 3. **Methods of studying progesterone receptor (PR) phosphorylation in rat gonadotropes.** Left panel: Immunoreactive products to PR10A9 antibody in the nulei of gonadotropes, the only rat pituitary cell expressing PR (Garrido-Gracia et al., 2008). Pituitaries were incubated with medium alone (A, DMEM) or progesterone (B). No differences were found between the number of PR positive gonadotropes. Immunohistochemical expression of phosphorylated PR gonadotropes (C, D) in anterior pituitaries from proestrous rats (Gordon et al., 2009b). Immunoreactive products to pSer294 antibody are observed only in gonadotropes of pituitaries incubated with progesterone (D). The relative expression of pSer294-positive gonadotropes and PR109A9-positive gonadotropes provides an approximation of the PR phosphorylation rate. Right panel: PR A and B isoforms and phosphorylated PR-B content in pituitaries from proestrous rats incubated either with medium alone (DMEM) or with progesterone (P 10^{-6} M). Only PR-B phosphorylated product is seen in pituitaries incubated with progesterone (Gordon et al., 2011).

In the first study, the PR phosphorylation protocol in pituitaries was optimized by adding progesterone to the incubation medium. Subsequently, pituitaries from rats treated with FSH or with anti-inhibin serum were immunostained with an antibody that recognizes the immunogen corresponding to amino acid residues 288–300 from human PR-B, Ser294 being phosphorylated (Clemm et al. 2000). All the experimental groups in which attenuin was increased and preovulatory secretion diminished showed a significant drop in the number of cells expressing pSer294 (Gordon et al., 2009b, 2010a; fig. 3, left panel).

The following study analyzed the *in vitro* effect of calyculin, a potent inhibitor of intracellular phosphatases (Condrescu et al. 1999), on GnRH-stimulated LH secretion and GnRH self-priming in FSH-treated rats. The results showed that this drug was able, albeit partially, to reverse GnRH-stimulated LH secretion in a dose-dependent manner (Gordon et al., 2009b). Altogether, these results suggest that the ovarian-dependent inhibitory effect of FSH injection on the preovulatory LH secretion in the rat may involve an imbalance between the activities of protein kinases and phosphatases, resulting in a dephosphorylation of pituitary PR (see fig. 4 for additional details). In the light of previous immunohistochemical data (Gordon et al., 2009b, 2010a; fig. 3, left panel), the preliminary results obtained using the western blot technique (Gordon et al., 2011; fig. 3 right panel) supported the hypothesis that attenuin produces an inhibiting effect on LH secretion by dephosphorylation of pituitary PR.

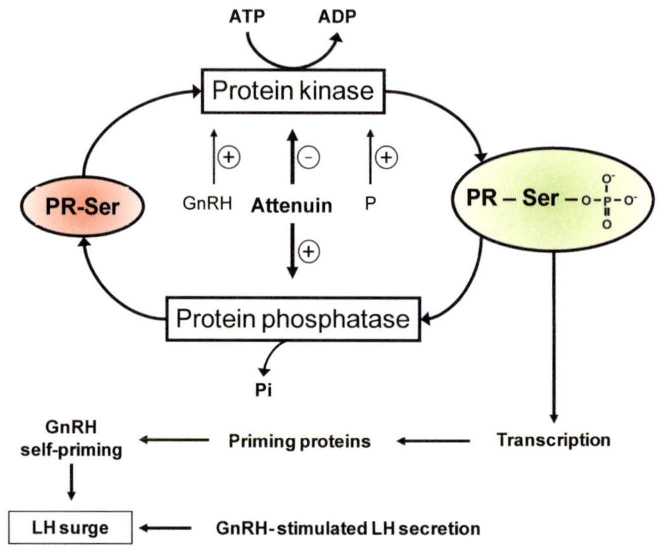

Fig. 4. **Proposed effects of attenuin on the LH surge**. GnRH: gonadotropin releasing hormone; PR-Ser: gonadotrope unphosphorylated progesterone receptor (PR); PR-Ser-PO_4^{2-}: gonadotrope phosphorylated PR. PR can be activated/phosphorylated in a ligand-dependent (progesterone) or independent (GnRH second pathways) manner. Attenuin reduces phosphorylation of Ser (serine) of the immunogen MAPGRS(p)PLATTV located in the N-terminal domain of PR-B. Activated PR-B transcribes "priming proteins" resulting in GnRH self-priming. This unique property of gonadotropes, together with estradiol sensitization of gonadotropes to GnRH, results first in GnRH-stimulated LH secretion and finally in the LH surge.

3.4 The relationship between attenuin and LH synthesis

The preovulatory secretion of LH is the result not only of increased LH synthesis (Tse et al., 1993) but also of increased LH secretion by gonadotropes (Ramey et al., 1987). While the effects of attenuin on LH secretion have been exhaustively studied, it is not known whether attenuin has any effect on LH synthesis. Fowler et al. (1995b), using rat pituitary cultures, studied the effects of steroid-free and inhibin-depleted hFF on GnRH- augmented LH synthesis and secretion in rat pituitary cultures. Results showed a decrease in both parameters, suggesting that this factor reduces pituitary responsiveness to GnRH by suppressing both the *de novo* synthesis and the acute and long term release of LH. However, there is no evidence to show how attenuin might effect this suppression. The present authors found that the addition of ionomycin (a calcium ionophore) to the incubation medium did not result, as expected, in a massive release of LH in pituitaries from FSH-treated rats. Moreover, no differences were found in LH secretion between calyculin plus GnRH and ionomycin, indicating a possible failure in LH synthesis (Gordon et al., 2009b). LH pituitary content and LHβ mRNA expression were therefore evaluated; results showed that FSH treatment decreased pituitary LH content in intact, but not in ovariectomized, rats injected with estradiol benzoate, without affecting LHβ mRNA levels. Altogether, these results suggest lower LH synthesis caused by attenuin, potentiating its inhibiting effects on LH secretion (Gordon et al., 2009a).

3.5 The relationship between attenuin, PR and LH synthesis

To determine whether pituitary PR was involved in LH synthesis inhibition by attenuin, cyclic rats were injected with different doses of FSH and progesterone. Results showed that while progesterone by itself had no effect (control groups), saturation of PR with the cognate ligand reversed the inhibitory effect of attenuin on LH protein levels, although not on LH secretion (Gordon et al., 2010b). Apart from these results showing that attenuin probably inhibits LH synthesis at post-transcriptional level, little is known about the mechanism involved in that inhibition - probably by increasing LH degradation (Kitahara et al., 1990) and/or decreasing GnRH-induced LH polypeptide glycosylation (Ramey et al., 1987) - except that, as indicated earlier, the inhibitory pathway in LH synthesis involves the gonadotrope PR. However, the detailed mechanism underlying the PR-mediated attenuin-induced inhibition of LH protein levels requires further detailed investigation. Even so, the available evidence supports the view of PR as a keystone in the neuroendocrine integrator at both hypothalamic and pituitary levels (Levine et al., 2001). In conclusion, it is postulated that, just as inhibin controls FSH synthesis and release (Attardi et al., 1991; Scott & Burger 1981), attenuin reduces proestrous GnRH-dependent LH secretion through a dual mechanism of action: inhibition of both LH synthesis and LH release.

4. The possible physiological role of attenuin

4.1 Humans

Menstrual cyclicity in women is highly dependent on positive and negative ovarian feedback mechanisms. During the follicular phase of the cycle, estradiol plays a key role in the control of both gonadotropins. Together with this steroid, low concentrations of circulating progesterone and inhibin B also contribute to the control of LH and FSH secretion, respectively. During the luteal phase, both estradiol and progesterone regulate secretion of the two gonadotropins, while inhibin A plays a role in FSH secretion. The transition from follicular to luteal phase involves a preovulatory secretion of both LH and FSH, helped by the estradiol positive mode (fig. 1, left panel). However, the change from negative to positive estradiol feedback at some threshold cannot entirely account for the change from pituitary insensitivity to the maelstrom of events leading to the LH surge. Although the question remains unresolved, there is evidence that estradiol and attenuin interact on the pituitary in the context of the positive feedback mechanism. It may be assumed that estradiol sensitizes the pituitary to GnRH, while attenuin antagonizes that sensitizing effect. Based on existing knowledge regarding attenuin action and its secretion pattern, it has been suggested that attenuin activity is greater during the early and midfollicular phases and lower both in the late follicular phase and at midcycle. Therefore, the pituitary LH response to GnRH is low during the early and midfollicular phase and is markedly enhanced during the late follicular phase, triggering the full expression of the preovulatory LH surge. According to this hypothesis, the role of attenuin in humans is to control the amplitude and not the onset of the LH surge (Messinis et al., 2006). It should be highlighted the possible role of attenuin in the polycystic ovary syndrome (PCOS). In PCOS, the mechanism responsible for abnormal gonadotropin secretion (elevated serum LH) has not been completely elucidated. One possible etiopathology mechanism is an increased of pituitary responsiveness to GnRH, caused by a decreased in attenuin production (Ruiz et al., 1996). This would offer an explanation for the most common endocrine disease that affects ovulation and fertility. At the same time, and once attenuin had been isolated, this peptide could be used as a GnRH antagonist and as a physiological contraceptive agent.

4.2 Rats

Administration of FSH during the diestrous phase prompts a reduction in proestrous LH secretion in the rat. It is worth noting that the effects of attenuin on proestrus can only be observed with this treatment (Culler, 1992; Geiger et al., 1980; Koppenaal et al., 1991). However, it is difficult to determine with any precision the role of attenuin in physiological conditions using this experimental model. Previous findings by the present authors (Gordon et al., 2010c) give grounds for speculation regarding the possible physiological role of attenuin. The incubation protocol for pituitary glands from intact cycling rats on each of the 4 days of the estrous cycle demonstrated the existence of GnRH self-priming in diestrous and proestrous phases. Subsequently, steroid-free inhibin-depeleted hFF was added to the medium. Results reported by Fowler et al. (Fowler et al., 1994b, 2001, 2003) suggest a reduction in attenuin synthesis and/or secretion when the ovarian follicle is close to preovulatory size. For this reason, we used hFF from follicles of two sizes: small (<15 mm in diameter) and large (>15 mm in diameter). Surprisingly, results in terms of secretion levels showed that only diestrous GnRH self-priming, but not proestrous self-priming as expected from the effects of injected FSH, was susceptible to the inhibiting action of attenuin contained in hFF. It should be noted that hFF from both large and small follicles had the same effects on all the LH and FSH secretion parameters so far studied. Nevertheless, the possibility that a different inhibitory bioactivity of hFF may be found using hFF from smaller follicles cannot be ruled out (Fowler et al., 2003; Fowler & Spears, 2004). Overall, these facts were interpreted as signifying that, during the normal estrous cycle, ovarian attenuin inhibited pituitary PR-dependent GnRH self-priming in diestrus only. Later on, in proestrus, pituitaries become either desensitized to the inhibitory bioactivity of attenuin and/or sensitized to the stimulatory activity of GnRH (fig. 1, right panel). By contrast, Tijssen et al. (1997) showed that attenuin was able to suppress both diestrous and proestrous GnRH self-priming. These discrepancies may be due to the different origins of FF (human vs. bovine), to the experimental model used (static vs. dynamic incubation) and to the absence or presence of inhibin. Previous results published by this research group (Tébar et al., 1996, 1998) support the hypothesis that the pituitary loses sensitivity to attenuin when follicles reach the preovulatory size, which would account for estradiol suddenly exerting a positive feedback. This intriguing mechanism, by which pituitaries become insensitive to attenuin and/or sensitive to the stimulatory action of GnRH, may provide an extra clue for understanding estrous cycle length regulation. This factor would limit the physiological timing (proestrous afternoon) as well as the magnitude (preovulatory secretion) of pituitary responsiveness to GnRH. This research thus shows how a decrease in endogenous FSH levels during diestrus, with a consequent reduction in attenuin production but no significant effect on estradiol levels, gives rise to a 1- or 2-day advancement of blunted preovulatory LH surges in 4- (Tébar et al., 1996, 1998) and 5-day (Sánchez-Criado et al., 1996) cyclic rats, respectively. This suggests that, in physiological circumstances, submaximal FSH-dependent ovarian attenuin bioactivity prevents the premature LH surge in diestrus by antagonizing the secretory effect of GnRH (Koppenaal et al., 1991; Tébar et al., 1998) and/or the sensitizing effect of estradiol on the pituitary (Schuiling et al., 1999). On the whole, all these findings, together with the existence of pituitary PR on diestrus, would suggest that PR-dependent GnRH self-priming in the diestrous phase in the 4-day cyclic rat is blocked by attenuin bioactivity.

5. Conclusions

Our work over the last few years suggests that attenuin is a FSH-dependent ovarian factor different from inhibin, which decreases preovulatory LH secretion in rats by activating gonadotrope membrane receptors, resulting in PR dephosphorylation. The reduction in PR activity is associated with a decrease in both LH secretion and LH synthesis.

The bioactivity of attenuin appears to play a major role in synchronizing physiological pituitary and ovarian events, so that preovulatory LH secretion is limited to proestrus, when the ovarian follicle and the oocyte are in optimal conditions to respond to the LH surge and to be fertilized, respectively.

However, all these findings must be viewed as speculative until experiments can be repeated using purified attenuin.

6. Acknowledgments

This review has been subsidized by grants BFU2008-00480 from DGICYT and P07-CVI2559 from CICE-Junta de Andalucia (Spain).

7. References

Arai K, Watanabe C, Taya K & Sasamoto S 1996 Roles of inhibin and estradiol in the regulation of follicle-stimulating hormone and luteinizing hormone secretion during the estrous cycle of the rat. Biology of Reproduction 55: 127–133.

Attardi B, Keeping HS, Winters SJ, Kotsuji F & Troen P 1991 Comparison of the effects of cycloheximide and inhibin on the gonadotropin subunit messenger ribonucleic acids. Endocrinology 128: 119–125.

Beck CA, Weigel NL & Edwards DP 1992 Effects of hormone and cellular modulators of protein phosphorylation on transcriptional activity, DNA binding, and phosphorylation of human progesterone receptor. Molecular Endocrinology 6: 607-620.

Busbridge NJ, Buckley DM, Cornish M & Whitehead SA 1988 Effects of ovarian hyperstimulation and isolated preovulatory follicles on LH responses to GnRH in rats. Journal of Reproduction and Fertility 82: 329-336.

Busbridge NJ, Chamberlain GV, Griffiths A & Whitehead SA 1990 Non-steroidal follicular factors attenuate the self-priming action of gonadotropin-releasing hormone on the pituitary gonadotroph. Neuroendocrinology 51: 493-499.

Byrne B, Fowler PA, Messinis IE & Templeton A 1993 Gonadotrophin surge-attenuating factor secretion varies during the follicular phase of the menstrual cycle of spontaneously cycling women. Journal of Endocrinology 139 (Suppl. p53).

Byrne B, Fowler PA, Fraser M, Culler MD & Templeton A 1995a Gonadotropin surge-attenuating factor bioactivity in serum from superovulated women is not blocked by inhibin antibody. Biology of Reproduction 52: 88-95.

Byrne B, Fowler PA & Templeton A 1995b GnSAF suppresses progesterone augmented GnRH self-priming. Journal of Reproduction and Fertility; Abstract Series 16: 3.

Byrne B, Fowler PA & Templeton A 1996 Role of progesterone and nonsteroidal ovarian factors in regulating gonadotropin-releasing hormone self-priming in vitro. Journal of Clinical Endocrinology and Metabolism 81: 1454–1459

Clayton RN, Solano AR, Garcia-Vela A, Dufau ML & Catt KJ 1980 Regulation of pituitary receptors for GnRH during the rat estrous cycle. Endocrinology 107: 699–706.

Clemm DL, Sherman L, Boonyaratanakornkit V, Schrader WT, Weigel NL & Edwards DP 2000 Differential hormone-dependent phosphorylation of progesterone receptor A and B forms revealed by a phosphoserine site-specific monoclonal antibody. Molecular Endocrinology 14: 52-65.

Condrescu M, Hantash BM, Fang Y & Reeves JP 1999 Mode-specific inhibition of sodium-calcium exchange during protein phosphatase blockade. Journal of Biological Chemistry. 274: 33279-33286.

Conneely OM, Kettelberger DM, Tsai MJ, Schrader WT & O'Malley BW 1989 The chicken progesterone receptor A and B isoforms are products of an alternate translation initiation event. Biological Chemistry 264: 14062-14064.

Cowking L, Fowler PA & Templeton A 1995 Acute exposure to ovarian steroids and a PKC activator do not overcome GnSAF bioactivity in vitro. Journal of Reproduction and Fertility; Abstract Series 15: 56-50.

Crowley WF Jr, Filicori M, Spratt DI & Santoro NF 1985 The physiology of gonadotropin-releasing hormone (GnRH) secretion in men and women. Recent Progress in Hormone Research 41: 473-531.

Culler MD 1992 In vivo evidence that inhibin is a gonadotropin surge-inhibiting/attenuating factor. Endocrinology 131: 1556-1558.

Danforth DR, Sinosich MJ, Anderson TL, Cheng CY, Bardin CW & Hodgen GD 1987 Identification of gonadotropin surge-inhibiting factor (GnSIF) in follicular fluid and its differentiation from inhibin. Biology of Reproduction 5: 1075-1082.

Danforth DR, Elkind-Hirsch K & Hodgen GD 1990 In vivo and in vitro modulation of gonadotropin-releasing hormone metabolism by estradiol and progesterone. Endocrinology 127: 319-324.

Danforth DR & Cheng CY 1995 Purification of a candidate gonadotropin surge inhibiting factor from porcine follicular fluid. Endocrinology 136: 1658-1665.

Denner LA, Weigel NL, Maxwell BL, Schrader WT & O'Malley BW 1990 Regulation of progesterone receptor-mediated transcription by phosphorylation. Science 250: 1740-1743.

van Dieten JA, Helder MN, van den Oever C & de Koning J 1999 Non-steroidal factors in bovine follicular fluid inhibit or facilitate the action of pulsatile administration of GnRH on LH release in the female rat. Journal of Endocrinology 161: 237-243.

Faus H & Haendler B 2006 Post-translational modifications of steroid receptors. Biomedicine and Pharmacotherapy 60: 520-528.

Ferraretti AP, Garcia JE, Acosta AA & Jones GS 1983 Serum luteinizing hormone during ovulation induction with human menopausal gonadotropin for in vitro fertilization in normally menstruating women. Fertility and Sterility 40: 742-747.

Fink G 1995 The self-priming effect of LHRH: a unique servomechanism and possible cellular model for memory. Frontiers in Neuroendocrinology 16: 183-190.

Fowler PA, Cunningham P, Fraser M, McGregor F, Byrne B, Pappa A, Messinis IE & Templeton A 1994a Circulating gonadotrophin surge-attenuating factor from superovulated women suppresses in vitro gonadotrophin releasing-hormone self-priming. Journal of Endocrinology 143: 45–54.

Fowler PA, Fraser M, Cunningham P, Knight PG, Byrne B, McLaughlin E, Wardle PG, Hull MGR & Templeton A 1994b Higher gonadotrophin surge-attenuating factor (GnSAF) bioactivity is found in small follicles from superovulated women. Journal of Endocrinology 143: 33–44.

Fowler PA, Bramley TA, MacGregor F & Templeton A 1994c Does GnSAF act through the pituitary protein kinase C pathway? Journal of Reproduction and Fertility; Abstract Series 13: 40.

Fowler PA, Fahy U, Culler MD, Knight PG, Wardle PG, McLaughlin EA, Cunningham P, Fraser M, Hull MG, Templeton A 1995a Gonadotrophin surge-attenuating factor bioactivity is present in follicular fluid from naturally cycling women. Human Reproduction 10: 68-74.

Fowler PA, Fraser M, Cunningham P & Templeton A 1995b GnSAF suppresses both the syntesis and release of LH induced by GnRH. Journal of Reproduction and Fertility; Abstract Series 15: 55-50.

Fowler PA & Templeton A 1996 The nature and function of putative gonadotropin surge-attenuating/inhibiting factor (GnSAF/IF). Endocrine Reviews 17: 103-120.

Fowler PA, Sorsa T, Harris WJ, Knight PG & Mason HD 2001 Relationship between follicle size and gonadotrophin surge attenuating factor (GnSAF) bioactivity during spontaneous cycles in women. Human Reproduction 16: 1353-1358.

Fowler PA, Sorsa-Leslie T, Cash P, Dunbar B, Melvin W, Wilson Y, Mason HD & Harris W 2002 A 60-66 kDa protein with gonadotrophin surge attenuating factor bioactivity is produced by human ovarian granulosa cells. Molecular Human Reproduction 8: 823-832.

Fowler PA, Sorsa-Leslie T, Harris W & Mason HD 2003 Ovarian gonadotrophin surge-attenuating factor (GnSAF): where are we after 20 years of research? Reproduction 126: 689-699.

Fowler PA & Spears N 2004 The cultured rodent follicle as a model for investigations of gonadotrophin surge-attenuating factor GnSAF production. Reproduction 127: 679-688.

Garrido-Gracia JC, Bellido C, Aguilar R & Sánchez-Criado JE 2006 Protein kinase C cross-talk with gonadotrope progesterone receptor is involved in GnRH-induced LH secretion. Journal of Physiology and Biochemistry 62: 35-42.

Garrido-Gracia JC, Gordon A, Bellido C, Aguilar R, Barranco I, Millán Y, Martín de las Mulas J & Sánchez-Criado JE 2007 The integrated action of oestrogen receptor isoforms and sites with progesterone receptor in the gonadotrope modulate LH secretion: evidence from tamoxifen-treated ovariectomized rats. Journal of Endocrinology 193: 107-119.

Garrido-Gracia JC, Gordon A, Aguilar R, Monterde JG, Blanco A, Martín de Las Mulas J & Sánchez-Criado JE 2008 Morphological effects of oestradiol-17beta, and selective oestrogen receptor alpha and beta agonists on luteinising hormone-secreting cells in tamoxifen-treated ovariectomised rats. Histology and Histopathology 23: 1453-1463.

Geiger JM, Plas-Roser S & Aron Cl 1980 Mechanisms of ovulation in female rats treated with FSH at the beginning of the estrous cycle: changes in pituitary responsiveness to luteinizing hormone releasing hormone (LHRH). Biology of Reproduction 22: 837-845.

Glasier A, Thatcher SS, Wickings EJ, Hillier SG & Baird DT 1988 Superovulation with exogenous gonadotropins does not inhibit the luteinizing hormone surge. Fertility and Sterility 49: 81-85.

Gordon A, Garrido-Gracia JC, Aguilar R, Bellido C, Velasco JA, Millan Y, Tena-Sempere M, Martín de Las Mulas J & Sánchez-Criado JE 2008 The ovary-mediated FSH attenuation of the LH surge in the rat involves a decreased gonadotroph progesterone receptor (PR) action but not PR expression. Journal of Endocrinology 196: 583-592.

Gordon A, Garrido-Gracia JC, Aguilar R & Sánchez-Criado JE 2009a Ovarian stimulation with FSH in the rat reduces proestrous GnRH-dependent LH secretion through a dual mechanism: inhibition of LH synthesis and release. Neuroscience Letters 460: 219-222.

Gordon A, Garrido-Gracia JC, Aguilar R, Guil-Luna S, Millán Y, de Las Mulas JM & Sánchez-Criado JE 2009b Ovarian stimulation with FSH reduces phosphorylation of gonadotrope progesterone receptor and LH secretion in the rat. Reproduction 137: 151-159.

Gordon A, Aguilar R, Garrido-Gracia JC, Guil-Luna S, Sánchez Cespedes R, Millán Y, Watanabe G, Taya K, Martín de Las Mulas J & Sánchez-Criado JE 2010a Immunoneutralization of Inhibin in Cycling Rats Increases Follicle-Stimulating Hormone Secretion, Stimulates the Ovary and Attenuates Progesterone Receptor-Dependent Preovulatory Luteinizing Hormone Secretion. Neuroendocrinology 91: 291-301.

Gordon A, Garrido-Gracia JC, Sánchez-Criado JE & Aguilar R 2010b Involvement of rat gonadotrope progesterone receptor in the ovary-mediated inhibitory action of FSH on LH synthesis. Journal of Physiology and Biochemistry In press.

Gordon A, Aguilar R, Garrido-Gracia JC, Bellido C, Millán Y, Guil-Luna S, García-Velasco JA, Bellido-Muñoz E, Martín de Las Mulas J & Sánchez-Criado JE 2010c Human follicular fluid (hFF) from superovulated women inhibits progesterone receptor (PR)-dependent GnRH selfpriming in an estrous cycle-dependent manner in the rat. Journal of Endocrinological Investigation 33: 564-570.

Gordon A, Garrido-Gracia JC, Aguilar R & Sánchez-Criado JE 2011 La atenuina (GnSI/AF) ovárica reduce la secreción preovulatoria de LH en la rata por desfosforilación de la isoforma B del receptor de progesterona. 53º Congress of Spanisn Society of Endocrinology and Nutrition, Santiago de Compostela, Spain.

Helder MN, van Eersel SE, van Heurn JW & de Koning J 1997 Gonadotrophin surge-inhibiting factor inhibits GnRH-stimulated mitogen-activated protein kinase activation. Human Reproduction 1: 67-68.

Ishigame H, Medan MS, Watanabe G, Shi Z, Kishi H, Aray KY & Taya K 2004 A new alternative method for superovulation using passive immunization agaist inhibin in adult rats. Biology of Reproduction 71: 236-243.

de Jong FH, Welschen R, Hermans WP, Smith SD & van der Molen HJ 1979 Effects of factors from ovarian follicular fluid and Sertoli cell culture medium on in-vivo and in-vitro release of pituitary gonadotrophins in the rat: an evaluation of systems for the assay of inhibin. Journal of Reproduction and Fertility (Suppl.) 26: 47-59.

de Jong FH 1988 Inhibin. Physiological Reviews 68: 555-607.

Karligiotou E, Kollia P, Kallitsaris A & Messinis IE 2006 Expression of human serum albumin (HSA) mRNA in human granulosa cells: potential correlation of the 95 amino acid long carboxyl terminal of HSA to gonadotrophin surge-attenuating factor. Human Reproduction 21: 645-650.

Kile JP & Nett TM 1994 Differential secretion of follicle-stimulating hormone and luteinizing hormone from ovine pituitary cells following activation of protein kinase A, protein kinase C, or increased intracellular calcium. Biology of Reproduction 50: 49-54.

Kita M, Taii S, Kataoka N, Shimatsu A, Nakao K & Mori T 1994 Changes of gonadotrophin surge inhibiting/attenuating factor activity in pig follicular fluid in relation to follicle size. Journal of Reproduction and Fertility 101: 59-66.

Kitahara S, Winters SJ, Attardi B, Oshima H & Troen P 1990 Effects of castration on luteinizing hormone and follicle-stimulating hormone secretion by pituitary cells from male rats. Endocrinology 126: 2642-2649.

Knobil E 1980 The neuroendocrine control of the menstrual cycle. Recent Progress in Hormone Research 36: 53-88.

de Koning J, Tijssen AM & van Rees GP 1987 The involvement of ovarian factors in maintaining the pituitary glands of female rats in a state of low LH responsiveness to LHRH. Journal of Endocrinology 112: 265-273.

de Koning J, Tijssen AM & van Rees GP 1989 The self-priming action of LHRH increases the low pituitary LH and FSH response caused by ovarian factors: observations in vitro. Journal of Endocrinology 120: 439-447.

de Koning J 1995 Gonadotrophin surge-inhibiting/attenuating factor governs luteinizing hormone secretion during the ovarian cycle: physiology and pathology. Human Reproduction 10: 2854-2861.

Koppenaal DW, Tijssen AM, van Dieten JA & de Koning J 1991 The self-priming action of LHRH is under negative FSH control through a factor released by the ovary: Observations in female rats in vivo. Journal of Endocrinology 129: 205-211.

Koppenaal DW, Tijssen AM & de Koning J 1992 The effect of gonadotrophin surge-inhibiting factor on the self-priming action of gonadotrophin-releasing hormone in female rats in vitro. Journal of Endocrinology 134: 427-436.

Koppenaal DW, van Dieten JA, Tijssen AM & de Koning J 1993 Induction of the gonadotrophin surge-inhibiting factor by FSH and its elimination: a sex difference in the efficacy of the priming effect of gonadotrophin-releasing hormone on the rat pituitary gland. Journal of Endocrinology 138: 191-201.

Levine JE, Chappell PE, Schneider JS, Sleiter NC & Szabo M 2001 Progesterone receptors as neuroendocrine integrators. Frontiers in Neuroendocrinology 22: 69-106.

Littman BA & Hodgen GD 1984 Human menopausal gonadotropin stimulation in monkeys: blockade of the luteinizing hormone surge by a highly transient ovarian factor. Fertility and Sterility 41: 440-447.

Messinis IE & Templeton A 1986 The effect of pulsatile follicle stimulating hormone on the endogenous luteinizing hormone surge in women. Clinical Endocrinology 25: 633-640.

Messinis IE, Templeton A & Baird DT 1986 Relationships between the characteristics of endogenous luteinizing hormone surge and the degree of ovarian hyperstimulation during superovulation induction in women. Clinical Endocrinology 25: 393-400.

Messinis IE & Templeton A 1987 Effect of high dose exogenous oestrogen on midcycle luteinizing hormone surge in human spontaneous cycles. Clinical Endocrinology 27: 453-459.

Messinis IE & Templeton A 1988 The endocrine consequences of multiple folliculogenesis. Journal of Reproduction and Fertility (Suppl.) 36: 27-37.

Messinis IE & Templeton A 1989 Pituitary response to exogenous LHRH in superovulated women. Journal of Reproduction and Fertility 87: 633-639.

Messinis IE, Hirsch P & Templeton A 1991 Follicle stimulating hormone stimulates the production of gonadotrophin surge attenuating factor (GnSAF) in vivo. Clinical Endocrinology 35: 403-407.

Messinis IE, Lolis D, Papadopoulos L, Tsahalina T, Papanikolaou N, Seferiadis K & Templeton A 1993 Effect of varying concentrations of follicle stimulating hormone on the production of gonadotrophin surge attenuating factor (GnSAF) in women. Clinical Endocrinology 39: 45-50.

Messinis IE, Lolis D, Zikopoulos K, Tsahalina E, Seferiadis K & Templeton AA. 1994 Effect of an increase in FSH on the production of gonadotrophin-surge-attenuating factor in women. Journal of Reproduction and Fertility 101: 689-95.

Messinis IE, Lolis D, Zikopoulos K, Milingos S, Kollios G, Seferiadis K & Templeton A 1996 Effect of follicle stimulating hormone or human chorionic gonadotrophin treatment on the production of gonadotrophin surge attenuating factor (GnSAF) during the luteal phase of the human menstrual cycle. Clinical Endocrinology 44: 169-175.

Messinis IE 2006 Ovarian feedback, mechanism of action and possible clinical implications. Human Reproduction Update 12: 557-571.

Mroueh JM, Arbogast LK, Fowler P, Templeton AA, Friedman CI & Danforth DR 1996 Identification of gonadotrophin surge-inhibiting factor (GnSIF)/attenuin in human follicular fluid. Human Reproduction 11: 490-496.

Muttukrishna S, Fowler PA, Groome NP, Mitchell GG, Robertson WR & Knight PG 1994 Serum concentrations of dimeric inhibin during the spontaneous human menstrual cycle and after treatment with exogenous gonadotrophin. Human Reproduction 9: 1634-1642.

Pappa A, Seferiadis K, Fotsis T, Shevchenko A, Marselos M, Tsolas O & Messinis IE 1999 Purification of a candidate gonadotrophin surge attenuating factor from human follicular fluid. Human Reproduction 14: 1449-1456.

Ramey JW, Highsmith RF, Wilfinger WW & Baldwin DM 1987 The effects of gonadotropin-releasing hormone and estradiol on luteinizing hormone biosynthesis in cultured rat anterior pituitary cells. Endocrinology 120: 1503-1513.

Ruiz A, Aguilar R, Tébar M, Gaytán F & Sánchez-Criado JE 1996 RU486-treated rats show endocrine and morphological responses to therapies analogous to responses of women with polycystic ovary syndrome treated with similar therapies. Biology of Reproduction 55: 1284-1291.

Sanchez-Criado JE, Ruiz A, Tebar M & Mattheij JA 1996 Follicular and luteal progesterone synergize to maintain 5-day cyclicity in rats. Revista Española de Fisiología 52: 223-229.

Sánchez-Criado JE, Garrido-Gracia JC, Bellido C, Aguilar R, Guelmes P, Abreu P, Alonso R, Barranco I, Millán Y & de Las Mulas JM 2006 Oestradiol-17beta inhibits tamoxifen-induced LHRH self-priming blocking hormone-dependent and ligand-independent activation of the gonadotrope progesterone receptor in the rat. Journal of Endocrinology 190: 73-84.

Sarkar D, Chiappa SA, Fink G & Sherwood NM 1976 Gonadotropin-releasing hormone surge in pro-oestrous rats. Nature 264: 461–463.

Schenken RS, Anderson WH & Hodgen GD 1984 Follicle-stimulating hormone increases ovarian vein nonsteroidal factors with gonadotropin-inhibiting activity. Fertility and Sterility 42: 785-790.

Schwartz NB 2000 Neuroendocrine regulation of reproductive cyclicity. En Neuroendocrinology in Physiology and Medicine, pp 135–145. Eds PMConn & ME Freeman. Totowa, NJ: Humana Press Inc.

Schuiling GA, Valkhof N & Koiter TR 1999 FSH inhibits the augmentation by oestradiol of the pituitary responsiveness to GnRH in the female rat. Human Reproduction 14: 21-26.

Scott RS & Burger HG 1981 Mechanism of action of inhibin. Biology of Reproduction 24: 541–550.

Seo SH & Danforth DR 1994 Porcine granulosa cells produce gonadotropin surge inhibiting factor (GnSIF) activity in vitro. Serono Symposia Xth Ovarian Workshop. Raven Press, New York, p 62.

Sopelak VM & Hodgen GD 1984 Blockade of the estrogen-induced luteinizing hormone surge in monkeys: a nonsteroidal, antigenic factor in porcine follicular fluid. Fertility and Sterility 41: 108-113.

Sorsa-Leslie T, Mason HD, Harris WJ & Fowler PA 2005 Selection of gonadotrophin surge attenuating factor phage antibodies by bioassay. Reproductive Biology and Endocrinology 3: 49.

Speight A, Popkin R, Watts AG & Fink G 1981 Oestradiol-17 beta increases pituitary responsiveness by a mechanism that involves the release and the priming effect of luteinizing hormone releasing factor. Journal of Endocrinology 88: 301-308.

Takimoto GS & Horwitz KB 1993 Progesterone receptor phosphorylation: Complexities in defining a functional role. Trends in Endocrinology and Metabolism 4: 1-7.

Tavoulari S, Frillingos S, Karatza P, Messinis IE & Seferiadis K 2004 The recombinant subdomain IIIB of human serum albumin displays activity of gonadotrophin surge-attenuating factor. Human Reproduction 19: 849-858.

Tebar M, Ruiz A, Bellido C & Sanchez-Criado JE 1996 Ovary mediates the effects of RU486 given during proestrus on the diestrous secretion of luteinizing hormone in the rat. Biology of Reproduction 54: 1266-1270.

Tebar M, Ruiz A & Sanchez-Criado JE 1998 Involvement of estrogen and follicle-stimulating hormone on basal and luteinizing hormone (LH)-releasing hormone-stimulated LH secretion in RU-486-induced 3-day estrous cycle in the rat. Biology of Reproduction 58: 615-619.

Tijssen AM, Helder MN, Chu ZW & de Koning J 1997 Intracellular antagonistic interaction between GnRH and gonadotrophin surge-inhibiting/attenuating factor bioactivity downstream of second messengers involved in the self-priming process. Journal of Reproduction and Fertility 111: 235-242.

Tio S, Koppenaal D, Bardin CW & Cheng CY 1994 Purification of gonadotropin surge-inhibiting factor from Sertoli cell-enriched culture medium. Biochemical and Biophysical Research Communications 199: 1229-1236.

Tse A, Tse FW, Almers W & Hille B 1993 Rhythmic exocytosis stimulated by GnRH-induced calcium oscillations in rat gonadotropes. Science 260: 82-84.

Turgeon JL & Waring DW 1994 Activation of the progesterone receptor by the gonadotropin-releasing hormone self-priming signaling pathway. Molecular Endocrinology 8: 860-869.

Vegeto E, Shahbaz MM, Wen DX, Goldman ME, O'Malley BW & McDonnell DP 1993 Human progesterone receptor A form is a cell- and promoter-specific repressor of human progesterone receptor B function. Molecular Endocrinology 7: 1244-55.

Waring DW & Turgeon JL 1980 Luteinizing hormone-releasing hormone-induced luteinizing hormone secretion in vitro: cyclic changes in responsiveness and self-priming. Endocrinology 106: 1430-1436.

Watanabe G, Taya K & Sasamoto S 1990 Dynamics of ovarian inhibin secretion during the oestrous cycle of the rat. Journal of Endocrinology 126: 151-157.

Wen DX, Xu YF, Mais DE, Goldman ME & McDonnell DP 1994 The A and B isoforms of the human progesterone receptor operate through distinct signaling pathways within target cells. Molecular and Cellular Biology 14: 8356-8364.

Whitehead SA 1990 A gonadotrophin surge attenuating factor? Journal of Endocrinology 126: 1-4.

Yen SS, Tsai CC, Vandenberg G & Rebar R 1972 Gonadotropin dynamics in patients with gonadal dysgenesis: a model for the study of gonadotropin regulation. Journal of Clinical Endocrinology and Metabolism 35: 897-904.

15

Calcitonin Functions Both as a Hypocalcemic Hormone and Stimulator of Steroid Production and Oocyte Maturation in Ovarian Follicles of Common Carp, *Cyprinus carpio*

Dilip Mukherjee, Sourav Kundu, Kousik Pramanick, Sudipta Paul and Buddhadev Mallick
Endocrinology Laboratory, Department of Zoology, University of Kalyani, West Bengal India

1. Introduction

Calcitonin (CT) is a calcium regulating hormone produced mainly by the parafollicular C cells of the thyroid gland in mammals. In lower vertebrates, these cells are concentrated primarily in a specialized gland, the ultimobranchial gland. The common structure of CT is 32-amino acid residues with a seven-residue cyclic loop formed by disulfide bond between cysteines at position 1 and 7 and prolinamide at carboxyl terminal.

Calcitonin in mammals and birds is acknowledged to be the principal hypocalcemic agent, but the situation in fish is less clear. Several laboratories although showed a hypocalcemic action of CT in fish, conflicting results are often reported. Moreover, fish have other hypocalcemic factor like Staniocalcin, a product of Corpuscles of Stannius, secretion of which is positively regulated by extracellular calcium levels. Control of calcium homeostasis in fish may likely to be different from that in terrestrial vertebrates because of the aquatic environment.

In addition to the involvement of CT in calcium homeostasis in mammals, an endocrine role of endogenous CT at brain, pituitary and gonad has also been suggested. Similarly, a role for CT in calcium ion regulation in fish may be subordinate to other functions which include acting as neurotransmitter or inducer of ovarian steroid hormone synthesis. A major question thus arises- what is the exact role of CT in fresh water teleost? Does it really has any role in calcium homeostasis or involved in many other functions including reproduction? The evolutionary history and functions of CT in aquatic vertebrate therefore require further investigation and as part of ongoing studies in to endocrine/paracrine factors involved in calcium homeostasis and the role of CT, if any, on reproduction in fish, we tried to answer these questions.

2. Work done so far

2.1 Calcium ion regulation

2.1.1 Mammals

The classic concept of CT function in mammals has focused on its effects on calcium homeostasis (Copp et al., 1967). In mammals, CT lowers serum calcium levels by its action on bone. Cellular activity of the skeleton is largely devoted to an orderly sequence of bone resorption and formation, called remodeling. CT receptors are found in high concentrations in mammalian osteoclast and the hormone exerts its control on serum calcium by inhibiting bone calcium resorption through its direct action on osteoclasts (Nicholson et al., 1986; Raisz et al., 1998; see review Zaidi et al., 2002).

As mammalian bone osteoclasts are characterized by high acid phosphatase activity, particularly, that of tartrate-resistant acid phosphatase (TRACP) and as collagen degradation in bone releases hydroxyproline (HYP) in circulation; these two parameters are used as reliable markers for bone resorption (Vaes, 1988; Raisz et al., 1998; Fujita et al., 1999). Available reports indicate that CT inhibits osteoclast secretory activity, particularly of TRACP in terms of both synthesis and release. It reduces osteoclastic acid secretion by altering Na^+-K^+-ATPase activity, and carbonic anhydrase localization, as well as direct H^+-ATPase inhibition (see review Zaidi et al., 2002). Available information shows that salmon CT is the most potent in hypocalcemic activity in terms of bone resorption determined in human and rat (Zaidi et al, 1988) and least potent is the human CT.

2.1.2 Non-mammalian vertebrates

Calcitonin has been identified from several species of birds including goose, duck, domestic fowl, and Japanese quail (Kenny, 1971; Boelkins & Kenny, 1973). Plasma content of CT is much higher in birds than normally observed in mammals. The role of CT in birds is controversial (Dacke, 2000; DeMatos, 2008) as conflicting accounts regarding the hypocalcemic effect of CT have been reported. Few investigators have found no effect after CT administration to birds (Urist, 1967; Dacke, 1979). On the other hand, positive responses of injected CT to birds have been reported by Calaney and Barket, (1970), on young cock and laying hen (Lloyd et al., 1970), in domestic fowl, Kraintz and Inscher (1969, in partially parathyroidectomized cockrels) and Swarup et al. (1980a, in parrots). Very recently, Yadav and Srivastava (2009) suggested a hypoclacemic role of CT in *Columba livia*. It is also reported that CT is very important during egg laying when it reduce excessive oscillation in blood plasma calcium levels and possibly influence calcium deposition in the egg.

Reptiles are the first vertebrates to be completely independent of the water environment by developing an egg shell and an amnion. This fact shows that reptiles can perform calcium metabolism of the terrestrial type different from that of amphibians. Calcitonin is present in the ultimobranchial gland and in plasma of reptiles (Kline & Longmore, 1986). But hypocalcemic function of CT in reptiles has not yet been demonstrated successfully in a variety of reptiles, including turtles, snakes, and lizards (Cope & Kline 1989). However, using salmon CT, a hypocalcemic effect of CT has been observed in *Iguana iguana* and in young Chuckwallas, *Sauromalus obesus* (Kline, 1981; 1982). Reptiles share with bird the problem associated with the production of large cleidoic eggs, which in many species are covered with a calcareous shell. Very little information is available on the role of calcemic hormones on reptilian bone and intestine.

Amphibians have a special position with regard to our understanding of vertebrate calcium metabolism, as in this group, parathyroid gland first appear on the phyletic scale. Well developed ultimobranchial gland is present in amphibians. Removal of ultimobranchial bodies in *Rana pipiens* results an initial elevation of plasma calcium levels which subsequently subsides and replaces by hypocalcemia (Robertson et al., 1975). Ultimobranchialectomized bullfrog tadpoles display deficiency in their ability to maintain plasma calcium levels when kept in solution containing high-calcium concentrations (Sasayama and Oguru, 1976).

Calcitonin has been identified in the plasma of *Rana pipiens* and the level increased when these frogs were kept in high-calcium water (Robertson, 1987). Srivastav and Rani (1989) reported that CT injection result in hypocalcemia in *Rana tigrina*, but it has no effect on either urinary excretion or plasma calcium concentrations in toad *Bufo arinus* (Bentley, 1983).
Information on the regulation of calcium ion metabolism in cartilaginous fish is very limited. Like most non-mammalian vertebrates, they have ultimobranchial bodies, which contain CT. High levels of CT is present in plasma of several species of sharks (Glowacki et al., 1985). Early observations using tetrapod CT failed to detect any effects of CT on calcium metabolism in cartilaginous fish. Salmon CT however, induced modest hypocalcemia in leopard shark (Glowacki et al., 1985). Information on the regulation of calcium homeostasis in bony fish is almost entirely limited to teleosts. Within this group, few species have been studied and considerable variation exists among the species. Ultimobranchial gland of teleost fish is a rich source of CT and circulatory level of this hormone is very high in this group of fish. CT has been extracted and purified from ultimobranchial gland of many fish (Niall et al., 1969; Noda and Narita, 1976; Ukawa et al., 1991; Sasayama et al., 1993). Several laboratories although have been able to show the hypocalcemic action of CT in fish (Chan et al., 1968; Lopez et al., 1976; Wendelaar-Bonga, 1981; Chakraborti and Mukherjee 1993; Srivastava et al., 1998; Suzuki et al., 1999), conflicting results are often reported (Wendelaar-Bonga and Pang 1991; Singh and Srivastava 1993). Calcitonin producing C cells in ultimobranchial gland of fish showed less distinct responses to changes in extracellular calcium levels than mammals (Ross et al., 1974). As such, establishing a clear and unequivocal role of CT in calcium homeostasis in fish seems to be extremely difficult. Moreover, in those experiments, where CT has been shown to function as a hypocalcemic hormone in fish, the way this is affected has been addressed in only few studies (Milhaud et al., 1977; Milet et al., 1979; Wagner et al., 1997; Mukherjee et al., 2004a, b). There may be two probabilities relating to hypocalcemic action of fish CT. Responses of fish to this peptide could involve either gills and gill-calcium (Ca^{2+}) transport (GCAT) or as in mammals, inhibition of bone calcium resorption or both. Experimental evidence in support of these probabilities is very limited. Calcitonin receptors have been identified in gills of teleosts (Fouchereau-Peron et al., 1987) and this hormone has been observed to decrease influx of calcium across the perfused gills of salmon and eels (Milhaud et al., 1977; Milet et al., 1979). Later on, an *in vivo* measurement of calcium uptake in intact young rainbow trout and fingerlings and adult fresh water air-breathing teleost, *Channa punctatus*, after salmon CT administration lend support in favor of gills and GCAT (Wagner et al., 1997; Mukherjee et al., 2004a). Since the endoskeleton of fish, at least in part, consists of cellular bones, which have the ability to remodel themselves (Mugiya & Watabe, 1977; Dacke, 1979), the probability of CT function on bone can not be ruled out.

2.2 Other function of CT in vertebrates

Calcitonin is reported to have a role to increase the concentration of insulin-like growth factor (IGF-I) in serum free-culture of human osteoblast-like cells (Farley et al., 2000). Calcitonin may also prevent osteoblast and osteocyte apoptosis (Plotkin et al., 1999). Calcitonin actions on brain, pituitary and gonads have been investigated in mammals. CT-like immunoreactivity has been found in human and rat pituitary gland (Cooper et al., 1980). Specific CT-binding sites have been found in brain and pituitary gland (Maurer et al., 1983) and in ovary and testis in mammal (Chausmer et al., 1982). Wang et al., (1994) found that

CT-like peptides, human CT, salmon CT and CT-gene related peptide inhibit spontaneous and gonadotropin-stimulated testosterone secretion by acing directly on testes and also by reducing the release of pituitary luteinizing hormone (LH). Inhibition of salmon CT on secretion of progesterone- and gonadatropin-releasing hormone (GnRH)-stimulated release of pituitary LH in rat also has been documented (Tsai et al., 1999). Very recently, we also reported for stimulation of salmon CT on secretion of 17β-estradiol by the ovarian follicles of common carp *C. carpio* (Paul et al., 2008). All these observations suggest an endocrine role of endogenous CT at brain, pituitary and gonads in vertebrates. Another interesting cellular action of CT involves the early demonstration of its effect on growth of breast cancer cells. CT retards cell division in CT receptor-transfected HEK cells (Piserchio et al., 2000).

3. Objective

The purpose of the present study was aimed: 1) to investigate the action of CT on hypocalcemic regulation in a fresh water teleost, *Cyprinus carpio* and its mode of action through inhibition of gill-Ca^{2+} transport and bone calcium resorption; 2) to examine the effects of CT on basal and hCG-stimulated *in vivo* release of 17β-estradiol (E_2) and *in vitro* production of E_2 and 17α,20β-dihydroxy-4-pregnen-3-one (17,20β-P) by the ovarian follicles; and finally 3) to find out the efficacy of CT alone or in combination with hCG on induction of oocyte maturation in post-vitellogenic ovarian follicles of *C. carpio.*

4. Materials and methods

4.1 Chemicals

Synthetic salmon calcitonin (sCT), all cold steroids and dibutyryl cyclic AMP (dbcAMP) were purchased from Sigma Chemicals. Analytical grade *p*-nitrophenol, *p*-nitrophenyl phosphate, ninhydrin and reference standard amino acid kit were purchased from Sisco Research laboratories, Mumbai, India. hCG was a gift from National Hormone and Pituitary Programm (Torrance, CA, USA). SQ 22536 (RBI, Natrick, MA, USA) and NPC-15437 dihydrochloride (Sigma) was a gift from Dr. Arun Bandopadhyay, Molecular Endocrinology Laboratory, Indian Institute of Chemical Biology, Kolkata, India. TRI reagent was purchased from Ambion Inc., USA. Smart-PCR cDNA synthesis kit was purchased from Clontech. RevertAid M-MuLV reverse transcriptase and deoxyNTPs were purchased from MBI Fermentas and Taq DNA polymerase from Invitrogen. Radiolabelled ^{45}Ca (specific activity 32.5 mCi/mg calcium), radiolabelled [^{3}H] estradiol 17β (specific activity 75.0 Ci/mmol), [^{3}H]testosterone (sp activity 95.0 Ci/mmol), 17α, Hydroxy [1,2,6,7-^{3}H]progesterone (sp activity 75 Ci/mmol) and [^{125}I]sCT (sp activity 2000 Ci/mmol)were purchased from Amersham Biosciences. The E_2 antibody was a gift from Prof. Gordon Niswender, Colorado State University, Fort Collins, USA. Labelled 17α,20β-P was prepared from labeled 17α, Hydroxy [1,2,6,7-^{3}H]progesterone by sodium borohydide reduction followed by chromatographic separation as described by Sen et al., (2002). 17α,20β-P antibody was obtained from Dr. A. P. Scott, Lowestoft, UK. All chemicals used were of analytical grade.

4.2 Calcitonin in calcium ion regulation in fish

4.2.1 Animals

For evaluation of CT action on calcium ion regulation, sexually mature (200-250 g body wt) and immature (30-35 g body wt) female *C. carpio* and fingerlings of this fish (3-4 g body wt) were obtained from local fish farm and maintained in re-circulating de-chlorinated normal tap water (300 L capacity; Ca, 0.15 mM; 24 ± 1°C) for 10 days prior to use. Groups of mature and immature fish as well as fingerlings were transferred to either low-Ca water (Ca, 0.05 mM) or normal tap water for 7 days prior to treatment. During the period of acclimatization, fish and fingerlings both were maintained on a daily commercial fish food (Shalimer Fish Food, Mumbai, India) and starved 24 h prior to use. Ultimobranchial glands (UBG) were removed from freshly collected female *C. carpio* and extract was prepared following the procedure described early (Chakraborty and Mukherjee, 1993). Briefly, ten glandular bodies were quickly homogenized in ice-cold saline and homogenate was centrifuged in cold condition for 10 min at 5000 x g. The supernatant was taken as UBG extract.

4.2.2 Time-course and dose-response effects of sCT and UBG extract on plasma calcium

Sexually mature and immature fish, kept either in normal tap water or low-Ca water received a single i.p injection of sCT (0.5 μg/100 g body wt) at 07.00 h in the morning for conducting time-course study or with increasing concentrations of sCT for dose-response study. Homologous UBG extract treatments were conducted in a similar way only with immature fish kept in low-Ca water. Controls were injected with similar volume of vehicle. A sham-injected control group was always included along with saline–control group to ensure that saline treatment evoked no stress on fish. Fish were sampled at different time intervals or 4 h after CT or UBG extract injection. In a separate experiment, sexually immature fish kept in low-Ca water were injected daily with sCT (0.5 μg/100 g body wt) for 15 days and sampling of fish was done at 4 h after last injection.

4.2.3 Effects of sCT on gill-calcium transport (GCAT)

Time-course and dose-response study of ^{45}Ca uptake in response to sCT was conducted with fingerlings and sexually immature fish, kept either in normal tap water or low-Ca water. After light anesthesia with MS222, both fingerlings and immature fish were given either single injection of sCT (0.5 μg/100 g body wt) for time-course study or with increasing doses of sCT in such a way that each fish received either 0.1 or 0.2 or 0.5, 1 or 2 μg sCT/100 g body wt. Immediately after injection fingerlings were transferred to individual glass tank (2 L capacity) each containing 1 liter ^{45}Ca (200 μCi) water and immature fish to individual glass aquarium (5 L capacity) each containing 3 liter ^{45}Ca (600 μCi) water. In both the treatment groups six individuals per tank or aquarium were kept. Fish were sampled at 1, 2, 4, 6, 8 and 12 h after sCT treatment.

4.2.4 Procedure for determination of whole body calcium uptake and calculation of GCAT

This has been done following the procedure described early (Mukherjee et al., 2004a). Briefly, fish were euthanized in 0.25% solution of benzocane followed by a wash with 0.1M HCl for 10 minutes to remove the externally bound ^{45}Ca. From each fish and fingerling, gut with its content was removed and weight of each fish/ fingerling was recorded. They were then placed in a muffle furnace at 600 °C to convert them to complete ash. The isotope content of ash was determined by scintillation counting of the dissolved ash. The rate of GCAT for each fish was calculated on the basis of isotope content of the fish/ fingerling and specific activity of ^{45}Ca and expressed as mmol Ca^{2+} transport /kg body weight per hour (Wagner et al., 1997; Mukherjee et al., 2004a).

4.2.5 Effects of sCT on plasma TRACP and ALP activities and urinary HYP content

This experiment was conducted with immature fish kept in normal tap water. Fish, after light anesthesia received either a single injection of sCT (0.5 μg/100 g body wt) or single injection of one of four different concentrations of sCT (0.01, 0.1, 0.5 or 1 μg/100 g body wt). Sampling of fish was done at 4 h of sCT injection. Calcium content of skeletal bones as well as plasma TRACP and ALP activities and urinary HYP content of immature fish adapted to normal tap water were measured after daily sCT treatment (0.5 μg/100 g body wt) for 15 days. Fish were sacrificed 4 h after last injection and skeletal bones were processed for quantification of calcium.

4.2.6 Estimation of plasma and bone calcium and determination of TRACP and ALP activities and urinary HYP

Immediately after sampling, blood was collected and processed for plasma separation. Aliquots of plasma samples were subjected to either separation of protein free ultrafiltrate (Chakraborty and Mukherjee, 1993) or determination of TRACP and ALP activities following the procedure described early (Mukherjee et al., 2004b). Ultrafiltrate samples were analyzed by atomic absorbance spectroscopy (Varian SpectrAA 250) for determination of calcium content. Skeletal bones of individual control and treated fish was processed for preparation of bone powder and calcium content was estimated following the procedure described early (Mukherjee et al., 2004b). Urine samples from control and treated fish were collected with the help of fine catheter (0.5 mm i.d) and HYP from the urine was extracted and estimated following the procedure described previously (Mukherjee et al., 2004b).

4.3 Effects of sCT on ovarian steroid production and oocyte maturation in fish

4.3.1 Animals

Adult female *C. carpio* (300-400g body wt) after collection during the month of September to November were maintained in re-circulating de-chlorinated normal tap-water in laboratory concrete tanks (300 L capacity, Ca^{2+}, 0.15 mM) at 23 ± 2 °C at least for 5 days prior to experiment. They were fed with commercial fish food. A group of vitellogenic and post-vitellogenic stage fish was transferred to high-calcium water (Ca, 0.4 mM) for 7 days for *in vivo* and *in vitro* experiments. Reproductive cycle and the method of categorization of different follicles in the ovary of *C. carpio* to different stages have been reported previously (Mukherjee et. al., 2006). To state briefly, during the months of September and October in the plains of West Bengal, India, ovary of female carp comprises mostly vitellogenic follicles (0.3 - 0.4 mm diameter) with oocytes containing centrally located germinal vesicle (GV). The cytoplasm was filled up with yolk granules and cortical granules were shown to cover the entire oocyte. In the month of November, ovaries mostly contain post-vitellogenic follicles (0.5 - 0.7 mm diameter) in which the oocytes were found to initiate coalescence of lipid droplets around a centrally located GV. Follicular developmental stage was determined by stripping out few follicles through the ovipore followed by examination under microscope after fixing them with a clearing solution of acetic acid-ethanol-formalin mixture (1: 6: 3 v/v) for 12 h.

4.3.2 Effects of sCT on plasma 17β-estradiol levels in vitellogenic stage fish

Vitellogenic stage *C. carpio* after maintaining seven days in high-Ca water were divided into two groups and following *in vivo* experiments were conducted: One group of fish received a single i.p injection of increasing concentration of sCT in such a way that each fish received

0.1, 0.5, 1.0 or 2.0 μg sCT/ 100 g body wt. Controls were injected with similar volume of solvent. Sampling of fish was done at 8 h after injection. Fish were lightly anaesthetized with MS222 before treatment. The second group of fish was given a single injection of sCT (0.5μg /100 g body wt) or hCG (0.5μg /100 g body wt) or hCG plus sCT at 07.00 h in the morning. Controls were injected with similar volume of solvent. Fish were sampled at 0, 2, 4, 8, 12, 16 and 24 h after injection. In both the experiments, immediately after sampling, blood was collected from caudal vein of the fish under light anesthesia and processed for plasma separation and kept at -20 °C until steroid analysis.

4.3.3 *In vitro* incubation of ovarian follicles

Vitellogenic and post-vitellogenic follicles after collection from the ovaries of respective stage fish were placed in ice-cold Idler's medium containing streptomycin (100 μg/ml) and penicillin (100 IU/ml) adjusted to pH 7.4 (Mukherjee et al., 2006). Follicles, after collection, were kept separately in ice-cold medium until use. Follicles weighing approximately 100 mg were initially placed in individual well of a 24-well culture plate (Tarson, India) for 2 h that contained 1.0 ml control medium. After 2 h, the medium was replaced by fresh medium containing effectors. Cultures were placed in a metabolic shaker bath at 23 ± 1°C under air. Viability of ovarian follicles was observed to be about 90% as detected using 0.1% Trypan blue dye exclusion. At the end of incubation, medium samples were aspirated, centrifuged (5000x g) and stored at - 20 °C for E_2 and 17, 20β-P measurement by specific RIA. The follicles were fixed for 12 h in clearing solution as mentioned and oocyte maturation was examined by scoring germinal vesicle breakdown (GVBD) under microscope (Bhattacharyya et. al., 2000).

4.3.4 RNA isolation, cDNA preparation and Reverse Transcriptase Polymerase Chain Reaction

Total RNA was extracted from isolated vitellogenic ovarian follicles using TRI reagent solution following the manufacturer's instruction and method described earlier (Chomzynski and Sacchi, 1987) and cDNA was synthesized using Smart-PCR cDNA synthesis kit. First strand cDNA synthesis was carried out with 2 μg total RNA and RT-PCR was performed following the procedure described early (Paul et al., 2008). The RT-PCR products were cloned, sequenced and used for the expression purpose. The primers (used for RT-PCR) of the respective genes with the accession number and their amplified segments are listed Table 1.

Gene product	Forward primer	Reverse primer	Size of amplicon (bp)
CYP19A (cytochrome P450 aromatase; DQ534411)	5′ TACACATTCTGGAGAGTTTTATCA 3′	5′ GGAAGTTGTCTAGACTGAACTCAT 3′	198
GAPDH (AJ870982)	5′ AGGGGCTCAGTATGTTGTGG 3′	5′ AGGAGGCATTGCTGACAACT 3′	185

Table 1. Primers used in semi-quantitative polymerase chain reaction

4.3.5 Preparation of oocyte membrane for sCT binding assay

Membrane from ovarian follicles was prepared using the method described previously (Mukherjee et al., 1994; Paul et al., 2008). Protein content of the preparation was measured according to the method of Lowry et al., (1951) using BSA as standard. Salmon CT binding assay was conducted following the procedure described early (Mukherjee et al., 1994; Paul et al., 2008). In brief, for [^{125}I]-sCT binding, membrane preparation (2.0 mg protein) was incubated with 20 µl [^{125}I]/-sCT solution (1x10^5 c.p.m.) in the absence (total binding) or presence of a 1000-fold excess of unlabelled sCT to measure nonspecific binding in a final assay volume of 500 µl at 23 °C. Incubation was terminated at 90 min by addition of γ globulin (0-1% v/v) or NaCl (0.1mol/L). Ice cold polyethylene glycol (PEG; 1 ml, 20% v/v) was then added to each tube. The final pellet was counted in a [^{125}I] gamma counter. Specific binding was estimated by subtracting non-specific binding from total binding.

4.3.6 Extraction and assay of steroids

The method of extraction and assay of E_2 and 17, 20β-P was similar to the previously described procedure for these steroids (Mukherjee et al., 2001, 2006).

4.3.7 Statistical analysis

Data were statistically analyzed by analysis of variance (ANOVA) followed by Duncan's multiple range test for experiments on calcium ion regulation and Bonferroni's multiple comparison tests for reproduction. Differences were considered significant at $p< 0.05$ and $p< 0.01$ as indicated in the text. Comparisons between sexually immature and mature fish were performed with student's t-test.

5. Results

5.1 Calcium ion regulation

5.1.1 Effects of sCT and UBG extract on calcium ion regulation

A single injection of sCT to sexually mature fish, kept in normal tap water (Fig. 1 A) or in low-Ca water (Fig. 1 B) reduced ultrafiltrable plasma calcium content within 2 h with a maximum at 4 h (p<0.01). This hypocalcemic effect was continued up to 8 h. There was no change between sham-control and saline-control group. Since there was significant short-duration hypocalcemic effect of sCT in sexually mature fish kept both in normal tap water and low-Ca water, an attempt has been made to examine whether the interference of endogenous sex steroid (s) was responsible. It is evident from a similar experiment with sexually immature fish kept in normal tap water (Fig. 1 C) and low-Ca water (Fig. 1 D) that a single injection of sCT was highly effective in reducing plasma calcium fraction within 2 to 8 h with a maximum at 4 h (p< 0.01). No changes in plasma calcium levels were noticed between sham- and saline-control groups. While comparing the degree of inhibitory response after 4 h of sCT injection, the immature fish was shown to be more responsive than mature fish.
Dose-response effect of sCT on plasma calcium was conducted with sexually immature fish kept in normal tap water and low-Ca water. Figure 2 A demonstrate that at increasing doses of sCT, a gradual and significant (p<0.01) reduction in plasma calcium fraction was recorded with a maximum at 0.5 µg dose in fish kept both in normal tap water and low-Ca water. Effects of repeated doses of sCT on plasma calcium levels were examined with sexually immature fish kept in low-Ca water and compared with the effects produced after single injection. Results in Fig. 2 B clearly shows that daily injection of sCT (0.5 µg/100g body wt) for 15 days caused significant reduction (p<0.01) in plasma calcium fraction as compared to saline control and the rate of inhibition was almost identical with that registered after single injection.

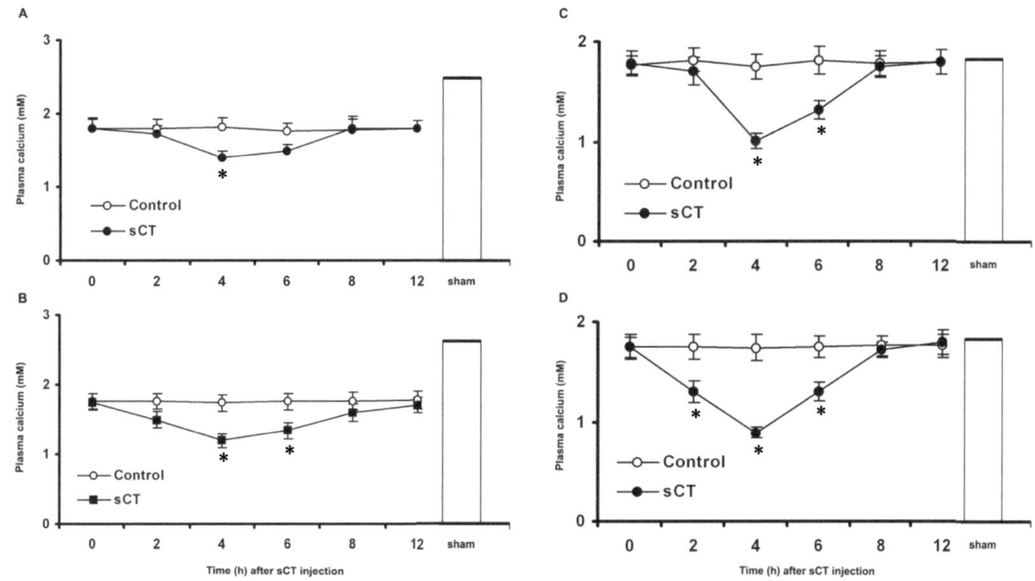

Fig. 1. Plasma calcium levels of sexually mature *Cyprinus carpio* kept in normal tap water (A) or low-Ca water (B) and immature fish kept in normal tap water (C) and low-Ca water (D) after a single sCT injection (0.5 µg/ 100 g body wt.). Data presented as mean ± SEM of five observations from five different fishes. [Asterisks significantly (p<0.01) different from those shown for sham- and saline control (ANOVA, Duncan's multiple range test).]

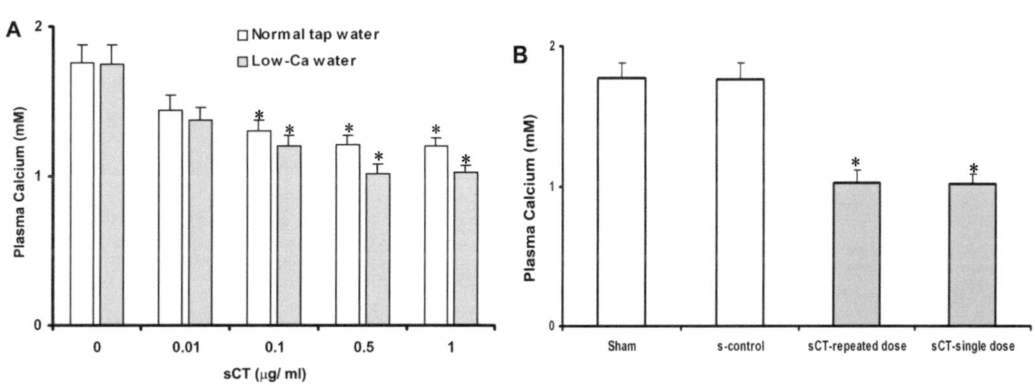

Fig. 2. Dose-response effects of SCT on plasma calcium levels of sexually immature fish kept in normal tap water or in low-Ca water (A) and of immature fish kept in low-Ca water (B) after daily injection of SCT (0.5 µg/ 100 g body wt.) or saline for 15 days. Fish were sacrificed at 4 h after last injection. Each value represents the ± SEM of five observations. Values were compared with those shown after single injection of SCT (B, 0.5 µg/ 100 g body wt.). [Asterisk indicates significant difference at p<0.01 from vehicle injected control. (ANOVA, Duncan's multiple range test).]

Results of the effects of homologous UBG extract on plasma calcium levels are depicted in Fig 3A and B. It appears from the Figure that UBG extract at the dose 0.5 UBG eq. /100 g body wt caused significant ($p<0.01$) reduction in plasma calcium levels at 4 h after injection both in normal tap water and low-Ca water adapted fish. Dose-response study to observe the effects of UBG extract was conducted in fish adapted only in low-Ca water. Fig. 3 C shows that UBG extract at increasing doses caused a gradual and significant reduction ($p<0.05$) in plasma calcium levels with a maximum at 0.5 UBG eq/100 g body wt.

5.1.2 Effects of sCT on gill-calcium transport (GCAT)

Results of the time-course tracer uptake study in response to sCT are depicted in Fig. 4. It is evident from the figure that a single injection of sCT (0.5 μg/100g body wt) to fingerlings, kept either in normal tap water (Fig. 4 A) and low-Ca water (Fig. 4 B) significantly ($p<0.05$) reduced GCAT between 2 to 6 h with a maximum at 4 h compared to their saline controls. No apparent changes in GCAT were noticed between sham-control and saline-control groups. Fig. 4 C depicts that reduction of GCAT was recorded at the dose of 0.1 μg sCT with a maximum at 0.5 μg sCT /100 g body wt compared to their respective control values. Here also no changes were observed between saline control group and sham control group.

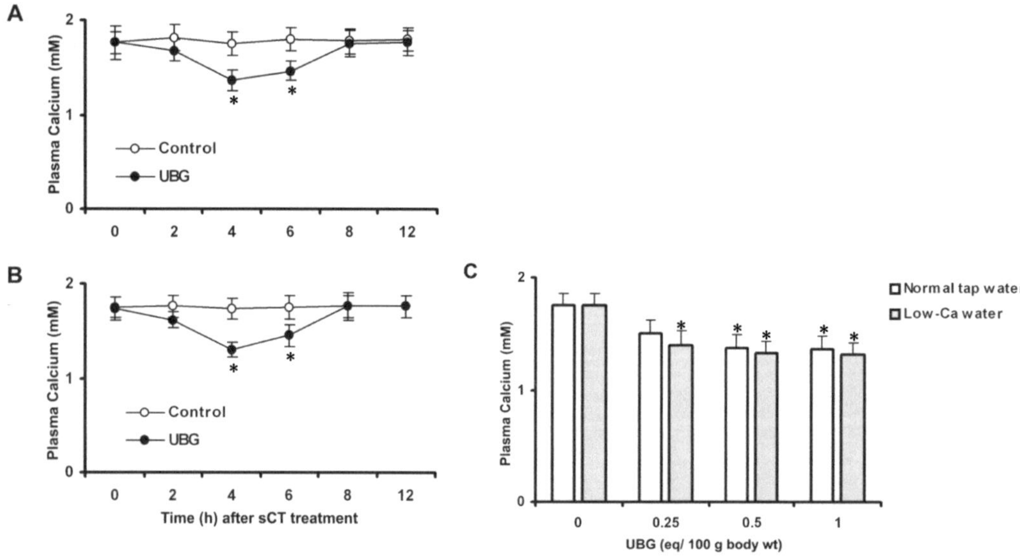

Fig. 3. Time course effects of UBG extracts on plasma calcium levels of sexually immature fish kept in normal tap water (A) or low Ca water (B). Dose response effects of UBG extracts on plasma calcium levels of sexually immature fish kept in normal tap water or low Ca water (C). Fish was sacrificed 4 h after last injection. Each value represents the mean ± SEM of five specimens. [Asterisk indicates significant difference at $p<0.05$ from sham, and saline injected control.]

It is evident that a single injection of sCT (0.5 μg/100 g body wt) to sexually immature fish, kept in normal tap water (Fig. 5 A) or in low-Ca water (Fig. 5 B) was able to reduce GCAT significantly ($p<0.05$) between 2 to 6 h with a maximum at 4 h, compared to saline control group. Beyond 6 h, inhibitory effects of sCT on GCAT were absent.

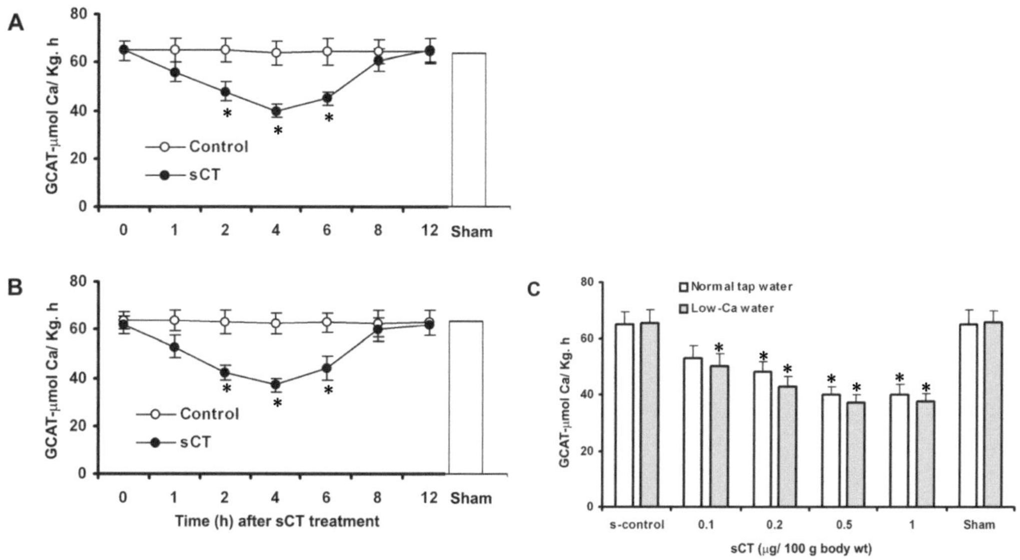

Fig. 4. Time-course study of the inhibition of gill Ca^{+2} transport (GCAT) in fingerlings of *C. carpio,* kept in normal tap water (A) or low-Ca water (B) after a single injection of sCT (0.5 μg/ 100 g body wt.). Dose response effects sCT on inhibition of GCAT in fingerlings kept either in normal tap water or low-Ca water (C). Values are mean of six fingerlings. [Asterisk indicates significantly (p<0.05) low value from these shown for sham and saline control (ANOVA, Duncan's multiple range test)]

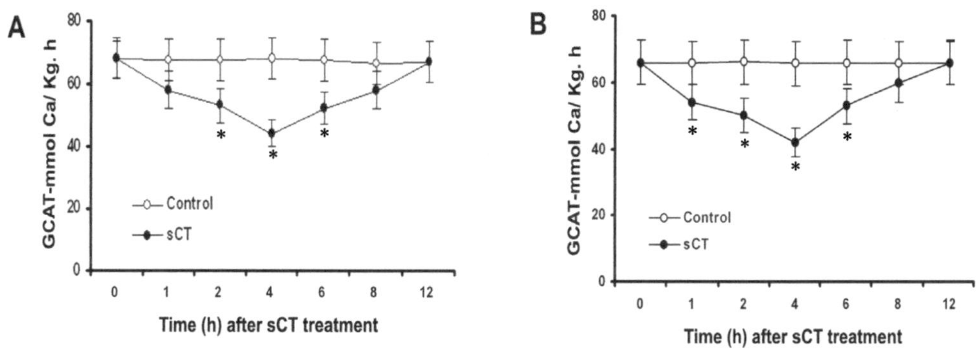

Fig. 5. Time-course study of the inhibition of gill Ca^{+2} transport (GCAT) in immature *C. carpio,* kept in normal tap water (A) or low-Ca water (B) after a single injection of sCT (0.5 μg/ 100 g body wt.). Values are mean of six fingerlings. Asterisk indicates significantly (P<0.05) low value from these shown for sham and saline control (ANOVA, Duncan's multiple range test).

5.1.3 Effects of sCT on plasma TRACP and ALP activities and urinary HYP content – a time-course and dose- response study

Since no differences were obtained between low-Ca water and normal tap water adapted fish in lowering plasma calcium levels and lowering GCAT after CT treatment, changes of plasma TRACP and ALP activities and excretion of urinary HYP in response to sCT was observed in fish adapted to normal tap water. A single injection of sCT to sexually immature fish kept in normal tap water was able to suppress both TRACP and ALP activities in plasma and HYP excretion in urine. Salmon CT-induced suppression of TRACP and ALP activities and reduction in urinary HYP extracts were noticed as early as 2 h and reached the lowest values ($p < 0.01$) at 4 h after treatment (Fig. 6 A, B and C). No changes in the activities of TRACP and ALP and excretion of urinary HYP were observed between sham-control and saline group.

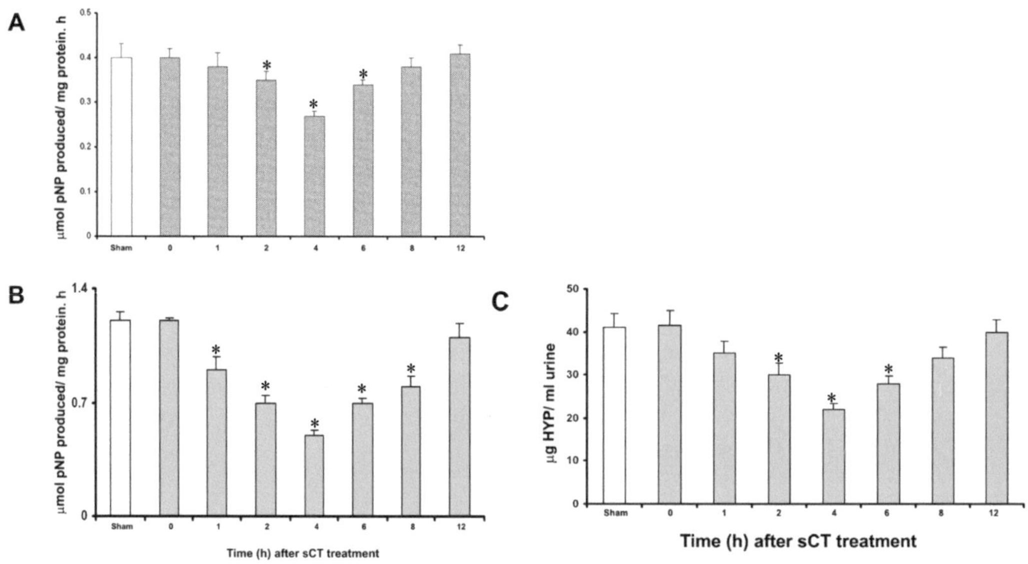

Fig. 6. Effects of sCT (0.5 µg/ 100 g body wt) and vehicle on TRACP (A) and ALP (B) activities in plasma and HYP (C) content in urine in sexually immature fish kept in normal tap water. Values of (A) and (B) are means of five specimens and (C) is of four observations. For each observation urine samples from three individual fish were pooled. [Asterisk indicates significant difference at $p<0.01$ from vehicle-injected control (ANOVA, Duncan's multiple range test)].

Result of increasing concentration of sCT administration to sexually immature fish is shown in Fig. 7. At a very low concentration (0.01µg /100 body wt) sCT was able to suppress plasma TRACP and ALP activities (Fig. 7 A and B) as well as urinary HYP excretion (Fig. 7 C). Increasing doses suppressed activities of both the enzymes and urinary HYP content gradually with a maximum ($p < 0.01$) at the dose 0.5 µg sCT/100g body wt.

Results of plasma TRACP and ALP activities and excretion of urinary HYP and calcium content of skeletal bone of sCT-, treated and -untreated fish are depicted in Fig. 8. It appears from the figure that daily injection of sCT for 15 days to sexually immature fish kept in normal tap water caused significant suppression ($p<0.01$) of the activities of both the enzymes in plasma and HYP content in the urine (Fig. 8 A, B and C). On the other hand, there was a significant increase ($p<0.01$) in the calcium content of skeletal bones of sCT-injected fish compared to control values (Fig. 8 D).

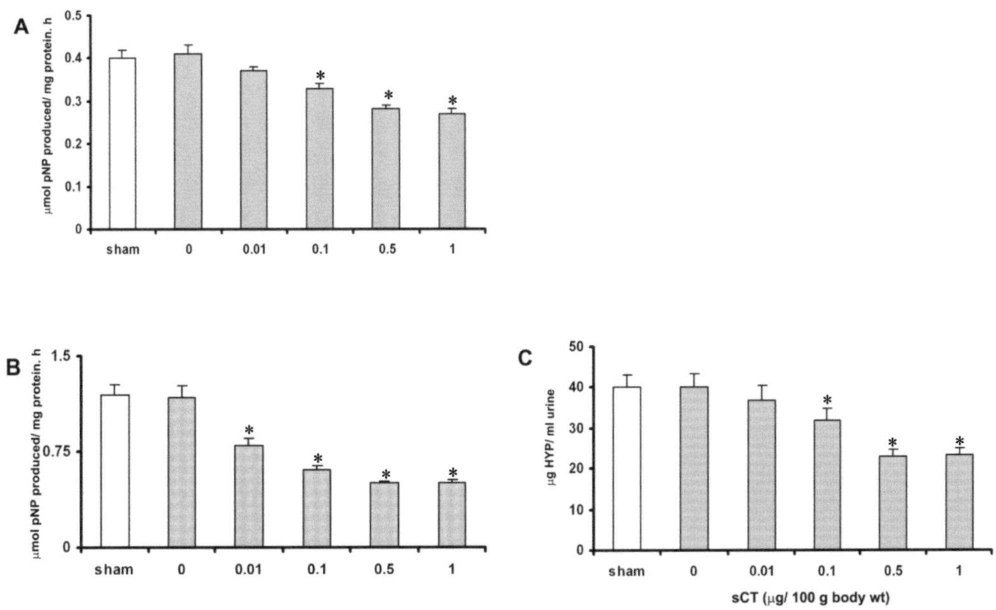

Fig. 7. Effects of increasing doses of sCT on TRACP (A) and ALP activities in plasma and HYP (C) content in urine in sexually immature fish kept in normal tap water. Each value of TRACP and ALP represents ± SEM of five specimens and HYP of four observations. [Asterisk indicates significant difference at $p<0.01$ from sham and saline control (ANOVA, Duncan's multiple range test)].

5.2 Effects of sCT on 17β-estradiol production by the vitellogenic follicles

5.2.1 Plasma 17β-estradiol levels in response to sCT and HCG

Results shown in Fig. 9 A demonstrates that sCT at increasing doses caused a gradual increase in plasma E_2 levels in carp, 8 h after injection. The maximum effective dose of sCT was 0.5 µg/ 100g body wt. The minimum dose at which sCT was able to induce increase in plasma E_2 levels was 0.1 µg. Injection of solvent did not alter the level of plasma E_2 in fish (Fig. 9 B). Injection of hCG (0.5 µg/ 100 g body wt) stimulated E_2 secretion and highest plasma concentrations of this steroid was recorded at 12 h (Fig. 9 B). Injection of hCG plus sCT (each 0.5 µg /100g body wt) resulted in a significantly ($p<0.05$) higher level of plasma E_2 at 8 h and 12 h after challenge compared with that induced by hCG alone (Fig. 9 B). Mean levels of ultrafiltrable plasma calcium in vitellogenic stage fish at all time points were 1.6 ± 0.17 mM, 1.6 ± 0.16 mM and 1.65 ± 0.17 mM respectively for the vehicle-, hCG- and sCT-injected group.

5.2.2 sCT binding to fish ovarian tissue

Fig. 10 shows that with increasing concentrations of [^{125}I] sCT, the specific binding increases until 2 nM and then saturation was reached. Scatchard plot analysis of the data (inset of Fig. 10) showed that Bmax (MBC) of ovarian follicular membrane preparation for [^{125} I] sCT was 1.2 pM/mg protein and *Kd* was 48.8 pM/ L.

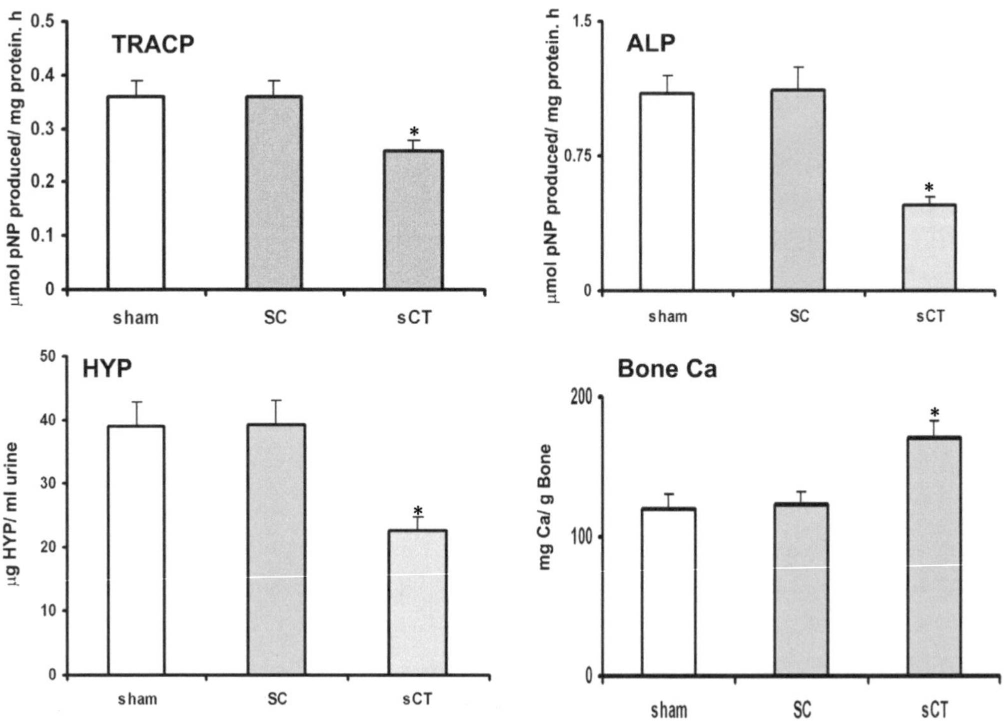

Fig. 8. Changes in plasma TRACP and ALP activities in plasma, HYP content in urine and calcium content of skeletal bones of sexually immature fish kept in normal tap water after daily injection of sCT (0.5 µg/100g body wt) for 15 days. Each value of TRACP and ALP of plasma and the bone calcium content represents the mean ± SEM of five and HYP of four observations. [Asterisk indicates significant differences (p<0.01) compared with the values in the normal control (ANOVA, Duncan's multiple range test)].

5.2.3 Effects of sCT on *in vitro* E_2 production by ovarian follicles

Since there was a significant increase in plasma E_2 levels in vitellogenic stage fish after sCT treatment, and since sCT binds with the ovarian membrane preparation with high-affinity, physiological importance of sCT binding to ovarian follicles was assessed by incubating follicles with varied concentrations of sCT with or without hCG and steroid production was measured.

The effect of sCT ranging from 25 to 200 ng /ml incubation on E_2 release by the ovarian follicles is illustrated in Fig. 11A. During a 12-h incubation, sCT at 50 ng dose released maximum quantity of E_2 in the medium (p<0.05). Incubation with increasing doses of hCG for 12 h caused a significant increase (p<0.05) of E_2 release at 25 ng dose and highest was recorded at the dose of 50 ng/ml incubation (Fig. 11 B). Ovarian follicles were incubated with sCT (0 to 100 ng/ ml) in presence of hCG (25 ng ml) for 12 h. Fig. 11 C shows that hCG-induced release of E_2 was significantly increased (p<0.05) by sCT ranging from 25 to 100 ng dose/ ml incubation. Ovarian follicles were incubated with sCT or hCG (each 50ng/ ml) for various length of time up to 16 h. It appears from Fig. 11 D that after addition of hormones, E_2 release increased steadily from 2 h and the maximum was recorded at 6 h by sCT and 12 h by hCG.

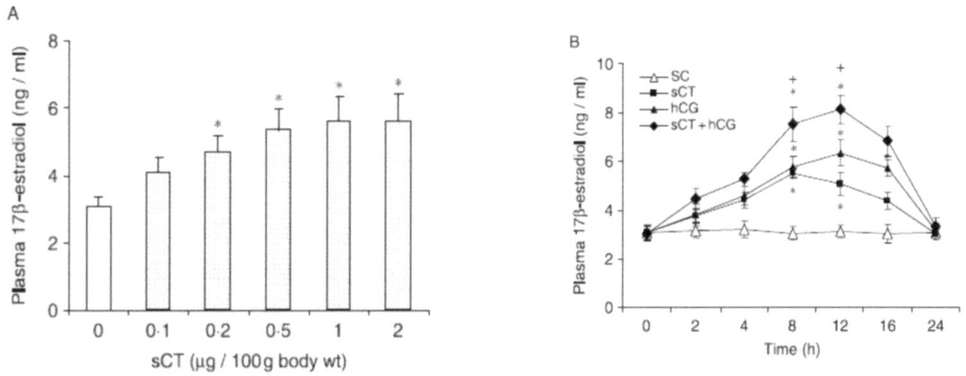

Fig. 9. Dose-response effects of sCT (A) and a time-course study on the effects of sCT (0.5 µg /100g body wt), human chorionic gonadotropin (hCG, 0.5 µg/100g body wt) and hCG + sCT (each 0.5 µg /100g body wt) (B) on plasma 17β-estradiol (E_2) levels in vitellogenic stage *C. carpio*. Fish were injected with increasing doses of sCT as indicated and sacrificed 8 h after injection (B). Fish were given a single intraperitoneal (i.p.) injection of sCT, hCG or sCT + hCG. Blood samples were collected at time indicated after hormone challenge (B). Each value (A and B) is mean ± SEM of five observations. SC, saline control, **p*< 0.05 vs. sCT at 0 µg /100g body wt, (A) + ^{+}p<0.05 vs. hCG at 0.5 µg /100g body wt (B).

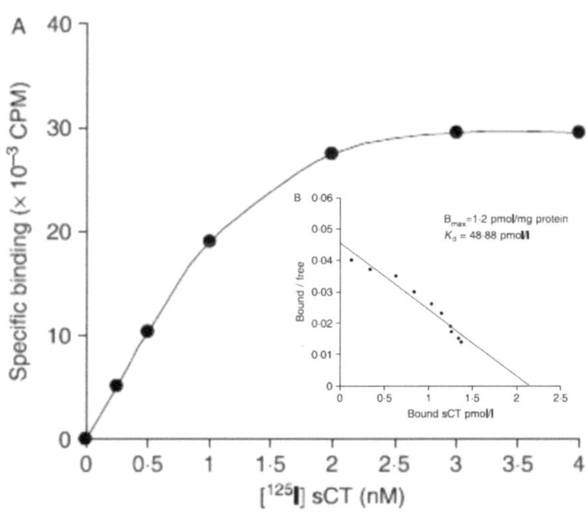

Fig. 10. Saturation curve of [^{125}I] sCT binding to membrane preparation of ovarian follicles of vitellogenic stage fish. Specific binding was determined by subtracting the nonspecific binding from the total binding. Inset shows Scatchard plot of [^{125}I] sCT binding to fish ovarian follicular membrane preparation. Values are mean ± SEM of four observations taking ovarian follicles in duplicate from four donor fish.

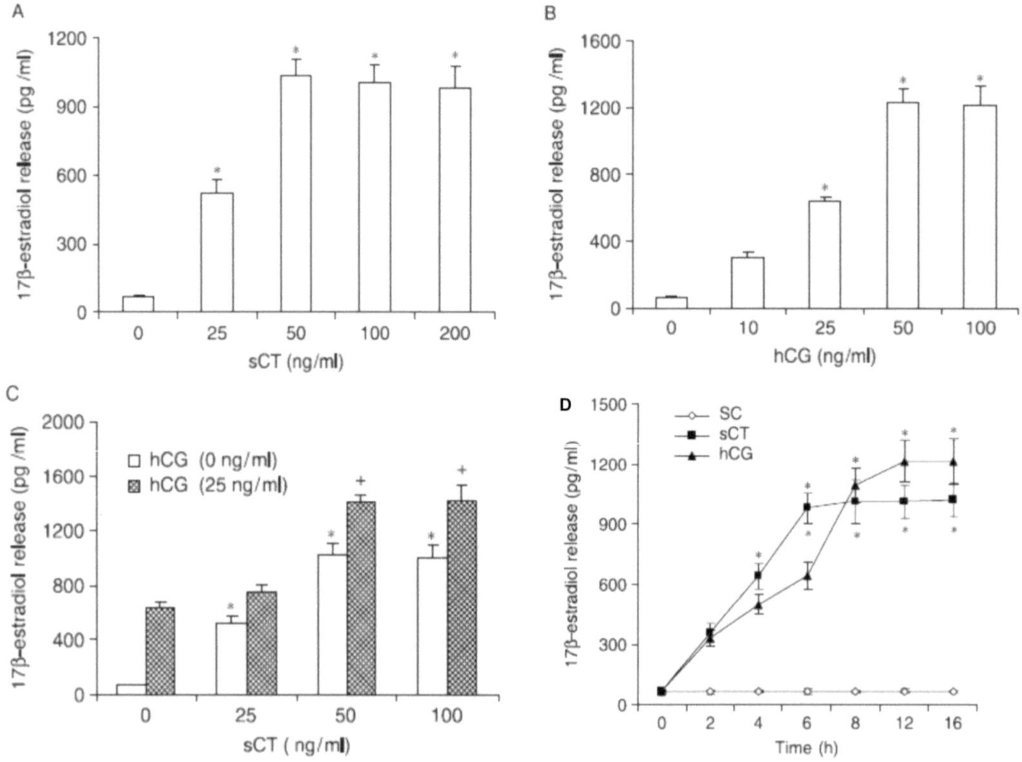

Fig. 11. Dose-response effects of sCT (A) and hCG (B) on *in vitro* production of 17β-estradiol by the vitellogenic follicles. Dose-response effects of sCT on basal (hollow bar) and hCG-stimulated (solid bar) *in vitro* production of 17β-estradiol by the vitellogenic follicles (C). Time-course effects of sCT and hCG (each 50 ng/ ml) on *in vitro* 17β-estradiol production by the vitellogenic follicles (D). All incubations (A, B and C) were terminated 12 h after addition of test compounds. Each value represents mean ± SEM of five incubations taking follicles in triplicate from five donor fish. *$p< 0.05$ vs. tissues incubated without hormone (0) (A and B), *$p<0.05$ verses hCG at 0 ng / ml (C). *$p< 0.05$ verses saline control (SC) at respective time period (D).

5.2.4 Effects of sCT on activity of P450arom

When ovarian follicles were incubated with [^{3}H] testosterone for 8 h in the presence of either sCT or hCG (each 50 ng/incubation), a significant increase ($p<0.05$) in [^{3}H]E_2 formation were noticed both in hCG and sCT administered incubations relative to their control values (Fig 12). These finding indicate that sCT-induced E_2 production in fish ovarian follicles like that of hCG was due to its stimulation of aromatase activity.

5.2.5 Effects of sCT and hCG on P450arom gene expression

Total mRNA was extracted from ovarian follicles exposed with or without sCT or hCG (each 50 ng/ml) for different time intervals and RT-PCR was performed using P450arom primer (CYP19A). Fig 13 A shows that both hCG and sCT stimulated P450arom gene expression in ovarian follicles incubated for 2 h and increased gradually and significantly (p<0.05) from 4 to 8 h. The expression of GAPDH was used as loading control (Fig. 13 B).

5.2.6 Effects of dbcAMP on sCT-stimulated E_2 release

To evaluate the role of intracellular cAMP in the regulation of E_2 release by sCT, the effects of dbcAMP and SQ22536 (a cell permeable selective adenylate cyclase inhibitor) on ovarian follicles were examined. Dibutyryl cyclic AMP at both the concentrations (0.5 mM and 1.0 mM) stimulated the release of E_2 by the ovarian follicles in a dose-dependent manner and addition of sCT (25 ng/ incubation) potentiated the effects of dbcAMP on E_2 release at all concentrations tested (Fig. 14 A). Administration of SQ22536 at increasing doses attenuated sCT-stimulated E_2 production in a concentration-dependent manner (Fig. 14 B). SQ22536 at increasing doses also gradually and significantly (p<0.05) attenuated hCG-stimulated E_2 production by the follicles (Fig. 14 C).

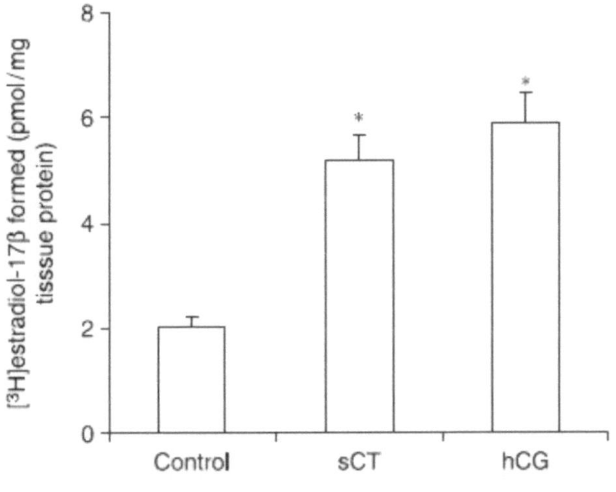

Fig. 12. Salmon CT- and hCG-stimulated conversion of $[^3H]$testosterone to $[^3H]$estradiol-17β in vitellogenic follicles. Follicles were incubated in the presence of $[^3H]$testosterone ($1x10^6$ c.p.m, 140 mmol) without or with sCT or hCG for 8 h. Each value is the mean ± SEM of five incubations taking follicles in triplicate from five donor fish). *p< 0.05 vs. saline control.

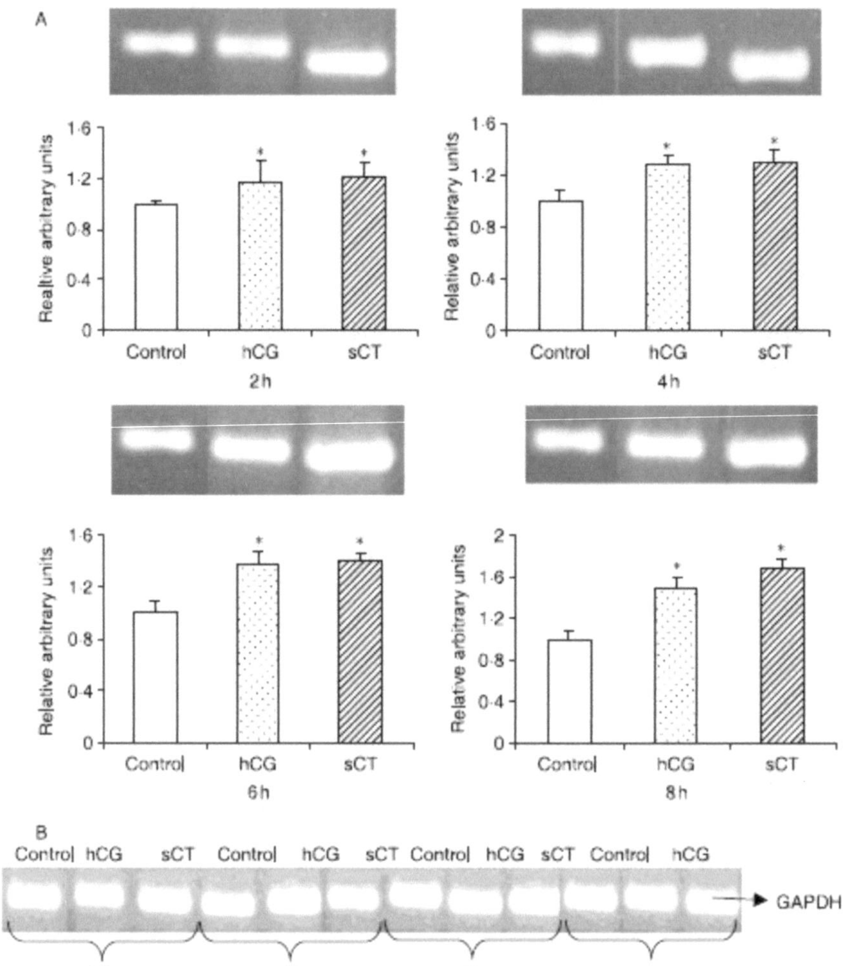

Fig. 13. Effect of hCG and sCT on the expression of P450arom mRNA in vitellogenic ovarian follicles. Follicles were incubated for 2, 4, 6 and 8 h without or with sCT or hCG (each 50 ng / ml). Total RNA was isolated from ovarian follicles and RT-PCR was performed using CYP19A gene specific primer. Amplified product was loaded in agarose gel as control, sCT and hCG treated samples. The pixel densities of the bands were quantified with ImageJ software[National Institute of Health (NIH)] and have been represented in bar diagram as relative arbitrary units considering the control value as 1 (A). The expression of GAPDH was used as a loading control (B). The experiments were performed three times in duplicate, and the values are mean ± SEM, * $p<0.05$.

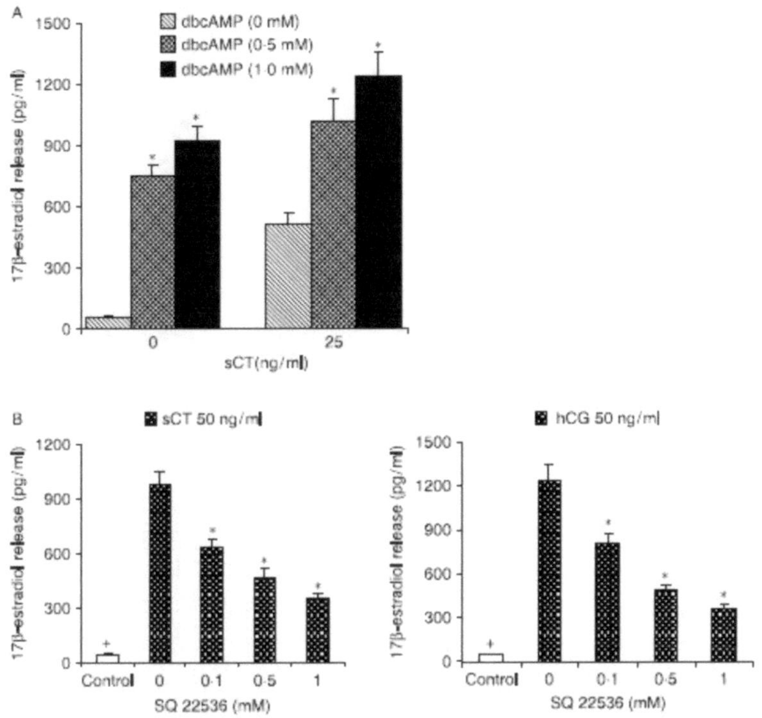

Fig. 14. Effects of sCT on *in vitro* production of 17β-estradiol by the vitellogenic ovarian follicles in absence (hatched bar) or presence of 0.5 mM (cross hatched bar) and 1.0 mM (solid bar) dbcAMP (A). Effects of SQ22536, a selective inhibitor of adenylate cyclase, on sCT- and hCG-stimulated *in vitro* 17β-estradiol production by the ovarian follicles (B). Ovarian follicles were incubated in the absence (control) or presence of sCT or hCG with increasing doses of SQ22536 for 12 h. Each value represents ± SEM of five incubations taking follicles in triplicate from five donor fish. (**p*< 0.05 vs. sCT corresponding control group. **p*<0.05 vs. hormone alone. +*p*<0.05 from those shown for tissues incubated with hormone alone).

5.2.7 Effects of PKC inhibitor on sCT- stimulated E_2 production

To ascertain the involvement of protein kinase C in the regulation of E_2 release by sCT, the effects of NPC-15437 dihydrochloride, a selective protein kinase C inhibitor, was examined. NPC-15437 at all concentration tested (0.1 mM to 1.0 mM) failed to attenuate sCT stimulated E_2 release in the medium (Fig. 15 A). PKC inhibitor, however attenuated hCG-stimulated E_2 release in a concentration-dependent manner (Fig 15 B; $p<0.05$).

5.2.8 Effects of sCT on 17, 20β-P production *in vitro*

Experiments were conducted to observe whether sCT is able to stimulate 17, 20β-P production *in vitro* in post-vitellogenic ovarian follicles of *C. carpio*. It appears from Fig. 16 A that sCT at increasing concentration during 24 h incubation was able to induce production of 17, 20β-P in a dose-dependent manner with a maximum at the dose 50 ng/ml. Higher doses over 50 ng/ml had no additive effect. hCG at increasing doses also produced 17, 20β-P almost in a dose-dependent manner with a maximum at the dose of 50 ng/ml (Fig. 16 B). In the next experiment, ovarian follicles were incubated with sCT (0-100 ng/ml) in presence

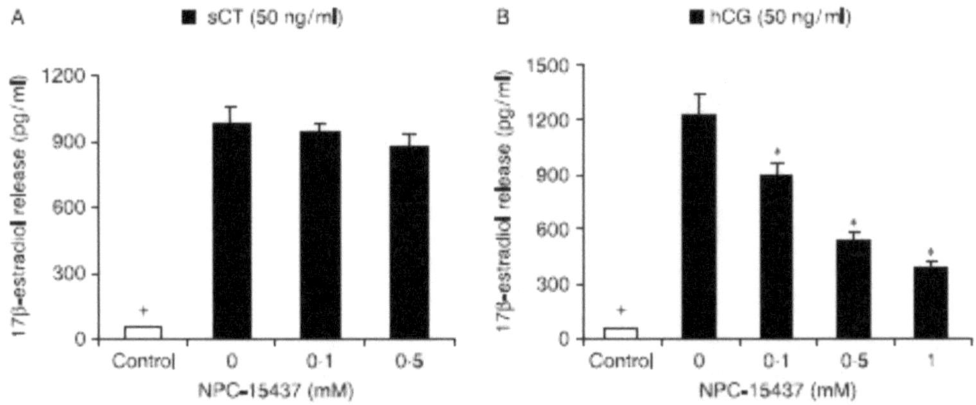

Fig. 15. Effects of NPC-15437 dihydrochloride, a selective inhibitor of PKC, on sCT- (A) and hCG-stimulated (B) *in vitro* production of 17β-estradiol by the ovarian follicles of *C. carpio*. Ovarian follicles were incubated in the absence (control) or presence of sCT or hCG with increasing doses of NPC-15437 dihydrochloride for 12 h. Each point represents mean ± SEM of five incubations, taking follicles in triplicate from five donor fish. (*$p < 0.05$ vs. hormone alone. +$p<0.05$ from those shown for tissues incubated with hormone alone).

of HCG (25 ng /ml) for 24 h and results depicted in Fig. 16 C shows that HCG-stimulated 17, 20β-P production was significantly increased ($p<0.05$) by sCT ranging from 25-100 ng dose/ml incubation. Ovarian follicles were incubated with sCT and hCG for various length of time up to 24 h. It appears from Fig. 17 that after addition of hormones, 17, 20β-P production increased steadily from 6 h and maximum was recorded at 16 h by sCT and hCG.

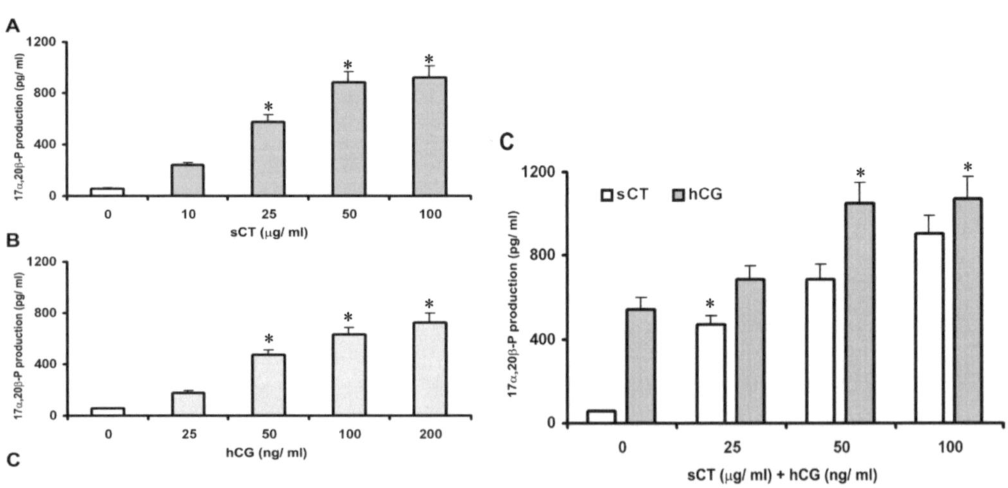

Fig. 16. Dose-response effects of sCT (A) and hCG (B) on *in vitro* production of 17, 20β-P by the post-vitellogenic follicles. Dose-response effects of sCT on basal (hollow bar) and hCG-stimulated (solid bar) *in vitro* production of 17, 20β-P by the follicles (C). All incubations were terminated 24 h after addition of test compounds. Each value represents mean ± SEM of five incubations, taking follicles in triplicate from five donor fish. (*$p < 0.05$ vs tissues incubated without hormone (0) (A and B), *$p < 0.05$ vs sCT at 0 ng /ml and *$p<0.05$ vs hCG at 0 ng /ml; C).

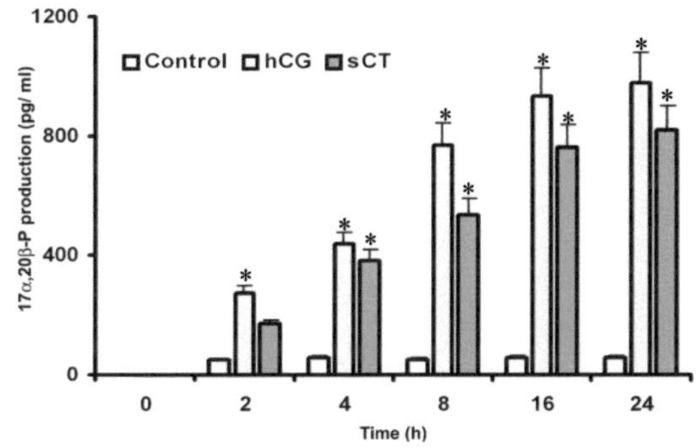

Fig. 17. Time-course effects of sCT and HCG (each at 50 ng/ml) on *in vitro* production of 17, 20β-P by the post-vitellogenic follicles. Each value represents ± SEM of five incubations taking follicles in triplicate from five donor fish. [*$p < 0.05$ vs tissues incubated without hormone (0)].

5.3 Effects of sCT on oocyte maturation

Experiments were also conducted to ascertain whether sCT can induce oocyte maturation in fish. For this, both intact follicles and denuded oocytes were incubated with test compounds. Increasing concentrations of either hCG (0-100 ng/ml) or sCT (10-100 ng /ml) for 24 h resulted induction of GVBD in intact follicles almost in a dose-response manner with maximum induction at the dose of 50 ng hCG/ml and 100 ng sCT/ml (Fig. 18 A, B). Higher doses had no additive effects in the induction of GVBD. Time-course effects of sCT and hCG on induction of GVBD shows that maximum induction of GVBD was recorded after 16 h after hormone treatments (Fig. 19). Interestingly, almost similar effects of sCT on GVBD induction was recorded in fully denuded oocyte with increasing concentrations of only sCT after 16 h incubation (Fig. 20). hCG had no effect on GVBD induction in fully denuded oocytes (data not shown).

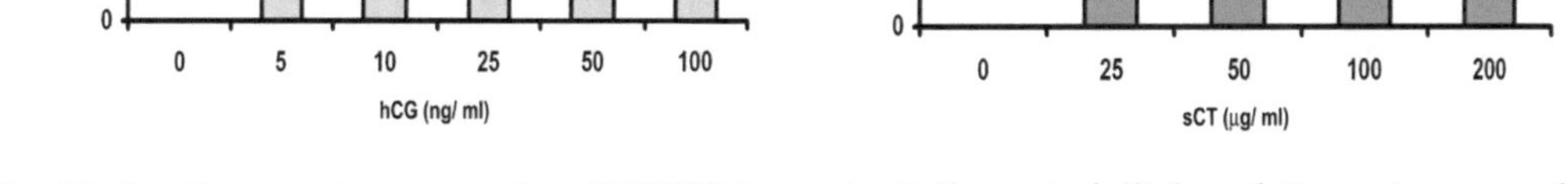

Fig. 18. *In vitro* oocyte maturation (GVBD) in post-vitellogenic follicles of *C. carpio* exposed to graded doses of hCG (A) and SCT (B) for 24 h. Each point represents mean of five incubations taking follicles from five donor fish. [Asterisks denote values significantly (p<0.05) different from those shown for tissue incubated without hormone (0)].

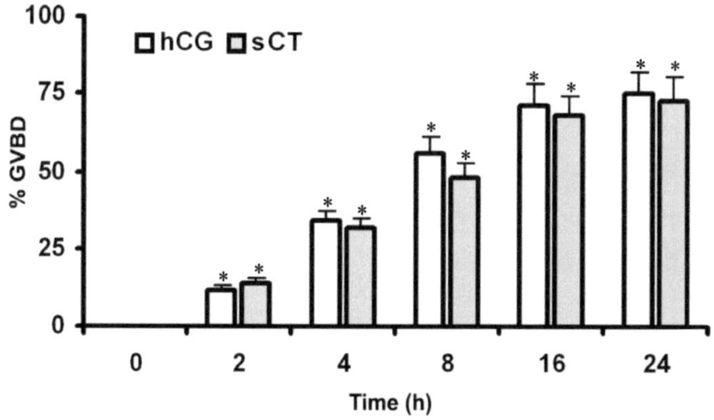

Fig. 19. Time-course effects of sCT (100 ng/ml) and hCG (50 ng/ml) on oocyte maturation in post-vitellogenic ovarian follicles. Each point represents the mean of five incubations taking follicles from five donor fish. [Asterisks denote values significantly (p<0.05) different from those shown for tissue incubated without hormone (0).]

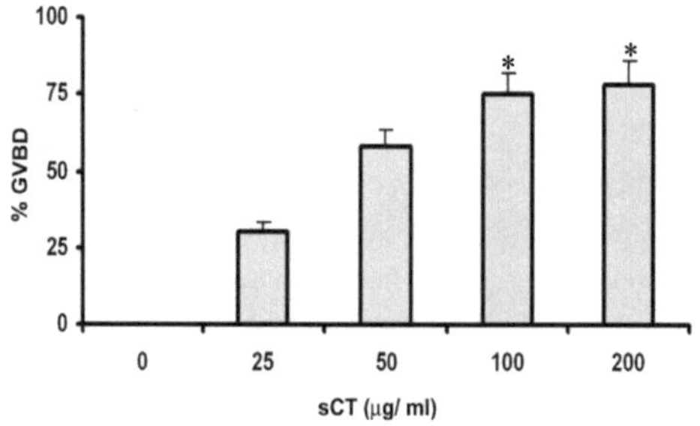

Fig. 20. Percent GVBD in denuded oocyte of post-vitellogenic follicles exposed to graded doses of sCT for 24 h. Each point represents the mean of five incubations taking follicles from five donor fish. [Asterisks denote values significantly (p<0.05) different from those shown for tissue incubation without hormone (0)].

6. Discussion

The present study demonstrate that administration of sCT and homologous UBG extract to sexually mature and immature *C. carpio* caused hypocalcemia within few hours. Salmon CT is capable of inhibiting both gill-Ca^{2+} transport (GCAT) and bone calcium resorption *in vivo* in this fish and the inhibitions were dose-, and time-related. We further described that carp ovarian follicles are equipped with CT receptors and demonstrated that administration of sCT to carp at vitellogenic stage significantly stimulated spontaneous and hCG-induced secretion of E_2 *in vivo* and *in vitro*. We also reported that sCT stimulated both aromatase activity and P450arom (CYP19A) gene expression and stimulatory action of sCT on ovarian E_2 secretion was mediated through cAMP pathway. In addition, sCT also stimulated 17, 20β-P (maturation inducing hormone of this fish) production *in vitro*. The most interesting aspect of this study was that sCT can induce carp oocyte maturation independent of MIH.

Calcitonin-induced short-duration reduction in plasma calcium levels in carp is in full agreement with earlier observations with some fresh water teleosts (Chan et al., 1968; Lopez et al., 1976; Wendelaar-Bonga, 1981; Chakraborti and Mukherjee 1993; Srivastava et al., 1998; Mukherjee et al., 2004a, b), marine bony fish (Glowacki et al., 1985) and elasmobranch *Dasyatis akajei* (Srivastava et al., 1998). Ultimobranchial gland of fish is a rich source of CT. In our present study we used crude extract of homologous UBG extract and observed good hypocalcemic potency. Since, the content of CT in UBG extract was not estimated; findings could only suggest effectiveness of native UBG extract of carp as a hypocalcemic factor and warrant further investigation on the nature and quantity of hypocalcemic factor present in UBG of this fish.

The present study demonstrates that sCT is capable of inhibiting gill Ca^{2+} transport (GCAT) *in vivo* in carp. This observation is in agreement with earlier studies on some other teleosts and also on carp (Wagner et al., 1997; Mukherjee et al., 2004 a). We, in our earlier studies and also in the present study observed that hypocalcemic effect of sCT is to be dependent on the levels of dissolved calcium in the surrounding water; in the sense that greater effects are observed if the fish are maintained in low-Ca water (Chakraborti and Mukherjee 1993; Mukherjee et al., 2004 a, b), findings that directly implicate the gills and changes in GCAT as an integral part of the response. Urist (1976) reported that teleosts have the ability to absorb most of the calcium from environment through gills. Salmon CT is reported to contribute to the calcium homeostasis in salmon and eel by preventing gill calcium influx (Milhaud et al., 1977; Milet et al., 1979). Wagner and his co-workers in 1997, considering whole body calcium uptake as a reliable indicator of GCAT, showed that sCT can inhibit GCAT in young rainbow trout. Our findings clearly indicate a dose- and time-related action of sCT in the inhibition of GCAT both in fingerlings and immature fish and this has been correlated with lowering of plasma calcium under identical situations. The dose and time required to produce maximum inhibition of GCAT as well as lowering plasma calcium levels in mature and immature fish was 0.5 μg/100 g body wt and 4 h respectively. In our study the estimated ED50 value for CT to evoke inhibition of GCAT and reduction of plasma calcium levels were ≈ 0.12 μg/100 g body wt). This value seems to be high as compared to the normal circulatory levels of CT in other teleosts studied (5 – 15 ng/ml) (Deftos et al., 1974; Sasayama et al., 1996). To get an exact idea of the pharmacological dose required for CT function in this fish, plasma CT value needs to be evaluated.

In the present study, tracer uptake rate in untreated fish has been found to be almost constant from 1 to 12 h indicating an efficient and steady-state maintenance of calcium homeostasis by the endogenous hormone (s), which may be either CT or STC or both. In CT-treated fish, a gradual inhibition of GCAT started from 1 h and achieved a maximum at 4 h irrespective of age and maturity. Such a short-duration inhibitory responses of this fish to sCT might be due to rapid metabolism of this hormone in fish blood. Similar short-duration GCAT inhibitory response of CT has been reported in young rainbow trout (Wagner et. al., 1997).

Calcitonin-induced tracer uptake in our study could not be attributed to changes in the intestinal absorption of ^{45}Ca, as fish were not fed during experiment and gut content of all the fish were excluded. Even externally bounded ^{45}Ca in fish was also removed. The present study therefore indicates that calcium measured in the fingerlings or sexually immature fish was the calcium uptake through gills. In our previous study (Chakraborti and Mukherjee 1993, Mukherjee et al., 2004 a) and also in the present study it has been shown that CT is more hypocalcemic when kept in either normal tap water or low-Ca water, than fish kept in high-Ca water. The findings therefore indicate an anti-hypercalcemic role of CT in this fish and suggest that GCAT is an integral part of this response to CT. GCAT inhibitory response in this fish in the present study seemed to be independent of age, since both fingerlings and sexually immature fish showed similar response. It may therefore be concluded that salmon CT is a potent inhibitor of GCAT in fresh water teleost *C. carpio* adapted to both low-Ca water and normal tap water and fish adapted to both the calcium environment are equally responsive to calcium regulating hormone.

In the present study using sexually immature and mature female fish, we observed a significant dose- and time-dependent suppression of plasma tartrate-resistant acid phosphatase (TRACP) and alkaline phosphatase (ALP) activities and excretion of urinary hydroxyproline (HYP) after a single injection of varied doses of sCT. It is known that in mammals TRACP is secreted by the osteoclasts in to serum and blood TRACP activity measurement is often used as a marker of bone resorption (Raisz et al., 1998). Collagen degradation in bone releases HYP in to circulation. As bone resorption is by far the largest contributor of collagen breakdown, urinary HYP excretion has also been considered as a measure of bone resorption (Raisz et al., 1998). In mammals, CT exerts its control on serum calcium and phosphate by inhibiting bone resorption and thus decreasing the loss of calcium from bone (Raisz et al., 1998). In our previous study with a fresh water air-breathing teleost, *Channa punctatus*, we reported significant suppression of plasma TRACP and urinary HYP after sCT treatment and suggested that like mammals, in *C .punctatus*, CT exerts its hypocalmecic function through bone Ca resorption (Mukherjee et al., 2004 b) and this was the first report of the action of CT through bone calcium resorption in any fresh water teleost. Our present study using sexually immature and mature carp also demonstrated that CT inhibited bone osteoclastic activity. The suppression of TRACP activity and urinary HYP content by sCT in carp was noticed from 2 h with a maximum at 4 h after sCT injection. Even effective dose and time at which sCT started its suppressive effects on plasma TRACP activity and excretion of urinary HYP were the same at which it caused reduction of plasma calcium levels and inhibition of GCAT of this fish. From all these findings it is clear that CT-induced reduction in plasma calcium may in part due to inhibition of bone calcium resorption.

Total plasma ALP was measured to monitor the osteoblastic activity and is used as a marker of bone formation in mammals (Raisz et al., 1998). In sCT-injected carp we observed dose-, and time-dependent suppression of the activity of plasma ALP, indicating an action of CT on osteoblast in fish bone. From histological observation by Wandelaar-Bonga and Lamers (1982), it seemed that CT has a stimulatory effect on the growth of bones and scales of fish, even though CT exerts no action on calcium and phosphate concentrations in the skeletal bone. In our earlier study by observing suppression of plasma ALP activity simultaneously with reduction in plasma Ca concentration in *C. punctatus* we reported for a osteoblastic activity after CT treatment (Mukherjee et al., 2004 b). In the present study a similar suppression in plasma ALP activity in carp also indicate an action of CT on osteoblast of this fish. Furthermore, we recorded considerably higher calcium concentration in skeletal bone in CT-treated fish, and from our findings it can be assumed that a relationship between bone osteoblast activity and plasma calcium levels exist in this fish and that is altered in presence of CT.

An important question may emerge from our findings as to what could be relevance of CT-induced inhibition of bone resorption when there are evidences that fish regulate hypocalcemia through inhibition of GCAT (Milhaud et al., 1977; Wagner et al., 1997; Mukherjee et al., 2004 b)? It is true that the skeleton of fresh water teleosts have cellular bones (Mugiya and Watabe, 1997; Dacke 1979), which have the ability to remodel themselves. In the light of these findings it appears most likely that in fish there might be some scope to find out a regulatory mechanism in bone remodeling. Since CT in carp as well as in *C. punctatus* is an effective regulator of plasma calcium, its action on bone calcium resorption is not unlikely.

In the present study, we found that administration of sCT to carp during vitellogenic stage significantly stimulated spontaneous and hCG-induced secretion of E_2 both *in vivo* and *in vitro*. We described that ovarian follicles are equipped with CT receptors as evidenced from the specific binding of sCT to the membrane preparation. We also reported that sCT stimulated the activity of cytochrome P450 aromatase and P450arom gene expression in the ovarian follicles. Furthermore, we suggested that stimulatory action of sCT on ovarian E_2 secretion was mediated through cAMP pathway.

Evidence for a physiological role of CT during teleost sexual maturation has now been available. Histological and ultrastructural studies of ultimobranchial glands of a number of fish show that this gland is maximally active in sexually mature preovulatory females (Oguri 1973; Yamane 1977, 1978; Yamane and Yamada, 1977). Plasma CT levels in coho salmon, Japanese eel and rainbow trout are higher in females during spawning season and reached a peak just before ovulation (Deftos et. al. 1974; Yamauchi et. al., 1976, 1978; Bjorsson et al., 1986; Norberg et al., 1989). 17β-estradiol (E_2) increases plasma CT levels in rainbow trout (Bjorsson et al., 1986, 1989) and a direct induction of estrogen on CT secretion from ultimobranchial glands in goldfish has also been suggested (Suzuki et al., 2004). Possible explanation for the hyperactivity of ultimobranchial gland and the rise in plasma CT levels during peak reproductive season in female fish has been put forwarded by many workers (Brown and Bern 1989; Bjorsson et al., 1989; Suzuki et al., 2004), but none of them were able to suggest an exact relationship between CT and reproduction in fish.

The present study provide evidence that sCT is effective in increasing plasma E_2 levels in vitellogenic stage fish and stimulating both spontaneous and hCG-induced secretion of E_2 by the ovarian follicles *in vitro*. For our *in vivo* experiment, we used fish kept in high-Ca water. As shown previously, hypocalcemic effects of sCT was less in fish kept in high-Ca water than in normal water (Chakraborti and Mukherjee, 1993; Mukherjee et al., 2004 a, b). In the present study, after sCT injection to vitellogenic fish, plasma calcium levels altered a little but the release of plasma E_2 was significantly increased. We concluded that the increase of plasma E_2 was independent of Ca-decreased effect of sCT. Effects of sCT on increased plasma E_2 levels might be due to its action either on high pituitary GtH release or its direct action on ovarian follicles. Intravenous infusion of CT in human caused a calcium-independent reduction in thyrotropin and LH secretion in response to hypothalamic releasing hormone (Leicht et al., 1974). Inhibition of sCT on secretion of progesterone and GnRH-stimulated pituitary LH has also been reported (Tan et al., 1994). Moreover, receptors of CT-designated C1a and C1b receptors have been identified in rat brain (Sexton and Hilton, 1992; Albrandt et al., 1993). All these information indicates a physiological role of CT at pituitary and ovarian levels in mammals. However, no such information is available in fish. Indeed we, in our present study, did not observe the pituitary LH release after sCT injection to fish. Therefore, possibility of a CT-regulated GtH release by the pituitary of fish can not be ruled out. In our *in vitro* observation as low as 25 ng sCT peptide per incubation is effective in stimulating spontaneous and hCG-induced release of E_2 by the vitellogenic ovarian follicles of fish. Therefore, the reason for sCT-induced rise in plasma E_2 levels is that sCT stimulated E_2 production by acting directly on ovarian follicular cells in fish.

Result of the present study shows that sCT can bind specifically to membrane preparation from ovarian follicles of carp indicating the presence of receptor molecules in the carp ovarian follicles which recognize sCT. Binding of CT with membrane receptors was found to be saturable with high affinity (*B*max, 1.2 pmol/mg protein, *K*d 48.8 pmol/L). Available information on the presence of CT-binding sites and sCT-induced inhibition of progesterone secretion in rat granulosa cells indicates a physiological role of CT at ovarian levels in mammals (Tsai et al., 1999). Our finding is the first report of the presence of sCT receptor in fish ovary apart from its presence in gills. Therefore, the presence of functional receptors for CT in the ovarian membrane preparation in vitellogenic follicles and sCT-induced *in vitro* production of E_2 by the ovarian follicles clearly indicate a functional link between binding and specific biological response.

In the present study, significant augmentation of aromatase activity both in hCG- and sCT-treated ovarian follicles is supported by a high rate of conversion of aromatizable androgen (testosterone to E_2) and enhanced synthesis and release of E_2 under stimulation of both the hormones. We also showed for the first time in teleost that sCT stimulated expression of P450arom gene in the ovarian follicles. It has been documented that the fish ovarian follicles possess aromatase enzyme participating in the conversion of aromatizable androgen to E_2 and P450arom mRNA levels are increased in association with the increase of enzyme activity under the stimulation of hCG (Gen et al., 2001; Kagawa et al., 2003, Paul et al., 2008, 2010).

It has been well established that in fish ovary, gonadotropin stimulates steroid production involving both PKA and PKC pathways (Nagahama, 1987; Srivastava and Van der Kraak, 1994). In our experiment, we found that in addition to lone effect of sCT on E_2 production, stimulatory effects of hCG on E_2 production *in vitro* was potentiated in presence of sCT in carp ovarian follicles. Results indicate that administration of dbcAMP stimulated sCT-induced E_2 production and cell permeable selective inhibitor of adenylate cyclase, SQ22536 attenuated both hCG- and sCT-induced E_2 production by the ovarian follicles in a concentration-dependent manner. Specific PKC inhibitor NPC-15437 dihydrochloride on the other hand had no inhibitory effects on sCT-stimulated E_2 release. We, therefore, suggest that signal for sCT-stimulated E_2 release might be transduced through cAMP pathway and interaction between sCT and hCG on the signal transduction in fish ovary is still open to elucidate. Increased production of cAMP caused by CT has been demonstrated in perfused rat bone, osteoblast like cell line, osteoclast, atria and aortic smooth muscle (Kubota et al., 1985; Sugimoto et al., 1986; Nicholson et al., 1987; Wang and Fiscus 1989; Iida-Klein 1992), and in rat testicular and anterior pituitary gland (Wang et al., 1994) substantiate the action of CT through cAMP path way in fish ovarian follicles.

Our present finding on the stimulatory role of sCT on basal and hCG-induced E_2 production by fish ovarian follicles is completely opposite to the observed action of CT in mammalian ovary and testes in the regulation of steroid production. Our unpublished data with ovarian follicles of perch *Anabas testudineus* also showed the same stimulatory action of sCT on E_2 production. Although the action of CT is well characterized in mammals, its action in fish, particularly with regard to calcium regulation is still controversial. Therefore, the observed stimulatory effect of CT on fish ovarian steroidogenesis, in contrast to mammals, is not unusual. It is most likely that CT has evolved distinct function in different lineage, which probably relates to its aquatic life and this needs further studies on higher group of vertebrates. It is also not clear the exact physiological relevance of the stimulation of E_2 production by sCT in fish ovary when GtH-stimulated E_2 production is normally operative. Researchers have become increasingly aware that the traditional concept of the action of GtH in the regulation of ovarian growth, maturation and steroidogenesis may no longer be tenable. Localization of several neuropeptides in the nerve that innervate the ovary, neuropeptide Y, substance P (SP), vasoactive intestinal polypeptide (VIP) and somatostatin in the ovary of mammals have already been reported (Ojeda et al. 1985; Ahmed et. al., 1986; McDonald et al., 1987). Function of most of these peptide in the ovary although remain unknown but stimulatory effects of VIP on estrogen and progesterone release from cultured granulosa cells have been reported. Reports are also available that the stimulatory action of VIP appears to be exerted at least, in part, through a direct stimulatory action of neuropeptide on the synthesis of cholesterol-side chain cleavage enzyme (Trzecizk et al., 1986; 87). Recently, Clark et al., (2002) reported for the expression of CT gene in the ovary of a teleost, *Fugu rubripes* and suggested that CT may act as a potential neuropeptide. Considering all these, it would appear that CT in fish may take some role, at least in part, to support the action of GtH on the ovary during vitellogenic growth by acting independently or synergistically with GtH. This assumption supports the high plasma CT levels in fish during this phase of gonadal growth (Deftos et al., 1974; Yamauchi et al., 1978; Bjorsson et al., 1986).

The present study show that sCT is also capable of stimulating 17, 20β-P production in vitro in postvitellogenic ovarian follicles and this fish and stimulation is dose- and time-dependant. Results show that 25 ng sCT peptide per incubation is effective in stimulating spontaneous and hCG-induced 17, 20β-P production by the postvitellogenic ovarian follicles. 17, 20β-P is considered to be the maturation-inducing hormone in most teleosts including *C. carpio* and is released by the postvitellogenic ovarian follicles by the induction pituitary gonadotropin (GtH-II) immediately before oocyte maturation (Nagahama et al., 1987, Paul et al., 2010). Apart from many other intra-ovarian factors shown to increase 17, 20β-P production in the fish ovarian follicles (Maestro et al., 1997; Weber and Sulivan, 2000; Mukherjee et al., 2006; Chourasia et al., 2008), CT-induced production of 17, 20β-P in fish ovarian follicles in our study is a new finding and warrant further study.

Meiotic cell division in fish oocyte is arrested at G2/M border of cell cycle and reenters cell division in response to MIH produced in the follicular cells by the induction of gonadotropins (see review Nagahama et al., 1997; Mukherjee et al., 2006; Paul et al., 2010). Apart from GtH, many other intra-ovarian peptides including IGFs also have the potentiality to induce oocyte maturation in fish (Kagawa et al., 1994; Weber and Sullivan, 2000; 2001; Mukherjee et al., 2006; Paul et al., 2010). Incidence of CT-induced oocyte maturation in carp ovarian follicles in the present study suggest the function of new peptide involved in fish oocyte maturation, origin of which is not the ovary itself. Most interestingly, sCT-induced occurrence of GVBD in carp oocytes also observed in fully denuded oocytes indicating that the action of CT may be via a steroid-independent pathway. Similar steroid-independent pathway of the action of IGF-I in fish oocyte maturation has been reported earlier (Mukherjee et al., 2006; Paul et al., 2010). Involvement of CT in oocyte maturation is thus a new finding and deserves further study to unfold the real picture on this aspect. One interesting cellular action of CT involves the demonstration of its effects on the growth of breast cancer. CT retards cell division in CT receptor infected HEK cells. It can affect cyclin-dependent kinase inhibitor, P21/WAF1/CIPI, which arrest cell cycle in G1 and G2 phases (Evdokion et al., 2000 and see review Zaidi et al., 2002). We do not know functional relevance of CT-induced oocyte maturation and its mechanism of action at the present moment and work is progressing to find out the mechanism of CT action in oocyte maturation in this fish.

7. Conclusion

In summary, the present findings suggest that salmon calcitonin would be an effective regulator of plasma calcium levels in fresh water teleost *C. carpio* adapted to water with different calcium concentrations, except a very high calcium level. Such effects of CT registered in *C. carpio* were shown to be dose- and time-dependent and may mediate at least in part, through inhibition of bone calcium resorption. Salmon CT is a potent inhibitor of GCAT in fresh water teleost adapted to both low-Ca and normal tap water. Fish were equally responsive to hormone at ages before attaining sexual maturity. From *in vivo* and *in vitro* study it may also suggest that sCT stimulates E_2 production in vitellogenic ovarian follicles and 17, 20β-P production in the post-vitellogenic ovarian follicle of *C. carpio* by acting directly on ovary, without altering plasma calcium level. Membrane preparation of ovarian follicles is equipped with CT receptor with high affinity. Salmon CT could stimulate both basal and hCG-stimulated E_2 and 17, 20β-P production. The stimulatory effect of sCT on E_2 production is associated with an increase in P450aromatase activities and P450arom gene expression in ovarian follicles. The signal transduction of the stimulatory effect of CT is mediated through cAMP pathway. The stimulatory effect of sCT on 17, 20β-P production is associated with oocyte maturation. Most interestingly, sCT-induced oocyte maturation also occurred independent of MIH action.

8. Acknowledgement

The authors are thankful for the supports from Council of Scientific and Industrial Research (CSIR), Govt. of India, New Delhi and from University of Kalyani, Kalyani, Nadia, India. There is no conflict of interest that would prejudice the impartiality of this work.

9. References

Albrandt, K., Mull, E., Brady, E.M.G., Herich, J., Moore, C.X., & Beaumont, K. (1993.) Molecular cloning of two receptors from rat brain with high affinity for salmon calcitonin. FEBS Letters Vol (325): 225–232.

Bentley, P. J. (1983.) Urinary loss of calcium in an anuran amphibian *(Bufo marinus*) with a note on the effects of calcemic hormones. *Comparative Biochemistry and Physiology B.* Vol (76): 717-719.

Bjorsson, B.T.H., Haux, C., Bern, H.A., & Deftos, L.J. (1989.) 17β-Estradiol increases plasma calcitonin levels in salmonid fish. *Endocrinology* Vol (125): 1754–1760.

Bjorsson, B.T.H., Haux, C., Forlin, L., & Deftos, L.J. (1986.) The involvement of calcitonin in the reproductive physiology of the rainbow trout. *Journal of Endocrinology* Vol (108): 17–22.

Boelkins, J. N., & Kenny, A. D. (1973.) Plasma calcitonin levels in Japanese quail. *Endocrinology* Vol (92): 1754-1760.

Brown, C.L., & Bern, H.A. (1989.) Thyroid hormones in early development, with special reference to teleost fishes. In *Development, Maturation and Senescence of neuroendocrine Systems: A Comparative Approach*, 289–306.Eds M Schreibman & C Scanes. New York: Academic Press.

Chakrabarti, P., & Mukherjee, D. (1993.) Studies on the hypocalcemic actions of salmon calcitonin and ultimobranchial gland extracts in the freshwater teleost *Cyprinus carpio*. *General and Comparative Endocrinology* Vol (90): 267–273.

Chan, D. K. O., Chester-jones, I., & Smith, R. N. (1968.) The effect of mammalian calcitonin on the plasma levels of calcium and inorganic phosphate in the European eel (*Anguilla anguilla* L). *General and Comparative Endocrinology* Vol (11): 243-254.

Chomczynski, P., & Sacchi, N. (1987.) Single step method of RNA isolation by acid guanidium thiocyanate–phenol–chloroform extraction. *Analytical Biochemistry* Vol (162): 156–159.

Chourasia, T.K., & Joy, K.P., (2008.) Estrogen-2/4 hydroxylase activity is stimulated during germinal vesicle break down induced by hCG,IGF,-I,GH and insulin in the catfish Heteropneustes fossilis. *General Comparative Endocrinology* Vol(155): 413-421

Cooper, C.W., Peng, T.C., Obie, J.F., & Garner, S.C. (1980.) Calcitonin-like immunoreactivity in rat and human pituitary glands: histochemical, *in vitro* and *in vivo*. *Endocrinology* Vol (107): 98–107.

Copp, D.H., Cockcroft, D.W., & Kueh, Y. (1967.) Calcitonin from the ultimobranchial glands of dogfish and chickens. *Science* Vol (158): 924-925.

Dacke, C. G. (1979.) Comparative nature of calcified tissue. Calcium regulation in sub-Mammalian vertebrates. *Academic Press*, London, pp 21-40.

Deftos, L.J., Watts, E.G., Copp, D.H., & Potts, J.T., Jr (1974.) Radioimmunoassay for salmon calcitonin. *Endocrinology* Vol (94): 155–160.

Evdokiou, A., Raggatt, L. J., Sakai, T., & Findlay, D. M. (2000.) Identification of a novel calcitonin response element in the promoter of the human p21 WAF1. CIP1.gene. *Journal of Molecular Endocrinology* Vol (25): 195-206.

Farley, J., Dimai, H. P., Sult-Coffing, B., Farley, PPham, T., & Mohan, S. (2000.) Calcitonin increases the concentration of insulin like-growth factor in serum free cultures of human osteoblast-like cells. *Calcified Tissue International* Vol (67): 247-254.

Fouchereau–Peron, M., Arlot-Bonnermains, Y., Moukhter M. S., Milhaud, G. (1987.) Calcitonin induces hypercalcemia in grey mullet and immature freshwater and sea-water adapted rainbow trout *Comparative Biochemistry & Physiology* Vol (87A): 1051-1053.

Fujita, T., Fuji, Y., Miyauchi, A., Takagi, Y. (1999.) Comparison of antiresorptive activities of ispriflavone, an isoflavone derivatives, and calcitonin an eel carbocalcitonin. *Journal of Bone and Mineral Metabolism* Vol (17): 289-295.

Gen, K., Okuzawa, K., Kumakura, N., Yamaguchi, Y., & Kagawa, H. (2001.) Correlation between messenger RNA expression of cytochrome P450aromatase and its enzyme activity during oocyte development in the red seabream (*Pagrus major*). *Biology of Reproduction* Vol (65): 1186–1194.

George, S.E., Bungay, P.J., & Naylor, L.H. (1997.) Functional coupling of endogenous serotonin (5-HT1B) and calcitonin (C1a) receptors in CHO cells to a cyclic AMP-responsive luciferase reporter gene. *Journal of Neurochemistry* Vol (69): 1278–1285.

Glowacki, J., O'Sullivan, J., Miller, M., Wilkje, D.W., & Deftos, L.J. (1985.) Calcitonin produces hypercalcemia in leopard sharks. *Endocrinology* Vol (166): 827-829.

Iida-Klein, A., Yee, C.D., Brandli, D.W., Mirikitani, E.J.M., & Hahn, T.J. (1992.) Effects of calcitonin on 30, 50 monophosphate and calcium second messenger generation osteoblast function in UMR 106-06 osteoblast-like cells. *Endocrinology* Vol (130): 81–388.

Kagawa, H., Gen, K., Okuzawa, K., & Tanaka, H. (2003.) Effects of luteinizing hormone and follicle-stimulating hormone and insulin-like growth factor-I on aromatase activity and P450 aromatase gene expression in the ovarian follicles of red seabream, Pagrus major, *Biology of Reproduction* Vol (68): 1562–1568.

Kagawa, H., Kobayashi, M., Hasegawa, Y., and Aida, K. (1994.) Insulin ans insulin-like growth factor I and II induced final oocyte maturation of oocyte of red seabream, *Pagrus major*, in vitro. *General Comparative Endocrinology* Vol (95): 293-300.

Kenny, A. D. (1971.) Determination of calcitonin in plasma by bioassay. *Endocrinology* Vol (89): 1005-1013.

Kline L.W. (1982.) An age-dependent response to synthetic salmon calcitonin in the chuckwalla, *Sauromalus obesus*. *Canadian Journal of Zoology* Vol (60): 1359-1361.

Kline, L. W. (1981.) A hypocalcemic response to synthetic salmon calcitonin in the green iguana, *Iguana iguana*. *General and Comparative Endocrinology* Vol (44): 476-479.

Kline, L.W., & Longmore, G.A. (1986.) Determination of calcitonin in reptilian serum by heterologus radioimmunoassay. *General and Comparative Endocrinology* Vol (61): 1-4.

Kubota, M., Moseley, J.M., Butera, L., Dusting, G.J., MacDonald, P.S., & Martin, T.J. (1985.) Calcitonin gene related peptide stimulates cyclic AMP formation in rat aortic smooth muscle cells. *Biochemical and Biophysical Research Communications* Vol (132): 88–94.

Leicht, E., Biro, G., & Weinges, K.F. (1974.) Inhibition of releasing-hormoneinduced secretion of TSH and LH by calcitonin. *Hormone and Metabolic Research* Vol (7): 410–414.

Lopez, E., Peignoux-Deville, J., Lallier, P., Martelly, E., Milet, C. (1976) Effects of calcitonin and ultimobranchialectomy (UBX) on calcium and bone metabolism in the eel, *Anguilla anguilla* L. *Calcified Tissue Research* Vol (20): 173-186.

Lowry, O.H., Rosebrough, N.J., Farr, A.L., & Randall, R.J. (1951.) Protein measurement with the folin phenol reagent. *Journal of Biological Chemistry* Vol (193): 265–275.

Maurer, R., Marbach, P., & Mousson, R. (1983.) Salmon calcitonin binding sites in rat pituitary. *Brain Research* Vol (261): 346–348.

Milet, C., Peignoux-Deville, J., & Martelly, E. (1979.) Gill calcium fluxes in the eel, *Anguilla anguilla* (L): Effects of stannius corpuscles and ultimobranchial body. *Comparative Biochemistry & Physiology* Vol (63A): 63-70.

Milhaud, G., Rankin, J.C., Bolis, L., & Benson, A.A. (1977.) Calcitonin: its hormonal action on the gill. *Proceedings of National Academy of Science* USA Vol (74): 4693-4696.

Mugiya, Y., & Watabe , N. (1977.) Studies of fish scale formation and resorption: II. Effects of estradiol on calcium homeostasis and skeletal tissue resorption in the goldfish, *Carassius aureatus* and the killifish, *Fundulus heteroclitus* . *Comparative Biochemistry & Physiology: PartA Molecular & Integrative Physiology* Vol (57): 197-202.

Mukherjee, D., Manna, P.R., & Bhattacharyya, S. (1994.) Functional relevance of lutinizing hormone receptor in mouse uterus. *European Journal of Endocrinology* Vol(131): 103-108.

Mukherjee, D., Mukherjee, D., Sen, U., Paul, S., & Bhattacharyya, S.P. (2006.) In vitro effects of insulin-like growth factors and insulin on oocyte maturation and maturation-inducing steroid production in ovarian follicles of common carp, Cyprinus carpio, *Comparative Biochemistry and Physiology, Part A* Vol (144): 63–77.

Mukherjee, D., Sen, U., Bhattacharyya, S.P., & Mukherjee, D. (2004.b) Inhibition of whole body Ca^{+2} uptake in fresh water teleosts, Channa punctatus and Cyprinus carpio in response to salmon calcitonin. *Journal of Experimental Zoology* Vol (301A): 882–890.

Mukherjee, D., Sen, U., Bhattacharyya, S.P., & Mukherjee, D. (2004.a) The effects of calcitonin on plasma calcium levels and bone metabolism in the fresh water teleost Channa punctatus, *Comparative Biochemistry and Physiology, Part A* Vol (138): 417–426.

Nagahama, Y. (1987.) Gonadotropin action on gametogenesis and steroidogenesis in teleost gonads. *Zoological Science* Vol (4): 209–222.

Niall, H. D., Keutmann, H. T., Copp, D.H., & Potts, J.T. Jr. (1969.) Amino acid sequence of salmon ultimobranchial calcitonin. *Proceedings of National Acadamy of Science* USA.Vol (64): 771-778.

Nicholson, G.C., Moseley, J. M., Sexton, P.M., Mendelshon, F. A. O., & Martin, T. J. (1986.) Abundant calcitonin receptors in isolated rat osteoclast. Biochemical and Autoradiographic Characterization. *Journal of Clinical Investigation* Vol (78): 355-360.

Nicholson, G.C., Mosley, J.M., Yatess, A.J.P., & Martin, T.J. (1987.) Control of cyclic adenosine 30, 50 monophosphate production activation and homologous desensitization of adenylate cyclase. *Endocrinology* Vol (120): 1902–1908.

Noda, T., & Narita, K. (1976.) Amino acid sequence of eel calcitonin. *Journal of Biochemtry* Vol (79): 353-359.

Oguri, M. (1973.) Seasonal histological changes in the ultomobranchial gland of the gold fish. *Bulletin of the Japanese Society of Scientific Fisheries* Vol 30 851–858.

Paul, S., Pramanick, K., Kundu, S., Kumar, D., & Mukherjee, D. (2010.) Regulation of ovarian steroidogenesis in vitro by IGF-I and Insulin in common carp *Cyprinus carpio*: Stimulation of aromatase activity and p450 arom gene expression. *Molecular and Cellular Endocrinology* Vol(315): 95-103.

Plotkin, L. L., Weinstein, R. S., Parfitt, A. M., Robertson P. K., Manolaga, S. C. & Bellido, T. (1999.) Prevention of osteocyte and osteoblast apoptosis by bisphophonates and calcitonin. *Journal of Clinical Investigation* Vol (104): 1363-1374.

Raisz, L.G., Kream, B. E., & Lorenzo, J. A. (1998.) Metabolic Bone Disease. In William Text Book of Endocrinology. 9th Edition (Eds. J. D. Wilson, D.W. Foster, M.D. Kronenberg, and P. R. Larsen P. R). Philadelphia, W. B. Saunders company pp 1211-1239.

Robertson, D.R. (1975.) Effects of ultimobranchial and parathyroid glands and vitamin D2, D3 and dihydrotachysterol2 on blood calcium and intestinal calcium transport in the frog. *Endocrinology* Vol (96): 934-940.

Robertson, D.R. (1987.) Plasma immunoreactive calcitonin in the frog (*Rana pipiens*). *Comparative Biochemistry & Physiology: A* Vol (88): 701-705.

Ross, B. A., Bundy, L. L., Baily, R., & Deftos, L. J. (1974.) Calcitonin secretion in vitro: 1. Preparation of monolayer C-cell culture. *Endocrinology* Vol (95): 1142-1149.

Sasayama, Y., & Oguro, C. (1976.) Effects of ultimobranchialectomy on calcium and sodium concentrations of serum and coelomic fluid in bullfrog tadpoles under high calcium and high sodium environment. *Comparative Biochemistry & Physiology: A* Vol (55): 35-37.

Sasayama, Y., Ukawa, K., Kaiya, H., Oguro, C., Takei, Y., Watanabe, T. X., Nakajima, K., & Sakakibara, S. (1993.) Goldfish calcitonin: Purification, characterization, and hypocalcemic potency. *General and Comparative Endocrinology* Vol (89): 189-194.

Sen, U., Mukherjee, D., Bhattacharyya, S.P., & Mukherjee, D. (2002.) Seasonal changes in plasma steroid levels in Indian major carp (Labeo rohita): influenceof homologous pituitary extract on steroid production and development of oocyte maturational competence. *General and Comparative Endocrinology* Vol (128): 123–134.

Sexton, P.M., & Hilton, J.M. (1992.) Biologically active salmon calcitonin-like peptide is present in rat brain. *Brain Research* Vol (596): 279–284.

Singh, S., & Srivastav, A. K. (1993.) Effects of calcitonin administration on serum calcium and inorganic phosphate levels of the fish, *Heteropneustes fossilis*, maintained either in artificial freshwater, calcium-rich freshwater, or calcium deficient freshwater. *Journal of Experimental Zoology* Vol (265): 35-39.

Srivastav, A. K., & Rani, L. (1989.) Influence of calcitonin administration on serum calcium and inorganic phosphate level in the frog, *Rana tigrina. General and Comparative Endocrinology* Vol (74): 14-17.

Srivastav, A. K., Sivastav, S. K., Sasayama, Y., & Suzuki, N. (1998.) Salmon calcitonin induced hypocalcemia and hyperphosphatemia in an elasmobranch, *Dasyatis akajei. General and Comparative Endocrinology* Vol (109): 8-12.

Srivastava, R.K., & Van Der Kraak, G. (1994.) Effects of activators of different intracellular signaling pathways on steroid production by goldfish vitellogenic ovarian follicles. *General and Comparative Endocrinology* Vol (93): 181–191.

Sugimoto, T., Fukase, M., Tsutsumi, M., Tsunenari, T., & Fujita, T. (1986.) Altered parathyroid hormone- or calcitonin - stimulated adenosine 30, 50-monophosphate release by isolated perfused bone from glucocorticoid treated rats. *Calcified Tissue International* Vol (38): 163–169.

Suzuki, N., Suzuki D., Sasayama Y., srivastava A, K., Kambegawa A., & Asshina, K. (1999.) Plasma calcium and calcitonin levels in eels fed a high calcium solution or transferred to sea water. *General and Comparative Endocrinology* Vol (114): 324-329.

Suzuki, N., Yamamoto, K., Sasayama, Y., Suzuki, T., Kurokawa, T., Kambegawa, A., Srivastav, A.K., Hayashi, S., & Kikuyama, S. (2004.) Possible direct induction by estrogen of calcitonin secretion from ultimobranchial cells in the goldfish. *General and Comparative Endocrinology* Vol (138): 121–127.

Tsai, S.C., Lu, C.C., Chen, J.J., Chiao, Y.C., Wang, S.W., Hwang, J.J., & Wang, P.S. (1999.) Inhibition of salmon calcitonin on secretion of progesterone and GnRH stimulated pituitary luteinzing hormone. *American Journal of Physiology, Endocrinology and Metabolism* Vol (277): 49–55.

Ukawa, K., Sasayama, Y., & Takei, Y. (1991.) Hypocalcemic potency of gold fish calcitonin. *In Current Themes in Comparative Endocrinology*. Proc. 2nd . Congr. AOSCE (Eds. R. N. Saxena, K. Muralidhar, L.Bhagat, N. Shegal, T. Saxena, P. Kaushal), pp. 304-305.

Urist, M. R. (1976.) Biogenesis of bone calcium and phosphorus in the skeleton and blood in vertebrate evolution. In: Aurbach G.D, ed. Handbook of physiology. American Physiological Society, Washington D.C. Vol(7): 183-213.

Vaes, G. F. (1998) Cellular Biology and Branchial mechanism of bone resorption. *Clinical Orthopaedics and Related Research* Vol (231): 239-271.

Wagner, G. F., Jaworski, E. M., & Radman D. P. (1997.) Salmon calcitonin inhibits whole body Ca^{+2} uptake in young rainbow trout *Journal of Endocrinology* Vol (155): 459-465.

Wang, P.S., Tsai, S.C., Hwang, G.S., Wang, S.W., Lu, C.C., Chen, J.J., Liu, S.R., Lee, Y., Chien, E.J., Chien, C.H., et al. (1994.) Calcitonin inhibits testosterone and luteinizing hormone secretion through a mechanism involving an increase in cAMP production in rats. *Journal of Bone and Mineral Research* Vol (9): 1583–1590.

Wang, X., & Fiscus, R.R. (1989.) Calcitonin gene related peptide increases cAMP tension, and rate in rat atria. *American Journal of Physiology. Regulatory, Integrative and Comparative Physiology* Vol (256): R421–R428.

Weber, G .M., & Sullivan, C. V. (2000.) Effects of insulin-like growth factor-I on in vitro final oocyte maturation and ovarian steroidogenesis in stripped bass , *Morone saxatilis. Biology of Reproduction*. Vol. (63):1049-1057.

Weber, G., & Sullivan, C. V. (2001.) *In vitro* hormone induction of final oocyte maturation in stripped bass *(Morone saxatilis)* follicles is inhibited by blockers of phosphatidylinositol 3-kinase activity. *Comparative Biochemistry and Physiology* Vol (129): 467-473.

Wedlaar-Bonga, S. E., & Lammers, P.I. (1982.) Effects of calcitonin on ultrastructure and mineral content of bone and scales of the cichlid teleost. Sarotherodon mosambicus. *General Comparative Endocrinology* Vol(48): 60-70.

Wendelaar- Bonga , S.E., & Pang, P.K.T. (1991.) Control of calcium regulating hormones in the vertebrates: parathyroid hormone, calcitonin, prolactin, and stanniocalcin. *International Review of Cytology* Vol (128): 139–213.

Wendlaar Bonga, S. E. (1981.) Effect of synthetic salmon calcitonin on protein-bound and free plasma calcium in the teleost *Gasterosteus aculeatus. General and Comparative Endocrinology* Vol (43): 123-126.

Yadav, S., & Srivastav, A. K. (2009.) Influence of calcitonin administration on Ultimobranchial gland and parathyroid glands of pigeon, *Columba livia. Microscopy Research and Techniques* Vol. (72): 380-384.

Yamane, S. (1977.) Sexual differences in histology and of the ultimobranchial gland of mature Japaneese eel (*Anguilla japonica*). *Zoological Magazine* Vol (86): 261–263.

Yamane, S. (1978.) Histology and fine structure of the ultomobranchial gland in the zebra fish, *Brachydanio rerio. Bulletin of the Faculty of Fisheries* Vol (29): 213–221.

Yamane, S., & Yamada, J. (1977.) Histological changes in the ultomobranchial gland through the life history of the Masu salmon. *Bulletin of the Japanese Society of Scientific Fisheries* Vol (43): 375–386.

Yamauchi, H., Matsuo, M., Yamauchi, K., Takano, K., Takahashi, H., & Orimo, H. (1976.) Studies on ultimobranchial calcitonin (4)- serum calcitonin levels in eel. *Igaku no Ayumi* Vol (99): 499–500.

Yamauchi, H., Orimo, H., Yamauchi, K., & Takahashi, H. (1978.) Increased calcitonin level during ovarian development in the eel, *Anguilla japonica, General and Comparative Endocrinology* Vol (36): 526–529.

Zaidi, M., Chambers, T.J., Bavis, P.J.R., Beacham, J.L., Gaines Das, R.E., & MacIntyre, I.(1988.) Effects of peptides from the calcitonin genes on bone and bone cells. *Journal of Experimental Physiology* Vol(73): 471-485.

Zaidi. M., Inzerillo, A. M., Moonga, B.S., Bevis, P. J. R., & Huang, C. L.-H. (2002.) Forty years of calcitonin -Where are we now? A tribute to the work of Iain Macintyre, FRS. *Bone* Vol 30(No.5): 655-663.

16

Ascidians: New Model Organisms for Reproductive Endocrinology

Honoo Satake, Tsuyoshi Kawada, Masato Aoyama,
Toshio Sekiguchi and Tsubasa Sakai
Suntory Institute for Bioorganaic Research
Japan

1. Introduction

Ovarian functions, including growth of oocytes and follicles, are believed to involve coordinated and multistep biological events that undergo functional regulation by a wide range of endogenous factors. Mammalian follicles consist of one oocyte surrounded by granulosa cells and theca cells (Orisaka et al., 2009). Mammalian follicular growth is basically classified into two phases: gonadotropin-independent and gonadotropin-dependent stages. The former includes early follicular growth stages, namely, primordial, primary, secondary, preantral, and antral stages, whereas follicle recruitment, selection, and ovulation occur during the latter. A great variety of intraovarian and extraovarian factors such as a pituitary hormone, gonadotropin, have been well structurally and functionally elucidated. In contrast, no signaling molecules responsible for gonadotropin-independent oocyte growth have ever been identified. "Neuropeptides" and "non-sexual peptide hormones" are promising candidates for regulators of early follicle growth, given that many of their receptors were found to be expressed in the ovary. Nevertheless, biological effects of neuropeptides and non-sexual hormones on the ovary still remain controversial or unknown. Such inconclusive data resulted primarily from the difficulty in elucidating *in vitro* and *in vivo* physiological functions of neuropeptides or non-sexual hormones in the mammalian ovaries due to heterogeneous quality of oocytes (the very small number of successfully growing oocytes), the low basal levels of receptor expression, and complicated sexual periods (Candenas et al., 2005; Satake & Kawada, 2006a; Debejuk, 2006; Wang & Sun 2007). Furthermore, most receptors of peptide ligands are not ubiquitously, but widely expressed, and thus, neuropeptides and peptide hormones have multiple biological roles, which frequently caused great difficulties in discriminating direct actions on the ovary from indirect actions of a peptide during functional analyses via *in vivo* administration or using a peptide- and/or a receptor-knockout mouse. In such cases, model studies using lower organisms, such as a fruitfly *Drosophila melanogaster* or a nematode *Caenorhabditis elegans*, may be useful as the primary step for studies on the biological sciences of mammals. Nevertheless, most invertebrate neuropeptides and hormones possess species-specific primary structures and biological activities. This has hindered comparative analysis and application of traditional invertebrate models to neuroscience and endocrinology research involving neuropeptides and hormones in mammals. These issues suggest a potential requirement for new approaches and model organisms for studies on biological roles of neuropeptides and non-sexual hormone peptides in the ovary. In this chapter, we propose an ascidian, *Ciona intestinalis*, as an emerging model organism for studies of endocrinology, in particular, reproductive biology of oocytes at early stages, and review a novel oocyte growth pathway revealed by studies on biological effects of *Ciona* homologs of mammalian neuropeptides on *Ciona* oocytes, and structures and functions of ascidian neuropeptides and hormone peptides which are highly likely to participate in growth of early-stage follicles and oocytes.

2. What is an "ascidian"?

2.1 Characteristics of an ascidian, *Ciona intestinalis*, and its utility in biological sciences

Ascidians (sea squirts), invertebrate deuterostome marine animals, belong to the subphylum Tunicata or Urochodata under the Chordata phylum (Burighel & Cloney, 1997). Their critical phylogenetic position as protochordates (Fig. 1) and their simple body plan (Fig. 2) and lifecycle have provided attractive and useful targets in research in embryogenesis,

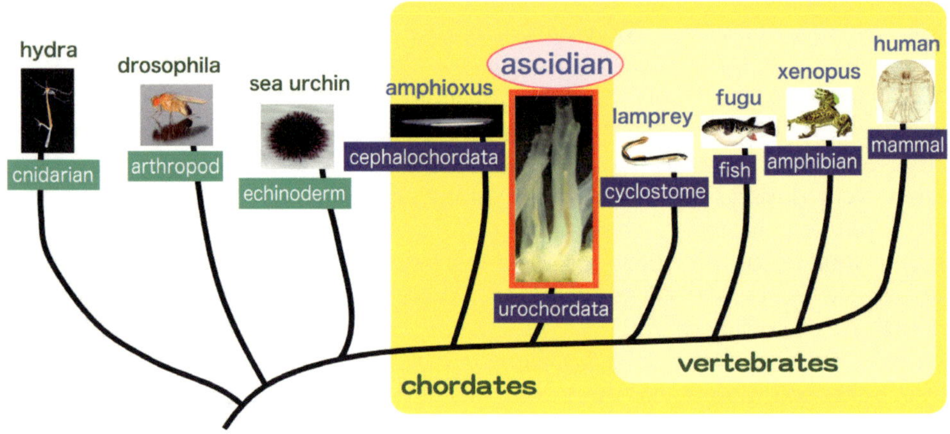

Fig. 1. Phylogenetic tree.

development, and evolution as a direct model or ancestor for vertebrates (Burighel & Cloney, 1997; Satoh, 2009). In 2002, a draft genome and expression sequence tags (ESTs) of the ascidian, *Ciona intestinalis*, (available at http://hoya.zool.kyoto-u.ac.jp/blast_kh.html http://genome.jgi-psf.org/Cioin2/Cioin2.home.html) revealed that the genome of *C. intestinalis* contains approximately 16000 protein-coding genes without the extensive gene duplications typical of vertebrates. Recently, most genes have been annotated by gene-model prediction and sequence homology analysis on the basis of 700,000 ESTs as well as genomic sequences, and the expression profiles of gene products are also available. Furthermore, the establishment of fundamental experimental methods such as morpholino DNA gene silencing and Minos transposon-based transgenic technology (Sasakura, 2007) has led to the post-genomic comprehensive studies in embryogenesis and development of whole chordates (Imai et al., 2006).

In addition to these advantages of *C. intestinalis*, characterization of *Ciona* peptide hormones and neuropeptides is expected to provide crucial clues to the elucidation of the molecular and functional evolution of endocrine, neuroendocrine and nervous systems of chordates as well as the biological roles of the *Ciona* neuropeptides and hormones. Despite these advantages in biological research, ascidian neuropeptides and hormones have received little attention. Moreover, as stated above, complexity of tissue organization and lifecycles of mammals frequently hinders advances in research for neuropeptidergic and hormonal systems. Therefore, molecular and functional characterization of neuropeptides and peptide hormones in *C. intestinalis* is expected to lead not only to investigation of structures and biological roles of ascidian bioactive peptides, but also to establishment of ascidians as novel deuterostome invertebrate models for research in the neuroscience and endocrinology of vertebrates.

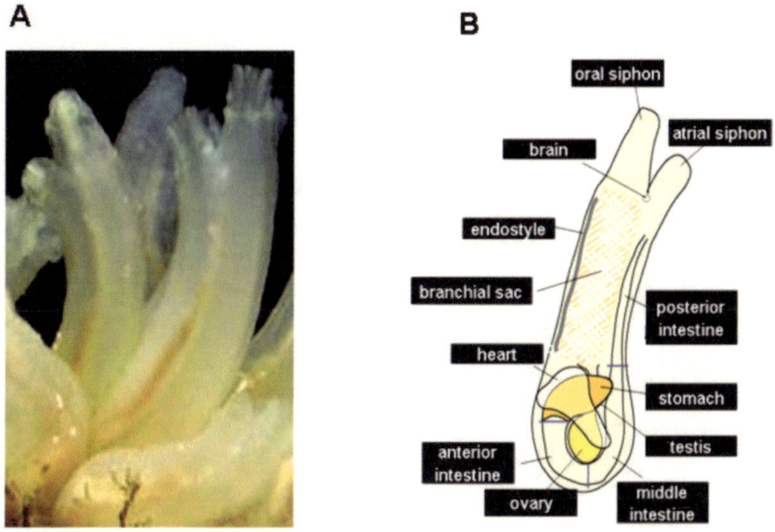

Fig. 2. *Ciona intestinalis* (A) and its tissue organization (B)

2.2 Biological aspects of *Ciona* oocytes and ovary

In the ovary of *C. intestinalis*, the large part is occupied by pre-germinal vesicle breakdown (GVBD) oocytes which are readily classified into three major growth stages on the basis of their diameter and organization of oocyte complexes (Fig. 3), even using 10-µm sections: stage I (pre-vitellogenic stage), stage II (vitellogenic stage), and stage III (post-vitellogenic stage). *Ciona* oocytes are equipped with test cells (TCs), which are believed to be functional

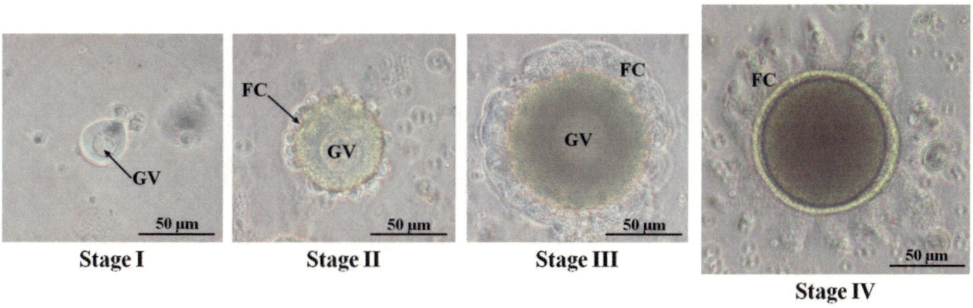

Fig. 3. *C. intestinalis* oocytes. Scale bar, 50 µm. GV, germinal vesicle; FC, follicular cells

and cytological counterparts for mammalian granulosa cells, an acellular vitelline coat, inner follicular cells, and outer follicular cells. Oocytes at stage I (less than 50 μm in diameter) contain the smallest GV and cytoplasm, and are surrounded by envelope organs consisting of undifferentiated primary follicular cells. Stage II oocytes (50-70 μm in diameter) have prominently individualized cube-shaped follicle cells surrounding the oocytes. Stage III oocytes (approximately 100 μm in diameter) have a larger cytoplasm and more outstanding inner follicle structure, and automatically cause GVBD when exposed to seawater (Burighel, & Cloney 1997; Prodon et al., 2006). In addition, stage IV (post-GVBD) oocyte (Fig.3), predominantly present in the oviduct, have the ability of fertilization (Burighel, & Cloney 1997; Prodon et al., 2006). *C. intestinalis* also displays advantages in study of reproductive biology of an ovary. Firstly, the *Ciona* ovary harbors numerous oocytes at each growth stage that are readily characterized and abundantly isolated. Secondly, numerous *Ciona* oocytes are normally grown at a high ratio or maintained for more than one week in sterile seawater. This advantage enables a variety of experiments for evaluation of biological effects of signaling molecules including neuropeptides and peptide hormones. Thirdly, ascidians are not endowed with an organ corresponding to a pituitary. This is in good agreement with the evolutionarily biological propensity of *C. intestinalis* that ascidians, unlike vertebrates, lack a complete circulation system. These findings indicate that the post-antral processes and hypothalamus-pituitary-ovary axis involving the secretion of gonadotropins in responsive to gonadotropin-releasing hormone (GnRH) has not been developed in ascidians, and reinforce the evolutionary scenario that the hypothalamus-pituitary endocrine system might have been established in concert with the acquisition of the closed circulation system in the evolutionary process of chordate invertebrates to vertebrates. Instead, as mentioned in the following sections, the functions of the *Ciona* ovary have been found to be regulated mainly by the neuroendocrine system and intraovarian paracrine system. Altogether, these findings lead to a presumption that whole *Ciona* oocyte growth process corresponds to the mammalian follicular growth process including the primordial to antral stages that is NOT subjected to the regulation by gonadotrpins, and thus, *Ciona* oocytes are excellent models for clarification of the molecular mechanisms underlying gonadotropin-independent follicular growth stages in vertebrates.

Despite these potentials of *C. intestinalis* as a novel model organism, this ascidian was not employed for study of endocrinology, neuroedocrinology, and neurology, given that only a few peptides had been identified in *C. intestinalis*. Over the past few years, however, various neuropeptides and/or hormone peptides have been characterized from *C. intestinalis*, which has paved the way for exploring the unprecedented regulatory systems for oocyte and follicle growth by neuropeptides and peptide hormones.

3. Novel oocyte growth pathway regulated by tachykinin and neurotensin

Recently, we have substantiated a novel oocyte growth pathway using *C. intestinalis.*, in which growth of vitellogenic oocytes to postvitellogenic oocytes is regulated via the regulation of protease activation by tachykinin (TK) and neurotensin-like peptide (NTLP) (Aoyama et al., 2008; Kawada et al., 2011). In this section, we provide basal knowledge concerning TKs and NTs followed by the clarification of the TK- and NTLP-directed oocyte growth.

3.1 TKs in C. *intestinalis*

TKs are vertebrate multi-functional brain/gut peptides involved in smooth muscle contraction, vasodilation, nociception, inflammation, neurodegeneration, and neuroprotection in a neuropeptidergic or endocrine fashion (Satake & Kawada, 2006a). All TKs are featured by the C-terminal consensus -Phe-X-Gly-Leu-Met-NH_2 (Satake & Kawada, 2006a). The mammalian TK family consists of four major peptides: Substance P (SP), Neurokinin A (NKA), Neurokinin B (NKB), and Hemokinin-1/Endokinins (HK-1/EKs), as shown in Table 1. TKs are encoded by three genes, namely *tac1* (or *pptA*), *tac3* (or *pptB*), or *tac4* (*pptC*) gene (Page, 2004; Satake & Kawada, 2006a). *tac1* generates four splicing variants which produce SP alone or SP and NKA. Similarly, several EK isoforms are produced from the *tac4* gene. The *tac3* gene yields only NKB.

TK receptors belong to the Class A (rhodopsin-like) G protein-coupled receptor (GPCR) family. Three subtypes of TK receptors, namely NK1, NK2, and NK3, have been identified in vertebrates (Satake & Kawada, 2006a). NK1, 2, and 3 were shown to induce both elevation of intracellular calcium and production of cAMP. NK1, 2, and 3 possess moderate ligand-selectivity: SP>NKA>NKB for NK1, NKA>NKB>SP for NK2, and NKB>NKA>SP for NK3, respectively (Page, 2004; Satake & Kawada, 2006a). HK-1 and the 10-amino acid C-terminal common sequence of EKA and EKB (EKA/B) were also found to exhibit potent binding activity on all NK1-3 with the highest selectivity to NK1 (Page 2004; Satake & Kawada, 2006a). In addition, EKC and EKD are devoid of any activity on NK1-3 (Page 2004; Satake & Kawada, 2006a).

In protostomes, TK-related peptides (TKRPs) exert a TK-like contractile activity and the expression of the *tkrp* gene is observed in the central nervous system (Satake et al, 2003; Satake & Kawada, 2006a). However, they contain the analogous Phe-Xaa1-(Gly/Ala)-Xaa2-Arg-NH_2 consensus (Table 1), and TKRP precursors encode multiple TKRP sequences (Satake et al., 2003; Satake and Kawada, 2006a), which are totally distinct from those of vertebrate TKs. These findings suggest that *tkrp* genes and *tk* genes diverged in distinct evolutionary lineages. TKRP receptors were characterized from several insects, an echiuroid worm and octopus (Kawada et al., 2002; Satake et al., 2003; Satake and Kawada, 2006a, Kanda et al., 2007). These GPCRs display high similarity to vertebrate TK receptors in the sequence and exon/intron organization (Kawada et al., 2002; Satake et al., 2003; Satake & Kawada, 2006a; Kanda et al., 2007). Consequently, TK receptors and TKRP receptors share the common original GPCR gene.

Moreover, TKRP receptors were shown to stimulate the increase in intracellular calcium or generation of cAMP (Satake et al., 2003; Satake & Kawada, 2006). Nevertheless, TKRP receptors, unlike NK1-3, exhibit no significant ligand selectivity to their cognate endogenous ligand peptides (Kawada et al., 2002; Satake et al., 2003; Satake & Kawada, 2006a; Kanda et al., 2007).

TKs were not identified in deuterostome invertebrates including ascidians till 2004. Two authentic TK peptides, Ci-TK-I and -II, were detected in the neural complex of *C. intestinalis* using a mass spectrometric analysis (Satake et al., 2004). The TK consensus motif is completely conserved in both the ascidian peptides (Table 1). Ci-TKs were found to elicit a TK-typical contraction of the guinea pig ileum, as seen in administration of SP. This data confirmed that Ci-TKs are conferred with the essential pharmacological characteristics of vertebrate TKs, given that protostome TKRPs are devoid of any effects on mammalian tissues (Satake et al., 2003; Satake & Kawada, 2006a). The Ci-TK precursor encodes both Ci-TK-I and Ci-TK-II, and shows structural organization similar to γ-*tac*1 (Satake et al., 2004;

Species	Peptide	Sequence
	Chordate tachykinins	
Mammals	Substance P	RPKPQQFFGLM-amide
	Neurokinin A	HKTDSFVGLM-amide
	Neurokinin B	DMHDFVGLM-amide
Rat and mouse	Hemokinin-1	SRTRQFYGLM-amide
Human	Endokinin A/B	GKASQFFGLM-amide
	Endokinin C	KKAYQLEHTFQGLL-amide
	Endokinin D	VGAYQLEHTFQGLL-amide
Ascidian (*Ciona intestinalis*)	**Ci-TK-I**	**HVRHFYGLM-amide**
	Ci-TK-II	**ASFTGLM-amide**
	Protostome tachykinin-related peptides	
Fruitfly	DTK-1	APTSSFIGMR-amide
Echiuroid worm	Uru-TK-I	LRQSQFVGAR-amide

Table 1. Tachykinins (TKs) and Tachykinin-related peptides (TKRPs). The TK and TKRP consensus moieties are underlined and dotted, respectively. *C. intestinalis* tachykinins (Ci-TK-I and -II) are indicated in boldface.

Satake & Kawada, 2006a). These findings provide evidence that the TK family is conserved as neuropeptides in chordates as well as in vertebrates, and indicate that the *ci-tk* gene is a direct prototype of vertebrate TKs. However, Ci-TK-I and -II sequences are located in the same exon, indicating that no alternative splicing of the *ci-tk* transcript occurs. Therefore, it is presumed that alternative production of TK peptides was established during the evolution of vertebrates (Satake et al., 2004). In combination, these findings indicate that the "prototype" *tk* gene, organized similarly to the *ci-tk*gene, originally encoded two TKs in the same exon, and then was divided by intron insertsion followed by acquirement of the alternative splicing system during the divergence of the ancestral gene into *tac*1, *tac*3, and *tac*4 during evolution of vertebrates.

The endogenous Ci-TK receptor, Ci-TK-R, was also identified in *C. intestinalis*. A sequence comparison verified that the transmembrane domain of Ci-TK-R displayed high sequence similarity (30-43%) to those of mammalian TK receptors (Satake et al., 2004). The phylogenetic analysis of TK receptors and TKRP receptors revealed that Ci-TK-R belongs to the vertebrate TK receptor clade (Satake & Kawada, 2006a). Moreover, *Ciona* database-searching for TK receptors detected only Ci-TK-R as an ortholog of TK receptors, indicating that ascidians possess one TK receptors (Satake et al., 2004). In combination, these findings suggest that Ci-TK-R is an ancestor of vertebrate TK receptors and that three vertebrate TK receptor genes were generated from a single common ancestor via gene duplication in the evolutionary process of vertebrates. Application of Ci-TK-I to Ci-TK-R evoked a typical intracellular calcium elevation (Satake et al., 2004). Additionally, SP and NKA also exhibited comparable responses to Ci-TK-I (Satake et al., 2004). These pharmacological analyses indicated that Ci-TK-R lacked the ligand selectivity typical of NK1-3 (Satake & Kawada, 2006a). Consequently, it is suggested that the ancestral TK receptor is highly likely to possess no significant ligand-selectivity and that the ligand-selectivity of TK receptors, along with the alternative production of TK ligands, were established during generation of NK1-3 in vertebrates.

3.2 NTLPs in *C. intestinalis*

Neurotensin (NT) is a vertebrate brain/gut peptide involved in dopamine transmission, pituitary hormone secretion, hypothermia, and analgesia as a neuromodulator (Evers, 2006). NT is yielded from a single precursor with a structurally related peptide, neuromedin N. These family peptides are featured by a Pro-Tyr-Ile-Ile C-terminal consensus sequence (Table 2). The NT family has so far been characterized only in mammals and birds (Evers, 2006). NT receptors, NTR1, 2, and 3 have been identified in mammals. NTR1 and -2 are Class A GPCRs, which trigger an elevation of intracellular calcium ion (Evers, 2006). NTR3 (or sortilin) is a non-GPCR membrane protein, and bound to NT. However, the resultant signal transduction has yet to be detected.

Peptide	Sequence
Neurotensin (rat)	pQLYENKPRRPYIL
Neurotensin (chicken)	pQLHVNKARRPYIL
Neuromedin N (rat)	KIPYIL
LANT 6(chicken)	KNPYIL
Ci-NTLP-1	**pQLHVPSIL**
Ci-NTLP-2	**GMMGPSII**
Ci-NTLP-3	**MMLGPGIL**
Ci-NTLP-4	**FGMIPSII**
Ci-NTLP-5	**NKLLYPSVI**
Ci-NTLP-6	**SRHPKLYFPGIV**

Table 2. Neurotesin (NT) and its related peptides. The NT consensus moiety is underlined. *C. intestinalis* NT-like peptides (Ci-NTLP-1 to -6) are indicated in boldface.

Quite recently, we have identified six *Ciona* NT-like peptides, Ci-NTLP-1 to -6, by a peptidomic approach (Kawada et al., 2011). As shown in Table 2, Ci-NTLPs share the Pro-Ser/Gly-Ile/Val-Ile-Leu, which is reminiscent of the NT C-terminal consensus (Table 2). Ci-NTLPs are encoded by two genes; Ci-NTLPs were encoded in two precursors; *ci-ntlp-A* encodes Ci-NTLP-1 to -4, while *ci-ntlp-B* encodes Ci-NTLP-5 and -6 (Kawada et al., 2011). Of particular interest is that *ci-ntlp-A* is expressed exclusively in neurons of the brain ganglion, whereas the abundant expression of *ci-ntlp-B* is detected in the ovary. Consequently, it is presumed that Ci-NTLP-1 to 4 serve as neuropeptides, while Ci-NTLP-5 and -6 are ovarian hormones. This is the first characterization of NT-related peptides in invertebrates.

3.3 The TK- and NTLP-regulated oocyte growth in *C. intestinalis*

The biological roles of TKs in the ovary remained to be elucidated. The ascidian ovary harbors numerous oocytes at each growth stage (Prodon et al., 2006; Aoyama et. al., 2008). Furthermore, *Ciona* oocytes are readily classified into four major growth stages on the basis of their dimeter and organization: previtellogenic (stage I), vitellogenic (stage II), postvitellogenic (stage III), and mature (stage IV) stages (Prodon et al., 2006). These advantages indicate the possibility that the *Ciona* ovary and oocytes are suitable models for functional analyses of ovarian TKs. The immunoreactivity of Ci-TK-R was detected exclusively in test cells residing in late stage-II oocytes (Aoyama et al., 2008), which are believed to be functional counterparts for mammalian granulosa cells and to be involved in growth of oocyte bodies and follicle cells (Burighel & Cloney, 1997).

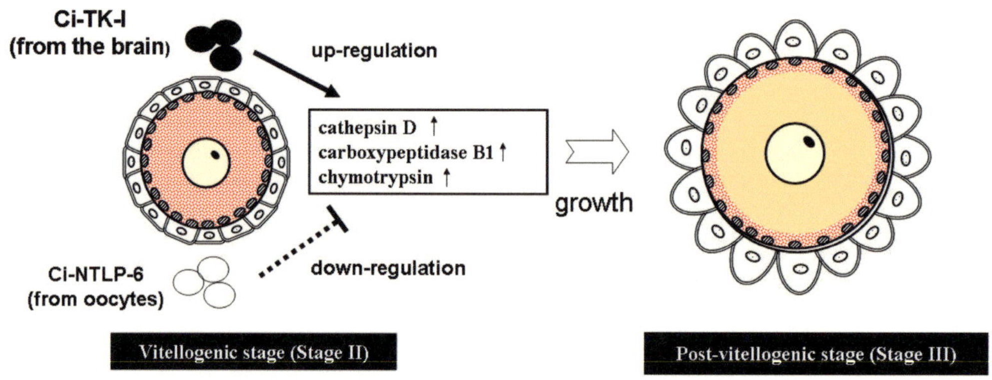

Fig. 4. Scheme of the oocyte growth regulated by Ci-TK-I and Ci-NTLP-6 in *C. intestinalis*.

Such specific expression of Ci-TK-R revealed that test cells of the late stage II oocytes are the sole targets of Ci-TK-I in the ovary. Comprehensive gene expression profiles between the untreated ovary and ovary treated with Ci-TK-I verified that the cathepsin D, chymotrypsin, and carboxypeptidase B1 genes are upregulated by Ci-TK-I (Aoyama et al., 2008). The enzymatic activities of these proteases were also shown to be enhanced by Ci-TK-I (Aoyama et al., 2008). Furthermore, treatment of *Ciona* late stage II oocytes with Ci-TK-I resulted in the growth to stage III, which was completely blocked by a Ci-TK-R antagonist or inhibitors of cathepsin D, chymotrypsin, and carboxypeptidase B1 (Aoyama et al., 2008). These findings revealed that Ci-TK-I is responsible for oocyte growth via the activation of the proteases. The involvement of these proteases in the *Ciona* oocyte growth is compatible with their functions in other species. For instance, leupeptin, which has the ability of inhibiting activity of chymotrypsin, was shown to suppress progression of oocyte growth at pre-GVBD stages in an ascidian *Halocynthia roretzi* (Sakairi and Shirai, 1991) and a starfish *Asterina pectinifera* (Takagi et al., 1989; Tanaka et al., 2000). In *Drosophila*, fluorescent-conjugated chymotrypsin inhibitors were localized to the growing oocyte-somatic follicle cells (Jakobsen et al., 2005). Carboxypeptidase B1 was also shown to play a crucial role in proteolytic processing of several component proteins for zona pellucida in mammalian oocytes at an early growth stage (Litscher et al., 1999). Cathepsin D was found to participate in production of yolk proteins and follicular component in various vertebrate oocytes at the stage prior to GVBD (Carnevali et al., 2006). Collectively, these results led to the conclusion that Ci-TK-I enhances growth of the vitellogenic oocytes via upregulation of gene expression and enzymatic activities of the proteases for vitellogenesis and oogenesis (Fig. 4), and suggested that the TK-regulated oocyte growth is an evolutionary origin of the TKergic functions in the ovary. More recently, a *Ciona* NT-like peptide, Ci-NTLP-6, has been shown to arrest the protease-associated oocyte growth at stage II via down-regulation of the gene expression of the Ci-TK-induced proteases (Kawada et al., 2011). It should be noteworthy that Ci-NTLP-6 serves as an oocytic hormone, given that the *ci-ntlp-B* gene expression was detected in the ovary (Kawada et al., 2011). This is the first clarification of the biological roles of TKs and NTs in the ovary and the underlying essential molecular mechanism, leading to a substantiation of a novel regulatory pathway for oocyte growth (Fig. 4). In addition, our preliminary work suggests that the protease-associated oocyte growth pathway is essentially conserved in mammals (unpublished data). Altogether, these data reinforce the view that ascidians are one of the most useful model organisms for functional analyses of neuropeptides and hormones conserved in vertebrates and ascidians.

4. Neuropeptides and peptide hormones in *C. intestinalis*

In addition to Ci-TKs and Ci-NTLPs, a wide variety of neuropeptides and peptide hormones have been identified in *C. intestinalis*. In this section, we present the *Ciona* homologs of mammalian peptides which are highly likely to be involved in ovarian functions due to the expression of several of their receptors or receptor candidates in the ovary or their potential reproductive functions.

4.1 Recent identification of *Ciona* neuropeptides and hormone peptides

Recently, two approaches for characterization of peptides and/or their genes are available. The first one is homology search on a genome/EST database of an organism of interest. This procedure is useful for detection of peptides containing long sequences and/or conserving consensus motifs. For instance, genes of *Ciona* GnRHs, calcitonin (CT), insulin-like peptides (INS-Ls), and corticotrophin-releasing factor (CRF) were identified by homology search on the *Ciona* genome/EST database (Adams et al., 2003., Olinski et al., 2006; Sekiguchi et al., 2009; Lovejoy & Barsyte-Lovejoy, 2010). In contrast, homology-based search is frequently useless for detection of small peptides or their genes, given that major neuropeptides and peptide hormones contain short sequences, and that their precursors have slight homology, even though homologous peptide hormones and neuropeptides harbor complete consensus motifs. Additionally, novel peptides or peptide homologs with partial consensus motifs cannot be detected by any form of homology search. The second one is mass spectrometry (MS)-based peptidomic analysis. This procedure enables direct characterization of peptide sequences present in the tissues of interest. The most important step in peptidomic analysis is to discriminate biologically significant peptides with protein fragments. In general, neuropeptide or peptide hormone precursors harbor a hydrophobic signal peptide sequence at the N-terminus, and the mature peptide sequences there are flanked by endoproteolytic mono- or dibasic sites (Lys-Lys / Lys-Arg / Arg-Arg / Arg). According to these criteria, authentic neuropeptides and peptide hormones can be discriminated from degraded protein fragments, when their precursors of candidates for neuropeptides and peptide hormones sequenced by peptidomic analysis are available. A genome/EST database allows us to detect precursor sequences of the peptide candidates by referencing the obtained sequences, but not by the cloning of their cDNAs. In conclusion, a combination of MS-based peptidomic analysis and database-referencing of the resultant sequence (Fig. 5) is the most reliable and efficient methods for characterization of neuropeptides and peptide hormones. Based on such a screening strategy, we eventually identified 33 *Ciona* peptides (Table 3).

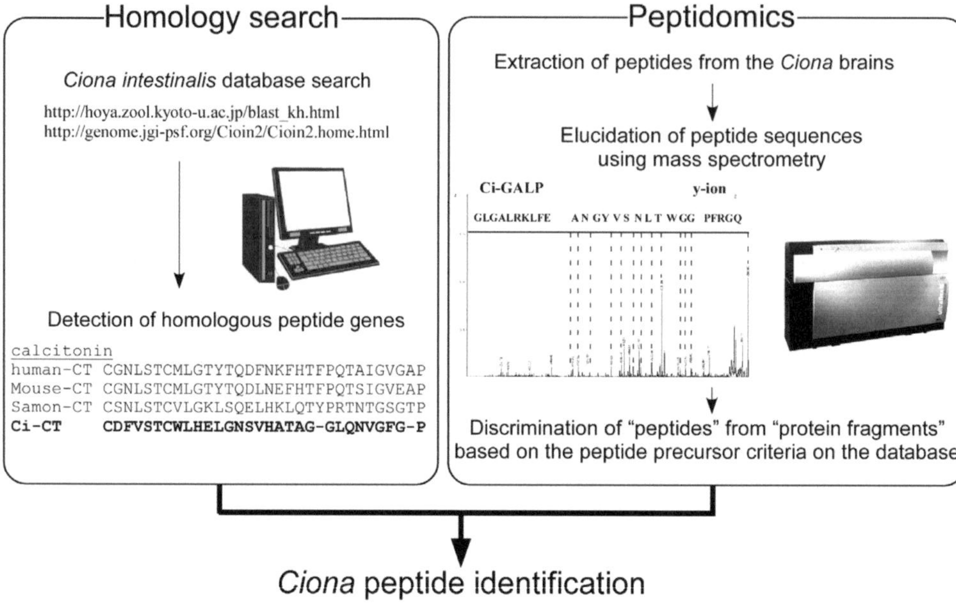

Fig. 5. Scheme of *Ciona* peptide identification

These *Ciona* peptides are largely classified into three categories: (i) prototypes and homologs of vertebrate peptides such as cholecystokinin (CCK), GnRHs, TK, CT, INS-Ls, CRF, galanin/galanin-like peptide (GALP), (ii) peptides partially homologous with vertebrate peptides including vasopressin (VP), GnRH-related peptide, NTLPs, (iii) novel peptides such as LF-family peptides and YFL/V peptides. Of particular significance is that *C. intestinalis* has been shown to possess the prototypes and homologs of vertebrate peptides, including CCK, TK, CT, CRF, galanin/GALP, and NTs, which have been never found in any other invertebrates including *Drosophila melanogaster, Caenorhabditis elegans* and *Stronglyocentrotus purpuratus* (Satake & Kawada, 2006b, Kawada et al., 2010). These findings provide indisputable evidence that *C. intestinalis* possesses a greater number of homologs to vertebrate peptides compared with other invertebrates, and suggest that many peptide prototypes originated from common ancestor chordates of ascidians and vertebrates, not from ancient vertebrates.

This view is compatible with the fact that ascidians occupy a phylogenetic position which is closer to vertebrates in evolutionary lineages of animals than any other invertebrates. It should be noteworthy that the *Ciona* homologs of vertebrate neuropeptides and/or peptide hormones from various glands including the hypothalamus have been identified, but no homologs of vertebrate pituitary hormones, such as ACTH, TSH, FSH, LH, GH, and PRL, have ever been reported (Kawada et al., 2010; Kawada et al., 2011). This is consistent with the fact that ascidians are not endowed with an organ corresponding to a pituitary (Burighel & Cloney, 1997). Collectively, these findings lead to a presumption that *C. intestinalis* shows applicability to the investigation of biological functions and their evolutionary aspects of neuropeptides and non-pituitary peptide hormones of vertebrates. In the following sections, we summarize *Ciona* homologs of vertebrate peptides, of which receptors or their candidates were shown to be expressed in the ovary.

Accession Number	Gene	Peptide	Peptide Sequence
BR000879	*ci-ntlp-B*	Ci-NTLP-5	NKLLYPSVI
		Ci-NTLP-6	SRHPKLYFPGIV
BR000880			AVLHLAINEFQRL
BR000876	*ci-ntlp-A*	Ci-NTLP-1	pQLHVPSIL
		Ci-NTLP-2	MMLGPGIL
		Ci-NTLP-3	GMMGPSII
		Ci-NTLP-4	FGMIPSII
BR000877	*ci-galp*	Ci-GALP	PFRGQGGWTLNSVGYNAGLGALRKLFE
BR000881	*ci-lf*	Ci-LF-1	*FQSLF*
		Ci-LF-2	YPGFQGLF
		Ci-LF-3	HNPHLPDLF
		Ci-LF-4	YNSMGLF
		Ci-LF-5	SPGMLGLF
		Ci-LF-6	SDARLQGLF
		Ci-LF-7	YPNFQGLF
		Ci-LF-8	GNLHSLF
BR000882			GFQNNAEGPV
			SADLFGAPMYII
AB219239	*ci-gnrh-x*	Ci-GnRH-X	pQHWSNWWIPGAPGYNG-amide
AY204706	*ci-gnrh-1*	t-GnRH-3	pQHWSKGYSPG-amide
		t-GnRH-5	pQHWSYEFMPG-amide
		t-GnRH-6	pQHWSYEYMPG-amide
BR000878			GEKESRPLSSYPGSV
BR000883			*DPLTNIM*
BR000884			WLRYDA
BR000885	*ci-yfv/l*	Ci-YFV-1	ELVVRDPYFV
		Ci-YFV-2	*NNQESYFV*
		Ci-YFV-3	DDEPRSYFV
		Ci-YFL-1	DAARPNYYFL
AB432887	*ci-vp*	Ci-VP	CFFRDCSNMDWYR
AB175738	*ci-tk*	Ci-TK-I	HVRHFYGLM-amide
		Ci-TK-II	SIGDQPSIFNERASFTGLM-amide
BR000886			NLLSLLQHAIETANNAYRSPR

Table 3. *C. intestinalis* peptides identified by a peptidomic approach.

4.2 GnRHs in *C. intestinalis*

GnRH (previously designated luteinizing-hormone-releasing hormone = LH-RH), has a critical role in reproductive development and function, which is released via the hypothalamic-hypophysial portal system to regulate the synthesis and release of pituitary gonadotropins that in turn trigger the steroidogenesis and stimulate gonadal maturation in vertebrates (Millar, 2005). Furthermore, GnRHs are involved in diverse neuroendocrine,

Peptide	Sequence
human GnRH-I	pQHWSYGLRPG-amide
human GnRH-II	pQHWSHGWYPG-amide
GnRH-III (fish)	pQHWSYGWLPG-amide
t-GnRH-3	**pQHWSYEFMPG-amide**
t-GnRH-4	**pQHWSNQLTPG-amide**
t-GnRH-5	**pQHWSYEYMPG-amide**
t-GnRH-6	**pQHWSKGYSPG-amide**
t-GnRH-7	**pQHWSYALSPG-amide**
t-GnRH-8	**pQHWSLALSPG-amide**
Ci-GnRH-X	**pQHWSNWWIPGAPGYNG-amide**
octopus-GnRH	pQNYHFSNGWHPG-amide

Table 4. GnRHs. The GnRH consensus moiety is underlined. *C. intestinalis* GnRH family peptides (t-GnRH-3 to -8 plus Ci-GnRH-X) are indicated in boldface.

paracrine, autocrine, and neurotransmitter/neuromodulatory functions in the central and peripheral nervous systems, and a wide range of peripheral tissues (Millar 2005). GnRH was isolated from protostomes, urochordates and vertebrates (Table 4). Vertebrate GnRHs are composed of 10 amino acids with the consensus sequences of pyro-Glu^{1}-His/Tyr^{2}-Trp^{3}-Ser^{4} and Pro^{9}-Gly^{10}-amide (Millar, 2005).

As shown in Table 4, two types of GnRH, GnRH-I and II were characterized in vertebrates, whereas GnRH-III was also found exclusively in teleosts (Millar, 2005). In lamprey GnRH, one GnRH-I orthlog (l-GnRH-II) and two paralogs (l-GnRH-I and –III) were identified (Kavanaugh et al., 2008). Protostome GnRHs were characterized from molluscs (Iwakoshi et al., 2002; Zhang et al, 2008). These molluscan GnRHs, composed of 12 amino acids, essentially conserve the GnRH consensus sequence (Table 4). All GnRHs are encoded as a single copy in the precursor, whose organization is conserved in vertebrates and protostomes (Iwakoshi-Ukena et al., 2004; Millar, 2005; Kavanaugh et al., 2008).

GnRH receptors (GnRHRs) belong to the class A (rhodopsin-like) GPCR family, and regulate elevation of intracellular calcium ion, generation and inhibition of cAMP production by coupling to different G-proteins (Millar et al., 2005). GnRHRs display some species-specific distribution, although at least one GnRHR was identified in all vertebrates (Kah et al., 2007). Mammalian type-I GnRHR completely lacks the C-terminal tail region which is found in non-mammalian counterparts (Millar et al., 2004; Millar 2005). Species-distribution of type-II GnRHR is relatively confounding; human, chimp, cow, and sheep type-II *gnrhr* gene is likely silenced due to deletion of functional domains or interruption of full-length translation by the presence of a stop codon, whereas a functional type-II GnRHR was identified in several monkeys, pigs, reptiles, and amphibians (Millar 2005; Kah et al., 2007). Moreover, type-II *gnrhr* genes have not been found in mouse and fish. Instead, fish possesses another GnRH receptor, type-III GnRHRs which are included in the subgroup separate from type-I and II GnRHRs (Millar 2005; Kah et al., 2007). Type-I GnRHRs show high affinity to both GnRH-I and II, whereas the type-II receptor is specific to GnRH-II. In protostomes, an octopus GnRHR was found to possess a C-terminal tail and to trigger mobilization of intracellular cellular calcium ions (Kanda et al., 2006).

In *C. intestinalis*, six authentic GnRH peptides (t-GnRH-3 to -8) and one structurally related peptide were identified (Adams et al., 2003; Kawada et al., 2009a). Of particular interest is that two *Ciona* GnRH genes, *ci-gnrh-1* and *-2*, encode three different GnRH peptide sequences (Adams et al., 2003): t-GnRH-3, -5, and -6 are encoded in *ci-gnrh-1*, whereas t-GnRH-4, -7, and -8 are encoded in *ci-gnrh-2*. All GnRH sequences are flanked by mono- or dibasic endoproteolytic sites at their N- and C-termini (Adams et al., 2003). These triplet GnRH sequence organizations were also observed in *cs-gnrh-1* and *2* of *Ciona savignyi*, an ascidan species closely related to *C. intestinalis* (Adams et al., 2003). These findings have established the basis that three copies of GnRH are present in one precursor in ascidians, unlike vertebrate and protostome GnRH precursors that encode only a single GnRH sequence, and that the structural organization of *Ciona gnrh* genes occurred from the ancestral GnRH gene during an ascidian-unique evolutionary process.

A novel GnRH-like peptide, Ci-GnRH-X (Kawada et al., 2009a), was also characterized from the neural complexes of adult *C. intestinalis*. The *Ciona* peptide was shown to contain the GnRH consensus sequences, such as the N-terminal pQHWS sequence and a C-terminal amidated Gly. However, Ci-GnRH-X, unlike the 10-residue chordate or 12-residue protostome GnRHs, is composed of 16 amino acid residues, and lacks the common Pro at position 2 from the C-termini of the GnRH family peptides (Table 4). It is noteworthy that the *t-gnrh-X* gene encodes only a single Ci-GnRH-X. This organization is closer to those of vertebrate *gnrh* genes than *ci-gnrh-1* and *-2*.

To date, four GnRH receptors, namely, Ci-GnRHR-1, -2, -3, and -4, have been identified in *C. inetestinalis* (Kusakabe et al., 2003; Tello et al., 2005). Ci-GnRHR-1 share 70%, 38%, and 36% sequence homology to Ci-GnRHR-2, -3, and -4, respectively, and all Ci-GnRHRs display approx. 30% sequence identity to human type-I GnRHR (Kusakabe et al., 2003; Tello et al., 2005). The phylogenetic analyses demonstrated that Ci-GnRHR-2, -3, and -4 are not homologs of vertebrate GnRHR subgroups but *Ciona*-specific paralogs of Ci-GnRHR-1 (Kusakabe et al., 2003; Tello et al., 2005). Of particular significance is the distinct ligand-selective production of second messengers mediated by Ci-GnRHRs. The elevation of intracellular calcium, which is typical of vertebrate and octopus GnRH and receptors (Millar 2005; Kanda et al., 2006), was only observed in administration of t-GnRH-6 to Ci-GnRHR-1, while other Ci-GnRHRs failed to stimulate the calcium elevation with any t-GnRHs (Tello et al., 2005). Instead, Ci-GnRHR-2 is responsive to t-GnRH-7, 8, 6 in this order of potency, while t-GnRH-3 and -5 specifically activate Ci-GnRHR-3 to a similar extent. Ci-GnRHR-4 exhibited neither elevation of intracellular calcium nor cAMP production (Tello et al., 2005). Instead, Ci-GnRHR-4 was shown to heterodimerize with Ci-GnRHR-1 and then potentiate the elevation of intracellular calcium, both calcium-dependent and –independent protein kinase C subtypes, and ERK phosphorylation in a ligand-selective fashion, verifying that Ci-GnRHR-4 serves as a protomer of GPCR heterodimers rather than a ligand-binding GPCR (Sakai et al., 2010). Intriguingly, Ci-GnRH-X was found to moderately (10-50%) inhibited the elevation of the intracellular calcium and cAMP production by t-GnRH-6 at Ci-GnRHR-1, and cAMP production by t-GnRH-3 and -5 via Ci-GnRHR-3 (Kawada et al., 2009a). In contrast, no inhibitory effect of Ci-GnRH-X at Ci-GnRHR-2 was observed (Kawada et al., 2009a). These findings provide evidence that t-GnRHs and Ci-GnRHRs have not redundant but specific biological roles. Adams et al. (2003) demonstrated that t-GnRH-3 and -5 elicited the efficient spawning activity. These findings provide evidence that a major function of t-GnRHs is the regulation of gamete release, suggesting that t-GnRHs plays a major role in gamete release in protochordates. Finally, t-GnRHs and Ci-GnRH-X were found to be expressed exclusively in neurons in the brain ganglion, whereas Ci-GnRHRs, including the Ci-GnRHR-1&R-4 heterodimer, were detected in test cells of vitellogenic oocytes as well as the brain ganglion (Adams et al., 2003, Kusakabe et al., 2003; Tello et al., 2005; Kawada et al., 2009a; Sakai et al., 2010). Altogether, it is concluded that *C. intestinalis* GnRHs participate in various reproduction-relevant functions as multifunctional neuropeptides. In other words, *C. intestinalis* has evolved neuropeptidergic GnRH-directed regulation of the ovary, which is highly likely to be a functional ancestor of vertebrate GnRHergic endocrine and neuroendocrine systems

4.3 Vasopressin/oxytocin in *C. intestinalis*

Oxytocin (OT) and vasopressin (VP) have so far been characterized from a great variety of animal species from protostomes to human (Kawada et al., 2009b). In mammals, it is well known that OT is responsible for reproductive behavior: uterine contraction, milk ejection, and male reproductive tract stimulation (Gimpl & Fahrenholz, 2001). On the other hand, VP plays a major part in osmoregulation including up-regulation of blood pressure and anti-diuretic effect (Frank & Landgraf, 2008). Moreover, a number of studies suggested that OT and VP served as multifunctional peptides in the central and peripheral tissues (Gimpl & Fahrenholz, 2001; Frank & Landgraf, 2008). OT and VP are likely to be also involved in highly advanced central functions and disorders including learning, social behavior, anxiety, and autism (Donaldson & Young, 2008; Frank & Landgraf, 2008).

OT and VP are composed of nine amino acids, and bear a circular structure formed by an intramolecular disulfide bridge between conserved Cys^1 and Cys^6 (Table 5). Moreover, Asn^5, Pro^7, Gly^9, and C-terminal amidation are conserved in most OT/VP superfamily peptides (Table 5). OT and VP are discriminated by an amino acid present at position 8; VP family peptides contain a basic amino acid (arginine or lysine), whereas a neutral amino acid (leucine, isoleucine, valine, or threonine) is located at this position of OT family peptides (Table 5). The sub-mammalian vertebrate VP homolog, vasotocin, also contains Arg at position 8, while the sub-mammalian vertebrate OT homologs, mesotocin and isotocin, harbor Ile at this position. Notably, one VP family peptide and one OT family peptide have been identified in most jawed vertebrates (Hoyle, 1998; Gimpl and Fahrenholz, 2001), although only one type of the OT/VP superfamily peptide has ever been found in cyclostomes and most invertebrates (Hoyle, 1998; Kawada et al., 2009b). Combined with the phylogenic position of cyclostomes as the stem species of vertebrates, the presence of vasotocin as the single member of the OT/VP superfamily in cyclostomes suggests that the OT family and VP family occurred via a gene duplication of the common ancestral gene during evolution from jawless fish to jawed fish. OT/VP superfamily peptides have also been identified in invertebrates: molluscs, annelids, insects, sea urchins, amphioxus, and ascidians (Hoyle, 1998; Kawada et al., 2009b). Protostome and non-ascidian deuterostome invertebrate OT/VP superfamily peptides are all composed of nine amino acids, and share the OT/VP consensus amino acids (Table 5).

Peptide	Sequence	Species
Protochordate		
Ci-VP	**CFFRDCSNMDWYR**	***Ciona intestinalis***
SOP	CYISDCPNSRFWST-amide	*Styela plicata*
Vertebrate		
oxytocin	CYIQNCPLG-amide	mammal
mesotocin	CYIQNCPIG-amide	non-mammalian tetrapod
isotocin	CYISNCPIG-amide	fish
vasopressin	CYFQNCPRG-amide	mammal
vasotocin	CYIQNCPRG-amide	non-mammalian vertebrates
Protostome		
Lys-conopressin	CFIRNCPKG-amide	*Lymnaea stagnail*
annetocin	CFVRNCPTG-amide	*Eisenia foetida*
octopressin	CFWTSCPIG-amide	*Octopus vulgaris*

Table 5. The oxytocin/vasopressin superfamily peptides. The *Ciona* peptide (Ci-VP) is indicated in boldface.

Both OT and VP precursors are composed of major three regions: a signal peptide, an OT or VP sequence flanked by a putative glycine C-terminal amidation signal and a dibasic endoproteolytic site, and a neurophysin featured by 14 highly conserved cysteines (Hoyle, 1998; Kawada et al., 2009b). Seven disulfide bridge pairs between each of the 14 cysteines are responsible for formation of correct tertiary structure to interact with OT/VP (Hoyle, 1998; Kawada et al., 2009b). This structural organization is conserved in all OT/VP superfamily peptide precursors with an exception of a *Ciona* counterpart as described later. Taken together, molecular characterstics of OT/VP superfamily peptides and their precursors are highly conserved in wide species from protostomes to human.

The OT/VP superfamily peptides manifest their activities through their receptors, which belong to the Class A GPCR family (Gimpl & Fahrenholz, 2001; Frank & Landgraf, 2008). The OT/VP superfamily peptide receptors display high sequence similarity with one another, indicating that they are included in a cognate GPCR superfamily. To date, three VP receptors (V1aR, V1bR, and V2R) and one OT receptor (OTR) have been identified in mammals. V1aR, V1bR and OTR have been shown to trigger an increase in the intracellular calcium ions (Gimpl & Fahrenholz, 2001; Frank & Landgraf, 2008), whereas V2R induces the production of cAMP (Frank & Landgraf, 2008).

The essential biological roles for the supefamily peptides are conserved in protostomes. An earthworm OT/VP superfamily peptide, annetocin, showed an OT-like physiological action. Injection of annetocin into the earthworm resulted in induction of the stereotyped egg-laying behavior (Oumi et al., 1996; Satake et al., 1999). Furthermore, the annetocin receptor gene was expressed specifically in the nephridia located in the clitellum region, suggesting that annetocin induced egg-laying behavior through the osmoregulatory action on the nephridia (Kawada et al., 2004). On the other hand, the osmoregulatory function was exhibited by inotocin that is an OT/VP superfamily peptide identified from a red flour beetle, *Tribolium castaneum*. Inotocin indirectly stimulated the Malpighian tubules through the central nervous system including the endocrine organs corpora cardiaca and corpora allata, leading to induction of the diuretic activity (Aikins et al., 2008).

OT/VP superfamily peptides were identified in different ascidians. Ci-VP is the first deuterostome invertebrate OT/VP family peptide from *C. intestinalis* (Kawada et al., 2008), and SOP was characterized from another ascidian, *Styela plicata* (Ukena et al., 2008). The most outstanding feature of the ascidian OT/VP superfamily peptide sequences is an elongation of the C-termini as compared with other OT/VP superfamily peptides (Table 5). Ci-VP and SOP are composed of 13 and 14 amino acids, respectively, whereas typical OT/VP superfamily peptides are comprised of 9 amino acids (Table 5). In particular, Ci-VP is the only OT/VP superfamily peptide that bears the non-amidated C-terminus (Table 5). Meanwhile, the N-termini of these ascidian peptides display high sequence homology to other OT/VP superfamily peptides (Table 5). Such unique forms of Ci-VP and SOP were presumed to have evolved in ascidian-specific evolutionary lineages.

OT/VP superfamily precursors harbor a neurophysin domain featured by 14 highly conserved cysteines including two doublet cysteines (Kawada et al., 2009b). The Ci-VP precursor also encoded a neurophysin-like domain, but the *Ciona* neurophysin was found to possess only 10 cysteines. However, 10 cysteines in the *C. intestinalis* neurophysin, including two cysteine doublets, are positioned almost identically to those of other neurophysin domains (Kawada et al., 2008). Additionally, the 13-residue and C-terminally non-amidated Ci-VP peptide and the 10-cysteine neurophysin domain were detected in the genome database of the closely related species, *Ciona savignyi*. In contrast, the 14-cysteine neurophysin domain is completely conserved in the SOP gene (Ukena et al., 2008). These findings indicate the intraphyletic molecular diversity of neurophysin domains as well as the hormone sequences within ascidian species.

C. intestinalis possesses the sole Ci-VP-receptor, Ci-VP-R, which displayed high amino acid sequence similarity (35–56%) to those of vertebrate and protostome OT/VP superfamily peptide receptors (Kawada et al., 2008). The molecular phylogenetic analysis also confirmed that Ci-VP-R belongs to the OT/VP superfamily peptide receptor family. Furthermore, Ci-VP-R specifically evoked an intracellular calcium elevation in response to Ci-VP (Kawada et al., 2008). These results lead to the conclusion that Ci-VP-R is an endogenous Ci-VP receptor in *C. intestinalis.*

The *ci-vp* gene was expressed predominantly in several neurons of the brain ganglion (Kawada et al., 2008). Ci-VP-R mRNA was detected in various tissues: the neural complex, alimentary tract, endostyle, heart, and ovary (Kawada et al., 2008). The distribution of Ci-VP and Ci-VP-R mRNAs suggested that Ci-VP served as a multifunctional neuropeptide and was transferred from the brain ganglion to target peripheral tissues followed by exertion of physiological functions. SOP mRNA was also distributed in the neural ganglion, and immunohistochemistry of SOP in the neural complex demonstrated that SOP was localized to the neuropil of the brain (Ukena et al., 2008). Intriguingly, the expression of SOP mRNA in hypotonic sea water was 2-fold greater than those in isotonic and hypertonic sea water (Ukena et al., 2008). Furthermore, SOP evoked contractions with increased tonus in the siphon of the ascidian (Ukena et al., 2008). These results proved the functional correlation of SOP with osmoregulation. Further studies are required for the elucidation of the physiological mechanism of ascidian OT/VP superfamily peptides.

4.4 Calcitonin in *C. intestinalis*

Calcitonin (CT) is a 32-amino acid peptide, and is synthesized mainly in the C cells of the thyroid gland in mammals and the ultimobranchial gland in non-mammalian vertebrates expect cyclostomes (Hull et al., 1998). CTs play a pivotal role in calcium metabolism via suppression of osteoclasts activity in bones and teleost scales. CTs conserve a C-terminal

Peptide	Sequence
	Vertebrate CT/CGRP family peptide
Human CT	CGNLSTCMLGTYTQDFNKFHTFPQTAIGVGAP-amide
Human CGRP	ACDTATCVTHRLAGLLSRSGGVVKNNFVPTNVGSKAF-amide
Human Adrenomeullin	YRQSMNNFQGLRSFGCRFGTCTVQKLAHQIYQFTDKDKDNVAPRSKISPQGY-amide
Human Amylin	KCNTATCATQRLANFLVHSSNNFGAILSSTNVGSNTY-amide
Pig CRSP	SCNTATCMTHRLVGLLSRSGSMVRSNLLPTKMGFKVFG-amide
	Ascidian CT/CGRP family peptide
Ci-CT	**CDGVSTCWLHELGNSVHATAGGKQNVGFGP-amide**

Table 6. The CT/CGRP superfamily peptides. The consensus motif is underlined. The *Ciona* peptide (Ci-CT) is indicated in boldface

amidated proline and N-terminal circular structure formed by a disulfide bridge between Cys[1] and Cys[7]. In vertebrates, CT, CT gene-related peptide (CGRP), Amylin (AMY), Adrenomedullin (AM), and CT receptor-stimulating peptide (CRSP) belong to the CT/CGRP family peptide (Hull et al., 1998; Katafuchi et al., 2003). Although they display low sequence similarity, they share the essential secondary structure with CTs (Table 6). CGRPs are yielded from the *ct* gene via alternative splicing (α-CGRP) and another CGRP gene (β-CGRP) in the central and peripheral neuron, and acts not only as a vasodilator but also as a neuromodulator (Hull et al., 1998). AMY is secreted from pancreatic β-cells, and inhibits insulin-induced glucose uptake and glycogen synthesis in the skeletal muscle (Cooper et al., 1988). AM is initially isolated from phaechromyctoma, and elicits a vasodilatory effect and reduces the blood pressure (Kitamura et al., 2002). CRSP was involved in suppression of food intake (Sawada et al., 2006). Although the CT/CGRP family peptides except CRSP were detected in most vertebrates, CRSP was identified in pigs and dogs of the Laurasiatheria (Katafuchi et al., 2003).

Ligand	Receptor	RAMP
Calcitonin	CTR	none
CRSP	CTR	none
CGRP and Amylin	CTR	RAMP1
Amylin	CTR	RAMP3
CGRP	CRLR	RAMP1
Adrenomedullin and CGRP	CRLR	RAMP2

Table 7. Ligand selectivity of CTR/RAMP and CRLR/RAMP complexes

Two Class B GPCRs, CT receptor (CTR) and CTR-like receptor (CRLR), have so far been shown to be the receptors for CT/CGRP family peptides (Conner et al., 2004). Furthermore, as summarized in Table 7, three receptor activity-modifying proteins (RAMPs), single-

transmembrane spanning proteins, have been shown to form a heterodimer with CTR or CRLR, and then to modulate the ligand-receptor specificity (Conner et al., 2004).
Although no CT/CGRP family peptide was identified in invertebrates till 2008, a *Ciona* CT (Ci-CT) gene was cloned from the adult *Ciona* neural complex (Sekiguchi et al., 2009). As summarized in Table 6, the deduced amino acid sequence of Ci-CT displays that the N-terminal circular region formed by a disulfide bond between Cys^1 and Cys^7 and the C-terminal amidated Pro are almost completely conserved, indicating that Ci-CT possesses the essential sequence characteristics of vertebrate CTs (Sekiguchi et al., 2009). In contrast, the *ci-ct* gene showed the four-exon/three-intron structure, whereas the most vertebrate *ct* genes are composed of six exons and five introns (Sekiguchi et al., 2009). CT or CGRP peptide is generated from the CT gene via alternative splicing (Hull et al., 1988), whereas the *ci-ct* gene encodes a Ci-CT peptide sequence alone, and no splicing variant was detected (Sekiguchi et al., 2009). No candidate for AM, AMY, CRSP, and beta CGRP genes was detected in the *Ciona* genome (Sekiguchi et al., 2009), suggesting that Ci-CT is the sole *Ciona* peptide of the CT/CGRP family peptides.
In *Ciona* juveniles, the transcript of Ci-CT was detected in the neural complex, stigumata cell of gill, gastrointestinal tract, blood cells, and endostyle (Sekiguchi et al., 2009). These multiple tissue-distribution implied that an original CT/CGRP family peptide might have played various physiological roles of current vertebrate CT/CGRP family peptides in common ancestral chordates, and current tissue-specific gene expressions and physiological roles of CT/CGRP family peptides diverged from those of a Ci-CT-like ancestor in concert with multiplication of the family gene members via gene duplications and advances of tissue organizations during evolution of protochordates to vertebrates. Ci-CT mRNA is localized to the neural gland, which is a non-neuronal ovoid body spongy texture lying immediately ventral to the brain ganglion, suggesting that Ci-CT serves as an endocrine/paracrine factor, not as a neuropeptide, in the neural gland of ascidians. Unfortunately, direct evidence for the interaction of Ci-CT with the endogenous receptor candidate, Ci-CT-R, has yet to be obtained (Sekiguchi et al., 2009). Further investigation of Ci-CT physiological activity will provide new insights into the functional evolution of chordate CT/CGRP family peptide.

4.5 Insulin and related peptides in *C. intestinalis*

The *Ciona* insulin-like peptides were also detected. Conserved synteny between the regions hosting the human insulin/relaxin (RLN) paralogs and the region hosting the three *Ciona* insulin-like proteins (INS-L1, -L2, and -L3) suggested that *Ciona* INS-Ls are putative orthologs of the vertebrate insulin–RLN family (Olinski et al., 2006a). Olinski et al. (2006b) also revealed that *Ciona* INS-L1 is orthologous to the vertebrate insulin-like/RLN genes, INS-L2 to insulin genes and INS-L3 to IGF genes by analysis of the gene structure, on the basis of the presence of the conserved protein motifs, the predicted maturation mode of the peptide precursors, putative receptor binding sites and the relative expression level of the *Ciona* INS-Ls. The ligand-receptor pairs and their biological actions await further study.

4.6 Galanin-like peptides in *C. intestinalis*

Galanin and galanin-like peptide (GALP) are vertebrate brain/gut peptides involved in reproduction and feeding (Lang et al., 2007). In particular, GALP is believed to stimulate LH secretion via up-regulation of GnRH secretion (Lang et al., 2007). The N-terminal region of

Peptide	Sequence
Galanin (quail)	GWTLNSAGYLLGPHAVDNHRSFNDKHGFTa
Galanin (goldfish)	GWTLNSAGYLLGPHAIDSHRSLGDKRGVAa
Galanin (human)	GWTLNSAGYLLGPHAVGNHRSFSDKNGLTSa
GALP (human)	PAHRGRGGWTLNSAGYLLGPVLHLPQMGDQDGKRETALEILDLWKAIDGLPYSHPPQPS
Ci-GALP	**PFRGQGGWTLNSVGYNAGLGALRKLFE**
	** ******* ** *

Table 8. The galanin/galanin-like peptide (GALP) family peptides. The *Ciona* peptide (Ci-GALP) is indicated in boldface. The galanin/GALP consensus motif is underlined. Asterisks denote amino acids highly conserved in vertebrate and *Ciona* galanin/GALP family peptides.

galanin is critical for its receptor binding and biological function, supported by the fact that the 13-amino acid N-terminal Gly-Trp-Thr-Leu-Asn-Ser-Ala-Gly-Tyr-Leu-Leu-Gly-Pro sequence is completely conserved in galanin of mammals, quail, and goldfish. On the other hand, GALP has thus far been characterized only in mammals. GALP also contains the identical consensus sequence in the N-terminal region. However, there are three different features between galanin and GALP sequences (Table 8). First, GALP has a longer sequence than galanin. Second, GALP is N-terminally elongated by a Pro-Ala-His-Arg-Gly-Arg-Gly sequence upstream of the consensus sequence, whereas galanin contains no amino acids at this region . Third, the C-terminus of galanin is amidated, while that of GALP is not. A single copy of galanin and GALP is encoded by a separate gene (Lang et al., 2007). Galanin and GALP share two Class A GPCRs, GLR1 and 2, while galanin- or GALP-specifc receptors have not ever been identified (Lang et al., 2007).

The peptidomic analysis also detected a *Ciona* galanin/GALP-related peptide, Ci-GALP (Kawada et al., 2011). The detected peptide sequence conserves the galanin/GALP consensus-like sequence, Gly-Trp-Thr-Leu-Asn-Ser-Val-Gly-Tyr-Asn-Ala-Gly-Leu, whereas it has a C-terminally truncated sequence compared with galanin and GALP (Table 8). Furthermore, the *Ciona* peptide possesses a Pro-Phe-Arg-Gly-Gln-Gly sequence at the N-terminus which is homologous with the Pro-Ala-His-Arg-Gly-Arg-Gly sequence in GALP (Table 8). Consequently, we designated the peptide as Ci-GALP. Intriguingly, the C-terminus of Ci-GALP, unlike GALP, is not amidated as it is in galanin (Table 8). In addition, no other homologous galanin/GALP-like peptide was found in *C. intestinalis*. These features support the notion that Ci-GALP is a prototype of galanin and GALP, and vertebrate galanin and GALP diverged from a Ci-GALP-like ancestor during the evolution. This is also the first characterization of galanin/GALP peptides in invertebrates.

5. Conclusion

As reviewed in this chapter, *C. intestinalis* has been found to conserve major homologs and prototypes of mammalian neuropeptides and peptide hormones, and *Ciona* oocytes and ovary have been shown to possess prominent advantages in studies of gonadotropin-independent growth stages regulated by neuropeptides and non-sexual hormones. Since peptide receptors are targets of various novel drugs, elucidation of biological functions of peptides in the ovaries is expected to lead to advances in peptidergic drug development in two regards: exploration of new drug targets in the ovary and reduction of side effects on ovarian functions. Consequently, functional analyses of *Ciona* peptides in oocyte growth as primary model studies, leading to the verification of biological actions of peptides on the ovary and oocytes in mammals, is expected to eventually construct diverse fundamentals on the development of novel clinical pharmaceuticals or health diets for reproductive diseases or deficiencies. Such research strategies are now being attempted in our laboratory.

6. Acknowledgment

We thank Ms. Kazuko Hirayama and all members of the Maizuru Fisheries Research Station for cultivation of the ascidians. All ascidians (*C. intestinalis*) were provided by Kyoto University through the National Bio-Resource Project of the MEXT, Japan. This study is in part financially supported by JSPS (to H. S., K.T., and T. Sa.) and JST (to H. S.).

7. References

Adams, B.A., Tello, J.A., Erchegyi, J., Warby, C., Hong, D.J., Akinsanya, K.O., Mackie, G.O., Vale, W., Rivier, J.E., & Sherwood, N.M. (2003) Six novel gonadotropin-releasing hormones are encoded as triplets on each of two genes in the protochordate, *Ciona intestinalis*. *Endocrinology* 144, 1907-1919

Aikins, M.J, Schooley, D.A., Begum, K., Detheux, M., Beeman, R.W. & Park, Y. (2008) Vasopressin-like peptide and its receptor function in an indirect diuretic signaling pathway in the red flour beetle. *Insect Biochem Mol Biol* 38, 740-748

Aoyama, M., Kawada, T., Fujie, M., Hotta, K., Sakai, T., Sekiguchi, T., Oka, K., & Satoh, N. Satake, H. (2008) A novel biological role of tachykinins as an up-regulator of oocyte growth: identification of an evolutionary origin of tachykininergic functions in the ovary of the ascidian, *Ciona intestinalis*. *Endocrinology* 149, 4346-4356

Burighel P, Cloney RA (1997) In: *Microscopic Anatomy of Invertebrates*, F.W. Harrison (Ed). Vol. 15, 221-347, Wiley-Liss, New York, U.S.A.

Candenas, L., Lecci, A., Pinto, F.M., Patak, E., Maggi, C.A., & Pennefather, J.N. (2005) Tachykinins and tachykinin receptors: effects in the genitourinary tract. *Life Sci* 76, 835-862

Carnevali, O., Cionna, C., Tosti, L., Lubzens, E., & Maradonna, F. (2006) Role of cathepsins in ovarian follicle growth and maturation. *Gen Comp Endocrinol* 146, 195-203

Conner, A.C., Simms, J., Hay, D.L., Mahmoud, K., Howitt, S.G., Wheatley, M., Poyner, D.R. (2004) Heterodimers and family-B GPCRs: RAMPs, CGRP and adrenomedullin. *Biochem Soc Trans* 32, 843-846

Cooper, G.J., Leighton, B., Dimitriadis, G.D., Parry-Billings, M., Kowalchuk, J.M., Howland, K., Rothbard, J.B., Willis, A.C. & Reid, K.B. (1988) Amylin found in amyloid deposits in human type 2 diabetes mellitus may be a hormone that regulates glycogen metabolism in skelet al. muscle. *Proc Natl Acad Sci USA* 85, 7763-7766

Debeljuk, L. (2006) Tachykinins and ovarian function in mammals. *Peptides* 27, 736-742

Deyts, C., Casane, D., Vernier, P., Bourrat, F., & Joly, J.S. (2006) Morphological and gene expression similarities suggest that the ascidian neural gland may be osmoregulatory and homologous to vertebrate peri-ventricular organs. *Eur J Neurosci* 24, 2299-2308

Donaldson, Z.R. & Young, L.J. (2008) Oxytocin, vasopressin, and the neurogenetics of sociality. *Science* 322, 900-904

Evers, B.M. (2006) Neurotensin and growth of normal and neoplastic tissues. *Peptides* 27, 2424-2433.

Frank, E. & Landgraf, R. (2008) The vasopressin system--from antidiuresis to psychopathology. *Eur J Pharmacol* 583, 226-242

Gimpl, G. & Fahrenholz, F. (2001) The oxytocin receptor system: structure, function, and regulation. *Physiol Rev* 81 629-683

Hoyle, C.H.V. (1998) Neuropeptide families: evolutionary perspectives. *Regul Pept* 73, 1-33

Hull, K.L., Fathimani, K., Sharma, P. & Harvey S (1998) Calcitropic peptides: neural perspectives. *Comp Biochem Physiol C Pharmacol Toxicol Endocrinol* 119, 389-410

Imai, K.S., Levine, M., Satoh, N. & Satou, Y. (2006) Regulatory Blueprint for a Chordate Embryo. *Science* 312, 1183-1187

Iwakoshi, E., Takuwa-Kuroda, K., Fujisawa, Y., Hisada, M., Ukena, K,. Tsutsui, K., & Minakata, H. (2002) Isolation and characterization of a GnRH-like peptide from *Octopus vulgaris*. *Biochem Biophys Res Commun* 291, 1187-1193

Jakobsen, R.K., Ono, S., Powers, J.C., & DeLotto, R. (2005) Fluorescently labeled inhibitors detect localized serine protease activities in *Drosophila melanogaster* pole cells, embryos, and ovarian egg chambers. *Histochem Cell Biol* 123, 51-60

Kah, O., Lethimonier, C., Somoza, G., Guilgur, L.G., Vaillant, C., & Lareyre, J.J. (2007) GnRH and GnRH receptors in metazoa: a historical, comparative, and evolutive perspective. *Gen Comp Endocrinol* 153, 346-364

Katafuchi, T., Kikumoto, K., Hamano, K., Kangawa, K., Matsuo, H. & Minamino N. (2003) Calcitonin receptor-stimulating peptide, a new member of the calcitonin gene-related peptide family. Its isolation from porcine brain, structure, tissue distribution, and biological activity. *J Biol Chem* 278, 12046-12054

Kavanaugh, S.I., Nozaki, M., & Sower, S.A. (2008) Origins of gonadotropin-releasing hormone (GnRH) in vertebrates: identification of a novel GnRH in a basal vertebrate, the sea lamprey. *Endocrinology* 149, 3860-3869

Kanda, A., Takahashi, T., Satake, H., & Minakata, H. (2006) Molecular and functional characterization of a novel GnRH receptor isolated from *Octopus vulgaris*. *Biochem J* 395, 125-135

Kanda, A., Takuwa-Kuroda, K., Aoyama, M., & Satake, H. (2007) A novel tachykinin-related peptide receptor of Octopus vulgaris: Evolutionary aspect of invertebrate tachykinin and tachykinin-related peptide. *FEBS J* 274, 2229-2239

Kawada, T., Furukawa, Y., Shimizu, Y., Minakata, H., Nomoto, K., & Satake H (2002) A novel tachykinin-related peptide receptor. Sequence, genomic organization, and functional analysis. *Eur J Biochem* 269, 4238-4246

Kawada, T., Kanda, A., Minakata, H., Matsushima, O. & Satake, H. (2004) Identification of a novel receptor for an invertebrate oxytocin/vasopressin superfamily peptide: molecular and functional evolution of the oxytocin/vasopressin superfamily *Biochem. J.* 382, 231-237

Kawada, T., Sekiguchi, T., Itoh, Y., Ogasawara, M., & Satake, H. (2008) Characterization of a novel vasopressin/oxytocin superfamily peptide and its receptor from an ascidian, *Ciona intestinalis*. *Peptides* 29, 1672-1678

Kawada, T., Aoyama, M., Okada, I., Sakai, T., Sekiguchi, T., Ogasawara, M., & Satake, H. (2009a) A novel inhibitory gonadotropin-releasing hormone-related neuropeptide in the ascidian, *Ciona intestinalis*. *Peptides* 30, 2200-2205

Kawada, T., Sekiguchi, T., Sugase, K., & Satake, H. (2009b) Evolutionary aspects of molecular forms and biological functions of oxytocin family peptides. In; *Handbook of Oxytocin Research: Synthesis, Storage and Release, Actions and Drug Forms*, H. Jastrow & D. Feuerbach (Eds.), 59-85, Nova Science Publishers Inc, ISBN 978-1-60876-023-7, New York, U.S.A.

Kawada, T., Sekiguchi, T., Sakai, T., Aoyama, M., & Satake, H. (2010) Neuropeptides, hormone peptides, and their receptors in *Ciona intestinalis*: an update. *Zool. Sci.* 27, 134-153

Kawada, T., Ogasawara, M., Sekiguchi, T., Aoyama, M., Hotta, K., Oka, K, & Satake, H. (2011) Peptidomic analysis of the central nervous system of the protochordate, *Ciona intestinalis*: homologs and prototypes of vertebrate peptides and novel peptides. *Endocrinology* 152, 2416-2427

Kitamura, K., Kangawa, K. & Eto, T. (2002) Adrenomedullin and PAMP: discovery, structures, and cardiovascular functions. *Microsc Res Tech* 57, 3-13

Kusakabe, T., Mishima, S., Shimada, I., Kitajima, Y., & Tsuda, M. (2003) Structure, expression, and cluster organization of genes encoding gonadotropin-releasing hormone receptors found in the neural complex of the ascidian *Ciona intestinalis*. *Gene* 322, 77-84

Lang, R., Gundlach, A.L. & Kofler, B. (2007) The galanin peptide family: receptor pharmacology, pleiotropic biological actions, and implications in health and disease. *Pharmacol Ther* 115, 177-207

Litscher, E.S., Qi, H., & Wassarman, P.M. (1999) Mouse zona pellucida glycoproteins mZP2 and mZP3 undergo carboxy-terminal proteolytic processing in growing oocytes. *Biochemistry* 38, 12280-12287.

Lovejoy, D.A. & Barsyte-Lovejoy, D (2010) Characterization of a corticotropin-releasing factor (CRF)/diuretic hormone-like peptide from tunicates: Insight into the origins of the vertebrate CRF family. *Gen Comp Endocrinol* 165, 330-336

Millar, R.P. (2005) GnRHs and GnRH receptors. *Anim Reprod Sci* 88, 5-28

Olinski, R.P., Lundin, L.G. & Hallböök F (2006a) Conserved synteny between the *Ciona* genome and human paralogons identifies large duplication events in the molecular evolution of the insulin-relaxin gene family. *Mol Biol Evol* 23, 10-22

Olinski, R.P., Dahlberg, C., Thorndyke, M., & Hallböök, F. (2006b) Three insulin-relaxin-like genes in *Ciona intestinalis*. *Peptides* 27, 2535-2546

Orisaka, M., Tajima, K., Tsang, B.K., & Kotsuji, F. (2009) Oocyte-granulosa-theca cell interactions during preantral follicular development. *J. Ovarian Res.* 2, 9

Oumi. T, Ukena, K., Matsushima, O., Ikeda, T., Fujita, T., Minakata, H. & Nomoto, K. (1996) Annetocin, an annelid oxytocin-related peptide, induces egg-laying behavior in the earthworm, *Eisenia foetida*. *J Exp Zool* 276, 151-156

Page, N.M. (2004) Hemokinins and endokinins. *Cell Mol Life Sci* 61, 1652-1663

Prodon, F., Chenevert, J., & Sardet, C. (2006) Establishment of animal-vegetal polarity during maturation in ascidian oocytes. *Dev Biol* 290, 297-311

Sakai, T., Aoyama, M., Kusakabe, T., Tsuda, M., & Satake, H. (2010) Functional diversity of signaling pathways through G protein-coupled receptor heterodimerization with a species-specific orphan receptor subtype. *Mol Biol Evol* 27, 1097-1106

Sasakura, Y. (2007) Germline transgenesis and insertional mutagenesis in the ascidian *Ciona intestinalis*. *Dev Dyn* 236, 1758-1767

Satake, H., Takuwa, K., Minakata, H., & Matsushima, O. (1999) Evidence for conservation of the vasopressin/oxytocin superfamily in Annelida. *J. Biol. Chem.* 274, 5605-5611

Satake, H., Kawada, T., Nomoto, K., & Minakata, H. (2003) Insight into Tachykinin-Related Peptides, Their Receptors, and Invertebrate Tachykinins: A Review. *Zool Sci* 20, 533-549

Satake, H., Ogasawara, M., Kawada, T., Masuda, K., Aoyama, M., Minakata, H., Chiba, T., Metoki, H., Satou, Y., & Satoh, N. (2004) Tachykinin and tachykinin receptor of an ascidian, *Ciona intestinalis*: evolutionary origin of the vertebrate tachykinin family. *J Biol Chem* 279, 53798-53805

Satake, H. & Kawada, T. (2006a) Overview of the primary structure, tissue-distribution, and functions of tachykinins and their receptors. *Curr Drug Targets* 7, 963-974

Satake, H. & Kawada, T. (2006b) Neuropeptides, hormones, and their receptors in ascidians-Emerging model animals. In; *Invertebrate Neuropeptides and Hormones: Basic Knowledge and Recent Advances*, H. Satake (Ed.), 253-276, Transworld Research Network, ISBN 81-7895-224-6, Kerala, India

Satoh, N. (2009) An advanced filter-feeder hypothesis for urochordate evolution. *Zool Sci* 26, 97-111

Sawada, H., Yamaguchi, H., Shimbara, T., Toshinai, K., Mondal, M.S., Date, Y., Murakami, N,, Katafuchi, T., Minamino, N., Nunoi, H., & Nakazato, M .(2006) Central effects of calcitonin receptor-stimulating peptide-1 on energy homeostasis in rats. *Endocrinology* 147, 2043-2050

Sekiguchi, T., Suzuki, N., Fujiwara, N., Aoyama, M., Kawada, M., Sugase, K., Murata, Y., Sasayama, Y., Ogasawara, M., & Satake, H. (2009) Calcitonin in a protochordate, *Ciona intestinalis*: the prototype of the vertebrate Calcitonin/Calcitonin gene related peptide family. *FEBS J* 276, 4437-4447

Takagi-Sawada, M., Someno, T., Hoshi, M., & Sawada, H. (1989) Inhibition of starfish oocyte maturation by leupeptin analogs, potent trypsin inhibitors. *Dev Biol* 133, 609-612

Tanaka, E., Takagi-Sawada, M., & Sawada, H. (2000) Enzymatic properties of the proteasome purified from starfish oocytes and its catalytic subunits involved in oocyte maturation. *Comp Biochem Physiol C Toxicol Pharmacol* 125, 215-223

Tello, J.A., Rivier, J.E., & Sherwood, N.M. (2005) Tunicate gonadotropin-releasing hormone (GnRH) peptides selectively activate *Ciona intestinalis* GnRH receptors and the green monkey type II GnRH receptor. *Endocrinology* 146, 4061-4073

Ukena, K., Iwakoshi-Ukena, E., & Hikosaka, A. (2008) Unique form and osmoregulatory function of a neurohypophysial hormone in a urochordate. *Endocrinology* 149, 5254-5261

Wang, Q. & Sun, Q.Y. (2007) Evaluation of oocyte quality: morphological, cellular and molecular predictors. *Reprod Fertil Dev* 19, 1-12

Zhang, L., Tello, J.A., Zhang, W., & Tsai, P.S. (2008) Molecular cloning, expression pattern, and immunocytochemical localization of a gonadotropin-releasing hormone-like molecule in the gastropod mollusk, *Aplysia californica*. *Gen Comp Endocrinol* 156, 201-209

17

Estrogen Receptors in Leukocytes - Possible Impact on Inflammatory Processes in the Female Reproductive System

Chellakkan Selvanesan Blesson
Karolinska Institutet
Sweden

1. Introduction

Estrogens carry out various reproductive and non-reproductive functions. Traditionally, estrogen action was thought to be solely mediated through its nuclear receptors - estrogen receptor (ER)α and ERβ (Deroo & Korach, 2006). However, recently a membrane bound G protein-coupled receptor-30, now designated as G protein-coupled estrogen receptor-1(GPER), has been described as a receptor for estrogen (Prossnitz et al., 2007). ERα and ERβ belong to the nuclear receptor superfamily and functions as ligand activated transcriptional factors. The classical mechanism of nuclear ER action involves ligand binding to receptors, dimerization and binding to specific response elements of the target genes to elicit a transcriptional response. Although estrogen action is mostly targeted towards reproductive tissues, they also act via ERs in non-reproductive target tissues (Diel, 2002; Manolagas & Kousteni, 2001; Walker & Korach, 2004). Estrogens can also act rapidly through non-genomic mechanisms by binding to membrane bound ERs (Deroo & Korach, 2006; Prossnitz et al., 2007). GPER is a member of the G protein-coupled receptor superfamily containing seven transmembrane helices and mediates estrogen-dependent kinase activation as well as transcriptional responses (Prossnitz et al., 2007). Receptors for estrogens are present in leukocytes and perform various functions. ERs and several of their splice variants have been identified in polymorphonuclear and mononuclear leukocytes isolated from peripheral blood of both men and women (Stygar et al., 2006). ERs are present in a variety of leukocytes like myeloid progenitor cells, neutrophils, lymphocytes, natural killer cells, macrophages, monocytes, mast cells etc. This chapter will summarize the publications on the role of estrogen in leukocytes and its implications in female reproduction.

2. Estrogen receptors in leukocytes

Leukocytes play a key role in several physiologically important processes like immunity, inflammation, extracellular matrix remodeling, wound healing, cardiovascular disorders, autoimmune diseases, menstruation, embryo implantation, cervical ripening, labor etc. They are involved in various functions during normal as well as pathological conditions. Estrogens act on leukocytes and influence their number and function (Bouman et al., 2005). In recent years, several investigations have focused on the action of estrogens in the immune system and inflammation. Clinical, epidemiological and immunological studies have shown that women are more prone to autoimmune disorders in comparison to men. Studies have shown that the incidence of cardiovascular disease is higher in men than in women and the incidence in women increases towards the level of men after menopause. There is clear sex bias in the disease presentation. Estrogens have been suggested to be responsible for these differences (Cutolo et al., 2010; Druckmann, 2001; Nalbandian & Kovats, 2005). These diseases are often associated with leukocyte infiltration and immune dysfunction. It has been hypothesized that estrogens alter the course of these disorders by modulating leukocyte function in various tissues. Although the exact mechanism by which estrogens modulates the immune cell function is not completely understood, these observations clearly show that leukocytes are estrogen targets.

2.1 Neutrophils

Neutrophils are the most abundant type of leukocytes and form an essential part of the immune system. Klebanoff demonstrated that estrogens specifically bind to neutrophils using ligand binding experiments (Klebanoff, 1977). It was further shown that estrogens influence the neutrophil count and women have a higher neutrophil count than men (Bain & England, 1975a). In women, the neutrophil number varies during the menstrual cycle (Bain & England, 1975b; Smith et al., 2007). Higher levels of neutrophil counts correlate to the elevated levels of estradiol in peripheral blood (Mathur et al., 1979). Recent studies showed that ERs are present in neutrophils and execute various direct or indirect functions. It was shown that polymorphonuclear cells express both ERα and ERβ and their various splice variants (Molero et al., 2002; Stygar et al., 2007). Molero et al, demonstrated that estradiol up-regulated both ERα and ERβ in women but only ERα in men (Molero et al., 2002). The functional signaling of ERs in neutrophils was further established by the induction of nNOS by estradiol (Garcia-Duran et al., 1999). Further, estradiol and ER specific agonists regulated physiologically relevant genes in polymorphonuclear cells in rats (Stygar et al., 2007). Recently, we have identified the presence of GPER in terminally differentiated neutrophil like HL-60 cells. The GPER agonist G1 could stimulate a transcriptional response indicating that GPER is functionally active in these cells (Blesson and Sahlin, unpublished). Neutrophils have a very short life span and they stay in circulation for 6 to 18 hours before undergoing apoptosis. Estradiol along with progesterone increases neutrophil survival by delaying apoptosis via decreasing the activities of caspases 3 and 9 (Molloy et al., 2003). Estrogens may also have a vital role in the regulation of genes that are associated with the immune and inflammatory response, like chemokines and cytokines. These genes are responsible for neutrophil recruitment and activation during normal as well as pathological conditions (Jabbour et al., 2009; Straub, 2007).

2.2 Lymphocytes

Lymphocytes express nuclear as well as membrane estrogen receptors. Studies on human peripheral blood lymphocytes showed the presence of ERα and ERβ in various lymphocyte subsets including natural killer (NK) cells (Curran et al., 2001). A smaller variant of ERα called ERα 46 appears to be the most abundant isoform of ERs in lymphocytes. This variant was localized to the cell surface and mediates estrogen induced proliferation of T lymphocytes and NK cells but not B lymphocytes (Pierdominici et al.,

2010). ERβ is expressed predominantly in secondary lymphoid tissues and plays an important role in the peripheral immune system (Shim et al., 2006). Both ERα and ERβ are expressed in the NK cells of mice and humans (Curran et al., 2001). In mice, estrogens act via ERβ to suppress NK cell activity by altering their ability to lyse target cells (Curran et al., 2001). Estradiol induces the proliferation of splenic NK cells and suppresses the cytotoxicity of these cells (Hao et al., 2007). However, *in vitro* studies on murine NK cells showed that estradiol reduces NK cell proliferative capacity and reduces cytotoxicity by influencing cytokine expressions (Hao et al., 2008). In humans, the number of NK cells was significantly altered during the different phases of menstrual cycle. The NK cell population in the periovulatory phase when the estrogen level is high was twice that in other phases indicating a positive effect on its number (Yovel et al., 2001). The ERβ1 variant could be localized to uterine NK (uNK) cells (Henderson et al., 2003). Hence, estrogens could act directly on uNK cells via the ERβ1 receptor.

2.3 Other mononuclear leukocytes

ERs are also expressed in monocytes, macrophages, dendritic cells and mast cells. Both ERα and ERβ are present in monocytes and are able to regulate the expression of CD16 (Kramer et al., 2007). Estrogens can act on monocytes to modulate apoptosis and cell cycle progression (Thongngarm et al., 2003). Monocytes are responsive to estrogens and may be important in modulating the immune response (Scariano et al., 2008). These cells are recruited into damaged tissue and undergo differentiation to become macrophages or dendritic cells. In macrophages derived from a human primary monocyte culture, ERα and ERβ mRNA were detected. However, only the ERβ protein could be seen (Kramer & Wray, 2002). Stygar and co-workers showed the presence of mRNA and protein of wild type ERα and ERβ and their splice variants in mononuclear cells purified from peripheral blood (Stygar et al., 2006). Recent reports have shown the presence of ERα and ERβ localized to the membrane and cytoplasm of macrophages derives from THP-1 cells (Subramanian & Shaha, 2009). Estradiol was shown to regulate the expression of several genes related to macrophage activation and apoptosis (Kramer & Wray, 2002; Subramanian & Shaha, 2009). Further, plasma membrane associated ERα and cytosolic ERβ oppose the function of each other thereby promoting cell survival suggesting the importance of both receptors (Kramer & Wray, 2002; Subramanian & Shaha, 2009). A recent study showed that estradiol suppresses LPS induced NFkB activation in primary human macrophages (Murphy et al., 2010). These reports indicate that estrogen dependent ER signaling is necessary to perform various important activities in monocytes and macrophages. Estrogens act via ERα on myeloid progenitor cells to regulate their differentiation into dendritic cells by increasing expression of the transcription factor IRF4 (Carreras et al., 2010). It has also been reported that estradiol may strengthen innate immunity by enhancing interferon-γ production in dendritic cell suggesting an active role played by ER in these cells (Siracusa et al., 2008). ERs have also been localized in mast cells (Zhao et al., 2001). In mast cells, estradiol acts via a membrane bound ERα and regulates calcium influx, which is a non-genomic signaling mechanism (Zaitsu et al., 2007). Estradiol also enhances IgE-dependent mast cell activation, resulting in a shift of the allergen dose response (Zaitsu et al., 2007).

These observations clearly show that in addition to their role in reproduction, estrogens appear to influence the immune system by targeting leukocytes. The presence of ERs indicates that estrogens could act directly on these cells regulating cellular functions. It could also explain the sexual dimorphism in the immune and inflammatory response.

3. Leukocyte mediated estrogen action in reproduction

Many normal female reproductive processes show classical signs of inflammation. It is now widely accepted that ovulation, menstruation, implantation, pregnancy, cervical ripening and parturition are governed by inflammatory processes. These events are often associated with expression of an array of inflammatory mediators including various cytokines and chemokines (Jabbour et al., 2009). Leukocytes are present in substantial numbers in the female reproductive tract and sex hormones directly or indirectly play a role in the recruitment and activation of these cells (Wira et al., 2010). Abnormal activation of inflammatory pathways leads to various pathological conditions like menstrual disorders, infertility, pregnancy loss, complicated labor, unripe cervix, reproductive tract cancers etc. (Jabbour et al., 2009). It appears that there is a coordinated attempt by the immune system to protect, maintain and repair the reproductive organs to perform its normal functions.

3.1 Reproductive cycle

The female reproductive cycle is highly controlled by reproductive hormones from hypothalamus, pituitary and ovary. The ovarian steroids not only perform their primary reproductive functions but are also involved in various functions related to immunity and inflammation. Innate and adaptive immunity are active throughout the menstrual cycle and ovarian estrogens act on epithelial cells and leukocytes of the female reproductive tract to offer protection against infection (Wira et al., 2010). Infiltration of leukocytes into the ovary is essential for ovulation. The invading leukocytes secrete proteases to weaken the follicular wall and thus aiding ovulation (Oakley et al., 2010). These leukocytes include macrophages and lymphocytes (Oakley et al., 2010). Leukocytes are present in great numbers and diversity in the reproductive tract throughout the reproductive cycle. The human endometrium undergoes constant remodeling during the course of the menstrual cycle and is infiltrated by leukocytes. A variety of leukocytes including uNK cells, neutrophils, eosinophils, lymphocytes, macrophages and mast cells invade endometrium (Salamonsen & Lathbury, 2000). Endometrial remodeling involves inflammatory factors like cytokines, chemokines and prostanoids (Jabbour et al., 2009). Estrogens regulate the inflammatory process in the endometrium which involves influx of leukocytes (King & Critchley, 2010). Infiltrating leukocytes not only provide protection against pathogens but also actively participate in the degradation and subsequent regeneration of endometrial tissue by secreting various proteases, cytokines and chemokines (Guo et al., 2011; Lathbury & Salamonsen, 2000). Various proteases like tryptase, chymase, chymotrypsin plasminogen activator, elastase, heparanase, cathepsin G, β-glucuronidase, aryl sulphatase, metalloelastase and several metalloproteases are secreted and regulated by leukocytes, thereby playing an active role in tissue degradation prior to menstruation (Salamonsen & Lathbury, 2000). Leukocytes also participate during the process of regeneration of the endometrium. Endometrial regeneration is an estrogen dependent process and the repair begins with the restoration of glands, stroma and epithelium along with endometrial angiogenesis. Leukocytes are abundantly present and could participate in the endometrial rebuilding process (Salamonsen & Lathbury, 2000). Neutrophils are present in large numbers during endometrial repair and play an important role. In a mouse model designed to mimic the events of menstruation, it was observed that when neutrophils were depleted, endometrial regeneration was severely affected suggesting that neutrophils along with the regulatory factors they produce contribute to the tissue repair (Kaitu'u-Lino et al., 2007). Macrophages, eosinophils and lymphocytes could also contribute in this process (Salamonsen & Lathbury, 2000). In humans, different subpopulations of leukocytes are present during the menstrual, proliferative, mid-secretory, and late-secretory phases (Jones et al., 2004). Certain chemokines like MDC, MCP-3, and FKN are abundant throughout the cycle. During the menstrual phase, IL-8 and HCC-4 mRNAs are up-regulated. In the proliferative phase, MIP-1β, HCC-4, and eotaxin are up-regulated in glands and vessels of endometrium, whereas MIP-1β, HCC-1, HCC-4 and 6Ckine were up-regulated during in the mid-secretory phase followed by the upregulation of HCC-1 and 6Ckine in the late secretory phase (Jones et al., 2004). It was also noticed that neutrophils, eosinophils and macrophages are present during menstrual phase, macrophages during proliferative phase, uNK cells, macrophages and T cells during mid-secretary phase and neutrophils, eosinophils and macrophages during late-secretory phase of the menstrual cycle (Jones et al., 2004).

3.2 Implantation and decidualization

A large number of leukocytes especially monocytes, macrophages and uNK cells infiltrate the implantation site, believed to be important modulators of trophoblast invasion and decidualization (Drake et al., 2001; Jones et al., 2004). If pregnancy does not occur another sub-population of leukocytes like neutrophils, eosinophils, and macrophages infiltrate and facilitate endometrial destruction (Jones et al., 2004). Decidualization is the process by which stromal cells differentiate into decidual cells. It involves an inflammatory type of reaction including leukocyte infiltration and cytokine production (Hess et al., 2007). Leukocytes are present in large amounts during decidualization indicating their participation in the process (Guo et al., 2011). Studies in mice showed that uNK cells promote uterine vascular cell remodeling that assist decidual growth (Blois et al., 2011). Certain uNK cell derived chemokines and cytokines can influence the gene expression profile of human endometrial fibroblasts *in vitro* suggesting that a similar mechanism could operate in the endometrium (Germeyer et al., 2009). uNK cells express ERβ and it may exert control over trophoblast invasion (Henderson et al., 2003; Kwak-Kim & Gilman-Sachs, 2008). They also promote uterine vascular modifications assisting decidual growth during early pregnancy (Blois et al., 2011). Regulation of inflammation during implantation may follow a sequential model in which pro-inflammation is followed by anti-inflammation or there may be a continuous balance between the pro- and anti-inflammatory environments (Jabbour et al., 2009). These observations imply that there are interactions between different types of invading leukocytes and the factors that they secrete in the endometrium are important in order to bring about a successful implantation.

3.3 Pregnancy

The level of serum estrogens peaks during pregnancy and may reach more than a hundred fold to that of normal non-pregnant levels (Tulchinsky & Hobel, 1973). At these high levels, estrogens can suppress many cytotoxic and innate immune responses, but stimulate antibody production, neo-angiogenesis and growth (Straub, 2007). Several chemokines and cytokines like TPO, VEGF, IL1α, ENA-78, IL-8, GM-CSF and GRO-α are upregulated in the first-trimester decidua (Segerer et al., 2009). These factors perform various functions including attracting a variety of leukocytes. Estrogens along with progesterone can regulate leukocyte number and activity. Studies indicate that neutrophils from women at term pregnancy have a significant delay in apoptosis inducing physiologic neutrophilia (Watson et al., 1999). This delay in apoptosis could be induced by estradiol and progesterone (Molloy et al., 2003). Along with the increase in neutrophil count, several metabolic changes including accumulation of myeloperoxidase take place in neutrophils to enhance cell metabolism and oxidant release during pregnancy (Kindzelskii et al., 2006; Muller et al., 2009). The symbiosis between mother and fetus during pregnancy is not due to immunological ignorance, but a complex transient modulation of the maternal immune response where the adaptive immunity is down-modulated and the innate immune response is enhanced (Muller et al., 2009). It has been reported that there is a temporary suppression of maternal T cell responses by arginase secreted by polymorphonuclear leukocytes in normal pregnancies (Kropf et al., 2007). Thus, there is interplay between the different types of leukocytes to protect the fetus from the maternal immune system. Early pregnancy also involves the action of dendritic cells. They control stromal cell proliferation, angiogenesis and the homing and maturation of NK cell precursors in the pregnant uterus (Blois et al., 2011). The number of uNK cells increase drastically during pregnancy. Precursors of uNK appear to be recruited from blood and this is promoted by rising levels of plasma estrogens and luteinizing hormone and limited by increasing progesterone (van den Heuvel et al., 2005). uNK cells promote vascular modifications during gestation which is vital for the formation of the placenta (Blois et al., 2011). Further, placenta and trophoblasts produce chemokines that may also recruit NK cells into the decidua during pregnancy (Chantakru et al., 2002; Drake et al., 2001).

3.4 Cervical ripening and parturition

Cervical ripening is an important event prior to parturition. It has been suggested that leukocytes could be responsible for the ripening of the cervix at term and these leukocytes express ERs (Junqueira et al., 1980; Osmers et al., 1992; Sahlin et al., 2008; Wang et al., 2001). Cervical ripening includes an inflammatory type of process and thus there is an infiltration of leukocytes. Both polymorphonuclear and macrophages migrate from blood vessels and accumulate in cervix before the onset of parturition (Osman et al., 2003; Stygar et al., 2001). The quantum of infiltrating leukocytes is modulated by inflammatory mediators like IL-8 and prostaglandins (Chwalisz et al., 1994; Luo et al., 2000). Cervical extracellular matrix is remodeled by the degradation of collagens and proteoglycans. Proteases like matrixmetalloprotease (MMP)-2 and MMP-9 were expressed during cervical ripening (Stygar et al., 2002). Cervical stromal fibroblasts and smooth muscle cells were identified as main sources of MMP-2, but MMP-9 protein was localized exclusively in invading leukocytes (Stygar et al., 2002). There are also reports showing that migrating leukocytes secrete collagenases that could play an important role in tissue remodeling during cervical ripening (Osmers et al., 1992). These data indicate the involvement of invading leukocytes in the cervical ripening process. It was observed that the influx of leukocytes were impaired in cervix of women post term not responding to prostaglandin priming, indicating that leukocytes are important for normal cervical ripening (Sahlin et al., 2008). Infiltrating leukocytes express ERs where estrogen may also act directly. ERβ expression in human cervix was significantly increased at term pregnancy when compared to non-pregnant controls, implying a role for ERβ in cervical ripening (Wang et al., 2001). Further, it was later shown that ERβ is expressed in invading leukocytes including macrophages (Stygar et al., 2001). In rats, estradiol and selective agonists regulate a number of genes related to inflammation and extra cellular matrix remodeling (Stygar et al., 2007). Thus ERβ might mediate the estrogen action leading to the activation of leukocytes facilitating cervical ripening. Leukocytes also infiltrate myometrium prior to parturition. Macrophages and neutrophils massively infiltrate the upper and lower segment of myometrium at term, suggesting that parturition is an inflammatory event (Thomson et al., 1999). Inflammatory genes are significantly regulated in human endometrium and cervix in association with parturition (Bollapragada et al., 2009). The inflammatory events are not limited to uterus and cervix but there are indications that peripheral blood leukocytes also actively participate in this process for a successful labor (Yuan et al., 2009). It has been suggested that inflammatory stimulus upregulate pro-inflammatory cytokines which may further upregulate prostaglandins, MMPs and attract leukocytes leading to myometrial contractility, rupture of membranes and cervical ripening (Challis et al., 2009).

4. Inflammatory pathologies regulated by estrogen

Abnormal regulation of the immune system could lead to various complications in female reproduction. Various autoimmune and inflammatory disorders have been reported (Cutolo et al., 2010; Deroo & Korach, 2006; Jabbour et al., 2009; Straub, 2007). Estrogens have been implicated directly in diseases like arthritis, osteoporosis, systemic lupus erythematosus, multiple sclerosis, preeclampsia, complications in fertility, pregnancy loss, post-term labor, labor complications, cancers of breast and reproductive tract. Estrogens also play a vital role in the pathophysiology of female reproduction mediated by leukocytes. There are ample evidences to indicate that aberrant inflammatory pathways are directly or indirectly regulated by estrogens, contributing to the cause of various diseases.

5. Conclusion

Estrogens act through ERs and regulate various aspects of the immune system directly or indirectly acting through various downstream mediators. ERs have been found on diverse types of leukocytes. Estrogens act directly via its different receptors and regulate various inflammatory functions mediated through different types of leukocytes. Estrogens are also able to regulate the number, migration and function of leukocytes involving complex mechanisms. There are several clues and confirmations; however the exact nature, timing and interactions are still to be explored. Considering the recent findings of the function of estrogens in various aspects of immune regulation and inflammation, it is difficult to consider estrogens just as a 'female reproductive hormone' anymore. The role of estrogens in various inflammatory processes and its significance is well accepted. Estrogens regulate normal and pathological inflammatory events in reproduction. However, the molecular mechanisms of these events are still being worked out and demand more attention.

Understanding the molecular mechanisms will enable us to know more about the normal and aberrant regulation of these reproductive events involving inflammation and their mediators. Both ERα and ERβ have several splice variants lacking different domains with possible different functions. The expression of these variants in different types of leukocytes is not known and warrants further investigation. With the identification of the new membrane bound GPER, the signaling mechanism has yet another layer of complexity and its presence or role in most of the leukocytes are yet to be established. Insights into the function and regulation of ERs in leukocytes could open up new possibilities for treatments for various diseases involving inflammation.

6. Acknowledgements

I wish to thank Dr. Lena Sahlin for her valuable comments on the manuscript. This work was supported by postdoctoral fellowships from Swedish Institute and The Swedish Research Council (Grant 20137) and research funding from Kronprinsessan Lovisas förening and Sällskapet Barnavård.

7. References

Bain, B. J. & England, J. M. (1975a) Normal haematological values: sex difference in neutrophil count. *British Medical Journal*, Vol.1, No.5953, pp. 306-309, ISSN 0007-1447

Bain, B. J. & England, J. M. (1975b) Variations in leucocyte count during menstrual cycle. *British Medical Journal*, Vol.2, No.5969, pp. 473-475, ISSN 0007-1447

Blois, S. M., Klapp, B. F. & Barrientos, G. (2011) Decidualization and angiogenesis in early pregnancy: unravelling the functions of DC and NK cells. *Journal of Reproductive Immunology*, Vol.88, No.2, pp. 86-92, ISSN 1872-7603

Bollapragada, S., Youssef, R., Jordan, F., Greer, I., Norman, J. & Nelson, S. (2009) Term labor is associated with a core inflammatory response in human fetal membranes, myometrium, and cervix. *American Journal of Obstetrics and Gynecology*, Vol.200, No.1, pp. 104 e101-111, ISSN 1097-6868

Bouman, A., Heineman, M. J. & Faas, M. M. (2005) Sex hormones and the immune response in humans. *Human Reproduction Update*, Vol.11, No.4, pp. 411-423, ISSN 1355-4786

Carreras, E., Turner, S., Frank, M. B., Knowlton, N., Osban, J., Centola, M., Park, C. G., Simmons, A., Alberola-Ila, J. & Kovats, S. (2010) Estrogen receptor signaling promotes dendritic cell differentiation by increasing expression of the transcription factor IRF4. *Blood*, Vol.115, No.2, pp. 238-246, ISSN 1528-0020

Challis, J. R., Lockwood, C. J., Myatt, L., Norman, J. E., Strauss, J. F., 3rd & Petraglia, F. (2009) Inflammation and pregnancy. *Reproductive Sciences*, Vol.16, No.2, pp. 206-215, ISSN 1933-7205

Chantakru, S., Miller, C., Roach, L. E., Kuziel, W. A., Maeda, N., Wang, W. C., Evans, S. S. & Croy, B. A. (2002) Contributions from self-renewal and trafficking to the uterine NK cell population of early pregnancy. *Journal of Immunology*, Vol.168, No.1, pp. 22-28, ISSN 0022-1767

Chwalisz, K., Benson, M., Scholz, P., Daum, J., Beier, H. M. & Hegele-Hartung, C. (1994) Cervical ripening with the cytokines interleukin 8, interleukin 1 beta and tumour necrosis factor alpha in guinea-pigs. *Human Reproduction*, Vol.9, No.11, pp. 2173-2181, ISSN 0268-1161

Curran, E. M., Berghaus, L. J., Vernetti, N. J., Saporita, A. J., Lubahn, D. B. & Estes, D. M. (2001) Natural killer cells express estrogen receptor-alpha and estrogen receptor-beta and can respond to estrogen via a non-estrogen receptor-alpha-mediated pathway. *Cellular Immunology*, Vol.214, No.1, pp. 12-20, ISSN 0008-8749

Cutolo, M., Brizzolara, R., Atzeni, F., Capellino, S., Straub, R. H. & Puttini, P. C. (2010) The immunomodulatory effects of estrogens: clinical relevance in immune-mediated rheumatic diseases. *Annals of the New York Academy of Sciences*, Vol.1193, pp. 36-42, ISSN 1749-6632

Deroo, B. J. & Korach, K. S. (2006) Estrogen receptors and human disease. *Journal of Clinical Investigation*, Vol.116, No.3, pp. 561-570, ISSN 0021-9738

Diel, P. (2002) Tissue-specific estrogenic response and molecular mechanisms. *Toxicological Letters*, Vol.127, No.1-3, pp. 217-224, ISSN 0378-4274

Drake, P. M., Gunn, M. D., Charo, I. F., Tsou, C. L., Zhou, Y., Huang, L. & Fisher, S. J. (2001) Human placental cytotrophoblasts attract monocytes and CD56(bright) natural killer cells via the actions of monocyte inflammatory protein 1alpha. *Journal of Experimental Medicine*, Vol.193, No.10, pp. 1199-1212, ISSN 0022-1007

Druckmann, R. (2001) Review: female sex hormones, autoimmune diseases and immune response. *Gynecological Endocrinology*, Vol.15 Suppl 6, pp. 69-76, ISSN 0951-3590

Garcia-Duran, M., de Frutos, T., Diaz-Recasens, J., Garcia-Galvez, G., Jimenez, A., Monton, M., Farre, J., Sanchez de Miguel, L., Gonzalez-Fernandez, F., Arriero, M. D., Rico, L., Garcia, R., Casado, S. & Lopez-Farre, A. (1999) Estrogen stimulates neuronal nitric oxide synthase protein expression in human neutrophils. *Circulation Research*, Vol.85, No.11, pp. 1020-1026, ISSN 0009-7330

Germeyer, A., Sharkey, A. M., Prasadajudio, M., Sherwin, R., Moffett, A., Bieback, K., Clausmeyer, S., Masters, L., Popovici, R. M., Hess, A. P., Strowitzki, T. & von Wolff, M. (2009) Paracrine effects of uterine leucocytes on gene expression of human uterine stromal fibroblasts. *Molecular Human Reproduction*, Vol.15, No.1, pp. 39-48, ISSN 1460-2407

Guo, Y., He, B., Xu, X. & Wang, J. (2011) Comprehensive analysis of leukocytes, vascularization and matrix metalloproteinases in human menstrual xenograft model. *Public Library of Science One*, pp e16840

Hao, S., Li, P., Zhao, J., Hu, Y. & Hou, Y. (2008) 17beta-estradiol suppresses cytotoxicity and proliferative capacity of murine splenic NK1.1+ cells. *Cellular & Molecular Immunology*, Vol.5, No.5, pp. 357-364, ISSN 1672-7681

Hao, S., Zhao, J., Zhou, J., Zhao, S., Hu, Y. & Hou, Y. (2007) Modulation of 17beta-estradiol on the number and cytotoxicity of NK cells in vivo related to MCM and activating receptors. *International Immunopharmacolgy*, Vol.7, No.13, pp. 1765-1775, ISSN 1567-5769

Henderson, T. A., Saunders, P. T., Moffett-King, A., Groome, N. P. & Critchley, H. O. (2003) Steroid receptor expression in uterine natural killer cells. *Journal of Clinical Endocrinology and Metabolism*, Vol.88, No.1, pp. 440-449, ISSN 0021-972X

Hess, A. P., Hamilton, A. E., Talbi, S., Dosiou, C., Nyegaard, M., Nayak, N., Genbecev-Krtolica, O., Mavrogianis, P., Ferrer, K., Kruessel, J., Fazleabas, A. T., Fisher, S. J. & Giudice, L. C. (2007) Decidual stromal cell response to paracrine signals from the trophoblast: amplification of immune and angiogenic modulators. *Biology of Reproduction*, Vol.76, No.1, pp. 102-117, ISSN 0006-3363

Jabbour, H. N., Sales, K. J., Catalano, R. D. & Norman, J. E. (2009) Inflammatory pathways in female reproductive health and disease. *Reproduction*, Vol.138, No.6, pp. 903-919, ISSN 1741-7899

Jones, R. L., Hannan, N. J., Kaitu'u, T. J., Zhang, J. & Salamonsen, L. A. (2004) Identification of chemokines important for leukocyte recruitment to the human endometrium at the times of embryo implantation and menstruation. *Journal of Clinical Endocrinology and Metabolism*, Vol.89, No.12, pp. 6155-6167, ISSN 0021-972X

Junqueira, L. C., Zugaib, M., Montes, G. S., Toledo, O. M., Krisztan, R. M. & Shigihara, K. M. (1980) Morphologic and histochemical evidence for the occurrence of collagenolysis and for the role of neutrophilic polymorphonuclear leukocytes during cervical dilation. *American Journal Obstetrics and Gynecology*, Vol.138, No.3, pp. 273-281, ISSN 0002-9378

Kaitu'u-Lino, T. J., Morison, N. B. & Salamonsen, L. A. (2007) Neutrophil depletion retards endometrial repair in a mouse model. *Cell and Tissue Research*, Vol.328, No.1, pp. 197-206, ISSN 0302-766X

Kindzelskii, A. L., Clark, A. J., Espinoza, J., Maeda, N., Aratani, Y., Romero, R. & Petty, H. R. (2006) Myeloperoxidase accumulates at the neutrophil surface and enhances cell metabolism and oxidant release during pregnancy. *European Journal of Immunology*, Vol.36, No.6, pp. 1619-1628, ISSN 0014-2980

King, A. E. & Critchley, H. O. (2010) Oestrogen and progesterone regulation of inflammatory processes in the human endometrium. *Journal of Steroid Biochemistry and Molecular Biology*, Vol.120, No.2-3, pp. 116-126, ISSN 1879-1220

Klebanoff, S. J. (1977) Estrogen binding by leukocytes during phagocytosis. *Journal of Experimental Medicine*, Vol.145, No.4, pp. 983-998, ISSN 0022-1007

Kramer, P. R., Winger, V. & Kramer, S. F. (2007) 17beta-Estradiol utilizes the estrogen receptor to regulate CD16 expression in monocytes. *Molecular and Cellular Endocrinology*, Vol.279, No.1-2, pp. 16-25, ISSN 0303-7207

Kramer, P. R. & Wray, S. (2002) 17-Beta-estradiol regulates expression of genes that function in macrophage activation and cholesterol homeostasis. *Journal of Steroid Biochemistry and Molecular Biology*, Vol.81, No.3, pp. 203-216, ISSN 0960-0760

Kropf, P., Baud, D., Marshall, S. E., Munder, M., Mosley, A., Fuentes, J. M., Bangham, C. R., Taylor, G. P., Herath, S., Choi, B. S., Soler, G., Teoh, T., Modolell, M. & Muller, I. (2007) Arginase activity mediates reversible T cell hyporesponsiveness in human pregnancy. *European Journal of Immunology*, Vol.37, No.4, pp. 935-945, ISSN 0014-2980

Kwak-Kim, J. & Gilman-Sachs, A. (2008) Clinical implication of natural killer cells and reproduction. *American Journal of Reproductive Immunology*, Vol.59, No.5, pp. 388-400, ISSN 1046-7408

Lathbury, L. J. & Salamonsen, L. A. (2000) In-vitro studies of the potential role of neutrophils in the process of menstruation. *Molecular Human Reproduction*, Vol.6, No.10, pp. 899-906, ISSN 1360-9947

Luo, L., Ibaragi, T., Maeda, M., Nozawa, M., Kasahara, T., Sakai, M., Sasaki, Y., Tanebe, K. & Saito, S. (2000) Interleukin-8 levels and granulocyte counts in cervical mucus during pregnancy. *American Journal of Reproductive Immunology*, Vol.43, No.2, pp. 78-84, ISSN 1046-7408

Manolagas, S. C. & Kousteni, S. (2001) Perspective: nonreproductive sites of action of reproductive hormones. *Endocrinology*, Vol.142, No.6, pp. 2200-2204, ISSN 0013-7227

Mathur, S., Mathur, R. S., Goust, J. M., Williamson, H. O. & Fudenberg, H. H. (1979) Cyclic variations in white cell subpopulations in the human menstrual cycle: correlations with progesterone and estradiol. *Clinical Immunology and Immunopathology*, Vol.13, No.3, pp. 246-253, ISSN 0090-1229

Molero, L., Garcia-Duran, M., Diaz-Recasens, J., Rico, L., Casado, S. & Lopez-Farre, A. (2002) Expression of estrogen receptor subtypes and neuronal nitric oxide synthase in neutrophils from women and men: regulation by estrogen. *Cardiovascular Research*, Vol.56, No.1, pp. 43-51, ISSN 0008-6363

Molloy, E. J., O'Neill, A. J., Grantham, J. J., Sheridan-Pereira, M., Fitzpatrick, J. M., Webb, D. W. & Watson, R. W. (2003) Sex-specific alterations in neutrophil apoptosis: the role of estradiol and progesterone. *Blood*, Vol.102, No.7, pp. 2653-2659, ISSN 0006-4971

Muller, I., Munder, M., Kropf, P. & Hansch, G. M. (2009) Polymorphonuclear neutrophils and T lymphocytes: strange bedfellows or brothers in arms? *Trends in Immunology*, Vol.30, No.11, pp. 522-530, ISSN 1471-4981

Murphy, A. J., Guyre, P. M. & Pioli, P. A. (2010) Estradiol suppresses NF-kappa B activation through coordinated regulation of let-7a and miR-125b in primary human macrophages. *Journal of Immunology*, Vol.184, No.9, pp. 5029-5037, ISSN 1550-6606

Nalbandian, G. & Kovats, S. (2005) Understanding sex biases in immunity: effects of estrogen on the differentiation and function of antigen-presenting cells. *Immunological Research*, Vol.31, No.2, pp. 91-106, ISSN 0257-277X

Oakley, O. R., Kim, H., El-Amouri, I., Lin, P. C., Cho, J., Bani-Ahmad, M. & Ko, C. (2010) Periovulatory leukocyte infiltration in the rat ovary. *Endocrinology*, Vol.151, No.9, pp. 4551-4559, ISSN 1945-7170

Osman, I., Young, A., Ledingham, M. A., Thomson, A. J., Jordan, F., Greer, I. A. & Norman, J. E. (2003) Leukocyte density and pro-inflammatory cytokine expression in human fetal membranes, decidua, cervix and myometrium before and during labour at term. *Molecular Human Reproduction*, Vol.9, No.1, pp. 41-45, ISSN 1360-9947

Osmers, R., Rath, W., Adelmann-Grill, B. C., Fittkow, C., Kuloczik, M., Szeverenyi, M., Tschesche, H. & Kuhn, W. (1992) Origin of cervical collagenase during parturition. *American Journal Obstetrics and Gynecology*, Vol.166, No.5, pp. 1455-1460, ISSN 0002-9378

Pierdominici, M., Maselli, A., Colasanti, T., Giammarioli, A. M., Delunardo, F., Vacirca, D., Sanchez, M., Giovannetti, A., Malorni, W. & Ortona, E. (2010) Estrogen receptor profiles in human peripheral blood lymphocytes. *Immunological letters*, Vol.132, No.1-2, pp. 79-85, ISSN 1879-0542

Prossnitz, E. R., Arterburn, J. B. & Sklar, L. A. (2007) GPR30: A G protein-coupled receptor for estrogen. *Molecular and Cellular Endocrinology*, Vol.265-266, pp. 138-142, ISSN 0303-7207

Sahlin, L., Stjernholm-Vladic, Y., Roos, N., Masironi, B. & Ekman-Ordeberg, G. (2008) Impaired leukocyte influx in cervix of postterm women not responding to prostaglandin priming. *Reproductive Biology & Endocrinology*, Vol.6, pp. 36, ISSN 1477-7827

Salamonsen, L. A. & Lathbury, L. J. (2000) Endometrial leukocytes and menstruation. *Human Reproduction Update*, Vol.6, No.1, pp. 16-27, ISSN 1355-4786

Scariano, J. K., Emery-Cohen, A. J., Pickett, G. G., Morgan, M., Simons, P. C. & Alba, F. (2008) Estrogen receptors alpha (ESR1) and beta (ESR2) are expressed in circulating human lymphocytes. *Journal of Receptors and Signal Transduction Research*, Vol.28, No.3, pp. 285-293, ISSN 1079-9893

Segerer, S., Kammerer, U., Kapp, M., Dietl, J. & Rieger, L. (2009) Upregulation of chemokine and cytokine production during pregnancy. *Gynecologic and Obstetric Investigation*, Vol.67, No.3, pp. 145-150, ISSN 1423-002X

Shim, G. J., Gherman, D., Kim, H. J., Omoto, Y., Iwase, H., Bouton, D., Kis, L. L., Andersson, C. T., Warner, M. & Gustafsson, J. A. (2006) Differential expression of oestrogen receptors in human secondary lymphoid tissues. *Journal of Pathology*, Vol.208, No.3, pp. 408-414, ISSN 0022-3417

Siracusa, M. C., Overstreet, M. G., Housseau, F., Scott, A. L. & Klein, S. L. (2008) 17beta-estradiol alters the activity of conventional and IFN-producing killer dendritic cells. *Journal of Immunology*, Vol.180, No.3, pp. 1423-1431, ISSN 0022-1767

Smith, J. M., Shen, Z., Wira, C. R., Fanger, M. W. & Shen, L. (2007) Effects of menstrual cycle status and gender on human neutrophil phenotype. *American Journal of Reproductive Immunology*, Vol.58, No.2, pp. 111-119, ISSN 1046-7408

Straub, R. H. (2007) The complex role of estrogens in inflammation. *Endocrine Reviews*, Vol.28, No.5, pp. 521-574, ISSN 0163-769X

Stygar, D., Masironi, B., Eriksson, H. & Sahlin, L. (2007) Studies on estrogen receptor (ER) alpha and beta responses on gene regulation in peripheral blood leukocytes in vivo using selective ER agonists. *Journal of Endocrinology*, Vol.194, No.1, pp. 101-119.

Stygar, D., Wang, H., Vladic, Y. S., Ekman, G., Eriksson, H. & Sahlin, L. (2001) Co-localization of oestrogen receptor beta and leukocyte markers in the human cervix. *Molecular Human Reproduction*, Vol.7, No.9, pp. 881-886, ISSN 1360-9947

Stygar, D., Wang, H., Vladic, Y. S., Ekman, G., Eriksson, H. & Sahlin, L. (2002) Increased level of matrix metalloproteinases 2 and 9 in the ripening process of the human cervix. *Biology of Reproduction*, Vol.67, No.3, pp. 889-894, ISSN 0006-3363

Stygar, D., Westlund, P., Eriksson, H. & Sahlin, L. (2006) Identification of wild type and variants of oestrogen receptors in polymorphonuclear and mononuclear leucocytes. *Clinical Endocrinology (Oxf)*, Vol.64, No.1, pp. 74-81, ISSN 0300-0664

Subramanian, M. & Shaha, C. (2009) Oestrogen modulates human macrophage apoptosis via differential signalling through oestrogen receptor-alpha and beta. *Journal of Cellular and Molecular Medicine*, Vol.13, No.8B, pp. 2317-2329, ISSN 1582-4934

Thomson, A. J., Telfer, J. F., Young, A., Campbell, S., Stewart, C. J., Cameron, I. T., Greer, I. A. & Norman, J. E. (1999) Leukocytes infiltrate the myometrium during human parturition: further evidence that labour is an inflammatory process. *Human Reproduction*, Vol.14, No.1, pp. 229-236, ISSN 0268-1161

Thongngarm, T., Jenkins, J. K., Ndebele, K. & McMurray, R. W. (2003) Estrogen and progesterone modulate monocyte cell cycle progression and apoptosis. *American Journal of Reproductive Immunology*, Vol.49, No.3, pp. 129-138, ISSN 1046-7408

Tulchinsky, D. & Hobel, C. J. (1973) Plasma human chorionic gonadotropin, estrone, estradiol, estriol, progesterone, and 17 alpha-hydroxyprogesterone in human pregnancy. 3. Early normal pregnancy. *American Journal Obstetrics and Gynecology*, Vol.117, No.7, pp. 884-893, ISSN 0002-9378

van den Heuvel, M. J., Xie, X., Tayade, C., Peralta, C., Fang, Y., Leonard, S., Paffaro, V. A., Jr., Sheikhi, A. K., Murrant, C. & Croy, B. A. (2005) A review of trafficking and activation of uterine natural killer cells. *American Journal of Reproductive Immunology*, Vol.54, No.6, pp. 322-331, ISSN 1046-7408

Walker, V. R. & Korach, K. S. (2004) Estrogen receptor knockout mice as a model for endocrine research. *Institute of Laboratory Animal Research Journal*, Vol.45, No.4, pp. 455-461, ISSN 1084-2020

Wang, H., Stjernholm, Y., Ekman, G., Eriksson, H. & Sahlin, L. (2001) Different regulation of oestrogen receptors alpha and beta in the human cervix at term pregnancy. *Molecular Human Reproduction*, Vol.7, No.3, pp. 293-300, ISSN 1360-9947

Watson, R. W., O'Neill, A., Brannigan, A. E., Coffey, R., Marshall, J. C., Brady, H. R. & Fitzpatrick, J. M. (1999) Regulation of Fas antibody induced neutrophil apoptosis is both caspase and mitochondrial dependent. *FEBS Letters*, Vol.453, No.1-2, pp. 67-71, ISSN 0014-5793

Wira, C. R., Fahey, J. V., Ghosh, M., Patel, M. V., Hickey, D. K. & Ochiel, D. O. (2010) Sex hormone regulation of innate immunity in the female reproductive tract: the role of epithelial cells in balancing reproductive potential with protection against sexually transmitted pathogens. *American Journal of Reproductive Immunology*, Vol.63, No.6, pp. 544-565, ISSN 1600-0897

Yovel, G., Shakhar, K. & Ben-Eliyahu, S. (2001) The effects of sex, menstrual cycle, and oral contraceptives on the number and activity of natural killer cells. *Gynecologic Oncology*, Vol.81, No.2, pp. 254-262, ISSN 0090-8258

Yuan, M., Jordan, F., McInnes, I. B., Harnett, M. M. & Norman, J. E. (2009) Leukocytes are primed in peripheral blood for activation during term and preterm labour. *Molecular Human Reproduction*, Vol.15, No.11, pp. 713-724, ISSN 1460-2407

Zaitsu, M., Narita, S., Lambert, K. C., Grady, J. J., Estes, D. M., Curran, E. M., Brooks, E. G., Watson, C. S., Goldblum, R. M. & Midoro-Horiuti, T. (2007) Estradiol activates mast cells via a non-genomic estrogen receptor-alpha and calcium influx. *Molecular Immunology*, Vol.44, No.8, pp. 1977-1985, ISSN 0161-5890

Zhao, X. J., McKerr, G., Dong, Z., Higgins, C. A., Carson, J., Yang, Z. Q. & Hannigan, B. M. (2001) Expression of oestrogen and progesterone receptors by mast cells alone, but not lymphocytes, macrophages or other immune cells in human upper airways. *Thorax*, Vol.56, No.3, pp. 205-211, ISSN 0040-6376

Part 3

Gynecological Endocrinology

18

Physiological Relevance of Pregnanolone Isomers and Their Polar Conjugates with Respect to the Gender, Menstrual Cycle and Pregnancy

Martin Hill, Antonín Pařízek, Radmila Kancheva,
David Cibula, Nikolaj Madzarov and Luboslav Stárka
*Institute of Endocrinology, Prague,
Czech Republic*

1. Introduction

5α/β-Reduced progesterone metabolites (PM) including pregnanolone isomers (PI) and their polar conjugates (PIC), are efficient neuromodulators operating in a number of physiological and pathological processes including psychiatric diseases or problems connected with pregnancy, parturition and postpartum period. The substances mostly belong to the group of neuroactive steroids.

The neuroactive steroids (including PI) originating directly in the central and peripheral nervous system are called neurosteroids. They have a wide variety of functions. Some neuroactive steroids are able to easily pass through the blood-brain barrier (Bixo, Andersson, Winblad, Purdy, & Backstrom, 1997; Kancheva, et al., 2010; M. D. Wang, Wahlstrom, & Backstrom, 1997). Disorders in their biosynthesis or malfunctions in interactions with the target sites can be the cause of many pathologies, including psychiatric illnesses (Backstrom, et al., 2003; Backstrom, Carstensen, & Sodergard, 1976). In contrast with the most common steroid hormones acting, neuroactive steroids largely affect non-genomic mechanisms and influence nerve excitability in both directions. Some neuroactive steroids, such as allopregnanolone and its derivates, also show neuro-protective effects (Ciriza, Azcoitia, & Garcia-Segura, 2004; Morfin & Starka, 2001; Shi, Schulze, & Lardy, 2000).

The enzymes involved in the neurosteroidogenesis can be classified in two main groups: the cytochrome P450 and the non-P450 group. Experiments proved the direct biosynthesis of steroids in the brain independent of the periphery (Corpechot, Leclerc, Baulieu, & Brazeau, 1985; Corpechot, Robel, Axelson, Sjovall, & Baulieu, 1981). Three years later, Harrison and Simmonds published their work on the anesthetic effect of the synthetic pregnane steroid ganaxalone through modulation of the stimulation of the γ-aminobutyric acid receptor (GABA-r) (Harrison & Simmonds, 1984). The following year Majewska and coworkers published the first study on the modulation effect of endogenous steroids on GABA-r, and thereby initiated an intense research effort focused on the mechanisms of action of neuroactive steroids (Majewska, Bisserbe, & Eskay, 1985).

This chapter is focused on the origin and the physiological impact of endogenous neuroactive PI and PIC in humans, respecting the status of sex, menstrual cycle and pregnancy. Particular attention is paid on the role of PI in pregnancy and parturition respecting their extensive production in this period.

2. The neuromodulating effects of 5α/β-reduced pregnanes

2.1 Effects of 5α/β-reduced pregnanes on γ-aminobutyric acid receptors

Pregnanolone isomers are known to modulate ionotropic receptors on neuronal membranes (Pisu & Serra, 2004). 3α-PI shorten the paradoxical sleeping, reduce the acetylcholine in neocortex and hippocampus, suppress the neurogenesis and deteriorate the spatial memory (Mayo, et al., 2003). From the membrane receptors influenced by PI, the most familiar are the type-A γ-aminobutyric acid receptors ($GABA_A$-r) that control the influx of chloride ions into the neuronal cells. 5α/β-Reduced pregnane (and androstane) steroids with a hydroxy-group in the 3α-position positively modulate the $GABA_A$-r. The maximum sensitivity to 3α-PI and namely to pregnanolone (3α-hydroxy-5β-pregnane-20-one, 3α,5β-THP) was observed in the receptor subtype $\alpha_4\beta_3\delta$ (A. J. Smith, et al., 2001). Alternatively, inactive 3β-PI compete with the 3α-PI on $GABA_A$-r (Lundgren, Stromberg, Backstrom, & Wang, 2003; Prince & Simmonds, 1992; M. Wang, et al., 2002). While the 3α-PI are potent endogenous neuroinhibitory substances, the PIC are their antagonists. Conjugation counteracts the effect of 3α-PI, and further amplifies the antagonistic effect of the 3β-PI on $GABA_A$-r (Park-Chung, Malayev, Purdy, Gibbs, & Farb, 1999).

2.2 Effects of 5α/β-reduced pregnanes on N-methyl-D-aspartate receptors

Further receptors, which are influenced by steroid polar conjugates, are the N-methyl-D-aspartate receptors (NMDA-r). The NMDA-r are responsible for Ca^{2+} influx into the neurons inducing their rapid activation. 5α-PIC operate as activators of NMDA-r like the sulfates of 3β-hydroxy-5-en-steroids but the 5β-PIC are the antagonists of 5α-PIC. Besides the effects on neuronal membranes, some PI bind to progesterone intracellular receptors and influence also the gene expression of $GABA_A$-r subunits (Dubrovsky, 2005). Apart from the central nervous system (CNS), both NMDA-r and GABA-r are present in the peripheral neurons (Leung, et al., 2002; Majewska, Falkay, & Baulieu, 1989).

2.3 Effects of 5α/β-reduced pregnanes on T-type calcium channels

5β-PM block calcium channels of T-type in the rat peripheral neurons playing a significant role in pain perception and transmission (Todorovic, et al., 2004). The aforementioned mechanism indicates an antinociceptive action of 5β-PM on the peripheral level.

2.4 Effects of 5α/β-reduced pregnanes on L-type calcium channels

Factors regulating intracellular calcium concentration are known to play a critical role in the brain function and neural development, including neural plasticity and neurogenesis. 3α,5α-THP-induced intracellular calcium concentration increase may serve as the initiation mechanism whereby 3α,5α-THP promotes neurogenesis. 3α,5α-THP induces a rapid, dose-dependent, stereo-specific, and developmentally regulated increase in intracellular calcium in (rat embryonic) hippocampal neurons via a mechanism that requires both the $GABA_A$-r and L-type calcium channels (J. M. Wang & Brinton, 2008).

3. 5α/β-Reduced pregnanes in non-pregnant subjects

3.1 Sources of 5α/β-reduced pregnanes in non-pregnant subjects

The results in the literature show the necessity to differentiate between men, women in follicular phase of the menstrual cycle (FP), women in luteal phase of the menstrual cycle (LP), and pregnant women when evaluating changes of circulating PI that are linked to various pathologies. The neuroexcitatory PIC (acting via $GABA_A$-r) strikingly prevail over the neuroinhibitory unconjugated 3α-PI irrespectively of the subject status. On the other hand, the proportions in the circulating levels of neuroactive steroids do not necessarily have to reflect steroid ratios at the sites where they have an effect. It is likely that the pronounced excess of polar PI conjugates in the circulation is principally connected to their higher solubility in comparison with their non-polar free analogs. However, the chances of overcoming the blood-brain barrier generally increase with the decreasing polarity of the substance (Oren, Fleishman, Kessel, & Ben-Tal, 2004). This means that the transport of free PI would be preferred over that of the conjugates, despite their striking excess as reported in the model focused on the transport of free and conjugated pregnenolone from circulation into the brain in rats (M. D. Wang, et al., 1997). The conjugation of PI is also important for regulating the proportion between neuroexcitatory and neuroinhibitory pregnane steroids or, at least as a key metabolic step responsible for the elimination of neuroactive PI. Figure 1 demonstrates a simplified scheme of the biosynthesis and catabolism of 5α/β-reduced pregnanes.

3.1.1 Biosynthesis of neuroactive steroids in the cells of neuronal system

The 3α,5α-THP is present in human post-mortem brain tissue at considerably higher concentrations than typically observed in blood (Marx, et al., 2006). These neurosteroids are synthesized in brain, peripheral glial cells and neurons (Schumacher, et al., 2000). As demonstrated on rats, the enzymes that are necessary for synthesis of neuroactive 5α/β-PM as type 2 3β-hydroxysteroid dehydrogenase (HSD3B2) and 5α-reductase of types 1 (SRD5A1) and 2 (SRD5A2) are present in the CNS. While the SRD5A1 was identified for the most part in glial cells of white matter, SRD5A2 was found in oligodendrocytes, neurons and astrocytes of the grey matter. The enzyme isoforms, which are effective as the 3α-hydroxysteroid dehydrogenase are present in oligodendrocytes, neurons and astrocytes of white and grey matter (Patte-Mensah, Penning, & Mensah-Nyagan, 2004; Schumacher, et al., 2004; Stoffel-Wagner, et al., 2000; Tsuruo, 2005). The important system mediating changes or even reversion of neuromodulating activity involves a steroid sulfatase (STS) and sulfotransferases controlling the balance between neuroinhibitory 3α-PI and PIC that exert an opposite effect. However, relatively high STS activity but very low sulfotransferase activity were detected in the brain (Compagnone, Salido, Shapiro, & Mellon, 1997; Kriz, Bicikova, Hill, & Hampl, 2005).

The GABAergic steroids can be inactivated by their 3α-oxidation to yield 5α-dihydroprogesterone (5α-DHP). It was found that 5α-DHP levels in HEK293 cells expressing type 10 17β-hydroxysteroid dehydrogenase (HSD17B10) increased as 3α,5α-THP was added to culture media. Brain astrocytes contain a moderate level of HSD17B10, which is elevated in activated astrocytes of brains with Alzheimer type pathology. Cerebral cortex has the lowest level of HSD17B10; whereas the hippocampus, hypothalamus, and amygdala possess relatively higher levels of this enzyme. The catalysis of HSD17B10 appears to be essential for maintaining normal functions of GABAergic neurons (He, Wegiel, & Yang, 2005).

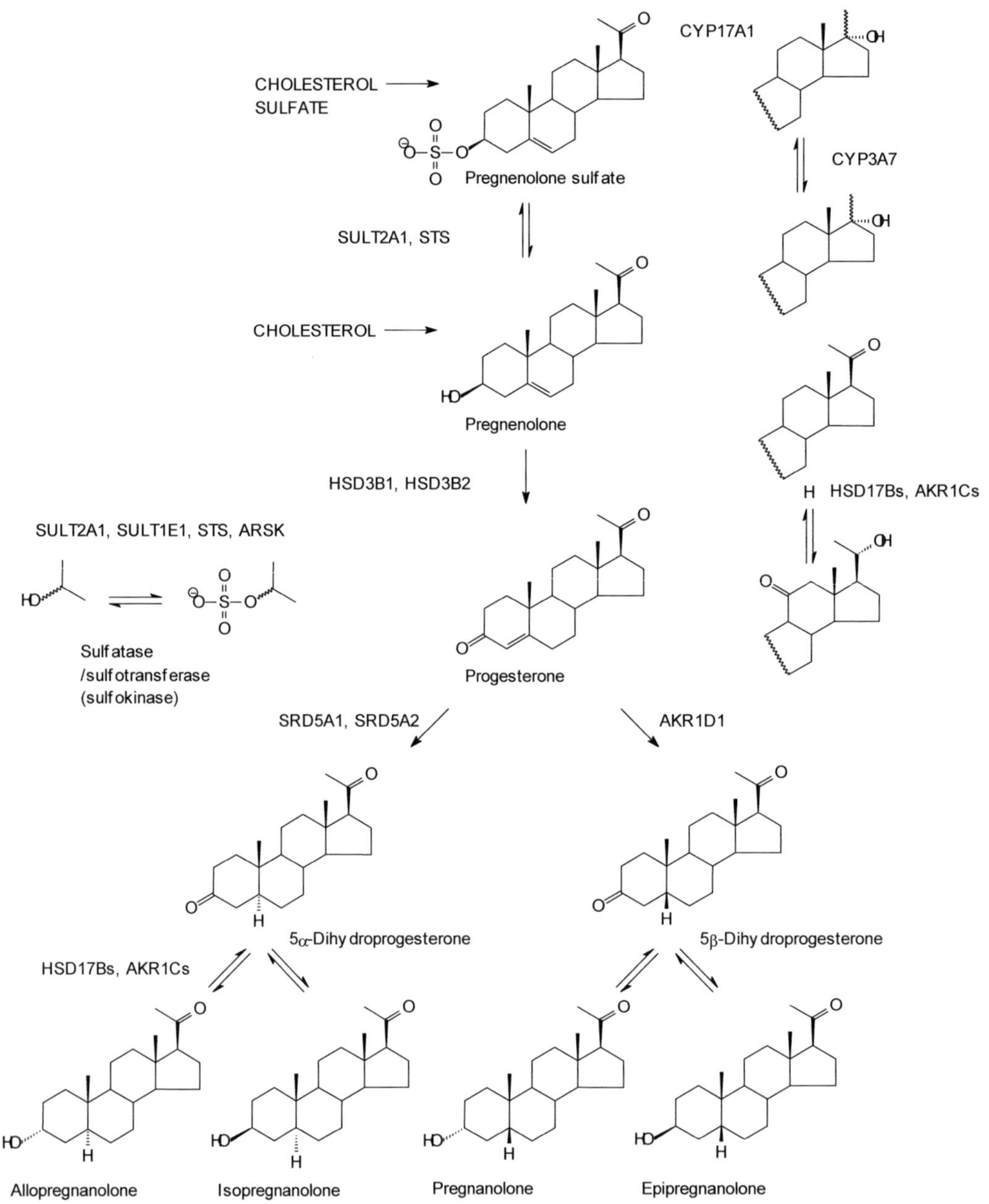

Fig. 1. Simplified scheme of the biosynthesis and catabolism of 5α/β-reduced pregnanes

3.1.2 Gonadal function and neuroactive steroids

The most part of neuroactive steroids in women in the luteal phase of menstrual cycle (LP) consists of metabolites of progesterone, which is formed in *corpus luteum* (Ottander, et al., 2005). The levels of PI and PIC strongly depend on the menstrual cycle, reflecting changes in progesterone formation. The mRNA of 5α-reductase (SRD5A), 5β-reductase (AKR1D1) and 3α-hydroxysteroid oxidoreductase (3α-HSOR) mRNA are all expressed in human *corpus luteum* and the release of 3α,5α-THP and 3α,5β-THP herein is stimulated by a trophic hormone. The dominant PI is the 3α,5α-THP (Havlikova, et al., 2006; M. Hill, et al., 2005). In women, progesterone and its reduced metabolites exhibit a decrease with increasing age and a qualitative change after menopause (Genazzani, et al., 1998). It is likely that the gonadal 5α/β-PM easily overcome the blood-brain-barrier (Bixo, et al., 1997; Kancheva, et al., 2010).

3.1.3 The role of adrenals in the biosynthesis of neuroactive steroids

Zona glomerulosa controlled by the renin-angiotensin axis produces deoxycorticosterone (DOC), the metabolites of which are neuroactive like the 3α,5α-tetrahydro-DOC (3α,5α-THDOC) and its isomers. However, DOC is produced in substantially greater quantities in *zona fasciculata,* which is controlled by the CRH-ACTH system. In contrast to the 3α,5α-THP reaching about 10% of progesterone concentration, the basal levels of DOC and 3α,5α-THDOC are almost comparable (<0.5 nmol/L) (Reddy, 2006).

Zona fasciculata primarily produces cortisol in relatively high amounts. 3α-5α/β-Reduced metabolites of cortisol are GABAergic such as the 3α-PI. The 3α,5α-tetrahydrocortisol and 3α,5α-THP posses a comparable activity on $GABA_A$-r (Stromberg, Backstrom, & Lundgren, 2005). In addition, adrenal *zona fasciculata* produces relatively abundantly pregnenolone sulfate (PregS) (20-400 nmol/l), which, like the cortisol, readily reacts to adrenocorticotropin (ACTH) stimulation (de Peretti, et al., 1986). PregS appears to be the most important precursor of progesterone and DOC of adrenal origin. Growing formation of PregS in adrenals that is further metabolized up to neuroactive PI may explain the increased levels of brain 5α/β-PM in patients with diagnoses associated with stress (Higashi, Takido, & Shimada, 2005). Increasing peripheral production of pregnane steroids and their precursors and their subsequent transport across the blood-brain-barrier could contribute to the physiological compensation of stress. Most probably, the peripheral levels of pregnane steroids primarily depend on adrenal activity in women in FP (Havlikova, et al., 2006; M. Hill, et al., 2005), postmenopausal women, children and men (Fig. 2A,B). However, the proportion of 5α/β-PM derived from the adrenal activity is pronouncedly lower compared to the quantity originating in the *corpus luteum* (Meczekalski, et al., 2000) (Fig. 2C).

3.2 Human CNS-related pathologies that are linked to the 5α/β-reduced pregnanes

3.2.1 Premenstrual syndrome

Changes in progesterone levels and respective changes in its neuroactive metabolites are apparently the cause of premenstrual dysphoric disorder in women (PMDD). Withdrawal effect in case of abrupt drop of steroid positive modulators rapidly supervenes like the addiction effect while increasing the steroid levels. Changing 5α/β-PI concentrations induce a decreased affinity of $GABA_A$-r for these steroids due to the changed expression of the receptor subunits and/or as a result of the changed phosphorylation status of the specific sites on the $GABA_A$-r (Brussaard, Wossink, Lodder, & Kits, 2000; Koksma, et al., 2003; Leng & Russell, 1999; Maguire & Mody, 2009). The aforementioned mechanism requires synchronization, the disturbances of which could have significant neuropsychiatric consequences in physiological and pathological situations like pregnancy, parturition, onset of menopause, traumas, endocrine diseases, and stress. Several $GABA_A$-r modulators, including 3α,5α-THP, exert biphasic effect. The low concentrations induce an adverse, anxiogenic effect whereas the higher concentrations decrease this effect and show calming properties (Andreen, et al., 2009). The severity of these mood symptoms is related to the

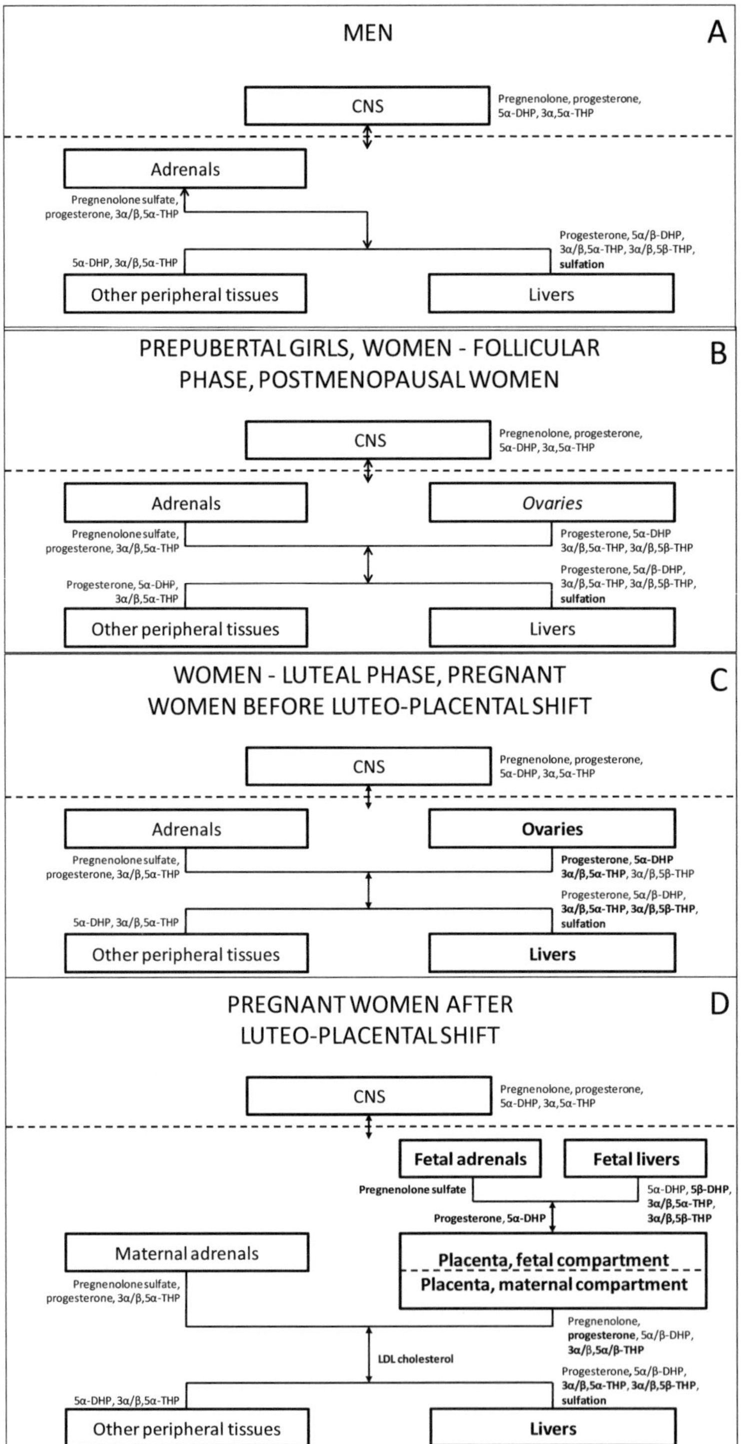

Fig. 2. Origin of pregnanolone isomers

3α,5α-THP serum concentrations in a manner similar to a bell-shaped curve. Negative mood symptoms occur when the serum concentration of 3α,5α-THP is similar to the endogenous LP levels, while low and high concentrations have no such effect. Progesterone/3α,5α-THP treatment in women increases the activity in the amygdala in a similar manner as the changes seen during anxiety reactions. Women with PMDD in LP show changes in $GABA_A$-r sensitivity and GABA concentrations that are related to the severity of the condition (Andreen, et al., 2009).

3.2.2 Chronic fatigue syndrome

Increased inhibition through $GABA_A$-r due to the accumulation of neuroinhibitory steroids may represent an important pathophysiological mechanism of fatigue in chronic liver diseases. The levels of 3α,5α-THP and 3β,5α-THP are increased in plasma of patients with chronic fatigue syndrome (Ahboucha, et al., 2008).

3.2.3 Depression

Antidepressants elevate 3α-PI levels in rodent brain (Uzunova, et al., 1998). However, recent studies suggest that changes in plasma neuroactive steroid levels may not be a general mandatory component of clinically effective antidepressant treatment *per se*, but may reflect distinct properties of pharmacotherapy only (Uzunova, Sampson, & Uzunov, 2006).

3.2.4 Epilepsy

Women with epilepsy show reduced progesterone levels in the LP. The progesterone deficit results in the debit of neuroinhibitory 3α-hydroxy- 5α/β-reduced progesterone metabolites (Stoffel-Wagner, 2001). Rat models of catamenial epilepsy exhibit an abstinence effect at lowered 3α,5α-THP concentrations, which however results in higher sensitivity after restitution of its original levels. Various authors demonstrate that catamenial epilepsy is linked to the disturbed biosynthesis of progesterone and its reduced metabolites (Backstrom, et al., 2003), particularly in the LP (Bonuccelli, et al., 1989).

3.2.5 Schizophrenia

GABAergic steroids may be candidate modulators for the pathophysiology of schizophrenia and bipolar disorder, and relevant to the treatment of these disorders. 3α,5α-THP levels tend to be decreased in parietal cortex in subjects with schizophrenia compared to control subjects (Marx, et al., 2006).

3.2.6 Neurodegenerative disorders

3α,5α-THP is reduced in prefrontal cortex in male patients with Alzheimer disease (AD) compared to male cognitively intact control subjects, and inversely correlated with neuropathological disease stage. 3α,5α-THP levels are reduced in temporal cortex in patients with AD compared to control subjects and inversely correlated with neuropathological disease stage. Patients carrying an APOE4 allele demonstrate reduced 3α,5α-THP levels in temporal cortex (Naylor, et al., 2010).

3.2.7 Eating disorders

Compared with healthy women, the patients with eating disorders exhibit increased plasma levels of 3α,5α-THP. However, the relevance of such hormonal alteration to the pathophysiology of eating disorders remains to be elucidated (Monteleone, et al., 2001) (Monteleone, et al., 2003).

4. 5α/β-Reduced pregnanes in human pregnancy

4.1 Fetal adrenal is the primary source of pregnancy steroids

4.1.1 Placental CRH controls the steroid biosynthesis in the fetal adrenal

The machinery regulating production of pregnancy steroids (including pregnanolone isomers and their polar conjugates) is based on the excessive placental production of corticoliberin (CRH) (Goland, Wardlaw, Stark, Brown, & Frantz, 1986; Rainey, Rehman, & Carr, 2004; R. Smith, et al., 2009). CRH in non-pregnant subjects is a hypothalamic hormone controlling the pituitary secretion of adrenocorticotropic hormone (ACTH) and, in turn, the corticosteroid production in adult adrenal. The hypothalamic-pituitary-adrenal axis in these subjects is based on a negative feedback loop between the final active hormone, ACTH and CRH. Alternatively, the pregnant women after luteo-placental shift produce CRH primarily in placenta and instead of the negative feedback loop cortisol-ACTH-CRH; there is a positive one between cortisol and CRH, while the ACTH production stagnates. The rising CRH levels in the last four weeks of pregnancy stimulate the synthesis of conjugated Δ^5 steroids (Sirianni, Mayhew, Carr, Parker, & Rainey, 2005; R. Smith, Mesiano, Chan, Brown, & Jaffe, 1998) in the fetal zone of the fetal adrenal (FZ), which is a specific transient tissue gradually converting to *zona reticularis* after labor. The excessive production of placental CRH is unique for primates and the boosting CRH production near term is exclusive for humans and great apes (Power & Schulkin, 2006).

The sulfated Δ^5 steroids, originating in the FZ represent the largest fraction of steroids in pregnancy (Ingelman-Sundberg, Rane, & Gustafasson, 1975; Lacroix, Sonnier, Moncion, Cheron, & Cresteil, 1997; Leeder, et al., 2005; Moghrabi, Head, & Andersson, 1997) (Fig. 2D). Sulfotransferase 2A1 (SULT2A1) transcript shows even 13-fold higher levels in the fetal adrenal. Alternatively, HSD3B2 mRNA expression in midgestation is 127-fold lower than the one in the adult adrenal due to preferential synthesis of the Δ^5 C-21 steroids over corticoids. The FZ is similar to the adult *zona reticularis* but unlike the adult *zona reticularis*, the FZ produces excessive amounts of sulfated C-21 Δ^5 steroids, including pregnenolone sulfate (PregS) (M. Hill, Parizek, Cibula, et al., 2010; M. Hill, Parizek, Jirasek, et al., 2010; Rainey, et al., 2004). The Δ^5 steroid sulfates (originating in the FZ) serve as precursors for the placental production of estradiol (Sirianni, et al., 2005; R. Smith, et al., 1998) and progesterone (M. Hill, Parizek, Jirasek, et al., 2010; Jaffe & Ledger, 1966; Komatsuzaki, et al., 1987; Walsh, 1988).

4.2 Steroid metabolism in the fetal and maternal liver

4.2.1 C-3, C-17 and C-20 oxidoreductive conversions

Human liver contains various isoforms of pluripotent aldoketo reductases (AKR1C1, AKR1C2, AKR1C3, and AKR1C4) with 20α-, 17β-, 3α- or 3β-hydroxysteroid dehydrogenase-like activity (Jin, et al., 2009; Penning, et al., 2001; Shiraishi, et al., 1998). The enzyme activities could control the occupancy of $GABA_A$-receptors (Penning, 1999) via reduction of oxo-groups in the steroid C3 position. *In vivo,* all AKR1Cs preferentially work as reductases (Steckelbroeck, Jin, Gopishetty, Oyesanmi, & Penning, 2004) and are capable of reducing estrone, progesterone, and 3-oxo- pregnane (androstane) steroids to estradiol, 20α-dihydroprogesterone, and GABAergic 3α-hydroxy-5α/β- pregnane (androstane) steroids, respectively. On the other hand, AKR1Cs may decrease the neurosteroid concentrations by inactivating 3α,5α-THP and eliminating the precursors like progesterone from the synthetic pathways via reduction of the 20-oxo-steroid group (Penning, et al., 2000; Usami, et al., 2002). The AKR1C2 preferring 3α-reduction over the 3β-reduction may catalyze 3α-, 17β-, and 20α-HSD reactions (Jin, et al., 2009; Jin, et al., 2001; Penning, et al., 2000; Usami, et al., 2002). From the family of short chain dehydrogenases (SDRs), type 7 17β-hydroxysteroid dehydrogenase (HSD17B7), preferring the reduction of the oxo-groups in 20-, 17- or 3-position to the corresponding 20α-hydroxy-, 17β-hydroxy- or 3α-hydroxy-counterparts, is also significantly expressed in the liver (Krazeisen, et al., 1999; Torn, et al., 2003).

Instead, other SDRs like type 2 HSD17B (HSD17B2), type 10 17β-HSD (HSD17B10) and type 11 17β-HSD (HSD17B11), which are also highly expressed in the liver, prefer the oxidative direction. HSD17B2 may contribute to the formation of 20-oxo- and 17-oxo-steroids from their 20α- and 17β- counterparts (Moghrabi, et al., 1997). Type 6 17β-HSD (HSD17B6) prefers oxidoreductase and 3(α-->β)-hydroxysteroid epimerase activities and acts on both C-19 and C-21 3α-hydroxysteroids (Huang & Luu-The, 2000). HSD17B10 being abundantly expressed in the liver, is capable of catalyzing the oxidation of steroid modulators of $GABA_A$-r (He, et al., 2001). HSD17B10 catalyzes the conversion of 3α,5α-THP and 3α,5α-THDOC to the corresponding inactive 3-oxo steroids (He, et al., 2003). The catalysis of HSD17B10 appears to be essential for maintaining normal functions of GABAergic neurons (Shafqat, et al., 2003).

4.2.2 5α/β-Reductases

The liver has also high activity of SRD5A and AKR1D1 (Charbonneau & The, 2001; Meikle, Stringham, Wilson, & Dolman, 1979). From the two isoforms of SRD5A, SRD5A1 is widely distributed in the body, with the highest levels in the liver and converts testosterone into 5α-dihydrotestosterone and progesterone, and corticosterone into their corresponding 3-oxo-5α-reduced steroids. In the androgen-dependent structures, 5α-DHT is almost exclusively formed by SRD5A2 (Poletti, et al., 1998). In the peripheral tissues, including the liver, SRD5A1 and 3α-HSD reductive AKR1Cs and HSD17Bs work consecutively eliminating the androgens, protecting against the hormone excess (Jin & Penning, 2001) and producing GABAergic steroids, which are, however, extensively sulfated in the liver.

Liver AKR1D1 efficiently catalyzes the reduction of both C-19 and C-21 3-oxo-Δ^4 steroids to the corresponding 5β-PM (Kochakian, 1983; Okuda & Okuda, 1984). The higher levels of 5β-PM in the fetus than in maternal compartment as well as the arteriovenous differences in the fetus indicate that steroid 5β-reduction in the fetal liver (but not in the placenta) is important for production of 5β-PM in both maternal and fetal compartment (M. Hill, Parizek, Cibula, et al., 2010).

4.2.3 Balance between polar conjugates and unconjugated steroids

The sulfotransferase SULT2A1 is highly expressed in human liver (Comer & Falany, 1992; Geese & Raftogianis, 2001; Meloche & Falany, 2001; Zhang, Varlamova, Vargas, Falany, & Leyh, 1998). However, the liver also strongly expresses the STS (Selcer, Difrancesca, Chandra, & Li, 2007) like the placenta. The formation of sulfated steroids with a 3α-hydroxy-5α configuration may account for 50% of the metabolism of progesterone in late pregnancy (Anderson, et al., 1990). The sulfation of 3β,5α-THP is an important metabolic step contributing to progesterone catabolism and significantly affecting the balance between neuroinhibitory steroids and their antagonists in pregnant women. The further major pathway of progesterone catabolism in the maternal compartment proceeds in the sequence progesterone → 5β-DHP → 3α,5β-THP→ conjugated 3α,5β-THP (Kancheva, et al., 2007), which is analogous to the situation out of pregnancy (Havlikova, et al., 2006). In this pathway, the 5β-reduction and the reduction of the 3-oxo-group in 5β-DHP, resulting in the synthesis of 3α,5β-THP, appear to be critical metabolic steps (Kancheva, et al., 2007). Humans with low progesterone production exhibit very low concentrations of unconjugated 3α,5β-THP (men, women in the FP). In these subjects, the 3α,5β-THP is rapidly conjugated. Alternatively, in woman in the LP and so much the more in pregnant women, the conjugation capacity for 3α,5β-THP may be limited. The increased conjugation of 5α-PI probably further diminishes the difference between the 3α,5α-THP and 3α,5β-THP levels in pregnant women and may also regulate the proportions between neuroinhibitory 3α,5α-THP and antagonistic conjugated 5α-PI (Kancheva, et al., 2007).

4.3 5α/β-Reductases in the liver, placenta and fetal membranes

Placental SRD5A1 and SRD5A1 may provide precursors for 3α,5α-THP synthesis in fetal brain (Vu, et al., 2009). Milewich, et al. reported *in vitro* synthesis of 5α-reduced pregnanes [3H]5α-DHP and [3H]3β,5α-THP from [3H]progesterone by a placental tissue (Milewich, Gant, Schwarz, Chen, & Macdonald, 1978). Although AKR1D1, catalyzing the 5β-reduction is primarily expressed in the liver, its activity was also detected in other tissues including placenta (Sheehan, Rice, Moses, & Brennecke, 2005). However, AKR1D1 activity in extrahepatic tissues appears to be minor in comparison with that found in the liver (M. Hill, Parizek, Cibula, et al., 2010; Milewich, Gant, Schwarz, Chen, & MacDonald, 1979).

4.4 Steroid metabolism in placenta

4.4.1 Steroid sulfatases and placental production of sex hormones

The principal metabolic step that is indispensable for placental metabolism of sulfated Δ^5 steroids originating in FZ is their desulfation, which is catalyzed by the placental STS. Placental STS activity is independent of substrate concentration (Watanabe, et al., 1990) and of gestational age (GA) (Fukuda, Okuyama, & Furuya, 1986; Ishida, et al., 1985; Leslie, et al., 1994). The placental STS expression in pregnancy explicitly outweighs the production in other tissues (Miki, et al., 2002) and allows access of Δ^5 steroids to the HSD3B1 and CYP19A1 within the syncytiotrophoblast layer and their conversion to estrogens (Siiteri, 2005) and progestogens (M. Hill, Parizek, Cibula, et al., 2010; M. Hill, Parizek, Jirasek, et al., 2010). The latter substances are subsequently converted to 5α/β-PM by placental and liver enzymes.

4.4.2 Reversible C-3, C-17 and C-20 oxidoreductive inter-conversions in placenta and fetal membranes

The cytoplasmic type 1 HSD17B (HSD17B1) is highly expressed in syncytiotrophoblast (Moghrabi, et al., 1997). Besides catalyzing the conversion of estrone and progesterone to estradiol and 20α-dihydroprogesterone, respectively, HSD17B1 may also catalyze the formation of 5-androstene-3β,17β-diol from dehydroepiandrosterone (Lin, et al., 2006; Peltoketo, Nokelainen, Piao, Vihko, & Vihko, 1999). Syncytiotrophoblast, coming directly into contact with maternal blood, converts estrone to estradiol. In contrast to HSD17B1 mRNA, HSD17B2 mRNA is not detectable in cell cultures of human cytotrophoblast nor syncytiotrophoblast (Bonenfant, Provost, Drolet, & Tremblay, 2000). Besides HSD17B1, the AKR1C3, HSD17B7 and type 12 HSD17B (HSD17B12) may also catalyze progesterone deactivation to 20α-dihydroprogesterone and conversion of inactive estrone to bioactive estradiol (Li, et al., 2005; Peltoketo, et al., 1999; Penning, et al., 2001; Sakurai, et al., 2006). AKR1C3 functions as a bi-directional 3α-, 17β- and 20α-HSD and can interconvert active androgens, estrogens, progestins and their 5α/β reduced metabolites with their cognate inactive metabolites. However, like other AKR1Cs *in vivo*, AKR1C3 preferentially works as a reductase (Matsuura, et al., 1998; Penning, et al., 2001; Steckelbroeck, et al., 2004). Although this enzyme is expressed in placenta, its importance appears to be secondary to the HSD17B1.

HSD17B2 (preferring the oxidative direction) converts inactive 20α-dihydroprogesterone to bioactive progesterone as well as the bioactive estradiol to inactive estrone (Moghrabi, et al., 1997). HSD17B2 may also convert the GABAergic 3α-hydroxy-5α/β-PM to inactive and antagonistic substances but, on the other hand, may transform the less active GABAergic 3α,20α-dihydroxy-5α/β-isomers to the more active 3α-hydroxy-5α/β-20-oxo-isomers. The site of expression of HSD17B2 was identified in endothelial cells of fetal capillaries and some stem villous vessels (Moghrabi, et al., 1997; Takeyama, et al., 1998) and in endothelial cells of villous arteries and arterioles (Bonenfant, Blomquist, et al., 2000) in the close proximity of the fetal circulation. The reversible oxido-reductive interconversion of GABAergic C21 and C19 3α-hydroxy-5α/β-reduced metabolites to the corresponding inactive 3-oxo-metabolites and antagonistic 3β-hydroxy-metabolites (catalyzed by HSD17Bs an AKR1C1s) may also influence the balance between neuroinhibitory and neuroexcitatory steroids (Lundgren, et al., 2003). While the reductive conversion in the C3 position produce GABAergic steroids, the conversion of 20-oxo- to 20α-hydroxy-group or a modification of the C17,20 side chain in the 3α-hydroxy-5α/β C21 steroids result in subtype dependent reduction of positive allosteric modulation of $GABA_A$-r (Belelli, Lambert, Peters, Gee, & Lan, 1996).

In all probability, the distribution of placental oxidoreductase isoforms controls the reductive and oxidative status of steroid inter-conversions in maternal and fetal compartment, respectively (Fig. 3). Therefore the difference between oxidative fetal- and reductive maternal steroid metabolomic status is the most apparent when comparing umbilical venous blood, containing placental steroids before their further metabolism in other fetal tissues and maternal venous blood. The umbilical venous blood contains higher proportions of 20-oxo-steroids including progesterone, 17-oxo steroids (e.g. estrone and dehydroepiandrosterone), 3-oxo-steroids like 5α/β-DHP, and 3β-hydroxy-steroids (3β,5α-THP and 3β,5β-THP), while maternal venous blood contains higher proportions of 20α-hydroxy-steroids (like 20α-dihydroprogesterone), 17β-hydroxy-steroids (such as estradiol and androstenediol) and 3α-hydroxy-5α/β-reduced steroids (like GABAergic 3α,5α-THP and 3α,5β-THP). Even the levels of conjugated 3α-hydroxy-5α/β-reduced-17-oxo C-19 steroids in maternal venous blood are pronouncedly higher than in the fetal circulation, while the 3β-isomers does not significantly differ (M. Hill, Parizek, Cibula, et al., 2010) (Fig. 3).

Some authors report that the metabolism of placental sex steroids in the reductive direction increases as pregnancy advances and significantly rises during human parturition (Diaz-Zagoya, Wiest, & Arias, 1979; Milewich, et al., 1978). This phenomenon may be of an importance in the mechanism of initiation and continuation of labor and might indicate a mechanism of progesterone withdrawal and estradiol rise in association with the onset of human parturition.

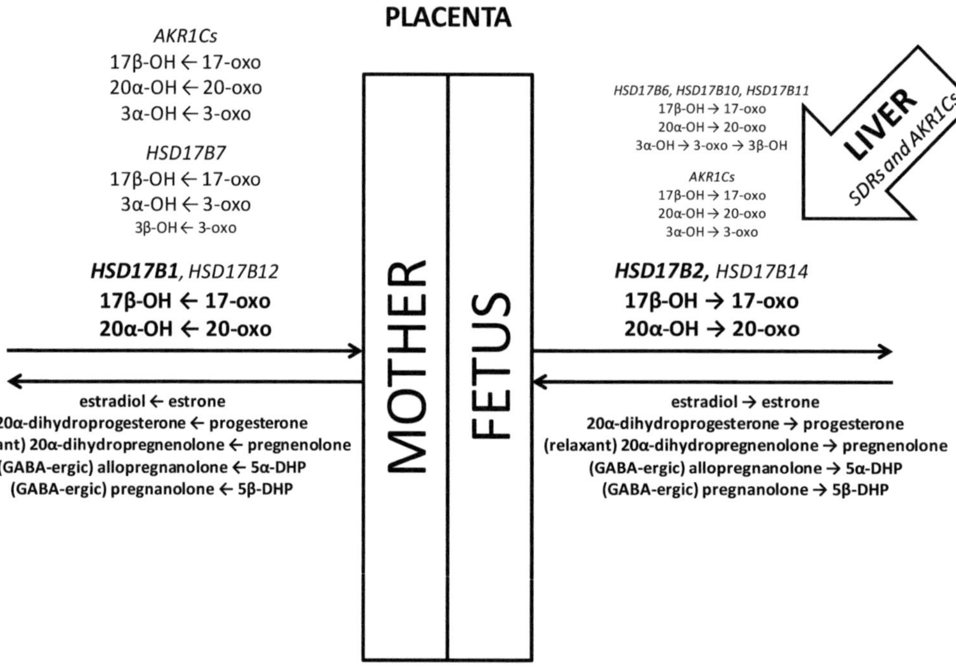

Fig. 3. Steroid conversion during the transplacental passage

4.5 Levels of 5α/β-reduced pregnanes in pregnant women and fetuses

4.5.1 5α/β-Reduced pregnanes in pregnant and non-pregnant women

In pregnant women, the levels of 5α/β-PM including the GABAergic 3α-PI are persistently elevated (M. Hill, et al., 2007; M. Hill, Parizek, Kancheva, et al., 2010; Kancheva, et al., 2007; Luisi, et al., 2000; Mickan & Zander, 1979; Parizek, et al., 2005; Pearson Murphy, Steinberg, Hu, & Allison, 2001). Their concentrations in women after luteo-placental shift reach values about two orders of magnitude higher than the concentrations detected in the FP (Parizek, et al., 2005). Pearson Murphy et al. show that the levels of C21 steroids including 5α/β-PM rise greatly during pregnancy, being the highest for progesterone (562-fold the FP level), 5α-DHP (161-fold), 3β,5α-THP (56-fold), 3α,5α-THP (37-fold), pregnenolone (30-fold), 5β-DHP (16-fold) and 3β,5β-THP (16-fold) at 37th week of gestation (Pearson Murphy, et al., 2001). As already mentioned, these conditions induce a decreased affinity of $GABA_A$-r for the 5α/β-PI.

4.5.2 5α/β-reduced progesterone metabolites around parturition

Pearson Murphy et al. demonstrate that during the period 2-7 day postpartum, the level of progesterone fall precipitously, whereas those of pregnenolone and the metabolites decrease more slowly and their levels are still elevated compared with FP levels 2 weeks after delivery. By the 7th week postpartum only 3α,5α-THP and 3β,5β-THP remains slightly elevated (Pearson Murphy, et al., 2001). Our recent report (M. Hill, Parizek, Cibula, et al., 2010; M. Hill, Parizek, Kancheva, et al., 2010) as well as our previous data for PI around parturition display significantly lower PIC/PI ratios in the umbilical venous plasma than in the maternal plasma (M. Hill, et al., 2001; Klak, et al., 2003). Changes in concentrations of PI in the maternal serum exhibit a similar pattern, falling mostly within the first hour after the delivery. The decrease in PIC is shifted to the interval within the first hour and first day after delivery (M. Hill, et al., 2001; Klak, et al., 2003). The PIC/PI ratios significantly decrease within the first hour and the first day after delivery in all PI (M. Hill, et al., 2001; Klak, et al., 2003). These results indicate an intensive sulfation of GABAergic substances in the maternal compartment during pregnancy but attenuating sulfation activity shortly after labor. The sulfation of GABAergic steroids (transforming them to antagonistic substances) might represent a mechanism counterbalancing their placental overproduction. The ratios of 3α/3β-PI decrease around parturition (M. Hill, et al., 2001; Klak, et al., 2003), which may indicate that the placental and possibly also the liver reductive conversion of the 3-oxo- and 3β-hydroxy-5α/β-PI to the 3α-isomers may be of importance for pregnancy sustaining.

4.6 Effects of 5α/β-reduced pregnanes in pregnant women and fetuses

4.6.1 The role of progestogens and their 5α/β-reduced metabolites in pregnancy sustaining and induction of labor

Pregnant women and fetuses have exceedingly elevated levels of steroids positively modulating NMDA-r (including the 5α-PIC) (M. Hill, et al., 2007; M. Hill, Parizek, Cibula, et al., 2010; M. Hill, Parizek, Kancheva, et al., 2010; Malayev, Gibbs, & Farb, 2002; Weaver, et al., 2000). On the other hand, the 5β-PIC exert an antagonistic effect on NMDA-r (Malayev, et al., 2002; Park-Chung, et al., 1997; Weaver, et al., 2000) and promote their desensitization (Kussius, Kaur, & Popescu, 2009). Like the levels of other PIC, the levels of conjugated 3α,5β-THP are also extremely elevated in pregnant women and (in contrast to slightly increasing, stagnating or even decreasing levels of GABAergic PI) pronouncedly rise in the late pregnancy (Gilbert Evans, Ross, Sellers, Purdy, & Romach, 2005; M. Hill, et al., 2007; M. Hill, Parizek, Cibula, et al., 2010; M. Hill, Parizek, Kancheva, et al., 2010; Luisi, et al., 2000; Parizek, et al., 2005; Pearson Murphy, et al., 2001). These findings allow a speculation whether the conjugated 3α,5β-THP might serve as an endogenous antinociceptive agent around parturition (Hering, et al., 1996; Kallela, Haasio, & Korttila, 1994).

On the other hand, rising steroid sulfation that catabolizes both 3α,5α-THP and 5β-reduced steroids, produces high amounts of PIC. PIC induce neuroexcitatory effect via $GABA_A$-r and may shift the biological activity towards induction of labor (Park-Chung, et al., 1999). Majewska and Vaupel (Majewska & Vaupel, 1991) reported that 3α,5α-THP interact with $GABA_A$-r to modulate uterine contractility: 3α,5α-THP inhibits while PregS increases contractions. Further, 3α,5α-THP rapidly antagonizes the stimulatory effect of PregS, but progesterone inhibits the contractions after a delay, suggesting that the known pregnancy sustaining effect of progesterone on the uterus is at least partly mediated via the metabolite 3α,5α-THP, which potentiates the neuroinhibitory function of $GABA_A$-r (Majewska & Vaupel, 1991). On the other hand, Lofgren et al. (Lofgren, Holst, & Backstrom, 1992) reported contradictory data. Concerning the 3α-hydroxysteroid oxidoreductase-mediated turnover of 5α-DHP and 5β-DHP to their metabolites 3α,5α-THP and 3α,5β-THP, respectively, which reflects the ratios between these GABAergic 3α-PI and their inactive precursors, Gilbert Evans et al. (Gilbert Evans, et al., 2005) reported that the turnover of 5α-DHP to 3α,5α-THP rise during pregnancy and drops at the late prenatal visit. At 6 weeks postpartum, all steroids are significantly reduced compared with late prenatal values. Although, we have found no significant change of the ratio 3α/3β-PI during pregnancy (Parizek, et al., 2005), our more recent study shows contradictory results to the data of Gilbert Evans et al. and demonstrates a moderate but significant shift from the 3α-PI to the-3-oxo-isomers (M. Hill, Parizek, Cibula, et al., 2010).

When testing the capacity to inhibit the *in vitro* motility of rat uterus, progestins with their ring A reduced in the 5β-position are significantly more potent than Δ^4-3-oxo and 5α-reduced progestins (Kubli-Garfias, Medrano-Conde, Beyer, & Bondani, 1979; Perusquia & Jasso-Kamel, 2001). The 5α/β-PM elicit an immediate relaxing effect that is dose-dependent. With the exception of two 5α/β-PM (5α-DHP and 3β,5α-THP), the remaining ones used in the present study are more potent than progesterone. It is important that when the tissues are washed, the contractile activity is recovered. This rapid and reversible relaxing effect is not blocked by antiprogestin RU 486, which suggests its independence of receptor-mediated genomic action (Perusquia & Jasso-Kamel, 2001).

Being already mentioned, the abundance of progesterone, 3α-hydroxy-5α/β-pregnane-steroids and estradiol levels in pregnancy is high. Some of them like 3α,5α-THDOC, 3α,5α-THP and progesterone induce opening of voltage-dependent K^+ channels and relaxes myometrium while estradiol is their antagonist (Knock, Tribe, Hassoni, & Aaronson, 2001; Perusquia & Jasso-Kamel, 2001; Yoshihara, et al., 2005). Therefore the ratios progesterone/estradiol and 3α-PI/estradiol may be of importance for sustaining the uterine quiescence. Whereas 3α,5α-THP stagnates from the 36th week of gestation (M. Hill, et al., 2007), estradiol still shows an increasing trend (Buster, et al., 1979; Parizek, et al., 2005; Turnbull, et al., 1974), which might induce uterine contractions resulting in parturition onset.

Whereas the turnovers of 5α-DHP/progesterone and 5β-DHP/progesterone in the 3rd trimester show that the metabolism of progesterone to 5α-DHP inconspicuously culminates in the 35th week, the conversion of progesterone to 5β-DHP significantly declines from the 31st week of gestation (M. Hill, et al., 2007). This is in accordance with results of other authors as well as with our current data (Gilbert Evans, et al., 2005; M. Hill, Parizek, Cibula, et al., 2010; M. Hill, Parizek, Kancheva, et al., 2010; Sheehan, 2006; Sheehan, et al., 2005). Besides the modulation of ionotropic receptors, the 5β-reduced metabolites of progesterone may act chronically in pregnancy as uterine relaxants through a mechanism mediated by pregnane X-type receptors. Moreover, acute *in vitro* treatment with 5β-DHP causes rapid uterine relaxation that is independent of pregnane X-type receptors (Mitchell, et al., 2005; Putnam, Brann, Kolbeck, & Mahesh, 1991). The aforementioned data demonstrate that the progesterone metabolite 5β-DHP is a potent tocolytic (Mitchell, et al., 2005). In the placenta and myometrium, the relative expression of AKR1D1 decreases in association with labor by about two-fold and 10-fold, respectively (Sheehan, et al., 2005). Therefore, it is likely that the decrease in AKR1D1 activity during the third trimester is associated with a reduced ability to sustain the pregnancy (Gilbert Evans, et al., 2005; M. Hill, et al., 2007; M. Hill, Parizek, Cibula, et al., 2010; M. Hill, Parizek, Kancheva, et al., 2010; Sheehan, et al., 2005). AKR1D1 activity participates in the formation of almost 40% of pregnancy- sustaining PI.

4.7 Effects of 5α/β-reduced pregnanes on pain perception, induction of tolerance, receptor plasticity

4.7.1 The effects of 5α/β-reduced pregnanes in the fetal CNS

3α,5α-THP may interact with $GABA_A$-r to inhibit fetal CNS activity from mid-gestation. This inhibition may contribute to maintaining the sleep-like behavior and low incidence of arousal-type activity typical of fetal life (Crossley, et al., 2003). Mellor et al. reviewed the role of endogenous neuro-inhibitors that contribute to fetal sleep states, and thus mediate the suppression of fetal awareness. The authors show that there are several suppressors *in utero*, which inhibits neural activity in the fetus to a far greater degree than is seen postnatally in the infant. The authors suggest that the uterus plays a key role in keeping the fetus continuously asleep. Despite the presence of intact nociceptive pathways from around mid-gestation, the critical aspect of cortical awareness in the process of pain perception is missing. The mechanism providing the permanent sleeping status in the fetus combines neuroinhibitory actions of a powerful EEG suppressor and sleep inducing agent (adenosine), two GABAergic steroids anesthetics (3α,5α-THP, 3α,5β-THP) and a potent sleep-inducing hormone (prostaglandin D2), acting together with a putative peptide inhibitor and other factors produced by the placenta (Mellor, Diesch, Gunn, & Bennet, 2005). Concerning the role of GABAergic steroids in suppressing the nociceptive pathways in the fetus, our current data shows 2-3 times lower 3α,5α-THP levels in the fetal circulation than in the maternal one, while 3α,5β-THP levels in UV exceed those in MV 1-2.5 times (M. Hill, et al., 2011). The total amount of GABAergic PI is only slightly higher in the fetal compartment than in the maternal, mainly due to the contribution of unconjugated 3α,5β-THP. These results indicate that the peripheral GABAergic steroids exert a comparable effect on the maternal and fetal CNS. Even when considering the 1.5-3 fold excess of progesterone in the fetal circulation when compared to the maternal blood, a possibility of progesterone transport into the brain, and its conversion to the GABAergic steroids herein, the resulting contribution of GABAergic steroids originating from peripheral sources do not pronouncedly differ between mother and fetus. Therefore the importance of GABAergic steroids for maintenance of permanent fetal sleeping is open to discussion.

4.7.2 The effects of 5α/β-reduced pregnanes in the maternal CNS

Increases in the brain levels of 5α/β-PM during pregnancy are causally related to changes in the expression of specific $GABA_A$-r subunits and the function of extrasynaptic $GABA_A$-r in the cerebral cortex and hippocampus (Concas, Follesa, Barbaccia, Purdy, & Biggio, 1999; Mostallino, Sanna, Concas, Biggio, & Follesa, 2009). Turkmen et al. demonstrated that 3α,5α-THP treatment induce a partial tolerance against acute 3α,5α-THP effects in the Morris water maze (Turkmen, Lofgren, Birzniece, Backstrom, & Johansson, 2006). Alterations in $\delta GABA_A$-r expression during pregnancy result in region-specific increases in neuronal excitability in brain that are restored by the high levels of 3α,5α-THP under normal conditions. On the contrary, under pathological conditions may result in neurological and psychiatric disorders associated with pregnancy and postpartum period (Maguire, Ferando, Simonsen, & Mody, 2009). Besides the GABAergic effects in the CNS and periphery, 5β-PM also exert peripheral analgesic effects via blockade of testosterone-type calcium channels controlling pain perception (Todorovic, et al., 2004). These data as well as those mentioned previously, allow a speculation, whether these steroids might operate as endogenous analgesics around parturition.

4.7.3 Neuroprotective and excitotoxic effects of 5α/β-reduced pregnanes

The synthesis of neurosteroids from cholesterol in late gestation persists into neonatal life but SRD5A expression is greater in the fetus compared to the neonate. Fetuses exposed to stress during labor produce higher progesterone, which may protect them against the sequelae of hypoxia (Antonipillai & Murphy, 1977; Shaxted, Heyes, Walker, & Maynard, 1982). It is likely that the increasing fetal progesterone levels in stressful situations are associated with increased activity of the FZ producing extreme amounts of PregS. Physiologic concentrations of progesterone metabolite 3α,5α-THP provide protection against both necrotic and apoptotic injury induced by NMDA excitotoxicity via positive modulation of $GABA_A$-r (Yawno, Hirst, Castillo-Melendez, & Walker, 2009). This modulation limits excitatory neurotransmission (Crossley, et al., 2003; Lockhart, et al., 2002). Growth restriction is a potent stimulus for neurosteroid synthesis in the fetal brain in late pregnancy. The low concentrations of 3α,5α-THP in the growth-restricted postnatal brain suggest a delay in the capacity of the adrenal gland or brain to synthesize pregnane steroids or their precursors and may render the postnatal brain vulnerable to hypoxia-induced injury (Westcott, Hirst, Ciurej, Walker, & Wlodek, 2008). At birth, the 3α,5α-THP concentrations in the brain fall markedly, probably due to the loss of placental precursors; however, stressors, including hypoxia and endotoxin-induced inflammation, lift up 3α,5α-THP concentrations in the newborn brain. (Hirst, Yawno, Nguyen, & Walker, 2006). Abrupt changes in neonatal levels of 3α,5α-THP could be related to the susceptibility to neurodevelopmental disorders (Darbra & Pallares, 2010).

GABAergic PI may reduce the excitotoxicity induced by N-methyl-D-aspartate (Lockhart, et al., 2002). In pregnant women and fetuses, this effect might be of importance when considering exceedingly elevated levels of steroids, which positively modulate N-methyl-D-aspartate receptors (NMDA-r). The positive NMDA-r modulators (like the sulfated Δ^5 steroids and sulfates of 5α-PI) may induce excitotoxic effect (Guarneri, et al., 1998; M. Hill, et al., 2007; M. Hill, Parizek, Cibula, et al., 2010; M. Hill, Parizek, Kancheva, et al., 2010; Malayev, et al., 2002; Weaver, et al., 2000). Moreover, the sulfated 5β-PI, 3α,5β-THP, the levels of which pronouncedly rise in the late pregnancy (M. Hill, et al., 2007; M. Hill, Parizek, Kancheva, et al., 2010), have also antagonistic effect on NMDA-r (Malayev, et al., 2002; Park-Chung, et al., 1997; Weaver, et al., 2000) and promote their desensitization (Kussius, et al., 2009).

5. Summary

Although the effects of bioactive reduced progesterone metabolites in human and laboratory animals were extensively studied, their physiological importance remains commonly uncertain due to the lack of metabolomic data. Therefore, we focused on the intersection between steroid metabolomics and neurophysiology so as to give a comprehensive insight into the physiological and pathophysiological relevance of the aforementioned compounds.

6. Acknowledgements

This contribution was supported by grant IGA MZ ČR NS/9790-4.

7. References

Ahboucha, S., Butterworth, R. F., Pomier-Layrargues, G., Vincent, C., Hassoun, Z., & Baker, G. B. (2008). *Neuroactive steroids and fatigue severity in patients with primary biliary cirrhosis and hepatitis C.* Neurogastroenterol Motil,Vol.20, No.6, pp. 671-679, Jun, ISSN 1365-2982

Anderson, R. A., Baillie, T. A., Axelson, M., Cronholm, T., Sjovall, K., & Sjovall, J. (1990). *Stable isotope studies on steroid metabolism and kinetics: sulfates of 3 alpha-hydroxy-5 alpha-pregnane derivatives in human pregnancy.* Steroids,Vol.55, No.10, pp. 443-457, Oct, ISSN 0039-128X

Andreen, L., Nyberg, S., Turkmen, S., van Wingen, G., Fernandez, G., & Backstrom, T. (2009). *Sex steroid induced negative mood may be explained by the paradoxical effect mediated by GABAA modulators.* Psychoneuroendocrinology,Vol.34, No.8, pp. 1121-1132, Sep, ISSN 1873-3360

Antonipillai, I., & Murphy, B. E. (1977). *Serum oestrogens and progesterone in mother and infant at delivery.* Br J Obstet Gynaecol,Vol.84, No.3, pp. 179-185, Mar, ISSN 0306-5456

Backstrom, T., Andersson, A., Andree, L., Birzniece, V., Bixo, M., Bjorn, I., et al. (2003). *Pathogenesis in menstrual cycle-linked CNS disorders.* Ann N Y Acad Sci,Vol.1007, pp. 42-53, Dec

Backstrom, T., Carstensen, H., & Sodergard, R. (1976). *Concentration of estradiol, testosterone and progesterone in cerebrospinal fluid compared to plasma unbound and total concentrations.* J Steroid Biochem,Vol.7, No.6-7, pp. 469-472, Jun-Jul, IS SN 0022-4731

Belelli, D., Lambert, J. J., Peters, J. A., Gee, K. W., & Lan, N. C. (1996). *Modulation of human recombinant GABAA receptors by pregnanediols.* Neuropharmacology,Vol.35, No.9-10, pp. 1223-1231

Bixo, M., Andersson, A., Winblad, B., Purdy, R. H., & Backstrom, T. (1997). *Progesterone, 5alpha-pregnane-3,20-dione and 3alpha-hydroxy-5alpha-pregnane-20-one in specific regions of the human female brain in different endocrine states.* Brain Res,Vol.764, No.1-2, pp. 173-178, Aug 1

Bonenfant, M., Blomquist, C. H., Provost, P. R., Drolet, R., D'Ascoli, P., & Tremblay, Y. (2000). *Tissue- and site-specific gene expression of type 2 17beta-hydroxysteroid dehydrogenase: in situ hybridization and specificenzymatic activity studies in human placental endothelial cells of the arterial system.* J Clin Endocrinol Metab,Vol.85, No.12, pp. 4841-4850, Dec, ISSN 0021-972X

Bonenfant, M., Provost, P. R., Drolet, R., & Tremblay, Y. (2000). *Localization of type 1 17beta-hydroxysteroid dehydrogenase mRNA and protein in syncytiotrophoblasts and invasive cytotrophoblasts in the human term villi.* J Endocrinol,Vol.165, No.2, pp. 217-222, May, ISSN

Bonuccelli, U., Melis, G. B., Paoletti, A. M., Fioretti, P., Murri, L., & Muratorio, A. (1989). *Unbalanced progesterone and estradiol secretion in catamenial epilepsy.* Epilepsy Res,Vol.3, No.2, pp. 100-106, Mar-Apr, ISSN 0920-1211

Brussaard, A. B., Wossink, J., Lodder, J. C., & Kits, K. S. (2000). *Progesterone-metabolite prevents protein kinase C-dependent modulation of gamma-aminobutyric acid type A receptors in oxytocin neurons.* Proc Natl Acad Sci U S A,Vol.97, No.7, pp. 3625-3630, Mar 28, ISSN 0027-8424

Buster, J. E., Chang, R. J., Preston, D. L., Elashoff, R. M., Cousins, L. M., Abraham, G. E., et al. (1979). *Interrelationships of circulating maternal steroid concentrations in third trimester pregnancies. II. C18 and C19 steroids: estradiol, estriol, dehydroepiandrosterone, dehydroepiandrosterone sulfate, delta 5-androstenediol, delta 4-androstenedione, testosterone, and dihydrotestosterone.* J Clin Endocrinol Metab,Vol.48, No.1, pp. 139-142, Jan

Ciriza, I., Azcoitia, I., & Garcia-Segura, L. M. (2004). *Reduced progesterone metabolites protect rat hippocampal neurones from kainic acid excitotoxicity in vivo.* J Neuroendocrinol,Vol.16, No.1, pp. 58-63, Jan, IS SN 0953-8194

Comer, K. A., & Falany, C. N. (1992). *Immunological characterization of dehydroepiandrosterone sulfotransferase from human liver and adrenal.* Mol Pharmacol,Vol.41, No.4, pp. 645-651, Apr

Compagnone, N. A., Salido, E., Shapiro, L. J., & Mellon, S. H. (1997). *Expression of steroid sulfatase during embryogenesis.* Endocrinology,Vol.138, No.11, pp. 4768-4773, Nov, ISSN 0013-7227

Concas, A., Follesa, P., Barbaccia, M. L., Purdy, R. H., & Biggio, G. (1999). *Physiological modulation of GABA(A) receptor plasticity by progesterone metabolites.* Eur J Pharmacol,Vol.375, No.1-3, pp. 225-235, Jun 30, ISSN 0014-2999

Corpechot, C., Leclerc, P., Baulieu, E. E., & Brazeau, P. (1985). *Neurosteroids: regulatory mechanisms in male rat brain during heterosexual exposure.* Steroids,Vol.45, No.3-4, pp. 229-234, Mar-Apr, IS SN 0039-128X

Corpechot, C., Robel, P., Axelson, M., Sjovall, J., & Baulieu, E. E. (1981). *Characterization and measurement of dehydroepiandrosterone sulfate in rat brain.* Proc Natl Acad Sci U S A,Vol.78, No.8, pp. 4704-4707, Aug, IS SN 0027-8424

Crossley, K. J., Nitsos, I., Walker, D. W., Lawrence, A. J., Beart, P. M., & Hirst, J. J. (2003). *Steroid-sensitive GABAA receptors in the fetal sheep brain.* Neuropharmacology,Vol.45, No.4, pp. 461-472, Sep, ISSN 0028-3908

Darbra, S., & Pallares, M. (2010). *Alterations in neonatal neurosteroids affect exploration during adolescence and prepulse inhibition in adulthood.* Psychoneuroendocrinology,Vol.35, No.4, pp. 525-535, May, ISSN 1873-3360

de Peretti, E., Forest, M. G., Loras, B., Morel, Y., David, M., Francois, R., et al. (1986). *Usefulness of plasma pregnenolone sulfate in testing pituitary-adrenal function in children.* Acta Endocrinol Suppl (Copenh),Vol.279, pp. 259-263, ISSN 0300-9750

Diaz-Zagoya, J. C., Wiest, W. G., & Arias, F. (1979). *20 alpha-Hydroxysteroid oxidoreductase activity and 20 alpha-dihydroprogesterone concentration in human placenta before and after parturition.* Am J Obstet Gynecol,Vol.133, No.6, pp. 673-676, Mar 15

Dubrovsky, B. O. (2005). *Steroids, neuroactive steroids and neurosteroids in psychopathology.* Prog Neuropsychopharmacol Biol Psychiatry,Vol.29, No.2, pp. 169-192, Feb, ISSN 0278-5846

Fukuda, M., Okuyama, T., & Furuya, H. (1986). *Growth and function of the placenta--with special reference to various enzymes involved in the biosynthesis of steroids in the human placenta.* Nippon Sanka Fujinka Gakkai Zasshi,Vol.38, No.3, pp. 411-416, Mar

Geese, W. J., & Raftogianis, R. B. (2001). *Biochemical characterization and tissue distribution of human SULT2B1.* Biochem Biophys Res Commun,Vol.288, No.1, pp. 280-289, Oct 19

Genazzani, A. R., Petraglia, F., Bernardi, F., Casarosa, E., Salvestroni, C., Tonetti, A., et al. (1998). *Circulating levels of allopregnanolone in humans: gender, age, and endocrine influences.* J Clin Endocrinol Metab,Vol.83, No.6, pp. 2099-2103, Jun

Gilbert Evans, S. E., Ross, L. E., Sellers, E. M., Purdy, R. H., & Romach, M. K. (2005). *3alpha-reduced neuroactive steroids and their precursors during pregnancy and the postpartum period.* Gynecol Endocrinol,Vol.21, No.5, pp. 268-279, Nov, ISSN 0951-3590

Goland, R. S., Wardlaw, S. L., Stark, R. I., Brown, L. S., Jr., & Frantz, A. G. (1986). *High levels of corticotropin-releasing hormone immunoactivity in maternal and fetal plasma during pregnancy.* J Clin Endocrinol Metab,Vol.63, No.5, pp. 1199-1203, Nov

Guarneri, P., Russo, D., Cascio, C., De Leo, G., Piccoli, T., Sciuto, V., et al. (1998). *Pregnenolone sulfate modulates NMDA receptors, inducing and potentiating acute excitotoxicity in isolated retina.* J Neurosci Res,Vol.54, No.6, pp. 787-797, Dec 15, ISSN 0360-4012

Harrison, N. L., & Simmonds, M. A. (1984). *Modulation of the GABA receptor complex by a steroid anaesthetic.* Brain Res,Vol.323, No.2, pp. 287-292, Dec 10, IS SN 0006-8993

Havlikova, H., Hill, M., Kancheva, L., Vrbikova, J., Pouzar, V., Cerny, I., et al. (2006). *Serum profiles of free and conjugated neuroactive pregnanolone isomers in nonpregnant women of fertile age.* J Clin Endocrinol Metab,Vol.91, No.8, pp. 3092-3099, Aug

He, X. Y., Merz, G., Yang, Y. Z., Mehta, P., Schulz, H., & Yang, S. Y. (2001). *Characterization and localization of human type10 17beta-hydroxysteroid dehydrogenase.* Eur J Biochem,Vol.268, No.18, pp. 4899-4907, Sep

He, X. Y., Wegiel, J., & Yang, S. Y. (2005). *Intracellular oxidation of allopregnanolone by human brain type 10 17beta-hydroxysteroid dehydrogenase.* Brain Res,Vol.1040, No.1-2, pp. 29-35, Apr 8, ISSN 0006-8993

He, X. Y., Yang, Y. Z., Peehl, D. M., Lauderdale, A., Schulz, H., & Yang, S. Y. (2003). *Oxidative 3alpha-hydroxysteroid dehydrogenase activity of human type 10 17beta-hydroxysteroid dehydrogenase.* J Steroid Biochem Mol Biol,Vol.87, No.2-3, pp. 191-198, Nov

Hering, W. J., Ihmsen, H., Langer, H., Uhrlau, C., Dinkel, M., Geisslinger, G., et al. (1996). *Pharmacokinetic-pharmacodynamic modeling of the new steroid hypnotic eltanolone in healthy volunteers.* Anesthesiology,Vol.85, No.6, pp. 1290-1299, Dec

Higashi, T., Takido, N., & Shimada, K. (2005). *Studies on neurosteroids XVII. Analysis of stress-induced changes in neurosteroid levels in rat brains using liquid chromatography-electron capture atmospheric pressure chemical ionization-mass spectrometry.* Steroids,Vol.70, No.1, pp. 1-11, Jan, ISSN 0039-128X

Hill, M., Bicikova, M., Parizek, A., Havlikova, H., Klak, J., Fajt, T., et al. (2001). *Neuroactive steroids, their precursors and polar conjugates during parturition and postpartum in maternal blood: 2. Time profiles of pregnanolone isomers.* J Steroid Biochem Mol Biol,Vol.78, No.1, pp. 51-57, Jul, ISSN 0960-0760

Hill, M., Cibula, D., Havlikova, H., Kancheva, L., Fait, T., Kancheva, R., et al. (2007). *Circulating levels of pregnanolone isomers during the third trimester of human pregnancy.* J Steroid Biochem Mol Biol,Vol.105, No.1-5, pp. 166-175, Jun-Jul, ISSN 0960-0760

Hill, M., Parizek, A., Cibula, D., Kancheva, R., Jirasek, J. E., Jirkovska, M., et al. (2010). *Steroid metabolome in fetal and maternal body fluids in human late pregnancy.* J Steroid Biochem Mol Biol, May 21, ISSN 1879-1220

Hill, M., Parizek, A., Jirasek, J. E., Jirkovska, M., Velikova, M., Duskova, M., et al. (2010). *Is maternal progesterone actually independent of the fetal steroids?* Physiol Res,Vol.59, No.2, pp. 211-224, ISSN 0862-8408

Hill, M., Parizek, A., Kancheva, R., Duskova, M., Velikova, M., Kriz, L., et al. (2010). *Steroid metabolome in plasma from the umbilical artery, umbilical vein, maternal cubital vein and in amniotic fluid in normal and preterm labor.* J Steroid Biochem Mol Biol,Vol.121, No.3-5, pp. 594-610, Aug, ISSN 1879-1220

Hill, M., Parizek, A., Velikova, M., Kubatova, J., Kancheva, R., Duskova, M., et al. (2011). *The distribution of placental oxidoreductase isoforms provides different milieus of steroids influencing pregnancy in the maternal and fetal compartment.* Horm Mol Biol Clin Invest,Vol.4, No.3, pp. 581–600, December 2010, ISSN 1868-1883

Hill, M., Popov, P., Havlikova, H., Kancheva, L., Vrbikova, J., Kancheva, R., et al. (2005). *Altered profiles of serum neuroactive steroids in premenopausal women treated for alcohol addiction.* Steroids,Vol.70, No.8, pp. 515-524, Jul, ISSN 0039-128X

Hirst, J. J., Yawno, T., Nguyen, P., & Walker, D. W. (2006). *Stress in pregnancy activates neurosteroid production in the fetal brain.* Neuroendocrinology,Vol.84, No.4, pp. 264-274, ISSN 0028-3835

Huang, X. F., & Luu-The, V. (2000). *Molecular characterization of a first human 3(alpha-->beta)-hydroxysteroid epimerase.* J Biol Chem,Vol.275, No.38, pp. 29452-29457, Sep 22

Charbonneau, A., & The, V. L. (2001). *Genomic organization of a human 5beta-reductase and its pseudogene and substrate selectivity of the expressed enzyme.* Biochim Biophys Acta,Vol.1517, No.2, pp. 228-235, Jan 26

Ingelman-Sundberg, M., Rane, A., & Gustafasson, J. A. (1975). *Properties of hydroxylase systems in the human fetal liver active on free and sulfoconjugated steroids.* Biochemistry,Vol.14, No.2, pp. 429-437, Jan 28

Ishida, T., Seo, F., Hirato, K., Fukuda, T., Yanaihara, T., Araki, H., et al. (1985). *[Changes in placental enzymatic activities in relation to estrogen production during pregnancy].* Nippon Sanka Fujinka Gakkai Zasshi,Vol.37, No.4, pp. 547-554, Apr

Jaffe, R. B., & Ledger, W. J. (1966). *In vivo steroid biogenesis and metabolism in the human term placenta. I. In situ placental perfusion with isotopic pregnenolone.* Steroids,Vol.8, No.1, pp. 61-78, Jul, ISSN 0039-128X

Jin, Y., Duan, L., Lee, S. H., Kloosterboer, H. J., Blair, I. A., & Penning, T. M. (2009). *Human cytosolic hydroxysteroid dehydrogenases of the aldo-ketoreductase superfamily catalyze reduction of conjugated steroids: implications for phase I and phase II steroid hormone metabolism.* J Biol Chem,Vol.284, No.15, pp. 10013-10022, Apr 10

Jin, Y., & Penning, T. M. (2001). *Steroid 5alpha-reductases and 3alpha-hydroxysteroid dehydrogenases: key enzymes in androgen metabolism.* Best Pract Res Clin Endocrinol Metab,Vol.15, No.1, pp. 79-94, Mar

Jin, Y., Stayrook, S. E., Albert, R. H., Palackal, N. T., Penning, T. M., & Lewis, M. (2001). *Crystal structure of human type III 3alpha-hydroxysteroid dehydrogenase/bile acid binding protein complexed with NADP(+) and ursodeoxycholate.* Biochemistry,Vol.40, No.34, pp. 10161-10168, Aug 28

Kallela, H., Haasio, J., & Korttila, K. (1994). *Comparison of eltanolone and propofol in anesthesia for termination of pregnancy.* Anesth Analg,Vol.79, No.3, pp. 512-516, Sep, ISSN 0003-2999

Kancheva, R., Hill, M., Cibula, D., Vcelakova, H., Kancheva, L., Vrbikova, J., et al. (2007). *Relationships of circulating pregnanolone isomers and their polar conjugates to the status of sex, menstrual cycle, and pregnancy.* J Endocrinol,Vol.195, No.1, pp. 67-78, Oct, ISSN 0022-0795

Kancheva, R., Hill, M., Novak, Z., Chrastina, J., Velikova, M., Kancheva, L., et al. (2010). *Peripheral neuroactive steroids may be as good as the steroids in the cerebrospinal fluid for the diagnostics of CNS disturbances.* J Steroid Biochem Mol Biol,Vol.119, No.1-2, pp. 35-44, Mar, ISSN 1879-1220

Klak, J., Hill, M., Parizek, A., Havlikova, H., Bicikova, M., Hampl, R., et al. (2003). *Pregnanolone isomers, pregnenolone and their polar conjugates around parturition.* Physiol Res,Vol.52, No.2, pp. 211-221, ISSN 0862-8408

Knock, G. A., Tribe, R. M., Hassoni, A. A., & Aaronson, P. I. (2001). *Modulation of potassium current characteristics in human myometrial smooth muscle by 17beta-estradiol and progesterone.* Biol Reprod,Vol.64, No.5, pp. 1526-1534, May

Kochakian, C. D. (1983). *Conversion of testosterone and androstenedione to 5 beta-androstanes by adult male hamster liver cytosol.* J Steroid Biochem,Vol.19, No.4, pp. 1521-1526, Oct, ISSN 0022-4731

Koksma, J. J., van Kesteren, R. E., Rosahl, T. W., Zwart, R., Smit, A. B., Luddens, H., et al. (2003). *Oxytocin regulates neurosteroid modulation of GABA(A) receptors in supraoptic nucleus around parturition.* J Neurosci,Vol.23, No.3, pp. 788-797, Feb 1, ISSN 1529-2401

Komatsuzaki, K., Kosaki, T., Hashino, M., Yanaihara, T., Nakayama, T., & Mori, H. (1987). *[Metabolism of pregnenolone sulfate in feto-placental unit].* Nippon Sanka Fujinka Gakkai Zasshi,Vol.39, No.7, pp. 1095-1102, Jul, ISSN 0300-9165

Krazeisen, A., Breitling, R., Imai, K., Fritz, S., Moller, G., & Adamski, J. (1999). *Determination of cDNA, gene structure and chromosomal localization of the novel human 17beta-hydroxysteroid dehydrogenase type 7(1).* FEBS Lett,Vol.460, No.2, pp. 373-379, Oct 29

Kriz, L., Bicikova, M., Hill, M., & Hampl, R. (2005). *Steroid sulfatase and sulfuryl transferase activity in monkey brain tissue.* Steroids,Vol.70, No.14, pp. 960-969, Dec 15, ISSN 0039-128X

Kubli-Garfias, C., Medrano-Conde, L., Beyer, C., & Bondani, A. (1979). *In vitro inhibition of rat uterine contractility induced by 5 alpha and 5 beta progestins.* Steroids,Vol.34, No.6 Spec no, pp. 609-617, ISSN 0039-128X

Kussius, C. L., Kaur, N., & Popescu, G. K. (2009). *Pregnanolone sulfate promotes desensitization of activated NMDA receptors.* J Neurosci,Vol.29, No.21, pp. 6819-6827, May 27, ISSN 1529-2401

Lacroix, D., Sonnier, M., Moncion, A., Cheron, G., & Cresteil, T. (1997). *Expression of CYP3A in the human liver--evidence that the shift between CYP3A7 and CYP3A4 occurs immediately after birth.* Eur J Biochem,Vol.247, No.2, pp. 625-634, Jul 15

Leeder, J. S., Gaedigk, R., Marcucci, K. A., Gaedigk, A., Vyhlidal, C. A., Schindel, B. P., et al. (2005). *Variability of CYP3A7 expression in human fetal liver.* J Pharmacol Exp Ther,Vol.314, No.2, pp. 626-635, Aug, ISSN 0022-3565

Leng, G., & Russell, J. A. (1999). *Coming to term with GABA.* J Physiol,Vol.516 (Pt 2), pp. vi, Apr 15

Leslie, K. K., Zuckerman, D. J., Schruefer, J., Burchell, M., Smith, J., & Albertson, B. D. (1994). *Oestrogen modulation with parturition in the human placenta.* Placenta,Vol.15, No.1, pp. 79-88, Jan

Leung, J. C., Travis, B. R., Verlander, J. W., Sandhu, S. K., Yang, S. G., Zea, A. H., et al. (2002). *Expression and developmental regulation of the NMDA receptor subunits in the kidney and cardiovascular system.* Am J Physiol Regul Integr Comp Physiol,Vol.283, No.4, pp. R964-971, Oct, ISSN 0363-6119

Li, Y., Isomaa, V., Pulkka, A., Herva, R., Peltoketo, H., & Vihko, P. (2005). *Expression of 3beta-hydroxysteroid dehydrogenase type 1, P450 aromatase, and 17beta-hydroxysteroid dehydrogenase types 1, 2, 5 and 7 mRNAs in human early and mid-gestation placentas.* Placenta,Vol.26, No.5, pp. 387-392, May

Lin, S. X., Shi, R., Qiu, W., Azzi, A., Zhu, D. W., Dabbagh, H. A., et al. (2006). *Structural basis of the multispecificity demonstrated by 17beta-hydroxysteroid dehydrogenase types 1 and 5.* Mol Cell Endocrinol,Vol.248, No.1-2, pp. 38-46, Mar 27

Lockhart, E. M., Warner, D. S., Pearlstein, R. D., Penning, D. H., Mehrabani, S., & Boustany, R. M. (2002). *Allopregnanolone attenuates N-methyl-D-aspartate-induced excitotoxicity and apoptosis in the human NT2 cell line in culture.* Neurosci Lett,Vol.328, No.1, pp. 33-36, Aug 2, ISSN 0304-3940

Lofgren, M., Holst, J., & Backstrom, T. (1992). *Effects in vitro of progesterone and two 5 alpha-reduced progestins, 5 alpha-pregnane-3,20-dione and 5 alpha-pregnane-3 alpha-ol-20-one, on contracting human myometrium at term.* Acta Obstet Gynecol Scand,Vol.71, No.1, pp. 28-33, Jan, ISSN 0001-6349

Luisi, S., Petraglia, F., Benedetto, C., Nappi, R. E., Bernardi, F., Fadalti, M., et al. (2000). *Serum allopregnanolone levels in pregnant women: changes during pregnancy, at delivery, and in hypertensive patients.* J Clin Endocrinol Metab,Vol.85, No.7, pp. 2429-2433, Jul, ISSN 0021-972X

Lundgren, P., Stromberg, J., Backstrom, T., & Wang, M. (2003). *Allopregnanolone-stimulated GABA-mediated chloride ion flux is inhibited by 3beta-hydroxy-5alpha-pregnan-20-one (isoallopregnanolone).* Brain Res,Vol.982, No.1, pp. 45-53, Aug 22

Maguire, J., Ferando, I., Simonsen, C., & Mody, I. (2009). *Excitability changes related to GABAA receptor plasticity during pregnancy.* J Neurosci,Vol.29, No.30, pp. 9592-9601, Jul 29, ISSN 1529-2401

Maguire, J., & Mody, I. (2009). *Steroid hormone fluctuations and GABA(A)R plasticity.* Psychoneuroendocrinology,Vol.34 Suppl 1, pp. S84-90, Dec, ISSN 1873-3360

Majewska, M. D., Bisserbe, J. C., & Eskay, R. L. (1985). *Glucocorticoids are modulators of GABAA receptors in brain.* Brain Res,Vol.339, No.1, pp. 178-182, Jul 22, IS SN 0006-8993

Majewska, M. D., Falkay, G., & Baulieu, E. E. (1989). *Modulation of uterine GABAA receptors during gestation and by tetrahydroprogesterone.* Eur J Pharmacol,Vol.174, No.1, pp. 43-47, Dec 12, ISSN 0014-2999

Majewska, M. D., & Vaupel, D. B. (1991). *Steroid control of uterine motility via gamma-aminobutyric acidA receptors in the rabbit: a novel mechanism?* J Endocrinol,Vol.131, No.3, pp. 427-434, Dec, ISSN 0022-0795

Malayev, A., Gibbs, T. T., & Farb, D. H. (2002). *Inhibition of the NMDA response by pregnenolone sulphate reveals subtype selective modulation of NMDA receptors by sulphated steroids.* Br J Pharmacol,Vol.135, No.4, pp. 901-909, Feb, ISSN 0007-1188

Matsuura, K., Shiraishi, H., Hara, A., Sato, K., Deyashiki, Y., Ninomiya, M., et al. (1998). *Identification of a principal mRNA species for human 3alpha-hydroxysteroid dehydrogenase isoform (AKR1C3) that exhibits high prostaglandin D2 11-ketoreductase activity.* J Biochem,Vol.124, No.5, pp. 940-946, Nov

Mayo, W., George, O., Darbra, S., Bouyer, J. J., Vallee, M., Darnaudery, M., et al. (2003). *Individual differences in cognitive aging: implication of pregnenolone sulfate.* Prog Neurobiol,Vol.71, No.1, pp. 43-48, Sep, ISSN 0301-0082

Meczekalski, B., Tonetti, A., Monteleone, P., Bernardi, F., Luisi, S., Stomati, M., et al. (2000). *Hypothalamic amenorrhea with normal body weight: ACTH, allopregnanolone and cortisol responses to corticotropin-releasing hormone test.* Eur J Endocrinol,Vol.142, No.3, pp. 280-285, Mar, ISSN 0804-4643

Meikle, A. W., Stringham, J. D., Wilson, D. E., & Dolman, L. I. (1979). *Plasma 5 alpha-reduced androgens in men and hirsute women: role of adrenals and gonads.* J Clin Endocrinol Metab,Vol.48, No.6, pp. 969-975, Jun

Mellor, D. J., Diesch, T. J., Gunn, A. J., & Bennet, L. (2005). *The importance of 'awareness' for understanding fetal pain.* Brain Res Brain Res Rev,Vol.49, No.3, pp. 455-471, Nov

Meloche, C. A., & Falany, C. N. (2001). *Expression and characterization of the human 3 beta-hydroxysteroid sulfotransferases (SULT2B1a and SULT2B1b).* J Steroid Biochem Mol Biol,Vol.77, No.4-5, pp. 261-269, Jun

Mickan, H., & Zander, J. (1979). *Pregnanolones, pregnenolone and progesterone in the human feto-placental circulation at term of pregnancy.* J Steroid Biochem,Vol.11, No.4, pp. 1461-1466, Oct, ISSN 0022-4731

Miki, Y., Nakata, T., Suzuki, T., Darnel, A. D., Moriya, T., Kaneko, C., et al. (2002). *Systemic distribution of steroid sulfatase and estrogen sulfotransferase in human adult and fetal tissues.* J Clin Endocrinol Metab,Vol.87, No.12, pp. 5760-5768, Dec

Milewich, L., Gant, N. F., Schwarz, B. E., Chen, G. T., & Macdonald, P. C. (1978). *Initiation of human parturition. IX. Progesterone metabolism by placentas of early and late human gestation.* Obstet Gynecol,Vol.51, No.3, pp. 278-280, Mar, ISSN 0029-7844

Milewich, L., Gant, N. F., Schwarz, B. E., Chen, G. T., & MacDonald, P. C. (1979). *5 alpha-Reductase activity in human placenta.* Am J Obstet Gynecol,Vol.133, No.6, pp. 611-617, Mar 15, ISSN 0002-9378

Mitchell, B. F., Mitchell, J. M., Chowdhury, J., Tougas, M., Engelen, S. M., Senff, N., et al. (2005). *Metabolites of progesterone and the pregnane X receptor: a novel pathway regulating uterine contractility in pregnancy?* Am J Obstet Gynecol,Vol.192, No.4, pp. 1304-1313; discussion 1313-1305, Apr

Moghrabi, N., Head, J. R., & Andersson, S. (1997). *Cell type-specific expression of 17 beta-hydroxysteroid dehydrogenase type 2 in human placenta and fetal liver.* J Clin Endocrinol Metab,Vol.82, No.11, pp. 3872-3878, Nov

Monteleone, P., Luisi, M., Colurcio, B., Casarosa, E., Ioime, R., Genazzani, A. R., et al. (2001). *Plasma levels of neuroactive steroids are increased in untreated women with anorexia nervosa or bulimia nervosa.* Psychosom Med,Vol.63, No.1, pp. 62-68, Jan-Feb, ISSN 0033-3174

Monteleone, P., Luisi, M., De Filippis, G., Colurcio, B., Genazzani, A. R., & Maj, M. (2003). *Circulating levels of neuroactive steroids in patients with binge eating disorder: a comparison with nonobese healthy controls and non-binge eating obese subjects.* Int J Eat Disord,Vol.34, No.4, pp. 432-440, Dec, ISSN 0276-3478

Morfin, R., & Starka, L. (2001). *Neurosteroid 7-hydroxylation products in the brain.* Int Rev Neurobiol,Vol.46, pp. 79-95, IS SN 0074-7742

Mostallino, M. C., Sanna, E., Concas, A., Biggio, G., & Follesa, P. (2009). *Plasticity and function of extrasynaptic GABA(A) receptors during pregnancy and after delivery.* Psychoneuroendocrinology,Vol.34 Suppl 1, pp. S74-83, Dec, ISSN 1873-3360

Naylor, J. C., Kilts, J. D., Hulette, C. M., Steffens, D. C., Blazer, D. G., Ervin, J. F., et al. (2010). *Allopregnanolone levels are reduced in temporal cortex in patients with Alzheimer's disease compared to cognitively intact control subjects.* Biochim Biophys Acta,Vol.1801, No.8, pp. 951-959, Aug, ISSN 0006-3002

Okuda, A., & Okuda, K. (1984). *Purification and characterization of delta 4-3-ketosteroid 5 beta-reductase.* J Biol Chem,Vol.259, No.12, pp. 7519-7524, Jun 25, ISSN 0021-9258

Oren, I., Fleishman, S. J., Kessel, A., & Ben-Tal, N. (2004). *Free diffusion of steroid hormones across biomembranes: a simplex search with implicit solvent model calculations.* Biophys J,Vol.87, No.2, pp. 768-779, Aug

Ottander, U., Poromaa, I. S., Bjurulf, E., Skytt, A., Backstrom, T., & Olofsson, J. I. (2005). *Allopregnanolone and pregnanolone are produced by the human corpus luteum.* Mol Cell Endocrinol,Vol.239, No.1-2, pp. 37-44, Jul 15

Parizek, A., Hill, M., Kancheva, R., Havlikova, H., Kancheva, L., Cindr, J., et al. (2005). *Neuroactive pregnanolone isomers during pregnancy.* J Clin Endocrinol Metab,Vol.90, No.1, pp. 395-403, Jan, ISSN 0021-972X

Park-Chung, M., Malayev, A., Purdy, R. H., Gibbs, T. T., & Farb, D. H. (1999). *Sulfated and unsulfated steroids modulate gamma-aminobutyric acidA receptor function through distinct sites.* Brain Res,Vol.830, No.1, pp. 72-87, May 29

Park-Chung, M., Wu, F. S., Purdy, R. H., Malayev, A. A., Gibbs, T. T., & Farb, D. H. (1997). *Distinct sites for inverse modulation of N-methyl-D-aspartate receptors by sulfated steroids.* Mol Pharmacol,Vol.52, No.6, pp. 1113-1123, Dec, ISSN 0026-895X

Patte-Mensah, C., Penning, T. M., & Mensah-Nyagan, A. G. (2004). *Anatomical and cellular localization of neuroactive 5 alpha/3 alpha-reduced steroid-synthesizing enzymes in the spinal cord.* J Comp Neurol,Vol.477, No.3, pp. 286-299, Sep 20, ISSN 0021-9967

Pearson Murphy, B. E., Steinberg, S. I., Hu, F. Y., & Allison, C. M. (2001). *Neuroactive ring A-reduced metabolites of progesterone in human plasma during pregnancy: elevated levels of 5 alpha-dihydroprogesterone in depressed patients during the latter half of pregnancy.* J Clin Endocrinol Metab,Vol.86, No.12, pp. 5981-5987, Dec, ISSN 0021-972X

Peltoketo, H., Nokelainen, P., Piao, Y. S., Vihko, R., & Vihko, P. (1999). *Two 17beta-hydroxysteroid dehydrogenases (17HSDs) of estradiol biosynthesis: 17HSD type 1 and type 7.* J Steroid Biochem Mol Biol,Vol.69, No.1-6, pp. 431-439, Apr-Jun

Penning, T. M. (1999). *Molecular determinants of steroid recognition and catalysis in aldo-keto reductases. Lessons from 3alpha-hydroxysteroid dehydrogenase.* J Steroid Biochem Mol Biol,Vol.69, No.1-6, pp. 211-225, Apr-Jun

Penning, T. M., Burczynski, M. E., Jez, J. M., Hung, C. F., Lin, H. K., Ma, H., et al. (2000). *Human 3alpha-hydroxysteroid dehydrogenase isoforms (AKR1C1-AKR1C4) of the aldo-keto reductase superfamily: functional plasticity and tissue distribution reveals roles in the inactivation and formation of male and female sex hormones.* Biochem J,Vol.351, No.Pt 1, pp. 67-77, Oct 1

Penning, T. M., Burczynski, M. E., Jez, J. M., Lin, H. K., Ma, H., Moore, M., et al. (2001). *Structure-function aspects and inhibitor design of type 5 17beta-hydroxysteroid dehydrogenase (AKR1C3).* Mol Cell Endocrinol,Vol.171, No.1-2, pp. 137-149, Jan 22

Perusquia, M., & Jasso-Kamel, J. (2001). *Influence of 5alpha- and 5beta-reduced progestins on the contractility of isolated human myometrium at term.* Life Sci,Vol.68, No.26, pp. 2933-2944, May 18, ISSN 0024-3205

Pisu, M. G., & Serra, M. (2004). *Neurosteroids and neuroactive drugs in mental disorders.* Life Sci,Vol.74, No.26, pp. 3181-3197, May 14, ISSN 0024-3205

Poletti, A., Coscarella, A., Negri-Cesi, P., Colciago, A., Celotti, F., & Martini, L. (1998). *5 alpha-reductase isozymes in the central nervous system.* Steroids,Vol.63, No.5-6, pp. 246-251, May-Jun

Power, M. L., & Schulkin, J. (2006). *Functions of corticotropin-releasing hormone in anthropoid primates: from brain to placenta.* Am J Hum Biol,Vol.18, No.4, pp. 431-447, Jul-Aug

Prince, R. J., & Simmonds, M. A. (1992). *5 beta-pregnan-3 beta-ol-20-one, a specific antagonist at the neurosteroid site of the GABAA receptor-complex.* Neurosci Lett,Vol.135, No.2, pp. 273-275, Feb 3

Putnam, C. D., Brann, D. W., Kolbeck, R. C., & Mahesh, V. B. (1991). *Inhibition of uterine contractility by progesterone and progesterone metabolites: mediation by progesterone and gamma amino butyric acidA receptor systems.* Biol Reprod,Vol.45, No.2, pp. 266-272, Aug

Rainey, W. E., Rehman, K. S., & Carr, B. R. (2004). *The human fetal adrenal: making adrenal androgens for placental estrogens.* Semin Reprod Med,Vol.22, No.4, pp. 327-336, Nov, ISSN 1526-8004

Reddy, D. S. (2006). *Physiological role of adrenal deoxycorticosterone-derived neuroactive steroids in stress-sensitive conditions.* Neuroscience,Vol.138, No.3, pp. 911-920, ISSN 0306-4522

Sakurai, N., Miki, Y., Suzuki, T., Watanabe, K., Narita, T., Ando, K., et al. (2006). *Systemic distribution and tissue localizations of human 17beta-hydroxysteroid dehydrogenase type 12.* J Steroid Biochem Mol Biol,Vol.99, No.4-5, pp. 174-181, Jun

Selcer, K. W., Difrancesca, H. M., Chandra, A. B., & Li, P. K. (2007). *Immunohistochemical analysis of steroid sulfatase in human tissues.* J Steroid Biochem Mol Biol,Vol.105, No.1-5, pp. 115-123, Jun-Jul

Shafqat, N., Marschall, H. U., Filling, C., Nordling, E., Wu, X. Q., Bjork, L., et al. (2003). *Expanded substrate screenings of human and Drosophila type 10 17beta-hydroxysteroid dehydrogenases (HSDs) reveal multiple specificities in bile acid and steroid hormone metabolism: characterization of multifunctional 3alpha/7alpha/7beta/17beta/20beta/21-HSD.* Biochem J,Vol.376, No.Pt 1, pp. 49-60, Nov 15

Shaxted, E. J., Heyes, V. M., Walker, M. P., & Maynard, P. V. (1982). *Umbilical-cord plasma progesterone in term infants delivered by caesarean section.* Br J Obstet Gynaecol,Vol.89, No.1, pp. 73-76, Jan, ISSN 0306-5456

Sheehan, P. M. (2006). *A possible role for progesterone metabolites in human parturition.* Aust N Z J Obstet Gynaecol,Vol.46, No.2, pp. 159-163, Apr

Sheehan, P. M., Rice, G. E., Moses, E. K., & Brennecke, S. P. (2005). *5 Beta-dihydroprogesterone and steroid 5 beta-reductase decrease in association with human parturition at term.* Mol Hum Reprod,Vol.11, No.7, pp. 495-501, Jul

Shi, J., Schulze, S., & Lardy, H. A. (2000). *The effect of 7-oxo-DHEA acetate on memory in young and old C57BL/6 mice.* Steroids,Vol.65, No.3, pp. 124-129, Mar, IS SN 0039-128X

Shiraishi, H., Ishikura, S., Matsuura, K., Deyashiki, Y., Ninomiya, M., Sakai, S., et al. (1998). *Sequence of the cDNA of a human dihydrodiol dehydrogenase isoform (AKR1C2) and tissue distribution of its mRNA.* Biochem J,Vol.334 (Pt 2), pp. 399-405, Sep 1

Schumacher, M., Akwa, Y., Guennoun, R., Robert, F., Labombarda, F., Desarnaud, F., et al. (2000). *Steroid synthesis and metabolism in the nervous system: trophic and protective effects.* J Neurocytol,Vol.29, No.5-6, pp. 307-326, May-Jun, ISSN 0300-4864

Schumacher, M., Guennoun, R., Robert, F., Carelli, C., Gago, N., Ghoumari, A., et al. (2004). *Local synthesis and dual actions of progesterone in the nervous system: neuroprotection and myelination.* Growth Horm IGF Res,Vol.14 Suppl A, pp. S18-33, Jun, ISSN 1096-6374

Siiteri, P. K. (2005). *The continuing saga of dehydroepiandrosterone (DHEA).* J Clin Endocrinol Metab,Vol.90, No.6, pp. 3795-3796, Jun, ISSN 0021-972X

Sirianni, R., Mayhew, B. A., Carr, B. R., Parker, C. R., Jr., & Rainey, W. E. (2005). *Corticotropin-releasing hormone (CRH) and urocortin act through type 1 CRH receptors to stimulate dehydroepiandrosterone sulfate production in human fetal adrenal cells.* J Clin Endocrinol Metab,Vol.90, No.9, pp. 5393-5400, Sep

Smith, A. J., Alder, L., Silk, J., Adkins, C., Fletcher, A. E., Scales, T., et al. (2001). *Effect of alpha subunit on allosteric modulation of ion channel function in stably expressed human recombinant gamma-aminobutyric acid(A) receptors determined using (36)Cl ion flux.* Mol Pharmacol,Vol.59, No.5, pp. 1108-1118, May

Smith, R., Mesiano, S., Chan, E. C., Brown, S., & Jaffe, R. B. (1998). *Corticotropin-releasing hormone directly and preferentially stimulates dehydroepiandrosterone sulfate secretion by human fetal adrenal cortical cells.* J Clin Endocrinol Metab,Vol.83, No.8, pp. 2916-2920, Aug, ISSN 0021-972X

Smith, R., Smith, J. I., Shen, X., Engel, P. J., Bowman, M. E., McGrath, S. A., et al. (2009). *Patterns of plasma corticotropin-releasing hormone, progesterone, estradiol, and estriol change and the onset of human labor.* J Clin Endocrinol Metab,Vol.94, No.6, pp. 2066-2074, Jun, ISSN 1945-7197

Steckelbroeck, S., Jin, Y., Gopishetty, S., Oyesanmi, B., & Penning, T. M. (2004). *Human cytosolic 3alpha-hydroxysteroid dehydrogenases of the aldo-keto reductase superfamily display significant 3beta-hydroxysteroid dehydrogenase activity: implications for steroid hormone metabolism and action.* J Biol Chem,Vol.279, No.11, pp. 10784-10795, Mar 12

Stoffel-Wagner, B. (2001). *Neurosteroid metabolism in the human brain.* Eur J Endocrinol,Vol.145, No.6, pp. 669-679, Dec, ISSN 0804-4643

Stoffel-Wagner, B., Beyenburg, S., Watzka, M., Blumcke, I., Bauer, J., Schramm, J., et al. (2000). *Expression of 5alpha-reductase and 3alpha-hydroxisteroid oxidoreductase in the hippocampus of patients with chronic temporal lobe epilepsy.* Epilepsia,Vol.41, No.2, pp. 140-147, Feb, ISSN 0013-9580

Stromberg, J., Backstrom, T., & Lundgren, P. (2005). *Rapid non-genomic effect of glucocorticoid metabolites and neurosteroids on the gamma-aminobutyric acid-A receptor.* Eur J Neurosci,Vol.21, No.8, pp. 2083-2088, Apr

Takeyama, J., Sasano, H., Suzuki, T., Iinuma, K., Nagura, H., & Andersson, S. (1998). *17Beta-hydroxysteroid dehydrogenase types 1 and 2 in human placenta: an immunohistochemical study with correlation to placental development.* J Clin Endocrinol Metab,Vol.83, No.10, pp. 3710-3715, Oct, ISSN 0021-972X

Todorovic, S. M., Pathirathna, S., Brimelow, B. C., Jagodic, M. M., Ko, S. H., Jiang, X., et al. (2004). *5beta-reduced neuroactive steroids are novel voltage-dependent blockers of T-type Ca2+ channels in rat sensory neurons in vitro and potent peripheral analgesics in vivo.* Mol Pharmacol,Vol.66, No.5, pp. 1223-1235, Nov

Torn, S., Nokelainen, P., Kurkela, R., Pulkka, A., Menjivar, M., Ghosh, S., et al. (2003). *Production, purification, and functional analysis of recombinant human and mouse 17beta-hydroxysteroid dehydrogenase type 7.* Biochem Biophys Res Commun,Vol.305, No.1, pp. 37-45, May 23

Tsuruo, Y. (2005). *Topography and function of androgen-metabolizing enzymes in the central nervous system.* Anat Sci Int,Vol.80, No.1, pp. 1-11, Mar, ISSN 1447-6959

Turkmen, S., Lofgren, M., Birzniece, V., Backstrom, T., & Johansson, I. M. (2006). *Tolerance development to Morris water maze test impairments induced by acute allopregnanolone.* Neuroscience,Vol.139, No.2, pp. 651-659, May 12, ISSN 0306-4522

Turnbull, A. C., Patten, P. T., Flint, A. P., Keirse, M. J., Jeremy, J. Y., & Anderson, A. B. (1974). *Significant fall in progesterone and rise in oestradiol levels in human peripheral plasma before onset of labour.* Lancet,Vol.1, No.7848, pp. 101-103, Jan 26, ISSN 0140-6736

Usami, N., Yamamoto, T., Shintani, S., Ishikura, S., Higaki, Y., Katagiri, Y., et al. (2002). *Substrate specificity of human 3(20)alpha-hydroxysteroid dehydrogenase for neurosteroids and its inhibition by benzodiazepines.* Biol Pharm Bull,Vol.25, No.4, pp. 441-445, Apr

Uzunova, V., Sheline, Y., Davis, J. M., Rasmusson, A., Uzunov, D. P., Costa, E., et al. (1998). *Increase in the cerebrospinal fluid content of neurosteroids in patients with unipolar major depression who are receiving fluoxetine or fluvoxamine.* Proc Natl Acad Sci U S A,Vol.95, No.6, pp. 3239-3244, Mar 17

Vu, T. T., Hirst, J. J., Stark, M., Wright, I. M., Palliser, H. K., Hodyl, N., et al. (2009). *Changes in human placental 5alpha-reductase isoenzyme expression with advancing gestation: effects of fetal sex and glucocorticoid exposure.* Reprod Fertil Dev,Vol.21, No.4, pp. 599-607

Walsh, S. W. (1988). *Progesterone and estradiol production by normal and preeclamptic placentas.* Obstet Gynecol,Vol.71, No.2, pp. 222-226, Feb, ISSN 0029-7844

Wang, J. M., & Brinton, R. D. (2008). *Allopregnanolone-induced rise in intracellular calcium in embryonic hippocampal neurons parallels their proliferative potential.* BMC Neurosci,Vol.9 Suppl 2, pp. S11, ISSN 1471-2202

Wang, M., He, Y., Eisenman, L. N., Fields, C., Zeng, C. M., Mathews, J., et al. (2002). *3beta - hydroxypregnane steroids are pregnenolone sulfate-like GABA(A) receptor antagonists.* J Neurosci,Vol.22, No.9, pp. 3366-3375, May 1, ISSN 1529-2401

Wang, M. D., Wahlstrom, G., & Backstrom, T. (1997). *The regional brain distribution of the neurosteroids pregnenolone and pregnenolone sulfate following intravenous infusion.* J Steroid Biochem Mol Biol,Vol.62, No.4, pp. 299-306, Jul

Watanabe, H., Hirato, K., Hashino, M., Kosaki, T., Kimura, T., Nakayama, T., et al. (1990). *Effects of DHA-S on placental 3 beta-hydroxysteroid dehydrogenase activity, progesterone and 20 alpha-dihydroprogesterone concentrations in placenta and serum.* Endocrinol Jpn,Vol.37, No.1, pp. 69-77, Feb, ISSN 0013-7219

Weaver, C. E., Land, M. B., Purdy, R. H., Richards, K. G., Gibbs, T. T., & Farb, D. H. (2000). *Geometry and charge determine pharmacological effects of steroids on N-methyl-D-aspartate receptor-induced Ca(2+) accumulation and cell death.* J Pharmacol Exp Ther,Vol.293, No.3, pp. 747-754, Jun

Westcott, K. T., Hirst, J. J., Ciurej, I., Walker, D. W., & Wlodek, M. E. (2008). *Brain allopregnanolone in the fetal and postnatal rat in response to uteroplacental insufficiency.* Neuroendocrinology,Vol.88, No.4, pp. 287-292, ISSN 1423-0194

Yawno, T., Hirst, J. J., Castillo-Melendez, M., & Walker, D. W. (2009). *Role of neurosteroids in regulating cell death and proliferation in the late gestation fetal brain.* Neuroscience,Vol.163, No.3, pp. 838-847, Oct 20, ISSN 1873-7544

Yoshihara, S., Morimoto, H., Ohori, M., Yamada, Y., Abe, T., & Arisaka, O. (2005). *A neuroactive steroid, allotetrahydrocorticosterone inhibits sensory nerves activation in guinea-pig airways.* Neurosci Res,Vol.53, No.2, pp. 210-215, Oct

Zhang, H., Varlamova, O., Vargas, F. M., Falany, C. N., & Leyh, T. S. (1998). *Sulfuryl transfer: the catalytic mechanism of human estrogen sulfotransferase.* J Biol Chem,Vol.273, No.18, pp. 10888-10892, May 1

19

Menstrual Cycle Disturbances at Reproductive Age

Skałba Piotr
Silesian Medical University, Katowice, Poland

1. Introduction

During the last decade, the rapidly expanding fields of molecular biology and genetics have allowed us to better understand the clinical symptoms of endocrine disorders, including menstrual cycle disturbances at reproductive age. This chapter is an attempt to combine the results of new research and hypotheses with the proven facts about disorders of the functioning of the hypothalamic-pituitary-ovary axis.

2. Menstrual cycle

The menstrual cycle, as defined in the introduction, is the complex of changes which are the result of functional integration of stimulatory and inhibitory signals from the hypothalamus, pituitary and ovary. At the reproductive age, from puberty to menopause, normal function in women involves repetitive cycles of follicle development, and ovulation. The average menstrual cycle is 28 days from the start of one to the start of the next, but it can range from 21 days to 35 days. The menstrual cycle is divided into three phases: the follicular phase (postmenstrual), ovulation, and the luteal phase (premenstrual). Menstrual cycles are counted from the first day of menstrual bleeding. The length of the follicular phase depends on the rate of growth of the ovarian follicles and is thus variable from one woman to another. In contrast, the length of the luteal phase depends on the life span of the corpus luteum (CL), and is thus less variable. The mean duration of the follicular phase is 15.4 + 2.5 days and the mean duration of the luteal phase is 13.6 + 1.2 days. The early follicular phase starts on the first day of the cycle and ends when estradiol begins to increase. It is characterized by increasing LH and FSH and constant low levels of estradiol. The late follicular phase starts with the increase in estradiol and ends at its preovulatory peak. It is characterized by increasing estradiol and decreasing FSH levels.

The average level of estradiol ranges from 48 pg/ml in the early follicular phase, up to 168 pg/ml in the late follicular phase. At the peak, the level can reach 250 pg/ml. The average LH level ranges from 3 IU/l in the early follicular phase up to 4,5 IU/l in the late follicular phase, with ovulation peak to 12 IU/ml. The average level of FSH ranges from 6 IU/l in the early follicular phase up to 4 IU/l in the late follicular phase.

Ovulation occurs about 36 h after the LH peak, which is preceded by the estradiol peak.

The early luteal phase starts on the day of ovulation (the day after the LH peak) and ends when progesterone has reached a plateau. It is characterized by increasing progesterone and decreasing LH and FSH levels. The mid-luteal phase corresponds to plateauing progesterone levels. It is characterized by constant elevated progesterone and constant low levels of LH and FSH. The late luteal phase starts when progesterone decreases and ends on the day preceding the next menses. It is characterized by decreasing progesterone and increasing LH and FSH levels. The average estradiol level in the mid-luteal phase is about 250 pg/l, and average progesterone level at the same time is 12 ng/ml.

3. Hypogonadotropic hypogonadism

Hypogonadotropic hypogonadism (HH) is characterized by absent or decreased function of the male testes or the female ovaries. It can be defined by inappropriately low serum concentrations of LH and FSH, which is an effect of GnRH deficiency. HH is most frequently acquired and caused by a number of pathological processes but it can also occur as part of various congenital syndromes. The terminology of HH has evolved with the increased understanding of reproductive physiology. Once functional and later genetic causes of central hypogonadism were identified, "idiopathic" or "isolated" HH (IHH) was then used to indicate cases in which secondary causes of HH had been excluded. Acquired and syndromic causes of HH include the following: CNS or pituitary tumors, brain/pituitary radiation, pituitary apoplexy, head trauma, drugs (GnRH agonists/antagonists, glucocorticoids, narcotics, chemotherapy), functional deficiency resulting from chronic systemic illness, eating disorders, hypothyroidism, hyperprolactinemia, diabetes mellitus, and Cushing's disease. Most of the above causes of HH will not be discussed because they do not fall within the scope of the chapter.

Idiopathic hypogonadotropic hypogonadism (IHH), also called isolated GnRH deficiency, is characterized by a failure of initiation of puberty due to insufficient gonadotropin release, thus resulting in the failure to develop secondary sexual characteristics and a mature reproductive system. Currently known genetic defects account for about 30% of all IHH cases. When embryonic migration of GnRH neurons from the nasal placode to their final destination in the hypothalamus is disrupted, the resulting phenotype is Kallmann syndrome, which is clinically characterized by hypogonadotropic hypogonadism and anosmia. Normosmic idiopathic hypogonadotropic hypogonadism (nIHH) resulting from Kallmann syndrome has been observed. Family members with the same genotype may display a range of features of the GnRH neurons that successfully completed their embryonic journey to the hypothalamus. The prevalence of IHH has been estimated at 1/4000 to 1/10 000 in males. It is reported to be between 2 and 5 times less frequent in females (Brioude, 2009).

The classification of IHH has recently been made on the basis of genetic and pathophysiological features. Now a division into two forms of IHH been proposed. The paradigm of this division is to define Kallmann syndrome as a form generally combined with anosmia. There is substantial variation in clinical expression of the same genetic defect in families of patients with complete anosmia and hypogonadotropic hypogonadism to less severe hypogonadotropic hypogonadism manifesting as delayed puberty.

3.1 Genetic basis for IHH

The genetic causes of Kallmann syndrome and nIHH are summarized in Table 1. Some genes (FGFR1, FGF8, PROKR2, PROK2, CHD7) have been associated with both Kallmann syndrome and nIHH.

Gene	Year linked to human HH	Syndrome name	Phenotypes	Inheritance	Comment
KAL1	1991	Kallmann Syndrome 1	KS	X-linked R	70% synkinesia 30% unilateral renal agenesis
FGFR1	2003	Kallmann Syndrome 2	KS nIHH	DA (AR) oligogenic	30% Cleft lip/palate common
PROKR2	2006	Kallmann Syndrome 3	KS nIHH	AR AD oligogenic	Weak reported association with epilepsy, sleep disorder, synkinesis, fibrous dysplasia, obesity
PROK2	2006	Kallmann Syndrome 4	KS nIHH	AR AD oligogenic	
CHD7	2004	Kallmann Syndrome 5	CHARGE syn KS	AD	Deafness and semicircular canal hypoplasia common
FGF8	2008	Kallmann Syndrome 6	KS nIHH	AD (AR) oligogenic	Cleft lip/palate relatively common
GNRHR	1997		nIHH	AR oligogenic	No accessory features
GNRH1	2009		nIHH	AR AD?	No accessory features
KISS1R	2003		nIHH	AR	No accessory features
TAC3	2009		nIHH	AR	Only 2 patients described to date, both with mild learning disability
TACR3	2009		nIHH	AR	No accessory features

KS, Kallmann syndrome; nIHH, normosmic isolated hypogonadotropic hypogonadism; AD, autosomal dominant; AR, autosomal recessive.

Table 1. Genetic defects causing idiopathic hypogonadotropic hypogonadism (IHH) (modified by Semple and Topaloglu 2010)

Kallmann syndrome 1, caused by mutation in the KAL1 gene, is inherited in an X-linked manner. Deletion of KAL1 is an extremely rare cause of this syndrome. The KAL1 gene encodes an extracellular glycoprotein called anosmin-1, which is an adhesion molecule responsible for the migration of GnRH neurons and formation of the olfactory bulb in the fetal period. The syndrome has not been described in women so far.
Kallmann syndrome 2 and 6 are caused by mutations of the FGFR1 (fibroblast growth factor receptor) and FGF8 (fibroblast growth factor 8) genes. FGFR1 requires heparin sulfate proteoglycans as co-receptors, and anosmin-1. Loss of FGFR1 function has been confirmed to produce reproductive abnormalities ranging from severe autosomal dominant Kallmann syndrome through autosomal dominant, fully penetrant nIHH to delayed puberty. Approximately 10% of patients with Kallmann syndrome were found to have loss of function mutations in FGFR1. FGF8 mutation patients exhibited various degrees of olfactory

function and GnRH function. In addition, cleft palate is found in up to 30% of patients, while cartilage abnormalities in either ear or nose and some digital anomalies have been reported (Tsai & Gill, 2006).

Kallmann syndrome 3 and 4 are caused by mutations in the PROKR2 (prokineticin receptor 2) and PROK2 (prokineticin 2) genes. Prokineticin 2 is an 81-amino acid peptide, which together with its receptor was recognized as a strong candidate for failed development of the olfactory bulb and migration of GnRH neurons. These syndromes were found in 9% of Kallmann syndrome patients, most of them being heterozygous; however, homozygous and compound heterozygous mutations were also described. Patients with PROK2 or PROKR2 mutations have considerable phenotypic variability ranging from Kallmann syndrome to nIHH. A variety of accompanying clinical features including fibrous dysplasia, synkinesia, and epilepsy have been reported in patients with PROK2 or PROKR2 mutations.

Kallmann syndrome 5 is caused by a mutation of the CHD7 gene, which encodes a chromatin-remodeling factor (chromodomain helicase DNA-binding protein 7) and is defective in CHARGE syndrome. Some patients also have IHH and hyposmia. On the basis of the hypothesis that Kallmann syndrome and nIHH may be a milder allelic variant of *CHARGE syndrome*, patients diagnosed with hypogonadotropic hypogonadism and anosmia should be screened for clinical features consistent with CHARGE syndrome.

The term "CHARGE syndrome" is used to describe a pattern of birth defects in children with coloboma, heart defects, atresia of the choanae, retardation of growth and development, genital anomaly and ear abnormality. The prevalence of CHARGE syndrome is approximately 1 in 10 000, and more than 400 patients have now been reported (Aminzadeh et al., 2010). The clinical criteria of CHARGE syndrome are summarized in Table 2.

GnRH and GnRHR gene defects cause nIHH. To date, many familial and some sporadic cases of GnRHR gene mutation have been reported. On the basis of a large series GnRHR mutations have been suggested to account for about 40–50% of familial nIHH, and around 17% of sporadic nIHH. In most early reports, the GnRHR defects consisted of point mutations leading to amino acid substitutions. Rarer mutations lead to frame-shifts or premature stop codons, resulting in a truncated protein, but no true GnRHR deletions have so far been described (Bouligand et al., 2009). The most consistent characteristic of patients with GnRHR mutation is their pituitary resistance to pulsatile GnRH administration when the phenotype is severe. Pregnancy has been obtained after pulsatile administration of GnRH. In addition, isolated cases of nIHH have presented with pregnancy after clomifene citrate administration (Brioude et al., 2009). The differentiated clinical expression of GnRHR mutation results in partial loss of the GnRHR function, and in one case this was attributed to interaction with a mutation in FGFR1, which produces different phenotypes (Pitteloud, 2007).

Recently, defects in the GNRH1 gene itself were reported for the first time. Chan et al. (2009) reported a homozygous mutation in a male patient with severe nIHH. This single base-pair deletion produces a frame shift that is predicted to disrupt the GnRH decapeptide. These authors also identified a rare heterozygous GnRH1 sequence variant in four patients with nIHH. Simultaneously, Bouligand et al. (2009) presented isolated familial nIHH and GnRH1 mutation. The case reports concerned two of four children of non-consanguineous parents who were found to have nIHH. Both the brother and his sister showed characteristics of severe nIHH, and simultaneously they had a blunted response to GnRH bolus administration (100 µg intravenously).

Major criteria	Minor criteria	Inclusion rule
Coloboma of the iris, retina, choroid or disc (75–90%) Microphthalmia	Hypoplastic genitalia - micropenis and cryptorchidism (80%) - hypoplastic labia (30–40%) HH (65–85%)	4 majors OR 3 majors + 3 minors
Choanal atresia (35–65%)	Developmental delay - delayed motor milestones - language delay - learning disability of varying degree	
Ear abnormalities (>95%) - external ear (lop or cup shaped) - middle ear (ossicular malformations; chronic serous otitis media) - inner ear (cochlear defects) - mixed deafness (60–90%)	Cardiovascular malformations - conotruncal defect, e.g. Fallot's tetralogy - AV canal defects - aortic valve or arch defects	
Cranial nerve dysfunction - unilateral or bilateral facial palsy - sensorineural deafness - swallowing problems	Growth deficiency - short stature - GH deficiency Orofacial cleft (15–20%) Tracheoesophageal fistula Characteristic facies	

Table 2. Clinical criteria of CHARGE Syndrome by Aminzadeh et al. (2010)

In 2003 there was described a mutation in the G-protein-coupled *receptor GPR 54* (de Roux, 2003). GPR 54 had previously been shown to be the receptor for a small peptide derived from the KISS1 gene (leading to its recent redesignation as KISS1R). Before this discovery, some cases of familial nIHH had been identified as resulting from defects of the short arm of chromosome 19 (Seminara et al., 2003). Two genetic studies performed in the USA and in France demonstrated that nIHH may be due to inactivation of KISS1R (Iovane, 2004). KISSR1 mutations are a rare cause of nIHH. Individuals with nIHH have been shown to have severely reduced LH pulse amplitude, but approximately normal pulse frequency. Successful pregnancy has been reported after specific stimulation of ovulation (Semple & Topaloglu, 2010).

Topaloglu et al. (2009) reported four human pedigrees with severe congenital gonadotropin deficiency and pubertal failure in which all affected individuals are homozygous for loss of function mutation in *TAC3* (encoding neurokinin B) or its receptor *TACR3* (encoding neurokinin B receptor). Gianetti et al. (2010) presented phenotypic information concerning seven females with coding sequence variants in TACR3/TAC3. None of the females had spontaneous thelarche, and five of them demonstrated evidence for reversibility of their hypogonadism after discontinuation of therapy. Neurokinin B, a member of the substance P related tachykinin family, is known to be highly expressed in hypothalamic neurons, especially in the actuate nucleus, and is co-expressed there with kisspeptin. Neurokinin B exerts an influence on reproductive function, but its importance in sustaining the integrity of the hypothalamic-pituitary-gonadal axis is expected to be elucidated over the next few years.

3.2 Clinical presentation

Kallmann syndrome may be suspected in a prepubertal patient with anosmia, especially when there is already a positive family history. Usually, however, a clear picture of the disorder is revealed in adolescence. Rarely, individuals have normal sexual maturation and develop IHH in adulthood. The majority of girls can be suspected of IHH when pubertal development is incomplete or absent after the age of 13 years. Primary amenorrhea occurs in approximately 90% of cases of IHH. Girls before puberty have normal growth of stature, but the pubertal growth spurt does not occur. Stature retardation is very rare, but in contrast the absence of long-bone epiphyseal closure explains these patients' frequent eunuchoid aspect and relative tallness. To distinguish nIHH from constitutional late puberty could be difficult when these reversible forms occur before 20 years of age.

Adult females have little or no breast development, although in some patients it may be almost normal. Since adrenal maturation proceeds normally, the low levels of androgen production in the adrenal glands may allow normal onset of pubic hair growth (adrenarche) and therefore the pubic hair may be absent, sparse, or even normal. Partial forms are frequent in women, while very mild form occurs in only a minority of women. This form of IHH can be revealed by isolated chronic anovulation, whereas estradiol secretion is adequate for endometrial development, and can be shown by onset of bleeding after progestin administration, as well as by oligomenorrhea. These attenuated forms have also been described as having conceived spontaneously.

Retarded bone maturation, osteopenia and osteoporosis are frequent when the gonadotropin deficiency is discovered in adulthood (Brioude, 2009).

3.3 Establishing the diagnosis

The diagnosis of IHH is established by the presence of both suggestive clinical findings and laboratory findings consistent with hypogonadotropic hypogonadism, and the absence of secondary causes of hypothalamic hypogonadism. The first step of the diagnostic procedure is a detailed physical examination with the assessment of development of the secondary sexual characteristics, and checking family history. Then it is necessary to perform a semi-quantitative assessment of olfaction to detect hyposmia. Examination of the outer ear and hearing is also useful to rule out mild CHARGE syndrome. In women without anosmia or hypoosmia or identified genetic anomalies, the diagnostic procedure should exclude eating disorders, excessive physical activity, and chronic underlying conditions. Body mass index and body fat should also be calculated. Laboratory tests should be limited to assessing the level of LH, FSH, PRL and estradiol. Plasma LH, FSH and estradiol concentrations are often low in women, sometimes being near the detection limit. In very mild form, which occurs in only a minority of women, nIHH can be revealed by isolated chronic anovulation, whereas estradiol secretion is almost normal. The test with intravenous administration of 100 µg GnRH provides no extra diagnostic information relative to baseline gonadotropic levels, but its outcome reflects the severity of the gonadotropin deficiency

The diagnostic procedures should also exclude hyperprolactinemia, global anterior pituitary insufficiency and an associated endocrine disorder that may be part of syndromic forms of IHH.
Magnetic resonance imaging (MRI) of the brain and olfactory bulbs is useful in IHH. MRI can rule out expansive, infiltrative, or malformative disorders, and can also be useful to analyze the olfactory bulbs. Renal ultrasound examination should be made in Kallmann syndrome, as it can reveal renal malformation or agenesis. Pelvic sonography, which is now a routine part of gynecological examination, should always be performed to determine the size of the uterus, endometrial thickness and ovary development. In adult women, especially whose with osteoporotic risk factors, such as glucocorticoid treatment and smoking, one should consider measuring bone mineral density.

3.4 Management

Treatment options for IHH include sex steroid, gonadotropins, and pulsatile GnRH administration. The choice of therapy is determined by the goal of treatment. The majority of young women have a lack of development of the secondary sexual characteristics, and they should be treated with estrogens, initially with low doses (1 mg/estradiol p.o.). After a period of approximately six months when breast development has been optimized, replacement doses of estradiol and progestagens should be implemented. In women with nIHH who wish to become pregnant pulsatile GnRH stimulation can be used. Intravenous pulsatile administration of GnRH mimics normal cycle dynamics with the resulting ovulation of a single follicle (Layendecker et al., 1980). This therapy offers a clear advantage over treatment with exogenous gonadotropins, which involves higher rates of both multiple gestation and ovarian hyperstimulation syndrome. For either approach, however, the rate of conception is approximately 30% per ovulation cycle (Brioude, 2009). Recently, in nIHH women in order to stimulate ovulation recombinant FSH is commonly used. Its use provides a low risk of hyperstimulation syndrome. But in the cases of severe form of IHH at a concentration of LH in the blood below 1.2 mIU/ml, it is necessary to add to the therapy recombinant hCG, or a preparation containing FSH and LH, or recombinant LH, since FSH administration itself does not lead to luteinization of granulosa cells. It is also recommended to follow it with administration of progesterone to maintain corpus luteum function. This therapeutic regimen is assessed to give 70% of pregnancies with the application of 6 cycles of treatment, but it increases the risk of ovarian hyperstimulation syndrome and the development of multiple pregnancies.

4. Nutritional hypothalamic dysfunction

Adaptation of a woman's body to starvation leads to menstrual and fertility disorders. A number of reproductive disorders have emerged that appear to be related to dieting and the desire for leanness. Adolescent girls who present with eating disorders before menarche have not only lost weight but are also stunted in growth (Swenne & Thurfjell, 2003). Girls first begin to develop a preoccupation with dieting for weight loss and to describe feelings and behaviors associated with dieting around the time of menarche. This concern is accentuated by the rapid increase in height, weight, and body fat that occurs just before menarche, but it is also related to a window of vulnerability to sociocultural influences that focus on body image and weight. Most eating disorders first develop in adolescence, with 90% of eating disorders present before age 25 (Andersen & Ryan, 2009). In healthy adult women, a short-term calorie restriction diet (800 - 1100 kcal/per day) does not change the menstrual rhythm. When dietary restriction persists for more than one cycle, it is followed by weight loss and suppression of ovulation. Moderate dietary restriction and weight loss in normal cyclic women are associated with a reduction of estradiol levels in the face of almost normal LH levels, α consequence of which is *functional hypothalamic amenorrhea (FHA)*. Severe starvation in healthy women for two and half weeks induces a reversal of LH pulses to prepubertal patterns (Yen, 1999). Women with FHA have reduced central GnRH drive, resulting in low FSH and LH levels, which causes anovulation.

The most serious eating disorders, such as anorexia nervosa, bulimia nervosa, and binge eating disorder, were recently classified as psychiatric illnesses, and therefore will not be discussed in this chapter.

5. Athletic amenorrhea

The physiological and psychosocial health benefits of exercise have been widely promoted by society, but we should not forget that intense exercise can cause adverse health effects. First described in 1997, the *female athletic triad* is a syndrome that includes disordered eating, amenorrhea and osteoporosis. Athletic amenorrhea has been described in women involved in long-distance running, rowing, skiing, high-performance gymnastics, volleyball, judo and ballet. It was found that the disorder may affect not only professional sportswomen, but also women practicing recreational exercises. Intense recreational exercises cause 1/3 of these women to develop ovulatory dysfunction. Female athletes are characterized by changes in metabolism in the form of intermittent or chronic imbalance due to increased energy expenditure or caloric intake. Another factor negatively affecting hypothalamic function is stress associated with competition and performances. Under normal conditions, after acute stress or energy demand passes, hormonal equilibrium is restored. In contrast, chronic stress can result in alteration of hormone secretion, and in particular it may damage hypothalamic secretory function. The important role played by energy imbalance and psychological factors in the pathogenesis of athletic amenorrhea should be stressed (Pauli & Berga, 2010).

Risk factors of athletic amenorrhea are age below 17 years, psychological factors and food restrictions. But the mechanism most likely to initiate development of the disorder is a disparity between the calorie intake and energy expenditure. FHA is estimated to affect up to 5% of women of reproductive age and is the underlying cause of 35% of women seeking evaluation for secondary amenorrhea.

This disorder of energy balance reduces the activity of the hypothalamic centers responsible for the secretion of GnRH. Reduction of central drive GnRH results in low FSH and LH levels, which causes anovulation. In FHA women the disruption of GnRH drive is also connected with activation of the hypothalamic-pituitary-adrenal (HPA) axis, and suppression of the hypothalamic-pituitary-thyroidal (HPT) axis. Changing functions of the two axes is due to the need to mobilize energy in response to stress. Other peripheral metabolic factors such as ghrelin, insulin, leptin and peptide YY also play a role in communicating energy status to the brain areas that modulate metabolism. Gut peptides and adipocytokines also appear to be altered in exercising women with FHA, and have been hypothesized to be involved in the etiology of this disorder. Ghrelin is produced by cells in the stomach and appears to be a signal of disordered eating independent of weight or body fat, such that elevated ghrelin may result in continuing suppression of the hypothalamic-pituitary-ovarian axis with amenorrhea despite normal body fat and leptin levels. Eating disorders are also characterized by elevations in corticotropin-releasing hormone and cortisol, along with loss of the normal circadian rhythm of cortisol. Neuropeptide Y is produced by nuclei in the hypothalamus and appears to have both stimulatory and inhibitory effects on GnRH secretion in response to leptin (Andersen, at al., 2009). A critical leptin level threshold is suggested to be necessary for regular menses. Additionally, in FHA elevated night time serum growth hormone levels and lower 24 h prolactin levels have been observed (Berga et al., 1989).

The prospective study of Rauh et al. (2010) showed that high school female athletes with disordered eating and oligomenorrhea/amenorrhea have a reduced BMD (bone mineral density). A BMD level below the expected range for age was associated with musculoskeletal injury. The authors conclude that BMD levels should begin to be closely monitored in adolescent female athletes.

6. Eating disorders and athletic amenorrhea treatment

Appropriate intervention depends on determining which behavior needs to be modified. Attention should be concentrated on the promotion of psychosocial harmony, restoring ovulation and menstrual cyclicity. Methods that are considered useful include a combination of cognitive behavior therapy with relaxation techniques coupled with adequate caloric intake. One should avoid extensive workups for physical causes when women have a clear fear of fatness, drive for thinness, preoccupation with weight, binging and purging, or compulsive exercise suggesting an eating disorder. The implementation of hormonal therapy to regularize menstrual cycles is not indicated when the patient is underweight, dieting despite normal weight range, or compulsively exercising. It is advisable to prescribe 1500 mg calcium citrate/400 units vitamin D per day in divided doses. Before the plan of ovulation stimulation in order to become pregnant, a healthy weight should be established. The patient should also be educated about the effect of underweight on ovulation and risks of eating disorders for pregnancy and offspring (Andersen, at al., 2009).

7. Hypopituitarism

Hypopituitarism is defined as a clinical syndrome of deficiency in pituitary hormone production. This may result from disorders involving the pituitary gland, hypothalamus, or surrounding structures. Panhypopituitarism refers to involvement of all pituitary hormones; however, only one or some pituitary hormones are often involved, resulting in partial hypopituitarism. The Regal et al. (2001) population-based study noted an incidence of hypopituitarism of 4.2 cases per 100 000 per year, increasing with age. It should be noted that the study involved an adult Caucasian population of northwestern Spain.

Pituitary hormones of clinical significance include adrenocorticotropic hormone (ACTH, i.e., corticotropin), follicle-stimulating hormone (FSH), luteinizing hormone (LH), growth hormone (GH), prolactin (PRL), thyroid-stimulating hormone (TSH, i.e., thyrotropin), and antidiuretic hormone (ADH) (Fig. 1). Presented symptoms of the disease depend on the specific pituitary hormone deficiency, as summarized in Table 3.

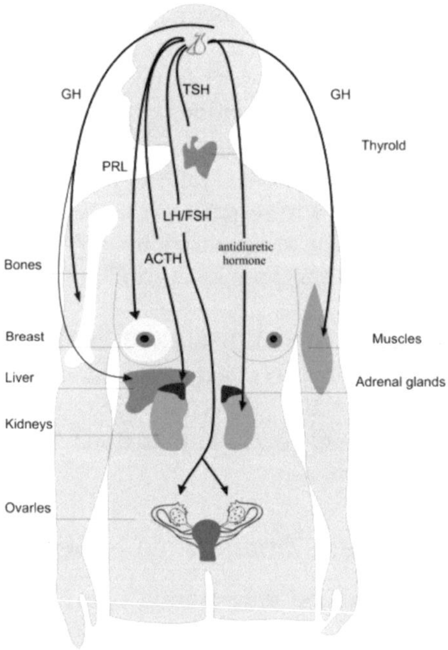

Fig. 1. Function of pituitary hormones.

Deficient hormone	Symptoms
GH	Growth retardation in children. Adults: excessive tiredness, muscle weakness, lack of drive, impaired quality of life scores
FSH/LH (women)	Amenorrhea, reduced libido, dyspareunia, and hot flashes
TSH	Weight gain, decreased energy, sensitive to cold, constipation, dry skin
ACTH	Pale appearance, weight loss, low blood pressure, dizziness, tiredness
AVP	Thirst, polyuria and nocturia - diabetes insipidus (pituitary adenomas themselves rarely cause diabetes insipidus unless it occurs after surgery. If it occurs spontaneously, usually some other sort of tumor or inflammation is present in the area)
PRL	The mother might not be able to breast feed following delivery.

Table 3. Symptoms of pituitary hormone deficiency (modification by The Pituitary Foundation 2010)

There are numerous causes of hypopituitarism (Table 4).
Traumatic brain injury (TBI) and subarachnoid hemorrhage have long been known to cause lesions in the hypothalamo-pituitary region. Therefore, it is considered that TBI is one of the main causes of hypopituitarism. TBI is also the main cause of death and disability in young

Brain damage*	Traumatic brain injury Subarachnoid hemorrhage Neurosurgery Irradiation Stroke
Pituitary tumors*	Adenomas Other
Non-pituitary tumors	Craniopharyngiomas Meningiomas Gliomas Chordomas Ependymomas Metastases
Infections	Abscess Hypophysitis Encephalitis
Infarction	Apoplexy Sheehan's syndrome
Autoimmune disorders	Lymphatic hypophysitis
Haemochromatosis, granulomatous diseases, histiocytosis Empty sella Perinatal insults Pituitary hypoplasia or aplasia Genetic causes Idiopathic causes	

*Pituitary tumors are classically the most common cause of hypopituitarism. However, new findings imply that causes related to brain damage might outnumber pituitary adenomas in causing hypopituitarism.

Table 4. Causes of hypopituitarism (by Schneider et al. 2007)

adults, with consequences ranging from physical disabilities to long-term cognitive, behavioral and social defects. Recently clinical evidence has demonstrated that TBI may frequently cause hypothalamic-pituitary dysfunction. Schneider et al. (2007) reported that the incidence is 31 cases of hypopituitarism per 100 000 cases of TBI and subarachnoid hemorrhage per year.

Changes in pituitary hormone secretion may be observed during the acute post-TBI phase, representing part of the acute adaptive response to the injury. Post-traumatic hypopituitarism is observed in about 40% of patients with a history of TBI (Bondanelli et al., 2005). In most cases there occurs an isolated deficiency of pituitary hormone (mainly gonadotropin and somatotropin).

The most common cause of hypopituitarism is a pituitary tumor (also known as a pituitary adenoma). Pituitary adenomas are almost invariably benign (not cancerous). However, the pituitary adenoma itself may put pressure on the remaining normal part of the pituitary gland and limit or even destroy its ability to produce hormones appropriately. Pituitary adenomas may exert mechanical compression of the portal vessels and the pituitary stalk and cause ischemic and necrotic damage of the anterior lobe of the pituitary. This mechanism is responsible for the occurrence of hypopituitarism.

Pituitary adenomas are classified according to the type of hormone secreted. The classification of pituitary adenomas is shown in Table 5.

Type of adenoma	Secretion	Pathology
Corticotropic adenomas	ACTH	Cushing's disease
Somatotropic adenomas	GH	Acromegaly
Thyrotrophic adenomas (rare)	TSH	Hyperthyroidism usually doesn't cause symptoms
Gonadotropic adenomas	LH, FSH and their subunits	Usually doesn't cause symptoms
Prolactinomas	PRL	Amenorrhea, infertility galactorrhoea
Null cell adenomas (Incidentalomas)	Do not secrete hormones	No symptoms

Table 5. Classification of pituitary tumors based on hormone levels

Hypopituitarism can also result from pituitary surgery, which might damage part of the normal pituitary. It can also result from radiation treatment. The pathway by which radiation induces hypopituitarism is largely unresolved. Attempts to explain the mechanism causing the damage take into account the direct neuronal damage, and altered neurotransmitter input from other brain centers. Other tumors that grow near the pituitary gland (e.g., craniopharyngioma, Rathke's cleft cyst) can cause hypopituitarism. In addition, tumors that metastasize from cancers elsewhere in the body can spread to the pituitary gland and can lead to hypopituitarism.

Inflammation of the pituitary can also cause hypopituitarism. Sarcoidosis and histiocytosis are types of chronic inflammation that also can result in hypopituitarism (Table 4).

Congenital hypopituitarism can range from mild, involving deficiency of a single hormone, through more severe phenotypes affecting multiple pituitary hormone axes, to panhypopituitarism.

Isolated growth hormone deficiency is the most common manifestation, affecting between 1 in 4000 and 10 000 live births. Normal anterior pituitary development is dependent upon a complex genetic cascade of signaling molecules and transcription factors. Mutations in several of these genes are associated with congenital hypopituitarism. In several cases, different mutations within the same gene have been reported to lead to variable phenotypes. Kelberman and Dattani (2006) presented details of the mutation and their consequences in their excellent review paper. For example, of interest is the detection of a new mutation of LHX3 presented by Rajab et al. (2008). They describe four patients from two unrelated consanguineous pedigrees with novel mutations in the LIM homeodomain transcription factor LHX3. All four patients presented with early-onset hypopituitarism and neonatal hypoglycemia. Subsequent clinical evaluation revealed that all four patients exhibited varying degrees of sensorineural hearing loss.

7.1 Diagnosis and clinical presentation

Hormone deficiency is diagnosed based on the patient's symptoms (Table 3). When a pituitary adenoma or other tumor is detected near the pituitary, or when a person is exposed to some other potential cause of hypopituitarism, the patients should be evaluated for hypopituitarism. Tumors in the sellar region with suprasellar extension can manifest with visual impairment. Headaches are another symptom of tumor masses. Infrequent symptoms of tumor expansion are oculomotor nerve impairment and damage to other cranial nerves. Brain damage can cause neurological deficits, weight changes, depression, sleep disturbances, and loss of drive (Schneider et al., 2007). Symptomatic patients should undergo blood and sometimes urine tests. The most important tests helping to determine specific pituitary hormone deficiencies are summarized in Table 6. Cranial and pituitary

Corticotropic function	
Morning cortisol	< 100 nmol/l: hypocortisolism > 500 nmol/l: hypocortisolism excluded
Morning ACTH	Below upper reference range secondary adrenal insufficiency
250 µg ACTH test	Cortisol < 500 nmol/l after 30 min
Thyrotropic function	
Free thyroxine	Low (<11 pmol/l)
TSH	Low or normal (occasionally slightly raised)
Gonadotropic function	
Estradiol	Low (< 100 pmol/l)
LH and FSH	Low (< 2 mIU/ml)
Postmenopausal	FSH inappropriate low
Somatotropic function	
IGF-1	Below or in the normal reference range
Insulin tolerance test	Adults: growth hormone < 3 µg/l Children: growth hormone <10 µg/l Transition phase: growth hormone < 5 µg/l
GHRH+arginine test	Underweight or normal weight (BMI<25): 11.5 µg/l Overweight (BMI >25 to <30): 8.0 µg/l Obese (BMI >30): 4.2 µg/l
GHRH+GHRP-6 test	Growth hormone <10 µg/l
Posterior pituitary function	
Basal urine and plasma sample	Urine volume (>40 ml/kg body weight per day) + urine osmolality <300 mOsm/kg water+ hypernatremia
Water deprivation test	Urine osmolality <700 mOsm/kg; Ratio of urine to plasma <2

Table 6. Criteria for pituitary hormone deficiency (modified by Schneider et al. 2007)

gland magnetic resonance imaging (MRI) should be performed to exclude tumors and other lesions of sellar and parasellar region. Diffusion-weighted MRI and perfusion MRI are advanced techniques that provide information not available from conventional MRI. In particular, these techniques have a number of applications with regard to characterization of tumors and assessment of tumor response to therapy (Provenzale, 2006). Contrast-enhanced images may be needed for the diagnosis of pituitary microadenomas (10 mm).

7.2 Treatment

If the hypopituitarism is caused by a lesion or tumors, removal of the tumor or radiation or both are treatment options. Patients who have a large pituitary tumor will occasionally develop a potentially life-threatening condition called pituitary apoplexy. Symptoms typically associated with pituitary apoplexy include sudden severe headache, decreased visual acuity, and ophthalmoplegia. Surgical decompression is an emergency procedure because permanent blindness may result if left untreated.

Transsphenoidal adenectomy surgery can often remove the tumor without affecting other parts of the brain. Endoscopic surgery has become common recently. External radiation is used to kill cancer cells and to shrink tumors. Stereotactic radiation therapy is a new procedure sending focused radiation directly into cancerous tissue. This is a precise technique that targets the cancer tumor, causing less damage to the surrounding tissues. Prolactinomas are most often treated with a dopamine agonist, as will be discussed in the next section of this chapter. Somatotropic adenomas respond to octreotide, a long-acting somatostatin analog, in many but not all cases. Unlike prolactinomas, thyrotrophic adenomas characteristically respond poorly to dopamine agonist treatment.

Hormone replacement therapy may be required after such a procedure.

Glucocorticoids are required if the ACTH-adrenal axis is impaired. This is particularly important in sudden collapse due to pituitary apoplexy or acute obstetric hemorrhage with pituitary insufficiency. In such circumstances, initiation of a possibly life-saving treatment pending a definitive diagnosis should not be delayed. The emergency measures apply hydrocortisone at a dose of 100-150 mg/day. In chronic treatment hydrocortisone 10-25 mg per day or 25-37.5 mg per day (usually 2-3 doses per day) is used.

Secondary hypothyroidism should be treated with thyroid hormone replacement. The dose of thyroxine should be adjusted so that the free thyroxine level is in the middle-upper normal range and tri-iodothyronine is normal.

In cases of gonadotropin deficiency, replacement therapy with estrogens and progestagens is used. The application of these hormones, as well as ways to induce ovulation with exogenous gonadotropin, are presented in section 3.4. (Hypogonadotropic hypogonadism/ management).

Growth hormone deficiency is treated with this hormone after dose adjustment to normal IGF-1 concentrations in the blood. Usually the dose for adults is 0.2-1 mg/day, and the dose for children is 25-50 μg/kg per day.

Diabetes insipidus is treated with desmopressin (0.3-1.2 mg/day oral, and 10-40 μg/day intranasal).

In most cases of hypopituitarism, the disorder is not preventable. Awareness of the risk allows early diagnosis and treatment. Hypopituitarism is usually permanent and requires life-long treatment. Adequate replacement of pituitary hormones can enhance quality of life, and reduces morbidity and mortality associated with this disorder.

8. Hyperprolactinemia

Hyperprolactinaemia is one of the most common endocrinological disorders affecting the hypothalamic-pituitary axis. The increase of prolactin level interrupts the pulsatile GnRH secretion and in turn causes disturbances of the menstrual cycle. Hyperprolactinaemia can occur in physiological and pathological conditions.

8.1 Prolactin secretion in physiological conditions

Prolactin (PRL) was originally identified as a neuroendocrine hormone of pituitary origin. PRL is a polypeptide hormone that as a result of posttranslational processes may take different forms. The monomeric form is a single chain polypeptide whose molecular weight is 23 kDa. PRL may occur in 50 kDa and 150 kDa molecular variants. These large PRL variants may be secreted predominantly; this condition is termed "macroprolactinemia". It is characterized by high immunological and normal biological serum levels of prolactin, and lack of clinical symptoms of hyperprolactinemia. Macroprolactin is formed by combination of the hormone with immunoglobulin IgG, or its autoantibodies. In normal conditions the monomeric isoform represents 75%-90% of the total hormone. The prolactin gene is located on chromosome 6 and contains 914 base pairs.

Prolactin receptor (PRLR) is a member of the cytokine receptor superfamily. The receptor is present in nearly all organs and tissues. Although the PRLR gene is unique in each species, alternative splicing generates different isoforms. A long PRLR isoform (long-R) and several short PRLR isoforms (short-R) have been detected. PRLR exists as seven recognized isoforms in humans. The role of prolactin in the mammary gland is largely the result of activity of the long-R isoform. It has been proposed that short-R isoforms inhibit the function of long-R, or act as positive regulators in the mammary gland. The mechanisms by which PRL signals through short-R isoforms remains unexplained. The long-R isoform is strongly expressed in the ovary, adrenal gland, kidney, mammary gland, small intestine, choroid plexus and pancreas, but other organs (e.g. liver) also express high levels of the short-R isoform. The various PRLR isoforms exhibit different signaling properties. It is also interesting to note that heterodimerization of different PRLR isoforms produces inactive complexes that might also be physiologically significant because PRL target cells usually express more than a single PRLR isoform.

The role of PRL in human ovarian function is unclear, in large part because no disruptive mutations of human PRL or the human PRLR have been identified. Furthermore, no study has yet compared the distribution of PRLR in human ovaries. Although it is not yet clear how PRL signals in the human ovary, signaling pathways induced by prolactin through its short-R isoform are very likely (Binart et al., 2010).

Hypothalamic regulation of PRL secretion mainly involves tonic inhibition via portal dopamine. This is in agreement with the fact that blockade of dopamine D2 receptors results in increased secretion of the hormone. Evidence suggests that prolactin secretion is regulated by three populations of hypothalamic dopaminergic systems: the tuberoinfundibular, tuberohypophyseal and periventricular hypophyseal dopaminergic neurons.

Prolactin secretion is also mediated by other factors, which stimulate prolactin gene transcription, synthesis of hormone, and its secretion. The most important and best studied of these are estradiol, TRH (thyrotropin releasing hormone), EGF (epidermal growth factor), and VIP (vasoactive intestinal peptide) (Binart et al., 2010). Serotonin (5-HT) has a stimulatory role in prolactin regulation by mediating suckling-induced rises. The stimulatory effect on prolactin secretion of estrogen is well known. The estrogen receptor binds directly to DNA, which contains an estrogen-responsive element, resulting in rapid stimulation of gene transcription. Estrogens act at the pituitary as well as at the hypothalamic level, affecting the secretion of GnRH by kisspeptin expressing cells. Estrogens can directly modify the neuronal activity of several brain regions which regulate reproduction. It should be emphasized that opioid peptides may mediate some effects of estrogen and thus affect the regulation of PRL secretion.

PRL is secreted in a pulsatile fashion, and it displays a circadian rhythm with nearly three times the increase of the hormone level at night, during sleep. The physiological causes of increased prolactin secretion are summarized in Table 7.

Although the pleiotropic actions of PRL are recognized, its role in regulating growth and differentiation of mammary tissues is better understood. PRL acts synergistically with steroid hormones, stimulates the growth and differentiation of mammary tissues (mammotrophic action), initiates the secretion of milk (lactotropic action), and sustains lactation (lactopoietic action). Experimental studies using animal models allow one to consider the participation of PRL in such physiological activities as behavior and in the brain in general metabolism, immune responses, and electrolyte balance. There are almost 300 functions or targets identified for this hormone in various species, but the question remains open as to which of them are really relevant in humans (Bernichtein et al., 2010). Unfortunately, until now there have not been found disorders related to the genes encoding human PRL or its receptor and therefore we lack a definitive clinical model of isolated PRL deficiency that could be used to completely identify the hormone function. The role of PRL in mammary cancer was suggested several decades ago, mainly based on observations involving animal models. However, a clinical and epidemiological study involving human patients failed to be conclusive. Nevertheless, studies on the role of PRL in breast tumorigenesis are constantly being developed. La Pensee and Ben-Jonathan (2010) in their elegant review presented the suggestion that a reduction in the ability of PRL and estrogens to confer chemoresistance should have several benefits for breast cancer patients, including an increase in the number as well as efficacy of valuable drugs. There is now clear evidence that high-normal circulating PRL levels increase breast cancer risk in both pre-menopausal and post-menopausal women (Bernichtein et al., 2010).

Type of stimulus	Additional explanations
Increased estrogen secretion	Pregnancy, puerperium, lactation, neonatal period
Nipple stimulation	Mechanical and during breast-feeding
Stimulation of the uterine cervix	Sexual intercourse
Sleep	Circadian rhythm
Stress, exercise and hypoglycemia	

Table 7. Physiological causes of increased PRL secretion

8.2 Hyperprolactinemia – laboratory results or pathology symptom?

Pathological hyperprolactinemia is defined as circulating PRL levels above the normal range, which occurs in conditions other than pregnancy and lactation, when hyperprolactinemia is due to physiological factors (Table 8).

Before a diagnosis of hyperprolactinemia can be made, it is necessary to exclude laboratory errors related to the technique for hormone assay, but also to the conditions of sampling. It is important that the sample of blood was collected in basal conditions after 11 o'clock in the morning, so as to eliminate early morning growth hormone associated with the circadian rhythm of secretion. In the final evaluation of the results it is important to incorporate three facts:

1. Hormone concentrations in blood (50-100 μg/L = average increase, > 100 μg/L = significant increase).
2. Presence or absence of circadian hormone secretion.
3. At high values, exclusion of macroprolactin.

Regardless of its cause, the degree of PRL increase correlates with the severity of hypogonadism. Serum concentrations of PRL greater than 100 μg/L are associated with amenorrhea. A PRL level of 50-100 μg/L can be associated with either amenorrhea or oligomenorrhea, and a level of 20-50 μg/L can result in shortening of the luteal phase (Helm et al., 2009). Absence of a circadian rhythm indicates tumors or macroprolactin as the cause of hyperprolactinemia. Macroprolactin diagnosis is based on the polyethylene-glycol (PEG) test.

In seeking the cause of pathological hyperprolactinemia, pharmacotherapy causing increased secretion of this hormone should be excluded. A significant increase in PRL is observed with therapeutic doses of neuroleptics, opiates, antidepressants, antihypertensives, antihistamines, and oral contraceptives. Low daily dosing regimens (e.g. 200 mg chlorpromazine), conventional antipsychotics or risperidone can cause significant prolactin elevations. A number of other agents are in development. Clozapine, quetiapine and olanzapine are reported either to cause no increase in prolactin secretion at all or to increase it only transiently and mildly. In contrast, risperidone and amisulpride cause a marked and sustained increase in serum prolactin levels. Conventional antipsychotic agents differ in their ability to pass the blood-brain barrier. Because the pituitary gland lies outside this barrier, one would expect that drugs with poor brain penetrability and higher serum concentrations such as sulpiride would have a greater effect on pituitary prolactin secretion. Antidepressants with serotonergic activity, including selective serotonin reuptake inhibitors, monoamine oxidase inhibitors and some tricyclic antidepressants, can cause modest elevations of prolactin levels and have the potential to elevate prolactin levels above the threshold (Wieck & Haddad, 2003). The main drugs that can cause hyperprolactinemia are summarized in Table 8.

The major cause of pathological hyperprolactinemia involves tumors of pituitary lactotroph cells (prolactinomas). Prolactin-secreting pituitary tumors also include GH-producing pituitary tumors, which in 25% of cases co-secrete PRL. Prolactinomas are classified as microadenomas (<10 mm) or macroadenomas (>10 mm).

Macroprolactinomas are frequently characterized by suprasellar penetration, and increased secretion of PRL. High PRL level may mean cavernous sinus invasion, and resistance to dopamine agonist. A serum cutoff level of 3300 μg/L predicts an invasive tumor with specificity of 91% (Helm et al., 2009).

Prolactinoma development is presently being studied employing molecular biological techniques; the question of whether tumorigenesis can be attributed to specific defects of gene regulation remains to be answered.

Neuroleptics	Phenothiazines Thioxanthenes Butyrophenones Atypical antipsychotics
Antidepressants	Tricyclic and tetracyclic antidepressants Monoamine oxidase inhibitors Selective serotonin reuptake inhibitors Other
Opiates and cocaine	
Antihypertensive medications	Verapamil Methyldopa Reserpine
Gastrointestinal medications	Metoclopramide Domperidone Histamine receptor blockers (?)
Protease inhibitors (?)	
Estrogens	

(?) - Case reports only

Table 8. Medication that may cause hyperprolactinemia (Helm et al. 2009)

Hyperprolactinemia also occurs in other types of adenomas, such as multihormonal adenomas, as well as in tumors of the pituitary stalk. Hyperprolactinemia accompanies diseases such as chronic renal failure, liver cirrhosis, epilepsy, polycystic ovary syndrome and chest injuries.

8.3 Treatment

The main goal of treatment of hyperprolactinemia is to eliminate symptoms through reduction of prolactin secretion. The largest group of patients needing treatment is that of women with micro- and macroprolactinoma. Treatment should lead to normalization of PRL levels, restoration of ovary function, reduction of tumor size, and recovery of pituitary function. Currently available medications to treat symptomatic hyperprolactinemia, mainly caused by prolactinomas, are dopamine agonists and include bromocriptine, quinagolide, and cabergoline. Pergolide is no longer used because of the finding that patients with Parkinson's disease who were treated with this dopamine agonist had increased risk of valvular heart diseases.

Bromocriptine (BEC) is generally considered to be the agent of choice in the treatment of prolactinomas, because it is well tolerated, and may be used chronically, over a long period of time. BEC is a safe medicine that effectively reduces the synthesis and secretion of PRL. Treatment begins with a low dose (1.25-2.5 mg/day) and then gradually increases to the minimum effective dose. The average daily dose is 2.5-15 mg, although about 30% of patients with macroadenomas require increased doses of 20-30 mg/day. It is usually used in 2-3 divided doses throughout the day. In approximately 80% of patients BEC effectively decreases the plasma PRL levels, and also reduces tumor size by 50% in 70% of cases. A limitation of the use of BEC is side effects such as dizziness, nausea, and vomiting. It is estimated that about 15% of patients are completely unable to tolerate therapeutic doses of BEC. In contrast to patients with microprolactinoma, in cases of macroprolactinoma the extent of reduction in tumor size is not well correlated with the change in plasma PRL levels which always precedes tumor shrinkage, and patients who do not show a drop in PRL do not have any tumor shrinkage (Babu Segu, 2011).

Another drug used in cases of hyperprolactinemia is the non-ergot dopamine agonist quinagolide, which has a long duration of action. The advantage of the drug is a lower number of adverse events than in the case of BEC with comparable efficacy. Tolerance of the drug may be reduced by alcohol. Treatment begins with a dose of 25 µg/day, which is increased in 3 consecutive days to 75 µg/day. In case of unsatisfactory results of treatment it can be increased to 150 µg/day. It is given as one dose per day.

In patients who do not respond to BEC or who cannot tolerate both the drugs mentioned above, a long-acting dopamine agonist, cabergoline, can be used. It is well tolerated, and its efficacy profiles are somewhat superior to those of BEC and quinagolide. It can be administered twice a week, with the usual starting dose of 0.25 mg biweekly to a maximum dose of 1 mg biweekly. As an adjunct or second line therapy of acromegaly, cabergoline has low efficacy in suppressing growth hormone levels and is highly efficient in suppressing the hyperprolactinemia that is present in 20-30% of acromegaly cases. It has at times been used as an adjunct to SSRI antidepressants as there is some evidence that it counteracts certain side effects of those drugs, such as reduced libido and anorgasmia. It has also been suggested that it has a possible use to control gynecomastia caused by elevated prolactin levels, through the use of anabolic steroids. Additionally, a systematic review and meta-analysis concluded that prophylactic treatment with cabergoline reduces the incidence, but not the severity, of ovarian hyperstimulation syndrome (Youssef et al., 2010).

Side effects are mostly dose dependent. Much more severe side effects are reported for treatment of Parkinson's disease with cabergoline, but when it is used for treatment of hyperprolactinemia and other endocrine disorders or gynecologic indications where the typical dose is significantly lower, the side effects are smaller. The list of possible, though rare side effects of treatment with cabergoline include nausea, constipation, dry mouth, vomiting, dyspepsia, insomnia, depression and very rarely dyskinesia and hallucinations. In two studies published in the New England Journal of Medicine on January 4, 2007, cabergoline was implicated along with pergolide in causing valvular heart disease (Schade et al., 2007; Zanettini et al., 2007). Both drugs are ergot-derived dopamine agonists, although their molecular skeletons are different. As a result of this, cabergoline is not approved in the U.S. for Parkinson's disease, but for hyperprolactinemia the drug remains on the market. The lower doses required for treatment of hyperprolactinemia have been found not to be associated with clinically significant valvular heart disease or cardiac valve regurgitation (Food and Drug Administration Public Health Advisory, 2007).

Transsphenoidal pituitary adenectomy is the preferred surgical treatment in patients with microprolactinoma and in most patients with macroprolactinoma. A transcranial approach is used in patients with large extrapituitary extension. Indications for neurosurgical treatment of prolactinoma are limited to specific clinical situations. These situations are: microadenoma in women desiring pregnancy and who cannot tolerate BEC, lack of consent of a patient with chronic long-term medication with BEC or other dopamine agonist, and lack of response to pharmacological treatment used, or occurrence of progression after an initial response.

Indications for emergency neurosurgical treatment are the states which were described in the section on hypopituitarism in this chapter. After surgical treatment the recurrence rate is about 15%-20%. Mortality and morbidity rates are less than 1% and 6%, respectively (Babu Segu , 2011). Pharmacological therapy of prolactinoma should be monitored for serial assay of plasma PRL levels, which should be repeated at least every two months. MRI, especially in cases of treated macroprolactinoma, should be repeated at least once a year.

9. Androgen excess in women

Androgen excess is one of the most common endocrine disorders of young women. According to the literature, these conditions apply to 7-10% of reproductive-aged women (Frank, 1995 ; Azziz et al., 2004 a; Abdel-Rahman & Hurd, 2010). Patients with androgen excess represent approximately 18% of hospitalizations in the department of gynecological endocrinology. The main reasons for the patients to undergo medical examinations are as follows: oligo/amenorrhea, ovulatory dysfunction, excess body and facial terminal hair growth, acne, alopecia, obesity and infertility. Many specific underlying disorders can be identified in androgen excess women. The above-mentioned causes are summarized in Table 9.

Polycystic ovary syndrome Hyperandrogenism, insulin resistance, and acanthosis nigrans (HAIR-AN) syndrome Ovarian hyperthecosis Androgen secreting ovarian tumors
Congenital adrenal hyperplasia (CAH) and nonclassic adrenal hyperplasia (NCAH) Cushing syndrome Androgen secreting adrenal tumors
Functional androgen excess Idiopathic hirsutism Hyperprolactinemia Pregnancy Exogenous androgens

Table 9. Cause of androgen excess in women

9.1 Androgens: definitions and sources of their synthesis

Chemical compounds called androgens stimulate growth of male genitals. According to another definition, androgens are hormones supporting male sexual behavior in castrated animals. These hormones can be defined as androgen receptor ligands that can regulate gene expression, thus affecting their own performance. The androgen receptor was discovered in 1970, and the gene that encodes it was cloned in 1988. The androgen receptor gene is located on the long arm of chromosome X. There are two isoforms of the androgen receptor (AR-A and AR-B). Both isoforms are present in almost all tissues and organs of the body. The highest affinity with the receptor is shown by dihydrotestosterone (DHT), lower by testosterone, and still lower by dehydroepiandrosterone and androstenedione. The adrenal glands and ovaries secrete five androgens through a similar pathway: testosterone, dehydroepiandrosterone sulfate (DHEAS), dehydroepiandrosterone (DHEA), androstenedione, and androstenediol, the latter of which has both androgenic and

estrogenic activity (Labrie, 2010). Testosterone and its biologically active metabolite dihydrotestosterone (DHT) are the only active androgens. DHEAS, DHEA, and androstenedione are all precursors of testosterone.
The ovaries produce 25% of circulating testosterone, whose secretion is controlled by LH. The ovaries also secrete 50% of the androstenedione and 20% of DHEA. The adrenal glands produce all the DHEAS, 80% of the DHEA, 50% of androstenedione and 25% of circulating testosterone, mainly via conversion of androstenedione to testosterone. DHEAS and 11-androstenedione are not secreted by the ovaries and therefore are used as markers of adrenal androgen secretion. Adrenal androgen secretion is controlled by ACTH. PRL and estrogen can affect adrenal androgen production (Abdel-Rahman & Hurd, 2010). Clinical manifestation of androgen excess may be the result of growth of androgen production, increase of receptor sensibility (receptor expression), and increased activity of 5-α-reductase (the enzyme responsible for converting testosterone to dihydrotestosterone).

9.2 Clinical features of androgen excess patients

The main symptoms of androgen excess in women are summarized in Table 10. Azziz et al. (2004 a) published a clinical study of over 1000 patients with symptoms of androgen excess. Complete relevant information could be obtained from the authors of 873 patients and they were included in the study. Oligo-ovulation was present in 88.2% of patients, most of whom showed menstrual disorders, mainly oligomenorrhea.

Defeminization symptoms	Oligo/amenorrhea, anovulation, infertility
Masculinization symptom	Hirsutism, acne, androgenic alopecia, clitoromegaly, increased muscle mass, lower tone of voice, masculine habitus
Metabolic disorders	Obesity, glucose intolerance, insulin resistance, lipid disorders, acanthosis nigricans

Table 10. Main symptoms of androgen excess in women

Most published studies support the view that the presence of hirsutism is a strong indicator of androgen excess (Azziz et al., 2006; Yidiz et al., 2010). Hirsutism refers to the occurrence in women of terminal hairs in characteristically masculine areas. Terminal hairs demonstrate regional morphological differences. Their growth and development is primarily stimulated by GH and thyroid hormones, and depending on body region, also by androgens (Yidiz et al., 2010). The optimal androgen effect requires the presence of normal androgen receptor and 5α-reductase function, although testosterone in sufficient concentration can also exert a direct effect on the hair follicle without the involvement of 5-α-dihydrotestosterone. 5-α-reductase, as both of its isoenzymes (type I and type II), is present in dermal papillae of the lower abdomen in hirsute women, and its activity was demonstrated to be regulated by androgens (Skalba et al., 2006).
The identification and assessment of the severity of hirsutism is determined visually using quantification of normal and abnormal hair growth in women. Ferriman and Gallwey (1961) evaluated eleven body areas in normal white women; each body area was scored on a scale

of 0-4. The authors observed that a score of >7, when summing the scores of all the body areas assessed with the exception of lower arms and legs, was observed in only 4.3% of their population. The results of most clinical studies suggest that 5-7% of unselected women of reproductive age have a point value according to the Ferriman Gallwey score >8, which can be used as the cut-off value to define hirsutism. It should be noted that hair is second only to skin color as a feature of racial difference. The number of hair follicles per unit skin area and the rate of hair growth vary among ethnic and racial groups. For example, in the population of Asian women (which includes Chinese, Japanese, Koreans, American Indians, and Eskimos) the overall density of facial and body terminal hair growth is lower, and the definition of hirsutism may therefore require a lower cut-off value (Yidiz et al., 2010). However, population studies involving 633 unselected women confirmed that the degree of facial and body terminal hair was similar in black and white women (De Ugarte et al., 2006). A modified Ferriman and Gallwey score, which evaluates nine body areas, is widely used by clinical endocrinologists, because it is a simple and practical method (Hatch et al., 1981). However, moderate to severe unwanted hair growth confined to one or two areas of the body, particularly the upper lip, chin, and lower abdomen, may be a sign of androgen excess (Fig. 2).

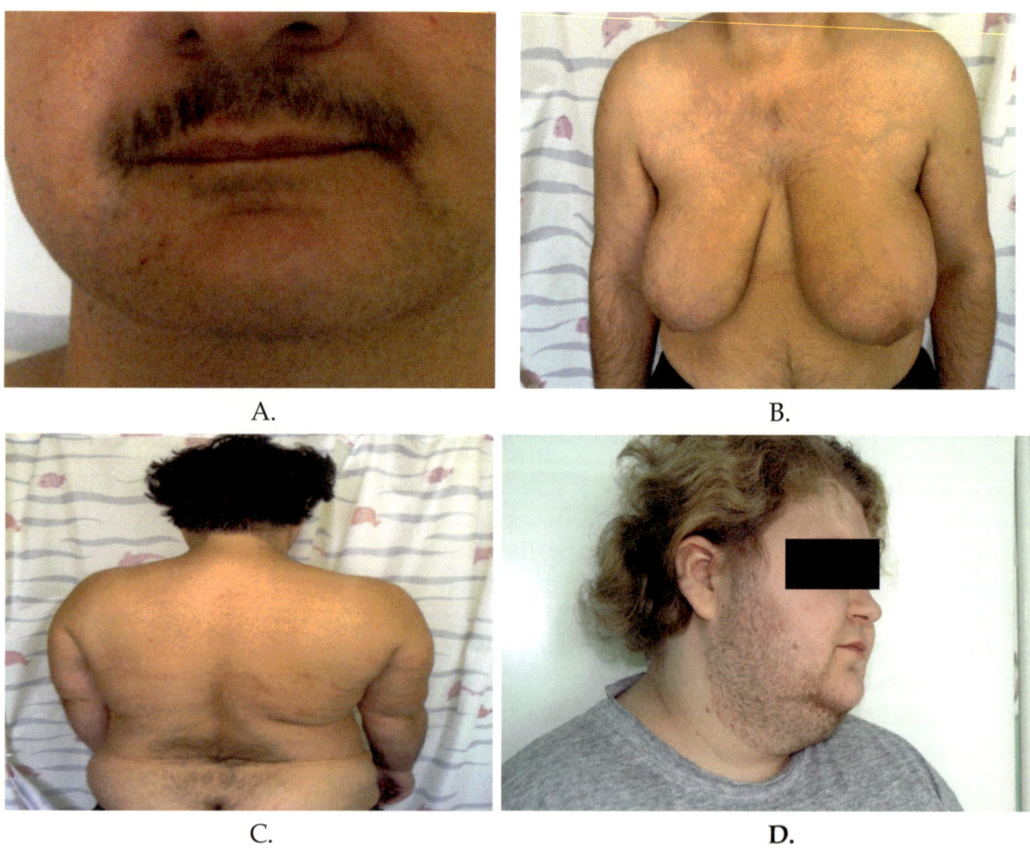

Fig. 2. Hirsutism in 37-year-old woman with diagnosed PCOS (A,B,C). Facial hirsutism in 25-year-old woman diagnosed with HAIR-AN syndrome (D).

According to studies cited above, 75.5% of patients with androgen excess had hirsutism, and 14.2% had acne, whereas 29.7% complained of infertility. Patients with infertility were more obese than their non-infertile counterparts (Azziz et al. 2004 a). Various studies have evaluated the impact of obesity on androgen excess in women. It was found that obese hyperandrogenic women are characterized by a significantly lower sex hormone binding globulin (SHBG) plasma level and more severe hyperandrogenemia, in comparison to their normal-weight counterparts. There is, therefore, consistent evidence that increasing body weight may favor a more severe form of disorders of hyperandrogenic women. Epidemiological studies show that the prevalence of obesity in women with androgen excess is within 40%-60% (Pasquali et al., 2007). These women have a tendency to visceral deposition of fat, mainly in the abdomen. Obesity in hypoandrogenic women is associated with metabolic changes, principally insulin resistance and metabolic syndrome. Metabolic syndrome is an integral part of androgen excess in women. In the typical form, it includes insulin resistance, obesity, and altered lipid profile. The molecular mechanism of insulin resistance in this disorder differs from those in other common insulin-resistance states, such as simple obesity, and type 2 diabetes mellitus. In these cases, hyperinsulinemia and subnormal insulin-mediated glucose uptake were observed. Insulin resistance in women with androgen excess is not observed in all tissues. Specifically, it is present in skeletal and adipose tissue, whereas insulin resistance is absent in the ovaries, adrenal glands, liver and skin. The cause of insulin resistance in polycystic ovary syndrome (PCOS) is considered to be a defect of the insulin receptor and insulin signaling in the post-receptor pathways. The defect lies in reduced autophosphorylation of the insulin receptor, secondary to excessive phosphorylation of serine residues of this receptor, which impairs its function and reduces further transmission of the signal. In addition, compensatory hyperinsulinemia exerts an androgen stimulatory effect on the ovaries and adrenal glands. Insulin resistance occurs more in obese hyperandrogenic women, but it can also occur in lean hyperandrogenic women. Dunaif et al. (1989) demonstrated that obese and lean hyperandrogenic women were both more insulin resistant than BMI-matched normal controls.

10. Polycystic ovary syndrome (PCOS)

10.1 PCOS – definition and epidemiology

PCOS is a very common endocrinopathy with heterogeneous presentation, whose etiology is unclear. The formulation of a precise definition is therefore difficult, and diagnostic criteria for PCOS remain controversial. After reviewing the literature, the most convincing seems to be the definition proposed by Azziz (Azziz, 2007): "Polycystic ovary syndrome (PCOS) is a heterogeneous disorder, whose principal features include androgen excess, ovulatory dysfunction, and/or polycystic ovaries".

Establishing the diagnosis of PCOS requires the exclusion of other androgen excess and ovulatory disorders of clearly defined etiologies. The list of disorders that require exclusion are nonclassic adrenal hyperplasia, which will be discussed later in this chapter, adrenal or ovarian androgen-secreting tumors, Cushing's disease and use or abuse of androgenic or anabolic drugs. The functional disorder resulting in clinical features suggestive of androgen excess, namely idiopathic hirsutism, should also be excluded. Causes of hyperandrogenism in women are shown in Table 9.

Ovulatory dysfunction is generally detectable by the presence of clinically evident oligo-amenorrhea, although about 20-30% of eumenorrhea PCOS women will present oligo-anovulation.

Ultrasound diagnosis of polycystic ovaries is often inconsistent with accepted criteria, and thus inappropriate. In addition, an ultrasound symptom of polycystic ovaries also occurs in other clinical situations.

It should be emphasized that PCOS is, by its nature, a set of symptoms, signs and biochemical features that can occur in various combinations. Deciding what combination of pathological features is sufficient for the diagnosis of PCOS was the subject of consultation of experts. The first definition of PCOS was determined by an expert conference sponsored by the US National Institutes of Health (NIH) in 1990 (Azziz, 2007). In May 2003 a group of experts in the field of PCOS, which gathered in Rotterdam for a conference sponsored jointly by the European Society for Human Reproduction and Embryology and the American Society for Reproductive Medicine, established the first agreed definition of PCOS (the Rotterdam ESHRE/ASRM-Sponsored PCOS Consensus Workshop Group 2004). The resulting statement of this conference constituted criteria, known as the "Rotterdam criteria", which are now commonly used in practice and the literature for defining PCOS. Some experts believe, however, that the Rotterdam Criteria do not resolve all controversies concerning the definition of PCOS (Franks, 2006). The discussion is whether hyperandrogenic women with polycystic ovaries and regular cycles should be included in the definition established in Rotterdam. Another, in my opinion, very important issue is to determine whether PCOS women with chronic anovulation without evidence of androgen excess should be defined as part of the syndrome. Opinions on this matter are varied. Certainly, the combination of hyperandrogenism and chronic anovulation provides a widely accepted basis for the diagnosis of PCOS. It was observed that PCOS women with hyperandrogenism and regular cycles are less likely to have insulin resistance and hyperinsulinemia than those with chronic anovulation (Franks, 2006). Obese women with PCOS are more likely to be anovulatory than lean hyperandrogenic subjects. These observations indicate the relationship between metabolic disorders and the maturation of ovarian follicles. With regard to the controversy over the definition of PCOS, the Androgen Excess Society (AES) recommend an evidence-based definition for this disorder. According to all available data, PCOS should be diagnosed according to the presence of three features: (a)androgen excess (clinical and/or biochemical hyperandrogenism), (b) ovarian dysfunction (oligo-anovulation and/or polycystic ovarian morphology), and (c) exclusion of other androgen excess or ovulatory disorders (Azziz et al., 2006). PCOS diagnostic criteria established by the three expert groups are summarized in Table 11.

According to the Rotterdam criteria there are four different phenotypes of PCOS patients, whereas in the AES criteria the phenotype of patients with PCOS is the only one (Figure 2).

New proposed additions to and at the same time simplifications of the diagnostic criteria for PCOS are the inclusion of plasma AMH levels, and calculation of the follicle number (Dewailly et al., 2010).

The prevalence of PCOS will depend to a degree on the criteria used to define this disorder. Using the NIH criteria in unselected women of reproductive age, the prevalence of clinically evident PCOS ranges from 6.5 to 8%. The racial difference was not statistically different (Azziz, 2007), although recently it has been suggested that PCOS is more prevalent in women of South Asian descent, based on clinical findings in South Asian immigrants and women in Britain (Chang 2009 a). The prevalence of PCOS according to the Rotterdam and AES criteria appears to be over 60% larger than the group classified as PCOS by the NIH definition. Approximately 80-90% of women with excess androgen have PCOS (Azziz et al., 2004 b; Dennedy et al., 2010). There are many factors influencing the prevalence of PCOS, such as metabolic disorders, premature adrenarche, and gestational diabetes.

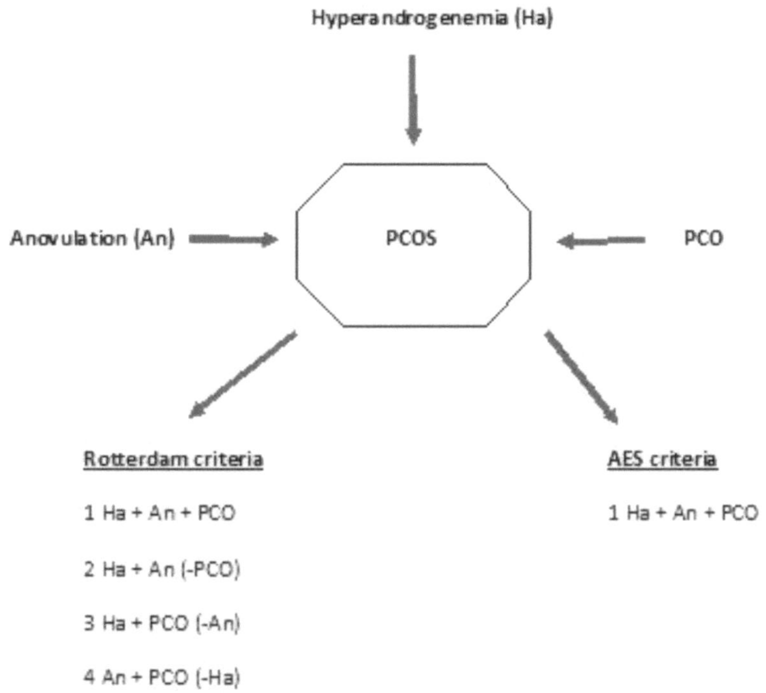

Fig. 3. PCOS phenotypes according to Rotterdam and AES criteria.

NIH 1990	**To include all of the following:** • Clinical hyperandrogenism and/or hyperandrogenemia • Chronic anovulation Exclusion of related disorders
ESHRE/ASRM (Rotterdam) 2003	**To include two of the following, in addition to exclusion of related disorders:** • Oligo-anovulation • Hyperandrogenism and/or hyperandrogenemia Exclusion of related disorders
AES 2006	**To include all of the following:** • Hyperandrogenism (hirsutism and/or hyperandrogenemia) • Ovarian dysfunction (oligo-anovulation and/or polycystic ovaries) • Exclusion of related disorders

NIH - US National Institutes of Health, ESHRE - European Society for Human Reproduction and Embryology, ASRM - American Society of Reproductive Medicine, and AES - Androgen Excess Society.

Table 11. Criteria for defining PCOS by Azziz (2007)

10.2 PCOS etiology

PCOS appears to have a complex, multifactorial etiology, wherein multiple predisposing genes interact with environmental and lifestyle factors responsible for the occurrence of disease symptoms constituting part of PCOS. Family studies demonstrate that PCOS is significantly more prevalent among family members than in the general population (Goodarzi, 2007). In both female and male first-degree relatives of patients with PCOS there occur more frequently than in the general population hormonal disorders, metabolic and phenotypic characteristics, such as premature balding in men and symptoms of hyperandrogenism in women. Hyperandrogenemia has been reported in 46% of sisters of PCOS women, of whom 22% were diagnosed with full-blown PCOS. Also in mothers of women with PCOS hyperandrogenemia was found. Moreover, in families of women with PCOS metabolic abnormalities are observed such as obesity, insulin resistance, and abnormal carbohydrate and lipid metabolism.

Numerous publications have allowed the compilation of a list of candidate genes responsible for different phenotypes of PCOS. The basis for creating a list of candidate genes is a hypothetical role of individual genes in PCOS, and the probability that polymorphisms are associated with the phenotype in populations or in families. These gene lists of candidates, constantly updated, can be found in numerous publications (Goodarzi, 2007 ; Wang et al., 2009; Panneerselvam, 2010). As a result, despite a large number of positive reports, no particular gene is universally recognized as significantly contributing to PCOS risk. The problem with PCOS is that the causes of it are still fundamentally unknown.

10.3 Clinical evaluation of PCOS

It has been estimated that approximately 75% of patients with PCOS have menstrual dysfunction, but approximately 20% of women diagnosed with PCOS will present with a history of apparent eumenorrhea. In most PCOS women with eumenorrhea anovulation occurs, but it may be prudent to confirm this in a repeated study.

Elevated circulating androgen levels are observed in approximately 60-80% of PCOS patients. The measurement of circulating androgen levels, including free testosterone and free androgen index (FAI), has been used only as an adjuvant for the diagnosis of hyperandrogenic disorders and never as the sole criterion for diagnosis. In fact, 20-40% of women with PCOS will have androgen levels within the normal range.

Clinical features of hyperandrogenism frequently seen in PCOS include hirsutism, acne, and androgenic alopecia. The diagnosis and assessment of severity of hirsutism are discussed above. Acne affects 15-25% of PCOS patients, although it is unclear whether the prevalence of acne is significantly increased in these patients compared to the normal population of similar age. Androgenetic alopecia is rare in patients with PCOS; possibly the incidence of this symptom is about 5% (Azziz et al., 2006).

Current data suggest that polycystic ovaries detected by ultrasound examination may be found in approximately 75% of PCOS women. This high percentage may be associated with false-positive test results. Ultrasound diagnosis of PCOS requires strict criteria. The criteria to define PCOS should include at least one of the following: either 12 or more follicles measuring 2–9 mm in diameter, or increased ovarian volume (>10 cm^3).

If there is a follicle >10 mm in diameter, the scan should be repeated at a time of ovarian quiescence in order to calculate the volume and area (Fig. 4).

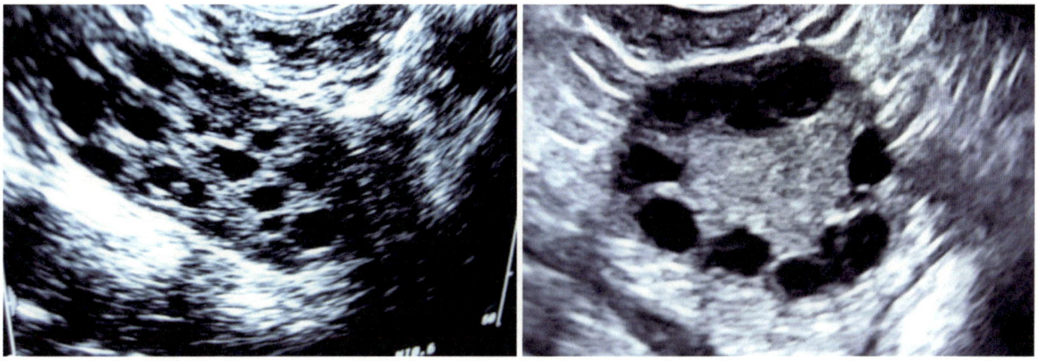

A. B.

Fig. 4. Sonography scans of polycystic ovaries (PCO)- A. central distribution of follicles, B. peripheral distribution of follicles.

The presence of a single polycystic ovary (PCO) is sufficient to establish the diagnosis. The distribution of follicles and a description of the stroma are not required in the diagnosis (Balen et al., 2003). However, note that PCO is a common, age-dependent finding among ovulatory women. The prevalence of PCO by AFC (antral follicle count) was 32% and decreased with age (Johnstone et al., 2010). Starting from the first descriptions of morphological changes in the ovary, we know that they are enlarged, with numerous peripheral small antral follicles and increased central stroma. It has been proposed that normal follicular growth appears to occur up to the mid-antral stage, after which maturation ceases. Stopping follicular maturation, however, does not prevent apoptosis, although it is not known if it will delay it. Several studies confirm that the plasma level of AMH in PCOS women is 2-3 times higher than in healthy women of similar age. We also know that this level correlates with the number of small antral follicles and plasma androgen levels. I have also observed that the characteristic reduction in AMH levels with age is delayed in PCOS women compared to their healthy peers (unpublished investigation). The evidence presented indicates the involvement of androgens in follicular development.

Obesity, insulin resistance and hyperinsulinism, the symptoms already discussed above, occur in a large proportion of PCOS patients. The PCOS-related insulin resistance state is associated both with decreased ability of insulin to stimulate glucose delivery to target cells and with reduction of glucose response to a given amount of insulin. In fact, a reduction of the transporter GLUT-4 expression in the insulin target tissues has been demonstrated (Palomba et al., 2009).

Abnormalities of lipid metabolism in PCOS include reduced levels of HDL cholesterol and increased LDL cholesterol and triglycerides. It seems that dyslipidemia develops secondary to insulin resistance, because insulin affects the regulation of lipoprotein lipase activity and lipid pathways of change.

10.4 PCOS laboratory and sonographic evaluation

Azziz (2007) proposes to divide the patients suspected of having PCOS into three subgroups, and for each of them to apply the appropriate diagnosis as follows.

a. Women with overt long-term oligomenorrhea and hirsutism: these women basically have PCOS, pending exclusion of related disorders. Circulating TSH, PRL, and 17OHP

(17-hydroxyprogesterone) levels should be determined. If these values are normal, then the patient is presumed to have PCOS. Androgen levels and ovarian ultrasonography, while of some value, are not critical to establish the diagnosis.

b. Women with overt long-term oligomenorrhea, but no obvious sign of androgen excess. Circulating androgen levels (total and free testosterone, and DHEAS) should be determined, and if elevated, assessment of TSH, PRL, and 17OHP should be made. If these latter values are normal, then the patient is presumed to have PCOS. In these women the use of ovarian ultrasonography will not alter the diagnosis.

c. Women with hirsutism but apparent eumenorrhea: these women should undergo confirmation of ovulation (determination of progesterone in the luteal phase). They should also undergo ovarian ultrasonography. If the patient is found to have anovulation or polycystic ovaries, they should have TSH, PRL and 17OHP assessed. If these values are normal, then the patient is presumed to have PCOS (classic if anovulatory, or ovulatory PCOS if she has polycystic ovaries but normal ovulation).

It seems obvious that PCOS cannot be diagnosed by symptoms alone. As is apparent from the above proposals of Azziz, depending on the symptoms, appropriate tests should be used. Most often, the following hormone levels are measured when considering a PCOS diagnosis: LH, FSH, PRL, total and free testosterone, FAI (free androgen index), DHEAS, androstenedione, progesterone, estradiol, TSH and 17OHP.

Correct values for levels of **LH, FSH**, estradiol and progesterone are presented in Section 2.3 (Menstrual cycle). In some PCOS women the LH level is about 18 IU/L and FSH is about 6 IU/L. This situation is called an elevated LH to FSH ratio or 3:1 ratio. This result is sufficient for ovulation inhibition. Currently, changes in pituitary gonadotropin plasma levels are not included in the diagnostic criteria, although they are still an important test for the evaluation of complex disorders associated with PCOS. LH excess worsens hyperandrogenism through ovarian stimulation of androgenesis. LH excess has long been considered the cause of increased ovarian androgen secretion, but presently its primary role is arguable. There is in fact evidence that ovarian theca cells are capable of androgen production regardless of the stimulation of LH. All observations suggest that dysregulation of androgen biosynthesis is an intrinsic property of PCOS theca cells, and excess LH may be a consequence of the metabolic alterations in PCOS (Doi, 2008).

There are two methods to measure testosterone levels: **total testosterone, and free testosterone.** Total testosterone refers to the amount of all testosterone, including free testosterone. The range for this is 6.0-86 ng/dl (according to some methods up to 100 ng/dl). Free testosterone refers to the amount of testosterone that is unbound and actually active in the body. This is usually in the range 0.7-3.6 pg/ml. PCOS women often have increased levels of both total and free testosterone (usually slightly, although sometimes up to the level of older men).

Information on the current circulating free androgens can be obtained by calculating the **free androgen index (FAI)**. FAI is the quotient of the plasma concentration of total testosterone to plasma concentration of sex hormone binding globulin (SHBG), multiplied by 100%. Normal values should not exceed 5%.

SHBG is a glycoprotein that binds reversibly and with high affinity to the main biologically active circulating androgen testosterone, and somewhat less well with active estradiol. Its plasma concentrations being regulated by, among other things, androgen/estrogen balance, thyroid hormones, insulin and dietary factors, it is involved in transport of sex steroids in plasma, and its concentration is a major factor regulating their distribution between the protein-bound and free states. It was originally described as a hepatically secreted protein, and it also functions as part of a novel steroid signaling system that is independent of the classical intracellular steroid receptors. Unlike the intracellular steroid receptors that are ligand-activated transcription factors, SHBG mediates androgen and estrogen signaling at the cell membrane by way of cAMP (Kahn, 2003).

SHBG may be important both physiologically and in a number of endocrine disorders including PCOS (Anderson, 1974). A little of the testosterone is bound to corticosteroid-binding globulins (CBG); however, the main fraction of testosterone in plasma is bound to SHBG. In female plasma the SHBG concentration is twofold higher and the testosterone concentration tenfold lower than in men. SHBG is a glycoprotein, and its molecular weight has been variously estimated at 95 000. It was proved that estrogens stimulate and androgens inhibit SHBG production in the liver. It appears that the balanced increase in estrogen and androgen production in PCOS women causes only a small fall in SHBG. In hirsute women regardless of their menstrual history, a reduction in plasma levels of SHBG takes place. In these women, SHBG concentration may be reduced in over 80%. This finding is independent of the presence or absence of polycystic ovaries (PCO). Low SHBG levels in PCOS are intimately associated with BMI, suggesting that some signals from the adipose tissue, independent of adiponectin and leptin, may regulate liver production of SHBG. In many cases low SHBG levels are associated with a rise in plasma testosterone and other 17β hydroxy-androgens. Measurement of SHBG is useful in the evaluation of mild disorders of androgen metabolism and enables identification of those women with hirsutism who are more likely to respond to estrogen therapy.

Evidence suggests that hyperinsulinemic insulin resistance may increase serum levels of ovarian androgens and reduce sex hormone-binding globulin (SHBG) levels in women. Reasoned opinions are, therefore, that a low SHBG level is a strong risk marker for dysglycemia in women, independently of both adiponectinemia and insulinemia (Bonnet et al., 2009). SHBG may therefore improve the identification of women at risk of diabetes. Metabolic syndrome in women is associated with lower SHBG levels (Brand et al., 2011). SHBG levels are low in myxedema, acromegaly, Cushing syndrome, hyperprolactinemia and in obese women.

SHBG levels rise markedly in pregnancy to some 5-10 times those in normal non-pregnant women. SHBG plasma levels are also higher in cases of cirrhosis and thyrotoxicosis (Anderson, 1974).

Thyroid hormones produce an elevation of SHBG in normal subjects and in hirsute women.

Dehydroepiandrosterone sulfate (DHEAS) is an androgen that is secreted by the adrenal glands. Normal hormone levels in women show a wide range between 35 and 430 µg/dl. DHEAS secretion decreases from the age of 30 years and is already decreased, on average, by 60% at the time of menopause. In addition, there is a large variability in the circulating levels of DHEAS and therefore recognition of the hormone deficit is difficult (Labrie, 2010).

Most PCOS women tend to have DHEAS levels greater than 200 µg/dl (Sterling, 2011). Values above 800 µg/dl show the need for more accurate diagnosis, because it may indicate an adrenal tumor. Elevated plasma DHEAS levels in PCOS women were associated with the presence of acne and a significantly reduced risk of abdominal obesity, independent of serum testosterone concentration and insulin resistance (Chen et al., 2011).

Androstenedione is a hormone that is produced by the ovaries and adrenal glands. Normal plasma levels of androstenedione in women of reproductive age in the early follicular phase of the menstrual cycle range between 0.9 and 3.4 µg/l. It is believed that determination of the hormone in the blood, as well as the assessment of the ratio of androstenedione to dehydroepiandrosterone, is more important for the differentiation of PCOS and nonclassic adrenal hyperplasia (NCAH) than to diagnose this first.

17-hydroxyprogesterone (17-HP) determination in the blood of patients with androgen excess is used as a screen for NCAH. The blood samples should be obtained in the morning, and, most importantly, in the follicular phase of the menstrual cycle. Before the 17-HP assay corticosteroids medication should be discontinued. If the screening 17-HP level is >1.7 µg/l an acute 30-60 min ACTH stimulation test is performed. Detailed test results will be discussed in the sections of the chapter concerning NC-CAH.

Prolactin is a pituitary hormone, discussed in Section 8. of this chapter. Some PCOS women have an elevated prolactin level, typically falling within 25-40 µg/l .

Thyrotropin (TRH) should be determined in the blood as a routine test of the pituitary thyroid axis. PCOS women usually have normal TSH levels (0.4-3.8 IU/l).

Anti-Müllerian hormone (AMH), which is produced by ovarian granulosa cells in women in reproductive age. Plasma levels of AMH in women with PCOS are significantly higher than in healthy subjects. In PCOS women the average plasma level of AMH is 10.5 (+/- 3.6) µg/l, and is 5 times higher than in healthy women of comparable age. Interestingly, the progressive decrease of hormone levels with age is slower in women with PCOS than in healthy controls. This may suggest a larger ovarian reserve in women with PCOS (Skałba P & Cygal A. 2011) (Fig. 5).

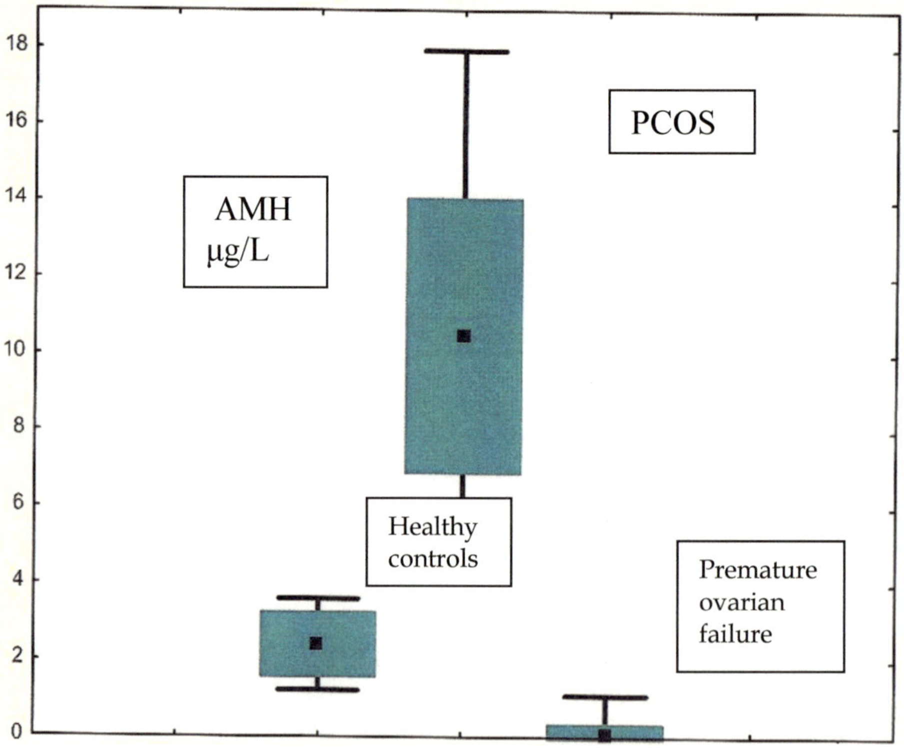

Fig. 5. AMH plasma level in healthy controls and women with PCOS and premature ovarian failure.

Insulin and glucose. PCOS is often accompanied by hyperinsulinism and insulin resistance, as mentioned above. Most PCOS women should have a fasting plasma glucose test and oral glucose tolerance test (OGTT). Both tests allow one to identify risk factors for insulin resistance and diabetes. For the precise diagnosis of insulin resistance, the glycemic clamp test is used. However, this method is very cumbersome and should be reserved for research purposes. The level of plasma fasting insulin is highly variable (15-25%). In women of normal weight it falls within the range of 5-15 μIU/ml. Simple tests of sufficient specificity allowing for assessment of insulin resistance are the following factors: glucose/insulin, HOMA and QUICKI. All results are based on determinations of fasting glucose and insulin.
The quantitative insulin sensitivity check index (QUICKI) is calculated from the mathematical formula:
QUICKI= 1/ (log (fasting glucose [mg/dl])+log (fasting insulin [μIU/ml])).
A value less than 0.357 demonstrates insulin resistance.
Homeostasis model assessment (HOMA) is calculated from the mathematical formula:
HOMA= (fasting glucose [mmol/l]). (fasting insulin [μIU/ml]) . 22.5.
A factor value greater than 2.5 indicates insulin resistance.
The fasting glucose-insulin ratio is simple to calculate, but also the least sensitive. The factor is calculated from the mathematical formula:
G/I= fasting glucose (mg/dl) / fasting insulin (μIU/ml).
An index value below 4.5 indicates reduced insulin resistance.

10.5 Clinical significance of obesity in PCOS

Compounds of obesity with androgen excess have already been discussed above in the section "Clinical features of androgen excess patients". It is estimated that nearly half of women with PCOS are obese. Obese PCOS women had a greater prevalence of hirsutism (73% compared with 56%) and menstrual disorders than non-obese subjects. Obesity causes changes in metabolism, including insulin resistance, glucose intolerance and metabolic syndrome. The concentration of total testosterone and androstenedione in the serum is similar in the two subgroups but SHBG concentration is significantly lower, and free testosterone levels higher, in obese PCOS women. In addition, concentration of androsterone glucuronide, a marker of peripheral 5α-reductase activity, is higher in obese PCOS women than in non-obese ones. Such observations may suggest impaired bio-availability of androgens to peripheral tissues and enhanced activity of 5-α-reductase in obese subjects (Kiddy et al., 1990).
Obese women with PCOS are less likely to become pregnant. In addition, compared to normal-weight women, obese PCOS women may have lower ovulatory responses to pulsatile GnRH administration and lower pregnancy rates after gonadotropin administration (Pasquali et al., 2007).
Low birth weight modifies the relationship between insulin resistance and PCOS and seems to increase the risk of developing PCOS. Diet composition, eating disorders, and psychological stress seem to be related to the syndrome, even if no causal link has been clearly demonstrated. Intriguingly, obesity has an important pathophysiological impact on PCOS. There is some evidence that the pathogenetic factors involved in determining hyperandrogenism and metabolic abnormalities may differ somewhat between obese and lean PCOS women. In women with PCOS there were found elevated levels of these markers of inflammation, such as C-reactive protein, fibrinogen, IL-6, TNF-α and IL-18. Despite

reports that chronic inflammation of moderate intensity could have a role in the development of PCOS, it seems that it is secondary to obesity.
Epidemiological studies indicate that women with PCOS are at increased risk of developing cardiovascular disease. A fourfold increased risk of cardiovascular events was found in women with this syndrome (Carmina & Lobo, 1999; Chang et al., 2009 b).

10.6 Ovarian hyperthecosis

Hyperthecosis refers to an unusual conditions in which the ovary contains nests of luteinized theca cells scattered throughout the stroma. The extent of theca cell involvement may vary from minimal to extensive. Severe hyperthecosis may be accompanied by extensive and dense fibroblast growth that results in an enlarged ovary of extremely firm texture. Morphology of the ovaries is therefore different from the classic PCOS, but this syndrome is considered to be a variety of PCOS, because its primary symptom is hyperandrogenism. Ovarian stromal hyperthecosis has variable sonographic features. Most commonly the affected ovaries are either normal or slightly enlarged. A solid mass may infrequently be visible, and PCOS changes may coexist with ovarian hyperthecosis. A possible association of hyperthecosis ovary with fibrothecoma was also noted (Brown, 2009). In this disorder, the cells that produce androgens are likely to be hypersensitive to the action of LH, because the plasma level of LH is generally normal, with high levels of androgens. Androgen excess causes severe hirsutism, insulin resistance and sometimes acanthosis nigricans and clitoromegaly. Androgen production may be resistant to oral contraceptive therapy, but administration of GnRH analogs causes it to decrease (Chang , 2009 a). In ovarian hyperthecosis the suggested treatment is ovarian wedge resection, although this method has already been eliminated as a means of treatment with classical PCOS.

11. Hyperandrogenic insulin resistance-acanthosis nigricans syndrome (HAIR-AN)

Hyperandrogenism, insulin resistance and acanthosis nigricans constitute HAIR-AN syndrome. It is estimated that this syndrome occurs in 1-3% of women with hyperandrogenism, often in black women and women with visceral obesity and type 2 diabetes. According to the large Azziz (2004 a) studies, already cited, HAIR-AN prevalence is 3.2% of the androgen excess population.
Each of these components of HAIR-AN syndrome may also occur in women with polycystic ovary syndrome. Acanthosis nigricans is a focal hyperkeratotic, mostly gray-brown, rarely black, hyperpigmentation and papillary hyperplasia of the skin. It is usually located in the vicinity of the neck, axilla, elbows, knees and groin, but may also affect the navel and the anus, and even, in rare cases, the entire skin. These changes result from prolonged exposure to high concentrations of insulin on keratinocytes (Fig. 6).
Treatment in these cases is difficult. It is logical to use drugs that improve insulin resistance, but a randomized study of 12-month treatment with metformin or rosiglitazone showed no effect on the severity of acanthosis nigricans (Palomba et al., 2009).

12. Idiopathic hirsutism

Idiopathic hirsutism (spontaneous, simple, peripheral) is hirsutism which is not accompanied by anovulation or menstrual disturbances, and serum androgen levels are

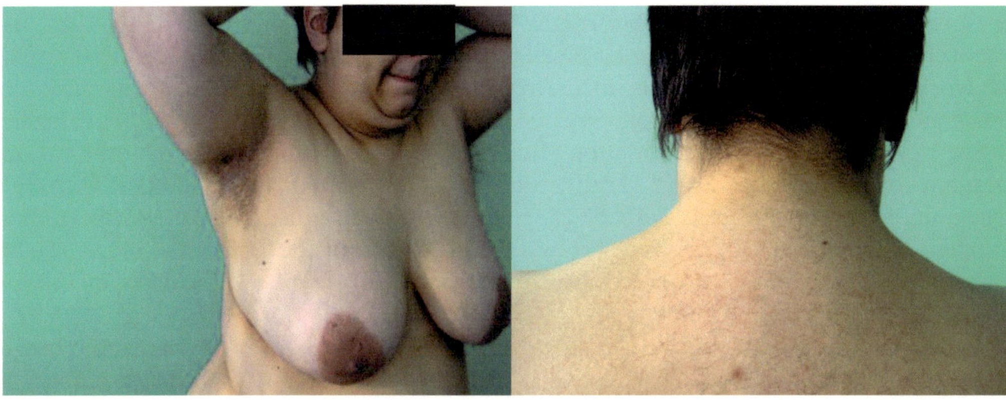

Fig. 6. 35-year-old woman diagnosed with HAIR-AN syndrome. Acanthosis nigricans in axilla and neck.

normal. It occurs in 15-20% of women with hirsutism. In some cases idiopathic hirsutism was found in a family. The pathogenesis of this type of hirsutism is believed to involve the role of increased activity of 5α-reductase in the skin, excessive sensitivity of androgen receptors to these hormones, and local effects of IGF-1, insulin, glucocorticoids, thyroid hormones and estrogen. In accordance with the recommendations of the Endocrine Society Clinical Practice Guideline Societies (Martin et al., 2008) detailed diagnosis of patients is essential in the following cases: (1). Hirsutism score is calculated as >15 points on the Ferriman and Gallwey scale. (2). Hirsutism occurs suddenly and is characterized by rapid progress. (3). Hirsutism is accompanied by at least one of the following symptoms: menstrual irregularities, infertility, central obesity, acanthosis nigricans, or clitoromegaly. Idiopathic hirsutism does not require medication, although if it is burdensome for the patient either pharmacological therapy or direct hair removal methods are recommended. For women who decide on treatment of hair removal, laser depilation is recommended (photoepilation), which can be further enhanced with the use of eflornithine cream (Martin et al., 2008).

13. Treatment of androgen excess

Appropriate and safe treatment depends on correct diagnosis of the cause of androgen excess. Such life-threatening diseases as ovarian and adrenal malignancy or Cushing syndrome need definitive treatment regardless of symptoms. Other more common disorders, such as PCOS, require treatment adapted to current needs, preferences and phenotype of the patient. Women with virilization require medical treatment, regardless of the identified cause, because of the dramatic and often irreversible cosmetic consequences and their psychological well-being (Abdel-Rahman & Hurd, 2010). The patient should be made aware that treatment requires prolonged and regular contact with a medical specialist. In adolescent girls the biggest problems associated with PCOS are oligo/amenorrhea, acne and hirsutism.

These patients most often respond to *oral contraceptives* (OCs). Both the estrogen and progestin components of OCs reduce androgen production by the ovary and adrenal glands. The estrogens increase SHBG production by the liver, and together with progestin work centrally by inhibiting pulsatile GnRH secretion. In addition, OCs containing the progestin drospirenone (17α-spironolactone derivate) block the androgen receptor.

For young patients who are overweight or obese, and who currently do not use contraception, insulin sensitizers may be proposed. *Metformin* is an oral antidiabetic drug that works by several mechanisms, including suppression of hepatic gluconeogenesis and gastrointestinal glucose absorption, and enhancement of insulin sensitivity, peripheral glucose uptake, and fatty acid oxidation (Tan et al., 2007). Metformin treatment of various symptoms of PCOS is the subject of numerous well-documented clinical studies. Currently metformin is commonly used to treat PCOS. It should be used as the first-choice agent in ovulation induction in PCOS women with insulin resistance (Palomba et al., 2009). Metformin freely crosses the placenta, resulting in exposure of the fetus to metformin therapeutic concentrations (Elliott et al., 1997).

According to experts, the use of metformin during pregnancy in PCOS women with previous miscarriage is safe and effective in reducing the rate of miscarriages (Glueck & Wang, 2007).

Metformin is indicated in patients over 10 years old, and the extended-release preparation is indicated in those over the age of 17 years (Palomba et al. 2009). It is believed that a dose of 1500-1700 mg/day is the optimal dose for induction of ovulation in PCOS women. Extremely variable target doses of 1500 to 2550 mg/day have been proposed. To minimize the drug-related adverse effects, metformin should be taken on an empty stomach, starting with a low dosage and gradually increasing over a period of 4-6 weeks. Nestler (2008) suggested administering immediate-release metformin initially at a low dose at meals, and increasing to the dose of 1000 mg twice daily.

Metformin is generally a well-tolerated drug. The most common side effect with metformin is gastrointestinal distress, which occurs in approximately 30% of patients taking metformin, limiting the compliance to treatment.

The list of gastrointestinal disorders consists of: abdominal discomfort, bloating, constipation, diarrhea, nausea and vomiting. Adverse events range from 3.3% (anovulatory bleeding) to 66% (nausea). The potential for serious side effects is estimated at 1%. Severe side effects of metformin treatment, such as lactic acidosis, can also be associated with high doses of metformin (higher than 3000 mg/d). Lactic acidosis is a rare complication of metformin administration (5.1 cases per 100 000 patient-years), although when it occurs, mortality of 50% has been observed (Palomba et al., 2009). The risk of occurrence of this severe complication increases in patients with hepatic or renal impairment, cardiac or respiratory insufficiency, severe infection, or alcoholism.

Most clinical studies indicate significant efficacy of metformin in the treatment of menstrual disorders. It is estimated that regular menstrual cycles and ovulation occur in between 35% and 90% of those treated with metformin. A meta-analysis comparing the effectiveness of PCOS treatment showed that metformin is less effective than OCs in improving the menstrual pattern (Costello et al., 2007). Effects of metformin compared with OCs are greater in the lowering of insulin and triglyceride levels but probably not in the cases of hirsutism and acne. Metformin treatment reduces the level of free testosterone, possibly due to the up-regulation of circulating levels of SHBG caused by improved insulin sensitivity, but there was not a significant treatment effect on total testosterone. It is therefore assumed that the effect of metformin on biochemical hyperandrogenism and its efficacy for clinical manifestation of hyperandrogenism are inconsistent (Palomba et al., 2009).

Other insulin-sensitizing agents include thiazolidinediones. The use of *troglitazone* at a dose of 600 mg/daily increased the ovulation rate, and reduced circulating insulin concentrations and the insulin response to an oral glucose challenge. There was also a decrease in circulating free testosterone concentrations and a rise in SHBG. Hepatic side effects were reported for troglitazone treatment. It was also found that *rosiglitazone* therapy improves insulin resistance and glucose tolerance in obese women with PCOS, decreases ovarian androgen production and hyperinsulinism, and short-term therapy helps restore spontaneous ovulation (Rautio et al., 2006; Sepilian,& Nagamani, 2005). Initial studies seemed to indicate that the treatment described above with the new insulin-sensitizing agents offers a new perspective of treatment for overweight anovulatory women with PCOS. But unfortunately, serious side effects, causing liver damage and increased risk of myocardial infarction, prevented the introduction of these drugs to the set of therapeutic agents in PCOS.

It should be emphasized that patients with symptoms related to PCOS increasingly demand treatment with metformin. A consensus of international experts (Thessaloniki, 2008) described the position of metformin in the treatment of infertility. The consensus is summarized in the following four points: (1) At present use of metformin in PCOS should be restricted to patients with glucose intolerance. (2) The decision about continuing insulin sensitizers during pregnancy in women with glucose intolerance should be left to obstetricians providing care and based on a careful evaluation of risk and benefits. (3) Metformin alone is less effective than clomifene citrate in inducing ovulation in women with PCOS. (4) There seems to be an advantage to adding metformin to clomifene citrate in women with PCOS. It should be noted that PCOS women treated with metformin are receiving treatment for an unlicensed indication. Therefore, *clinicians must counsel women appropriately before the initiation of metformin therapy* (Harborne et al., 2003).

Anti-androgens are another group of agents used as a first line therapy for hirsutism. However, the teratogenic potential of these drugs means that they should be used in conjunction with adequate contraception in women of reproductive age.

Spironolactone, an aldosterone antagonist, competes with testosterone and dihydrotestosterone at the androgen receptor. Although it primarily acts as a potassium-sparing diuretic, a dose of 50-200 mg per day will reduce facial hair growth in most patients after 6 cycles of treatment. Patients with hirsutism who take OCs with added spironolactone for 6 months achieve better results in reducing hirsutism. The drug is not devoid of side effects such as uterine bleeding, mastodynia, hair loss and fatigue. These symptoms do not occur often (less than 15% of patients).

A derivative of 17α-spironolactone is *drospirenone,* having drug action as an anti-androgen, anti-mineralocorticoid and progestin. Drospirenone has a high affinity for the progesterone and mineralocorticoid receptors and a low affinity for the androgen receptor. The drug is used in the contraceptive pill with 20 mg and 30 mg of ethinylestradiol. OCs with drospirenone are recommended for overweight PCOS women, and in the treatment of premenstrual syndrome.

Neither of the drugs mentioned above should be used in women with impaired renal function. During treatment, periodic checks of electrolyte levels, especially potassium, should be performed.

Cyproterone acetate is an anti-androgen as well as a progestin. The drug has strong progestational and anti-gonadotropic activity and is also a weak glucocorticoid. There is evidence that the drug inhibits the activity of 5-α reductase in the skin. So cyproterone acetate has an anti-androgenic effect both centrally and peripherally. The drug can be used in women with hyperandrogenism in doses ranging from 25 to 100 mg/day. It is also available in OCs as cyproterone acetate (2 mg) with ethinyl estradiol (35 µg). This drug is not currently available in the U.S. but in Europe OCs with cyproterone acetate have been widely used for many months in young women with hirsutism and acne. In more severe cases of these disorders cyproterone acetate can be used in a so-called reverse cycle. The reverse cycle is to add 25 or 50 mg of cyproterone acetate in the first 10 days of a 21-day cycle of application of OCs. Treatment should be discontinued for about 3 months before becoming pregnant.

Flutamide is an anti-androgen used for treatment of prostate cancer. Flutamide is very effective in treating hirsutism, but it is associated with frequent side effects and low long-term compliance. Hepatic cell damage, the major complication of flutamide, may be fatal (Abdel-Rahman, 2010). Consequently the drug is rarely used, is considered a second-line treatment, and is not approved by the FDA for treatment of hirsutism.

Finasteride selectively inhibits type 2 isoenzyme of 5-α-reductase to prevent the formation of 5-α-dihydrotestosterone. The drug is intended to treat benign prostatic hyperplasia and male pattern baldness. The FDA has not approved finasteride for treatment of hirsutism.

14. Infertility treatment related to PCOS

Before any intervention is initiated, preconceptional counseling should be provided emphasizing the importance of life style, especially weight reduction and exercise in overweight women, smoking and alcohol consumption.

According to the Thessaloniki ESHRE/ASRM-Sponsored PCOS Consensus Workshop Group (2007) first-line treatment for ovulation induction remains the anti-estrogen clomifene citrate (CC). The mechanism of drug action is not completely understood, but it is assumed that it increases the secretion of FSH. There are no specific criteria for PCOS women who have normal FSH and estradiol levels. Note also that in women with an increased ovarian volume and serious hyperandrogenism the response to CC is worse. Therefore, most clinicians recommend reducing plasma androgen levels before the start of ovulation stimulation. Patients with high BMI and older age also respond less well to CC, which is why their treatment with gonadotropins is justifiable.

The recommended dose is 50-150 mg of CC per day. The size of the initial dose is 50 or 100 mg/day depending on body weight. The maximum daily dose is 150 mg; higher doses do not increase efficacy. It is given for 5 days, starting from cycle day 2-5. If ovulation cannot be achieved within 6 months, further treatment is considered to be ineffective.

Hot flushes and visual complaints are well-recognized side effects during CC treatment, but they are rare, and the drug is considered safe. Metformin alone and in combination with CC were discussed above.

Recommended second-line treatment intervention, should CC fail to result in pregnancy, is either exogenous gonadotropin or laparoscopic ovarian surgery (LOS). Taking into account the risk of ovarian hyperstimulation syndrome (OHSS) in women with PCOS, low-dose protocols (37.5-75 IU FSH/day) are recommended. Currently two low-dose regimens are used:

1. Step-up regimens are based on the principle of stepwise increases in FSH supply to determine the FSH threshold for follicular development. If after use and treatment for a week there is no follicle increase, the dose should be increased.
2. The step-down regimen is designed to achieve the FSH threshold through a loading dose of FSH with subsequent stepwise reduction as soon as follicular development is observed on ultrasound.

It was proved that the step-up regimen is safer in terms of monofollicular development.
FSH treatment must be monitored, by serial ovarian ultrasound, and estradiol concentrations in the blood. Measurement of circulating estradiol levels has been used to cancel ovulation induction. Overall, ovulation induction (representing CC and FSH) is reported to be highly effective, with a cumulative singleton life birth rate of 72% (Thessaloniki Consensus, 2008).
The main indication for LOS is CC resistance in women with anovulatory PCOS. LOS also may be recommended for patients with hypersecretion of LH and patients who have experienced OHSS. Commonly employed methods for LOS include monopolar electrocautery (diathermy) and laser (ovarian drilling). Ovarian wedge resection is now rarely performed. A laser fiber or electrosurgical needle is used to puncture the ovary. Most authors use between four and ten punctures; however, more punctures have been associated with premature ovarian failure (Malkawi et al., 2003). There can be found in the literature very optimistic opinions, evaluating the efficacy of LOS obtained in 40-60% of pregnancies. However, according to experts, in 50% of LOS-treated patients, adjuvant therapy is required. In addition, five studies compared the effectiveness of LOS with that of gonadotropins for women with CC-resistant PCOS and did not find a difference in the ongoing pregnancy rate (Thessaloniki Consensus, 2008).
The recommended third-line treatment is in vitro fertilization.

15. Nonclassic congenital adrenal hyperplasia

One of the frequent causes of hyperandrogenism in young women is nonclassic congenital adrenal hyperplasia (NC-CAH). Whereas 21-hydroxylase (21-OH) deficiency accounts for the vast majority of NC-CAH, deficiency in 11-β-hydroxylase (11-OH) and 3--β-hydroxysteroid dehydrogenase (3-β-HSD) may result in the disorder (Azziz et al., 1994). The 21-OH genes are duplicated genes located on chromosome 6. The CYP21 gene (also designated CYP21B) is active, whereas CYP21A is inactive due to various nucleotide insertion, deletion, and point mutations. Approximately 90% of NC-CAH patients have one or more CYP21 mutations. Whereas NC-NAH is considered a homozygous recessive disorder, in most cases the same mutation does not affect both CYP21 alleles, and many patients have one mild and one severe CYP21 mutation (Azziz et al., 1994). Prevalent allelic mutations and genotypes were found to vary significantly among ethnic groups. There are ethnic-specific mutations in the CYP21A2 gene (for example, the mutation V281L is prevalent in Ashkenazi Jews). The phenotype of patients and severity of endocrine disorders depends on the specific genotype of patients, but assessment of the genotype is not possible on the basis of clinical manifestations (Bided et al., 2009).

15.1 Prevalence, clinical and biochemical features

NC-CAH appears to affect 1-2% of Caucasian hyperandrogenic women. In the Gynecological-Endocrinology Department of the Medical University of Silesia in the years 2003-2009, 2553 hyperandrogenic patients were hospitalized, and in 1.2% of them NC-CAH was identified (Franik & Skalba, 2011). It is estimated that in the populations of Central European countries, including Poland, and in the U.S. the incidence of NC-CAH is 1-2%. In contrast, studies from France, Italy, Croatia, and Canada have indicated prevalence of 3% to 6%, and studies from Israel, India and Jordan found prevalence of 6% to 10% (Romaguera, 2000). NC-CAH occurs much more frequently in the population of Ashkenazi Jews, Iranians and Yupik-speaking Eskimos of Western Alaska.

The symptoms of hyperandrogenism most often manifest peripubertally, frequently coinciding with the onset of adrenarche. In contrast, patients with classic adrenal hyperplasia have clinical features at birth or shortly thereafter. NC-CAH patients may exhibit short stature, premature development of pubic hair, insulin resistance and acne. Androgenic symptoms are usually mild, but hirsutism is often more pronounced (Franik & Skalba, 2011). However, clitoromegaly (but not true genital ambiguity), male habitus and temporal baldness are infrequent findings (Fig. 7). Menstrual disorders (oligo-/amenorrhea) and infertility occur in most patients. Ultrasonographic examination reveals PCO in the ovaries in about one third of patients. It should be stressed that symptoms of NC-CAH are very similar to those of PCOS, and on the basis of the clinical presentation patients suffering from these two disorders cannot be distinguished. As with other hyperandrogenic disorders, it is probable that NC-CAH is a progressive disorder, with symptoms becoming worse with age. Some women with NC-CAH may not show obvious symptoms. The disease is detected in them unintentionally, and it is also possible that it is not disclosed at all.

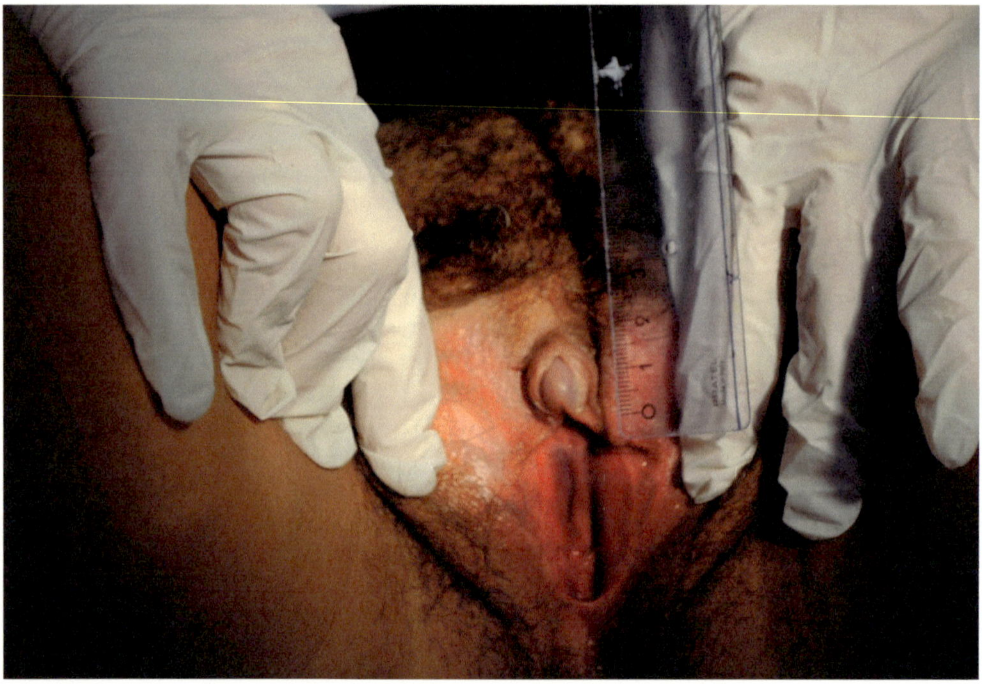

Fig. 7. 18-year-old woman diagnosed with NC-CAH with clitoromegaly.

Circulating testosterone and DHEAS are not different from ovarian hyperandrogenism, and DHEAS levels are often normal. It is important that circulating androstenedione is usually higher than in PCOS women, but the overlap between the two populations is too great to be of use as an effective marker. Patients with NC-CAH do not usually have an abnormally elevated LH/FSH ratio, although nor do many patients with ovarian hyperandrogenism (Azziz et al., 1994). It is interesting that the plasma level of estradiol in NC-CAH women is higher than in PCOS women, although the mechanism of increased production of estradiol in the ovaries in this disorder is not understood (Franik & Skalba, 2011). NC-CAH patients do not generally show ACTH oversecretion and cortisol deficiency (Raquel et al., 2000).

The standard diagnostic test for NC-CAH is the ACTH stimulation test. The test should be performed in patients with features of hyperandrogenism, when the 17OHP plasma concentration is above 1.7 µg/l. A blood sample for testing must be taken in the early morning in the early days of the menstrual cycle. The test involves intravenous administration of 0.25 mg of ACTH (for example, Synacthen), and collecting blood samples 30 minutes and 60 minutes after injection. In all blood samples 17OHP is determined. If the concentration of the hormone prior to administration of ACTH, or 60 minutes after injection, is equal to or greater than 10 µg/l, NC-CAH should be diagnosed.

15.2 Treatment of NC-CAH

The primary goal of treatment is to reduce hyperandrogenism. This applies to both glucocorticoids as well as anti-androgens. In special cases, a combination of the two groups of drugs may be used. Generally, very low doses of dexamethasone are needed (0.25-0.5 mg nightly). Anti-androgens were described in the above section of the chapter. In subfertile NC-CAH women, ovulatory function may be restored by dexamethasone treatment. In some patients, especially those who have symptoms of PCO, dexamethasone treatment may not be sufficient. For them, there are other ways to stimulate ovulation. In fact, many NC-CAH patients become pregnant without special treatment. During pregnancy in patients with NC-CAH "in utero" virilization may occur because of CAH in the fetus. Such a situation may arise if the father is a carrier for CAH, and the mother is a compound heterozygote. The risk of being a carrier is between 1/20 and 1/50 in the general Caucasian population. In pregnant NC-CAH cases, where the father's carrier status is not known, performance of prenatal testing and possible prenatal administration of dexamethasone should be considered.

16. Conclusion

The pattern of normal menstrual cycles is achieved through functional integration of stimulatory and inhibitory signals from the hypothalamus, pituitary and ovary. The important menstrual cycle disturbances concern primary or secondary amenorrhea. Disorders of the hypothalamic-pituitary-ovary axis arise from genetic defects, functional disorders and organic changes. Disorder treatment includes pharmacological, surgical and psychological methods. Improved treatment results should be sought in the development of research on the nature of the mechanisms of hormonal disorders.

17. References

Abdel-Rahman, M.Y., & Hurd, W.,W., (2010) *Androgen excess.* E-Medicine 2010 (http:// emedicine.com/aricle/273153-)

Aminzadeh, M., Kim, H.,G., Layman, L.,C.,& Cheetham, T.,D.,(2010). Rarer Syndromes Characterized by Hypogonadotropic Hypogonadism. *Front Horm Res. Basel, Karger,* Vol. 39, pp. 154-167, Eupub 2010 Apr 8

Andersen, A.,E., Ginny, L.,& Ryan, M.,D. (2009). Eating Disorders in the Obstetric and Gynecologic Patient Population. *Obstetrics & Gynecology,* Vol. 114, No.6, pp.1353-1367

Anderson, D.,C., (1974). Sex Hormone-Binding Globulin. *Clinical Endocrinology,* Vol. 3, No. 1, pp. 69-96.

Azziz, R. (2007). Definition, and Diagnosis, and Epidemiology of Polycystic Ovary Syndrome, In: *The Polycystic Ovary Syndrome: Current Concepts on Pathogenesis and Clinical Care,* Azziz,R., pp.1-16, Springer, ISBN 13:978-0-387-69246-3 , New York

Azziz, R., Carmina, E., Denwailly, D., Diamanti-Kandarakis, E., Escobar-Moreale, H.,F., Futterweit, W., Janssen, O.,E., Legro, S.,S., Norman, R.,J., Taylor, A.,E., & Witchel, S.,F. (2006). Position Statement: Criteria for Defining Polycystic Ovary Syndrome as a Predominantly Hyperandrogenic Syndrome; an Androgen Excess Society Guideline. *J Clin Endocrinol Metab,* Vol. 91, No. 11, pp. 4237-4245

Azziz, R., Dewailly, D., & Owerbach, D. (1994). Clinical Review 56 Nonclassic Adrenal Hyperplasia: Current Concepts. *J Clin Endocrin Metab, Vol.* 78, No. 4, pp. 810-815

Azziz, R., Sanchez, L.,A., Knochenhauer, E.,S., Moran, C., Lazenby, J., Stephens, K.,C., Taylor, K.,& Boots. L.,R. (2004 a). Androgen Excess in Women: Experience with over 1000 Consecutive Patients. *J Clin Endocrinol Metab,* Vol. 89, No. 2, pp. 453-462

Azziz, R., Woods, K.,S., Reyna, R., Key, T.,J., Knochenhauer, E.,S., & Yildiz, B.,O. (2004 b).The Prevalence and Features of the Polycystic Ovary Syndrome in an Unselected Population. *J Clin Endocrinol Metab,* Vol. 89, No. 6, pp. 2745-2749

Babu Segu, V. (2011) Prolactinoma: Treatment & Medication (http//emedicine.meddscape.com/article/124634-treatment)

Balen, A.,H., Laven, J.,S.,E., Lin Tan, S.,& Dewailly, D. (2003). Ultrasound Assessment of the Polycystic Ovary: International Consensus Definitions. *Human Reproduction Update,* Vol. 9, No. 6, pp.505-514

Berga, S.,L., Mortola, J.,F., Girton, L., Suh, B., Laughin, G., Pham, P., & Yen, S.,S. (1989). Neuroendocrine Aberrations in Women with Functional Hypothalamic Amenorrhoea *J Clin Endocrinol Metab,* Vol. 68, No. 2, pp.301-308

Bernichtein, S., Touraine, P., & Goffin, V. (2010). New Concepts in Prolactin Biology. *Journal of Endocrinology,* Vol. 206, No. 1, pp. 1-11.

Bidet, M., Bellanne-Chntelot, C., Galand-Portier, M.B., Tardy, V., Billaud, L., Laborge, K., Coussieu, C., Morel, Y., Vaury, C., Golmard, J.L., Claustre, A., Mornet, E., Chakthtoura, Z., Mowszowicz, I., Bachelot, A., Touraine, P., & Kuttenn, F. (2009). Clinical and Molecular Characterization of a Cohort of 161 Unrelated Women with Nonclassical Congenital Adrenal Hyperplasia Due to 21-hydroxylase Deficiency and 330 Family Members. *J Clin Endocrinol Metab,* Vol. 94, No. 5, pp. 1570-1576

Binart, N., Bachelot, A., & Bouilly, J. (2010). Impact of Prolactin Receptor Isoforms on Reproduction. *Trends in Endocrinology and Metabolism,* Vol. 21, No. 6 , pp. 362-368

Bondanelli, M., Ambrosio, M.R., Zatelli, M.C., de Marinis, L., & Uberti, E.C. (2005). Hypopituitarism after Traumatic Brain Injury. *European Journal of Endocrinology,* Vol. 152, No. 5, pp. 679-691

Bonnet, F., Balkau, B., Malécot, J.M., Picard, P., Lange, C., Fumeron, F., Aubert, R., Raverot, V., Déchaud, H., Tichet, J., Lecomte, P., & Pugeat, M. (2009). DESIR Study Group. Sex Hormone-Binding Globulin Predicts the Incidence of Hyperglycemia in Women: Interactions with Adiponectin Levels. *European Journal of Endocrinology* Vol. 161, No. 1, pp. 81-85

Bouligand, J., Ghervan, C., Tello, J.A., Brailly-Tobard, S., Salenave, S., Chanson, P., Lombes, M., Millar, R.P., Guiochon-Mantel, A., & Young, J. (2009). Isolated Familial Hypogonadotropic Hypogonadism and a GNRH1 Mutation. *New Engl J Med* , Vol. 360, No. 26, pp. 2742-2748

Brand, J.S., van der Tweel, I., Grobbee, D.E., Emmelot-Vonk, M.H., & van der Schouw Y.T. (2011). Testosterone, Sex Hormone-Binding Globulin and the Metabolic Syndrome: a Systematic Review and Meta-analysis of Observational Studies. *Int J Epidemiol,* Vol. 40,No. 1, pp. 189-207

Brioude, F., Bouligand, J., Trabado, S., Francou,B., Salanave, S., Kamenicky, P., Brailly-Tabard, S., Chanson, P., Guiochon-Mantel, A., & Young, J. (2009). Non-Syndromic Congenital Hypogonadotropic Hypogonadism: Clinical Presentation and Genotype-Phenotype Relationships. *European Journal of Endocrinology,* Vol. 162, No. 5, pp. 835-851

Brown, D.L., Henrichsen, T.L., Clayton, A.C., Hudson, S.B.A., Coddington,C.C., & Vella, A. (2009). Ovarian Stromal Hyperthecosis: Sonographic Features and Histologic Associations. *J Ultrasound Med.,* Vol. 28, No. 5, pp. 587-593

Carmina, E., & Lobo, R.A. (1999). Polycystic Ovary Syndrome (PCOS): Arguably the Most Common Endocrinopathy is Associated with Significant Morbidity in Women. *J Clin Endocrinol Metab,* Vol. 84, No. 6, pp. 1897-1899

Chan, Y.M., de Guillebon, A., Lang-Muritano, M., Plummer, L., Cerrato, F., Tsiaras, S., Gaspert, A., Lavoie, H.B., Wu, C-H., Crowley, W.F., Amory, J.K., Pitteloud, N., & Seminara, S.B. (2009). GnRH1 Mutations in Patients with Idiopathic Hypogonadotropic Hypogonadism. *PNAS,* Vol. 106, No. 28, pp. 11703-11708

Chang, R.J. (2009 a) Polycystic Ovary Syndrome and Hyperandrogenic States, In: *Reproductive Endocrinology,* Yen, S.S.C., Jaffe, R.B., Barbieri, R.L., pp. 30-81, W.B. Saunders Company, ISBN 0-7216-6897-6, Philadelphia, London, Toronto, Montreal, Sidney, Tokyo

Chang, A.Y., & Wild, R.A. (2009 b). Characterizing Cardiovascular Risk in Women with Polycystic Ovary Syndrome: More than the Sum of Its Parts? *Semin Repro Med.,* Vol. 27, No. 4, pp. 299-305

Chen, M.J., Chen, C.D., Yang, J.H., Chen, C.L., Ho, H.N., Yang, W.S., & Yang, Y.S. (2011). High Serum Dehydroepiandrosterone Sulfate is Associated with Phenotypic Acne and a Reduced Risk of Abdominal Obesity in Women with Polycystic Ovary Syndrome, *Hum. Reprod.,* Vol. 26, No. 1, pp. 227-234

Consensus on Infertility Treatment Related to Polycystic Ovary Syndrome. The Thessaloniki ESHRE/ASRM - Sponsored PCOS Consensus Workshop Group (2008). *Fertil Steril,* Vol. 89, pp. 505-522

Costello, M.F., Shrestha, B., Eden,J., Johnson, N.P., & Sjoblon, P. (2007). Metformin Versus Oral Contraceptive Pill in Polycystic Ovary Syndrome: a Cochrane Review. *Hum Reprod.,* Vol. 22, No. 5, pp. 1200-1209

De Roux, N., Genin, E., Carel, J.C., et al. (2003). Hypogonadotropic Hypogonadism Due to Loss of Function of the KiSS1-Derived Peptide receptor GPR54. *Proceedings of the National Academy of Sciences of the United States of America 2003,* Vol. 100, pp. 10972-10976

De Ugarte, C.M., Woods,K.S., Bartolucci, A.A.,& Azziz,R. (2006). Degree of Facial and Body Terminal Hair \growth in Unselected Black and White Women: Toward a Population Definitione of Hirsutism. *J Clin Endocrinol Metab,* Vol.91, No. 4, pp. 1345-1350

Dennedy, M.C., Smith, D., O'Sheba, D., & Mc Kenna, T.J. (2010). Investigation of Patients with Atypical or Severe Hyperandrogenaemia Including Androgen-Secreting Ovarian Teratoma. *Eur J Endocrinol,* Vol. 162, No. 2, pp.213-220

Dewailly, D., Pigny, P., Soudan, B., Catteau-Jonard, S., Decanter, C., Poncelet, E., & Duhamel, A. (2010). Reconciling the Definitions of Polycystic Ovary Syndrome: The Ovarian Follicle Number and Serum Anti-Müllerian Hormone Concentrations Aggregate with the Markers of Hyperandrogenism. *The Journal of Clinical Endocrinology & Metabolism,* Vol. 95, No. 9, pp. 4399-4405

Dunaif, A., Segal, K.R., Futerweit, W., et al. (1989). Profound Peripheral Insulin Resistance, Independent of Obesity in Polycystic Ovary Syndrome. *Diabetes,* Vol. 38, No. 9, pp. 1165-1174

Doi S.A. (2008) Neuroendocrine Dysfunction in PCOS: A Critique of Recent Reviews. *Clinical Medicine & Research,* Vol. 6, No 2, pp. 47 -53

Elliott, B.D., Langer,O., & Schuessling, F. (1997). Human Placenta Glucose Uptake and Transport are not Altered by the Oral Antihyperglycemic Agent Metformin. *Am J Obstet Gynecol,* pp. 176527-176530

Ferriman, D., & Gallway, J.D. (1961). Clinical Assessment of Body Hair Growth in Women. *J Clin Metab,* Vol. 21, pp.1440-1447

Franik, G., & Skałba, P. (2011). Clinical Observations and Hormone Secretings of Ill Patients with the Syndrome of Non-Classic Hypertrophy of Adrenal Cortex. *Endokrynologia Polska,* Vol. 62, pp 230-237

Frank, S. (1995). Polycystic Ovary Syndrome. *N Engl J Med,* Vol. 333, pp. 853-861

Frank, S. (2006). Controversy in Clinical Endocrinology. Diagnostic of Polycystic Ovary Syndrome: In Defense of the Rotterdam Criteria. *J Clin Endocrinol & Metabolism,* Vol. 91, No. 3, pp. 786-789

Gianetti, E., Tusset, C., Noel, S.C., Au, M.G., Dwyer, A.A., Hughes, V.A., Abreu, A.P., Carroll, J., Trarbach, E., Silveira, L.F., Costa, E.M., de Mendonca, B.B., de Castro, M., Lofrano, A., Hall, J.E., Bolu, E., Ozata, M., Quinto, R., Amory, J.K., Stewart, S.E., Arlt, W., Cole, T.R., Crowley, W.F., Kaiser, U.B., Latronico, A.C., & Seminara, S.B. (2010). TAC3/TACR3 Mutations Reveal Preferential Activation of Gonadotropin-Releasing Hormone Release by Neurokinin B in Neonatal Life Followed by Reversal in Adulthood. *J Clin Endocrinol Metab,* Vol. 95, No. 6, pp. 2857-2867

Glueck, C.J., & Wang, P. (2007). Metformin Before and During Pregnancy and Lactation in Polycystic Ovary Syndrome. *Expert Opin Drug Saf,* Vol. 6, pp. 191-198

Goodarzi, M. (2007). Genetics of PCOS, In: *The Polycystic Ovary Syndrome: Current Concepts on Pathogenesis and Clinical Care,* Azziz, R., pp. 392-396, Springer, New York

Harborne, L., Fleming, R., Lyall, H., Norman, J., & Naveed, S. (2003). Descriptive Review of the Evidence for the Use of Metformin in Polycystic Ovary Syndrome. *The Lancet,* Vol. 361, No. 9372, pp. 1894-1901

Hatch, R., Rosenfield, R.L., Kim, M.H., & Tredway, D. (1981). Hirsutism: Implication, Etiology and Management. *Am J Obstet. Gynecol,* Vol. 140, No. 7, pp. 815-830

Helm, K.D., Nass, R.M., & Evans, W.S. (2009). Physiologic and Pathophysiologic Alternation of the Neuroendocrine Components of the Reproductive Axis, In: *Reproductive Endocrinology,* Yen, S.S.C., Jaffe, R.B., Barbieri, R.L., pp. 30-81, W.B. Saunders Company, ISBN 0-7216-6897-6, Philadelphia, London, Toronto, Montreal, Sidney, Tokyo

Iovane, A., Aumas, C., de Roux, N. (2004). New Insights in the Genetics of Isolated Hypogonadotropic Hypogonadism. *European J Endocrin,* Vol. 151, pp. U83-U88

Johnstone, E.B., Rosen, M.P., Neril, R., Trevithick, D., Sternfeld, B., Murphy, R., Addauan-Andersen, C., McConnell, D., Reijo Pera, R., & Cedars, M.L.(2010) The Polycystic Ovary Post-Rotterdam: A Common, Age-Dependent Finding in Ovulatory Women without Metabolic Significance. *The Journal of Clinical Endocrinology and Metabolism,* Vol. 95, No. 11, pp. 4965-4972

Kahn, S.M., Hryb, D.J., Nakhla, A.M., Romas, N.A., & Rosner, W. (2003). Sex Hormone-Binding Globulin is Synthesized in Target Cells. BEYOND CARRIER PROTEINS. *The Journal of Clinical Endocrinology and Metabolism,* Vol. 88, No. 8, pp. 3626-3631

Kelberman, D. & Dattani, M.T. (2006). The role of transcription factors implicated in anterior pituitary development in the aetiology of congenital hypopituitarism. *Ann Med,* Vol. 38, No. 8, pp.560-77

Kiddy, D.S., Sharp, P.S., White, D.M., Scalon, M.F., Mason, H.D., Bray, S.C., Polson, D.W., Reed, M.J., & Franks, S. (1990). Differences in Clinical and Endocrine Features between Obese and Non-Obese Subjects with Polycystic Ovary Syndrome: an Analysis of 263 Consecutive Cases. *Clin Endocrinol,* Vol. 32, No. 2, pp. 213-220

Labrie, F. (2010). DHEA, Important Source of Sex Steroids in Men and Even More in Women. *Prog Brain Res,* Vol. 182, pp. 97-148

LaPensee, E.W., & Ben - Jonathan, N. (2010). Novel Roles of Prolactin and Estrogens in Breast Cancer: Resistance to Chemotherapy. *Endocrine-Related Cancer,* Vol. 17, No. 2, pp. R91-R107

Layendecker, G., Wild, L., & Hansman, M. (1980). Pregnancies Following Intermittent (Pulsatile) Administration of GnRH by Means of Portable Pumps (Zyklomat): a New Approach to the Treatment of Infertility in Hypothalamic Amenorrhoea. *J Clin Endocrinol Metab,* Vol. 51, pp. 1214-1216

Malkawi, H.Y., Qublan, H.S., Hamaideh, A.H. (2003). Medical vs. surgical treatment for clomiphene citrate-resistant women with polycystic ovary syndrome. *J Obstet Gynaecol,* Vol. 23, No. 3, pp.289-93

Martin, K.A., Chang, J.R., Ehrmann, D.A., Ibanez, L., Lobo, R.A., Rosenfield, R.L., Shapiro, J., Montori, V.M., & Swiglo, B.A. (2008). Evaluation and Treatment of Hirsutism in Premenopausal Women: An Endocrine Society Clinical Practice Guideline. *The Journal of Clinical Endocrinology and Metabolism,* Vol. 93, No. 4, pp. 1105-1120

Nestler, J.E. (2008). Metformin in the treatment of infertility in polycystic ovarian syndrome: an alternative perspective. *Fertil Steril,* Vol. 90, No. 1, pp.14-6

Palomba, S., Falbo, A., Zullo, F., & Orio, F. (2009). Evidence-Based and Potential Benefits of Metformin in Polycystic Ovary Syndrome: a Comprehensive Review. *Endocrine Rev,* Vol. 30, No. 1, pp. 1-50

Panneerselvam, P., Sivakumari, K., Jayaprakash, P., & Srikanth, R. (2010). SNP Analysis of Follistatin Gene Associated with Polycystic Ovarian Syndrome. *Advances and Applications in Bioinformatics and Chemistry,* Vol. 3, pp. 111-119

Pasquali, R., Patton, L., Diamanti-Kandarakis, E., & Gambineri, A. (2007). Role of Obesity and Adiposity in PCOS, In: *The polycystic ovary syndrome: current concepts on pathogenesis and clinical care,* Azziz, R., Springer Science+Business Media, New York

Pauli, S.A., & Berga, S.L. (2010). Athletic Amenorrhea: Energy Deficit or Psychogenic Challenge? *Ann NY Acad Sci,* Vol. 1205, pp. 33-38

Pitteloud,N., Quinton, R., Pearce et al. (2007). Digenic Mutations Account for Variable Phenotypes in Idiopathic Hypogonadotropic Hypogonadism. *Journal of Clinical Investigation,* Vol. 117, No. 2, pp.457-463

Provenzale, J.M., Mukundan, S., Barboriak, D.P., & Daniel, P. (2006). Diffusion-weighted and Perfusion MR Imaging for Brain Tumor Characterization and Assessment of Treatment Response. *Radiology,* Vol. 239, No. 3, pp. 632-649

Rajab, A., Kelberman, D., de Castro, S.C., Biebermann, H., Shaikh, H., Pearce, K., Hall, C.M., Shaikh, G., Gerrelli, D., Grueters, A., Krude, H., Dattani, M.T. (2008). Novel mutations in LHX3 are associated with hypopituitarism and sensorineural hearing loss. *Hum Mol Genet,* Vol. 17, No. 14, pp.2150-9

Raquel, H., Dewailly, D., Decanter, C., Knochenhauer, E., Boots, L., & Azziz, R. (2000). Adrenocortical Hyperresponsitivity to Adrenocorticotropic Hormone: Mechanism Favoring the Normal Production of Cortisol in 21-Hydroxylase-Deficient Nonclassic Adrenal Hyperplasia. *Fertility and Sterility,* Vol. 74, No. 2, pp. 329-334

Rauh, M.J., Nichols, J.F., & Barrack, M.T. (2010). Relationship Among Injury and Disordered Eating, Menstrual Dysfunction and Low Bone Mineral Density in High School Athletes: a Prospective Study. *Journal of Athletic Training,* Vol. 45, No. 3, pp. 243-252

Rautio, K., Tapanainen, J.S., Ruokonen, A., & Morin-Papunen, L.C. (2006). Endocrine and Metabolic Effects of Rosiglitazone in Overweight Women with PCOS: a Randomized Placebo-Controlled Study. *Human Reproduction,* Vol. 21, pp. 1400-1407

Regal, M., Paramo, C., Sierra, S.M., & Garcia-Maryor, R.V. (2001). Prevalence and Incidence of Hypopituitarism in an Adult Caucasian Population in Northwestern Spain. *Clin Endocrinol,* Vol. 55, No. 6, pp. 735-740

Romaguera, J., Moran, C., Diaz-Montes, T., Hines, G., Cruz, R., & Azziz, R. (2000). Prevalence of 21-Hydroxylase-Deficient Nonclassical Adrenal Hyperplasia and Insulin Resistance Among Hirsute Women from Puerto Rico. *Fertility and Sterility,* Vol. 74, No. 1, pp. 59-62

Schade, R., Andersohn, F., Suissa, S., Haverkamp, W., & Garbe, E. (2007). Dopamine Agonists and the Risk of Cardiac-Valve Regurgitation. *New England Journal of Medicine,* Vol. 356, No. 1 pp. 29-38.

Schneider, H.J., Almaretti, G., Kreischmann-Andermahr, I., Stalla, G.K., & Ghigo, E. (2007). Hypopituitarism. *Lancet,* Vol. 369, pp. 1461-1470

Seminara, S.B., Messager, S., Chatzidaki, E.E., et al. (2003). The GPR 54 Gene as a Regulator of Puberty. *New England Journal of Medicine*. Vol. 349, No. 17, pp. 1614-1627.

Semple, R.K., & Kemal Topaloglu, A. (2010). The Recent Genetics of Hypogonadotrophic Hypogonadism - Novel Insights and New Questions. *Clin Endocrinol*, Vol. 72, No. 4, pp. 427-435

Sepilian, V., & Nagamani, M. (2005). Effects of Rosiglitazone in Obese Women with Polycystic Ovary Syndrome and Severe Insulin Resistance. *The Journal of Clinical Endocrinology & Metabolism*, Vol. 90, No. 1, pp. 60-65

Skałba, P., Dąbkowska-Huć, A., Kazimierczak, W., Samojedny, A., Samojedny, M.P., & Chełmicki Z. (2006). Content of 5-alpha-reductase (type 1 and type 2) mRNA in dermal papillae from the lower abdominal region in women with hirsutism. *Experimental Dermatology*, Vol. 31, pp. 564-570

Skałba P, Cygal A. (2011). Anti- Mullerian Hormone: plasma level in women with polycystic ovary syndrome and with premature ovarian failure. *Przegląd Menopauzalny* (Menopause Review) Vol. 55, pp. 232-236

Sterling E. Understanding tests and hormone levels for PCOS. 2011 (www.soulcysters.net/showthread.php 239340-Understanding....)

Swenne, I. & Thurfjell, B. (2003). Clinical Onset and Diagnosis of Eating Disorders in Premenarcheal Girls is Preceded by Inadequate Weight Gain and Growth Retardation. *Acta Paediatrica*, Vol. 92, No. 10, pp. 1133-1137

Tan, S., Hahn, S., Benson, S., Dietz, T., Lahner, H.,& Moeller, L.C. (2007). Metformin Improves Polycystic Ovary Syndrome Symptoms Irrespective of Pre-Treatment Insulin Resistance. *European Journal Endocrinology*, Vol. 157, No. 5, pp. 669-676.

The Rotterdam ESHRE/ASRM- Sponsored PCOS Consensus Workshop Group (2004). Revised 2003 Consensus on Diagnostic Criteria and Long-Term Health Risks Related to Polycystic Ovary Syndrome (PCOS). *Fertil Steril* , Vol. 81, No. 1, pp. 19-25

Topaloglu, A.K., Reimann, F., Guclu, M., Yalin, A.S., Kotan, L.D., Porter, K.M., Serin, A., Mungan, N.O., Cook, J.R., Ozbek, M.N., Imamoglu, S., Akalin, N.S., Yuksel, B., O'Rahilly, S., Semple, R.K. (2009). TAC3 and TACR3 mutations in familial hypogonadotropic hypogonadism reveal a key role for Neurokinin B in the central control of reproduction. *Nat Genet*, Vol. 41, No. 3, pp.354-8

Tsai, P.S., & Gill, J.C. (2006). Mechanisms of Disease: Insights into X-linked and Autosomal-Dominant Kallmann Syndrome. *Nat Clin Pract Endocrinol Metab*, Vol. 2, No. 1, pp. 160–171

Wang, J., Tang, J., Wang, B., Song, J., Liu, J., Wei, Z., Zhang, F., Ma, X., & Cao, Y. (2009) FABP4: A Novel Candidate Gene for Polycystic Ovary Syndrome. *Endocrine*, Vol. 36, No. 3, pp.392-396

Wieck, A., & Haddad, P.,M. (2003). Antipsychotic-Induced Hyperprolactinaemia in Women: Pathophysiology, Severity and Consequences. *The British Journal of Psychiatry*, Mar 182, pp. 199-204

Yen, S.S.C. (1999). Neuroendocrine of Reproduction, In: *Reproductive Endocrinology*, Yen, S.S.C., Jaffe, R.B., Barbieri, R.L., pp. 30-81, W.B. Saunders Company, ISBN 0-7216-6897-6, Philadelphia, London, Toronto, Montreal, Sidney, Tokyo

Yidiz, B.O., Bolour, S., Woods, K., Moore, A., & Azziz, R. (2010) Visually Scoring Hirsutism. *Hum Reprod Update,* Vol. 16, No. 1, pp.51-64

Youssef, M.A., van Wely, M., Hassan, M.A., et al. (2010). Can dopamine agonists reduce the incidence and severity of OHSS in IVF/ICSI treatment cycles? A systematic review and meta-analysis. *Hum Reprod Update,* Vol. 16, No. 5, pp. 459-466

Zanettini, R., Antonini, A., Gatt, G., Gentile, R., Tese, S., & Pezzoli, G. (2007).Valvular heart disease and the use of dopamine agonists for Parkinson's disease. *New England Journal of Medicine,* Vol. 356, No. 1, pp. 39–46

20

Primary and Secondary Amenorrhea

Valentina Chiavaroli, Ebe D'Adamo, Laura Diesse,
Tommaso de Giorgis, Francesco Chiarelli and Angelika Mohn
*Department of Pediatrics, University of Chieti, Chieti,
Italy*

1. Introduction

Puberty represents a particular period of life characterized by hormonal changes and physical and psychological modifications leading children from childhood to adolescence. During this period, menarche represents the most important event in females. Age of menarche is different among populations and has been recognized as an useful marker of socio-economic status, as well as dietary and environmental patterns (Chumlea et al., 2003; Swenson & Havens, 1987; Thomas et al., 2001). Generally, the first menstrual cycle takes place between 12 and 13 years of age, with 98% of girls having menarche by 15 years of age (Diaz, 2006). The normal range for menstrual cycles is between 21 and 45 days, with flow length varying from 2 to 7 days (Flug et al., 1984; World Health Organization Task Force on Adolescent Reproductive Health, 1986). During the first 2 years after menarche, menses length is often abnormal due to immaturity of the hypothalamic-pituitary-ovarian axis (Diaz, 2006); however, cycles range can be regular also in the first gynecologic year (Flug et al., 1984; World Health Organization Task Force on Adolescent Reproductive Health, 1986).
Amenorrhea is defined as the complete absence or anomalous cessation of menstrual cycles in females during reproductive years. Just in three situations amenorrhea is considered physiological: during pregnancy, lactation and menopause. In all other situations, amenorrhea can be due to many pathological conditions and merits a careful assessment. Amenorrhea is classified as primary and secondary according to its occurrence before or after menarche, respectively (The Practice Committee of American Society for Reproductive Medicine, 2008). Amenorrhea is defined primary when menarche does not occur by the age of 16 years in a girl with complete secondary sexual development, or by the age of 14 years in a girl without secondary sexual development. Amenorrhea is defined secondary when menstrual cycles disappear for 6 consecutive months in a girl with irregular menses or for 3 consecutive months in a girl with regular menses (Deligeoroglou et al., 2010). According to the American Society for Reproductive Medicine, currently in literature many causes of amenorrhea have been recognized (The Practice Committee of American Society for Reproductive Medicine, 2008), including:

- anatomic defects of the genital tract
- hypothalamic/pituitary causes
- ovary insufficiency
- endocrinopathies
- chronic oligo- or anovulation

Treatment of amenorrhea depends on the aetiology and consists of specific diagnostic and therapeutic procedures. The aim of the present chapter is to summarize the most important and recent findings regarding primary and secondary amenorrhea.

2. Epidemiology of amenorrhea

It has been estimated that amenorrhea not due to physiological conditions has a prevalence ranging from 3% to 4% (Bachmann & Kemmann, 1982; Pettersson et al., 1973). The most frequent causes of amenorrhea are four: hypothalamic amenorrhea, hyperprolactinemia, ovarian failure, and polycystic ovary syndrome (The Practice Committee of American Society for Reproductive Medicine, 2008).

3. Causes of primary and secondary amenorrhea

The main causes of primary and secondary amenorrhea include anatomic defects of the genital tract, hypothalamic/pituitary causes, ovary insufficiency, endocrinopathies and chronic oligo- or anovulation (Table 1).

Anatomic genital defects	Hypothalamic causes	Pituitary causes	Ovary insufficiency	Endocrine diseases	Chronic oligo- or anovulation
Vaginal agenesis	Functional hypothalamic amenorrhea	Prolactinomas	Gonadal agenesis	Adrenal diseases •17aHydroxylase deficiency •17,20Lyase deficiency •Aromatase deficiency	Polycystic ovary syndrome
Transverse vaginal septum	• Psychogenic stress • Intensive physical activity • Nutritional disorders	Tumours secreting • FSH • LH	Gonadal dysgenesis		
Imperforate hymen	Isolated gonadotropin deficit	• GH • TSH • ACTH	Premature ovarian failure	Thyropathies	
Cervical agenesis or dysgenesis	• Kallman syndrome • Idiopathic hypogonadotropic hypogonadism		Enzymatic deficits	Poorly controlled diabetes	
Endometrial hypoplasia or aplasia		Inflammatory and infiltrative disorders		Ovarian tumours	
Intrauterine synechiae	Chronic diseases	Empty sella			
Mayer-Rokitansky-Küster-Hauser syndrome	Infections	Panhypopituitarism			
	Tumours	Sheehan syndrome			
Androgen insensitivity syndrome					

Table 1. Etiopathology of primary and secondary amenorrhea

3.1 Anatomic defects of the genital tract

Anatomic genital defects include vaginal agenesis, transverse vaginal septum, imperforate hymen, cervical agenesis or dysgenesis, endometrial hypoplasia or aplasia, Mayer-Rokitansky-Küster-Hauser syndrome, and androgen insensitivity syndrome.

Vaginal agenesis should be suspected in all girls with primary amenorrhea suffering frequent abdominal and pelvic pain due to the anatomic barrier which obstacles blood flow. Furthermore, the amassing of blood in the uterus (hematometra) can provoke retrograde menstruation leading to the development of adherences and endometriosis (The Practice Committee of American Society for Reproductive Medicine, 2008).

Transverse vaginal septum represents a congenital vaginal obstruction. There are two variety of transverse septum: partial and total; only the total variety is responsible for amenorrhea (Deligeoroglou et al., 2010). The obstruction can be located in the inferior (16%), central

(40%) or superior (46%) vaginal portion (Rock et al., 1982). Similarly to vaginal agenesis, also this defect is responsible for recurring abdominal and pelvic pain coming from blood accumulation in the uterus and vagina (hematocolpos) (Deligeoroglou et al., 2010).

Imperforate hymen has been estimated having an incidence of 1/1000 (Deligeoroglou et al., 2010). The diagnosis is uncommon during infancy because this condition is usually asymptomatic, although in rare cases neonates can suffer marked abdominal enlargement. More commonly, girls with amenorrhea will receive diagnosis of imperforate hymen after having abdominal pain, hematometra or hematocolpos during the pubertal period (Ameh et al., 2011).

Cervical anatomic defects represent another important cause of primary amenorrhea. There are two types of cervical abnormality: agenesis and dysgenesis. Both these defects can be associated with a normal development of the vagina. In details, while in the dysgenesis a partial cervical development is observed, in the agenesis patients are likely to present earlier with a history of primary amenorrhea and severe lower abdominal pain occurring at irregular intervals (Deligeoroglou et al., 2010).

Endometrial hypoplasia or aplasia represent the partial development or the congenital absence of endometrium.

Intrauterine synechiae, also named Ashermann syndrome, is a condition very unusual among adolescents, while represents the most frequent cause of secondary amenorrhea in women of reproductive age. In fact, abortion, postpartum curettage for haemorrhage, or postpartum endometritis can provoke the development of intrauterine synechiae leading to cessation of menses (Deligeoroglou et al., 2010).

Mayer-Rokitansky-Küster-Hauser syndrome is a congenital defect of the genital tract recognized as the more common cause of amenorrhea after gonadal dysgenesis, having an incidence of 1/5.000 (Fedele et al., 1996). This syndrome is also called "Müllerian agenesis" because is characterized by absence or hypoplasia of the Müllerian ducts derivatives. In fact, the main features of Mayer-Rokitansky-Küster-Hauser syndrome are the following: normal ovaries, anomalies of the uterine development ranging from absence to rudimentary residues of uterus and aplasia of the upper two thirds of the vagina. Furthermore, affected women show the development of secondary sexual characteristics with a female 46, XX karyotype (Bean et al., 2009; Morcel et al., 2007). There are two types of Mayer-Rokitansky-Küster-Hauser syndrome (Morcel et al., 2007): type 1 represents the isolated variety, while type 2 is associated with several organic abnormalities involving upper urinary tract (40% of cases), skeleton (10-12% of cases) (American College of Obstetricians and Gynecologist Committee on Adolescent Health Care, 2006), auditory system (10-25% of cases) (Cremers et al., 1995; Strübbe et al., 1994), and more rarely heart. The aetiology of Mayer-Rokitansky-Küster-Hauser syndrome is still uncertain: although at the beginning it was supposed that this syndrome was the result of sporadic abnormality, it has been recently assumed a genetic background on the basis of a growing amount of familial cases (Morcel et al., 2007). Clinically, the most common presentation is characterized by primary amenorrhea in adolescents with normal secondary female characteristics. Just in few cases, where patients have rudimentary residues of uterus with a normal endometrial function, there is a history of recurring severe lower abdominal pain; furthermore, some adolescents can suffer psychological distress from unsuccessful sexual life (Deligeoroglou et al., 2010). Endocrine evaluation shows normal levels of basal plasma gonadotropin and sex steroid (estradiol), without biochemical signs of androgen excess (Carranza-Lira et al., 1999).

Androgen insensitivity syndrome is a rare X-linked recessive androgen receptor defect having an incidence of 1/20.000-99.000 (Boehmer et al., 2001; Grumbach et al., 2003). The gene responsible for this condition has been mapped to chromosome Xq11-12 (Brinkmann et al., 1989), and about 30% of mutations are the result of sporadic anomalies (Hughes & Deeb, 2006). Nowadays, three variants of androgen insensitivity syndrome have been recognized based on the inactivity of androgen receptor: complete androgen insensitivity syndrome, with a phenotype characterized by normal female external genitalia; mild androgen insensitivity syndrome, with a phenotype characterized by normal male external genitalia; partial androgen insensitivity syndrome, with a phenotype characterized by partial masculinization of external genitalia (Hughes & Deeb, 2006). In details, complete androgen insensitivity syndrome has an incidence of 1/60.000 (Jorgensen et al., 2010) and is characterized by congenital agenesis of the uterus and absent or rudimentary vagina in women showing normal development of secondary sexual characteristics in presence of a 46,XY karyotype (Oakes et al., 2008). In addition, these patients present cryptorchidism, with gonads situated in the inguinal canal or abdominal cavity; testicles are functional and produce normal testosterone and dihydrotestosterone levels. Although usually patients affected by complete androgen insensitivity syndrome present primary amenorrhea together with scarce or absent pubic and axillary hair, girls can also present an inguinal hernia during infancy or childhood. In addition, since the incidence rate of complete androgen insensitivity syndrome has been reported to be 1%-2% in subjects with inguinal hernia, some authors have suggested to consider a karyotype in every girl with inguinal masses (Hughes & Deeb, 2006; Sarpel, 2005). The incidence of testes malignancy has been estimated to be 22%, although it is infrequent in subjects younger than 20 years of age (Manuel et al., 1976). Usually, endocrine evaluation shows high levels of basal plasma testosterone and luteinizing hormone, frequently in association to high levels of estradiol (Hughes & Deeb, 2006).

3.2 Hypothalamic causes

Hypothalamic diseases represent the most frequent cause of amenorrhea in adolescents (Deligeoroglou et al., 2010). In fact, girls with disorders of the hypothalamus are susceptible to the development of chronic anovulation, due to an insufficient secretion of gonadotropin-releasing hormone leading to low levels of basal plasma gonadotropins and estradiol. However, after stimulation with exogenous gonadotropin-releasing hormone, the secretion of gonadotropins is in the physiological range. Hypothalamic amenorrhea has frequently a dysfunctional origin, although in rare cases it can be due to other conditions including the isolated deficit of gonadotropins, chronic diseases, infections, and tumours (Deligeoroglou et al., 2010).

Dysfunctional causes of hypothalamic amenorrhea include psychogenic stress, excessive physical activity and nutritional disorders. Actually the precise mechanisms through which excessive stress and weight loss influence negatively gonadotropin-releasing hormone secretion are still uncertain (Golden & Carlson, 2008). However, in these girls the impaired production of gonadotropin-releasing hormone may have several implications on luteinizing hormone secretion, coming from absent or reduced pulses to normal or elevated pulses (Deligeoroglou et al., 2010).

Psychogenic stress seems to induce the secretion of high levels of corticotrophin-releasing hormone, which inhibits gonadotropin-releasing hormone pulses (Deligeoroglou et al., 2010).

Also girls performing excessive physical activity are prone to present hypothalamic amenorrhea and short luteine phases. These abnormalities are induced by the strenuous physical activity and the restricted caloric intake requested to maintain leanness. In fact, athletes show frequently a strong disproportion among nutritional intake and real energy expenditure, especially in disciplines where low body weight for performance and aesthetics is needed (Golden & Carlson, 2008). In particular, in athletes there is a risk of amenorrhea three times higher than in general population, with predominance between long-distance runners (Warren & Goodman, 2003). Interestingly, a peculiar condition called the "female athlete triad" has been recognized as the result of an inadequate caloric intake. This condition includes amenorrhea, eating disorders, and osteoporosis, and athletes can present one or more components of the triad. Therefore, all these alterations should be screened in order to perform an early diagnosis and to improve quality life of women involved in competitive sports (Mendelsohn & Warren, 2010).

Eating disorders represent another common cause of functional hypothalamic amenorrhea. Unfortunately, these disorders are increasing worldwide and the effects on reproduction are more than negative. In particular, in females the reproductive axis is strongly related to the nutritional status and is highly responsive to external stimuli due to the high energy expenditure during pregnancy and lactation. Therefore, in condition of undernutrition, the female reproduction can be interrupted and continued in better periods to preserve vital functions. In fact, a decrease of 10%-15% in normal body weight seems to be able to cause amenorrhea (European Society of Human Reproduction and Embryology Capri Workshop Group, 2006). Up to now, it has been estimated that about 1%-5% of women are affected by the "weight related amenorrhea" (Laughlin et al., 1998). Although the responsible mechanisms are not entirely clear, it has been proposed a minimal body weight of 47 kg for the onset or maintenance of menstrual cycles (Frisch & McArthur, 1974; Frisch, 1987). Among the most important eating disorders, anorexia nervosa and bulimia nervosa affect up to 5% of women of reproductive age causing amenorrhea and infertility (European Society of Human Reproduction and Embryology Capri Workshop Group, 2006). In details, anorexia nervosa has been defined as body weight less than 85% of expected weight or body mass index less than 17.5 kg/m^2, caloric restriction, fear of weight gain and an impaired perception of body image. Bulimia nervosa has been defined as binge eating followed by vomiting, intense physical activity and other compensatory actions (Becker et al., 1999). Approximately 15%-30% of girls affected by anorexia nervosa present amenorrhea (Miller et al., 2005; Watson & Andersen, 2003), while girls with bulimia may present oligoamenorrhea also in presence of a normal body mass index (European Society of Human Reproduction and Embryology Capri Workshop Group, 2006). The mechanisms underlying preservation or discontinuation of the physiological neuroendocrine regulation of ovarian function in girls with anorexia or bulimia are still unknown. However, it has been supposed the occurrence of impaired gonadotropin-releasing hormone secretion with alterations in dopaminergic and opioid systems. Recently, low levels of luteinizing hormone and estradiol have been demonstrated in women with hypothalamic amenorrhea, togheter with gonadotropins pulses insufficient to protract the development of follicles until ovulation (Welt et al., 2004). Furthermore, the lately discovered leptin, one of the most important adipose derived hormones which plays a key role in regulating energy intake and expenditure, seems to be strictly involved into the mediation of reproductive axis (Brennan & Mantzoros, 2006). In fact, low levels of leptin have been reported in women with hypothalamic amenorrhea (Welt et al., 2004). Although it is still unclear if leptin has direct hypothalamic effects or augments the metabolic substrates availability, it is probable that this hormone mediates both these effects.

Isolated deficit of gonadotropins represents a rare cause of hypothalamic amenorrhea, including the Kallman syndrome and the idiopathic hypogonadotropic hypogonadism.

The *Kallman syndrome* represents a genetic heterogeneous developmental disease characterized by gonadotropin-releasing hormone deficiency and defective development of olfactory nerves, bulbs and sulci, with an incidence of 1/40000 girls and 1:8000 boys (Dodé & Hardelin, 2009). This disorder can be autosomal-dominant with incomplete penetrance, autosomal-recessive, X-linked recessive, or can have an oligogenic/digenic inheritance pattern (Dodé & Hardelin, 2009; Jana & Kumar, 2010). Up to now, five genes have been implicated into the pathogenesis of the disease: KAL1 (Franco et al., 1991; Hardelin et al., 1992), FGFR1 (Dodé et al., 2003), FGF8 (Falardeau et al., 2008), PROKR2 and PROK2 (Dodé et al., 2006). However, a smaller amount (around 30%) of affected subjects present mutations in any of these genes. Affected women present hypogonadotropic hypogonadism, amenorrhea and absence of secondary sexual characteristics together with hyposmia or anosmia (Seminara et al., 1998). Generally, the diagnosis is performed during adolescence on the basis of reproductive and olfactory disorders. However, patients with Kallman syndrome can present further characteristics as well as mental retardation, cerebellar ataxia, cardiovascular anomalies, cranio-facial alterations, renal agenesis, hearing impairment, and abnormal visual spatial alterations (Quinton et al., 2001).

The *Idiopathic Hypogonadotropic Hypogonadism* is a rare genetic disease caused by a deficiency of hypothalamic gonadotropin-releasing hormone release; however, this disorder can be also caused by an impaired action of gonadotropin-releasing hormone on gonadotropes cells in the pituitary (Bianco & Kaiser, 2009). Idiopathic hypogonadotropic hypogonadism has been suggested to be the result of isolated functional anomalies of the neuroendocrine signals for release of gonadotropin-releasing hormone or gonadotropins. In fact, in these subjects no developmental or anatomical alterations of the hypothalamus-pituitary-gonadotropin axis have been described; the affected patients present a normal olfaction in presence of a phenotype deriving from pre- and postnatal gonadotropins and sex steroid deficiency (Brioude et al., 2010). Hypogonadotropic hypogonadism may be also due to mutations in gonadotropin-releasing hormone receptor genes (Layman et al., 2001).

Active, uncontrolled or untreated chronic diseases responsible for hypothalamic amenorrhea include malabsorption, acquired immune deficiency syndrome, diabetes, and kidney disorders (The Practice Committee of American Society for Reproductive Medicine, 2008).

Infections include meningitis, encephalitis, syphilis, and tuberculosis (The Practice Committee of American Society for Reproductive Medicine, 2008).

Possible *tumours* causing hypothalamic amenorrhea include craniopharyngioma, Langerhans cell histiocytosis, hamartoma, germinoma, endodermal sinus tumor, teratoma, metastatic carcinoma (The Practice Committee of American Society for Reproductive Medicine, 2008).

3.3 Pituitary causes

The main pituitary disorders responsible for amenorrhea include tumours, inflammatory/infiltrative disorders, panhypopituitarism and empty sella syndrome (Deligeoroglou et al., 2010).

Possible pituitary *tumours* causing amenorrhea include prolactinomas, and other tumours secreting hormones such as adrenocorticotropic hormone, thyrotropin-stimulating hormone, growth hormone, gonadotropins (luteinizing hormone, follicle-stimulating hormone).

Hyperprolactinemia represents the most frequent cause of amenorrhea of pituitary origin, being responsible for 1% of cases of primary amenorrhea (Patel & Bamigboye, 2007). In fact, high levels of prolactin suppress hypothalamic gonadotropin-releasing hormone release determining a reduction of estradiol levels. It is fundamental to recognize the origin of prolactin hypersecretion. In fact, in women with hyperprolactinemia it has been estimated a prevalence of pituitary tumours of approximately 50-60% (Brenner et al., 1985). However, it is important to rule out also any other cause responsible for rise in prolactin levels, including macroprolactinemia, hypothyroidism, stress, antipsychotics and masses reducing dopamine release; in fact, prolactin pituitary release is principally inhibited by dopamine (Asa & Ezzat, 2009). Furthermore, in women with mild prolactin increase it is common to find altered inhibiting systems (Deligeoroglou et al., 2010).

Among the pituitary disorders responsible for amenorrhea, Sheehan's syndrome represents a form of hypopituitarism resulting from ischemic pituitary necrosis caused by severe postpartum haemorrhage, especially in developing countries (Kelestimur, 2003). Up to now the pathogenesis of this syndrome is still unknown although it has been proposed that during pregnancy the enlarged pituitary gland, small sella dimension, autoimmunity and disseminated intravascular coagulopathy could play a pivotal role. A variety of signs and symptoms have been described in women affected by Sheehan's syndrome, including tiredness, weakness, agalactia, amenorrhea and partial to total hypopituitarism. The majority of affected women show empty sella on computer assisted tomography or magnetic resonance imaging. It has been recommended to consider primary empty sella syndrome and lymphocytic hypophysitis among differential diagnosis.

Systemic inflammatory/infiltrative diseases, like hemocromatosis and sarcoidosis, represent less frequent pituitary causes of amenorrhea (Deligeoroglou et al., 2010).

3.4 Ovary insufficiency

Ovary insufficiency includes a wide spectrum of diseases characterized by hypergonadotropic hypogonadism due to an insufficient production of sex steroids in presence of high follicle-stimulating hormone and luteinizing hormone levels. Hypergonadotropic hypogonadism can be due to several conditions including gonadal agenesis or dysgenesis, premature ovarian failure and enzymatic deficits; each of these conditions includes many other disorders (Deligeoroglou et al., 2010).

Gonadal dysgenesis includes those situations characterized by anomalous development causing streak gonads. These conditions can take place in patients with abnormal as well as normal karyotype.

Turner Syndrome represents the most frequent chromosomal abnormality responsible for gonadal dysgenesis, having an incidence of approximately 1/2500 live female births (Nielsen & Wohlert, 1991). The diagnosis of Turner syndrome is performed on the basis of typical phenotypic characteristics in phenotypic girls females (Turner, 1938; Ullrich, 1930) having partial or total absence of one X chromosome, with or without mosaicisms (Ferguson-Smith, 1965). The key features of Turner syndrome are webbing of the neck, misshapen ears, broad chest, widely spaced nipples, cubitus valgus, cardiac malformations, renal diseases and short stature (Morgan, 2007). Furthermore, one of the most frequent characteristics of Turner syndrome is the lack of pubertal development. In fact, although the ovaries develop normally, they degenerate during intrauterine life and infancy, and more than 90% of females will present gonadal failure (Bondy et al., 2007). However, approximately 30% of these patients will present natural pubertal development (Boechat et

al., 1996; Pasquino et al., 1997), and menses will occur in 2-5% of girls having 46,XX/45,X mosaicism due to a normal oocytes amount; furthermore, about 5% of girls with Turner syndrome will present spontaneous pregnancy (Hovatta, 1999).
Gonadal dysgenesis can happen also in subjects with 46,XY or 46,XX karyotype. In particular, subjects with 46,XY karyotype are known to be affected by Swyer syndrome. These subjects present female external or ambiguous genitalia with normal development of vagina and uterus due to the absent or inadequate production of anti-Mullerian hormone and testosterone (Barbaro et al., 2007). It has been estimated that approximately 25% of subjects with diagnosis of Swyer syndrome develop gonadal tumours; for this reason, it is necessary to remove gonads at the diagnosis (Manuel et al., 1976).
Premature ovarian failure refers to primary ovarian defect occurring in women younger than 40 years of age. This condition can be responsible for primary amenorrhea, or secondary amenorrhea when there is premature oocytes depletion and/or reduced folliculogenesis (Santoro, 2003; Timmreck & Reindollar, 2003). It has been estimated a premature ovarian failure incidence of approximately 1/1000 women under the age of 30 years, 1/250 around the age of 35 years and 1/100 at the age of 40 years (Timmreck & Reindollar, 2003). Furthermore, it has been described a familial form of premature ovarian failure which accounts for 4-31% of cases (Conway et al., 1996; Cramer et al., 1995; Torgerson et al., 1997). Premature ovarian failure can have different causes: iatrogenic after surgery or treatment of cancer (Santoro, 2003), autoimmune, infective (mumps oophoritis, cytomegalovirus, herpes zoster) and metabolic (galactosemia) (Beck-Peccoz & Persani, 2006). However, the major part of all cases of premature ovarian failure is idiopathic, and a genetic aetiology has been suggested on the basis of candidate genes found in some families (Van Kasteren & Schoemaker, 1999). In fact, disorders of the X chromosome have been found to be related with premature ovarian failure in women with Turner syndrome, partial X deletions or translocation, or presence of an extra X chromosome (Goswami & Conway, 2007). In particular two genes, respectively POF1, localised on Xq21.3–Xq27, and POF2, localised on Xq13.3–q21.1, have been found to be associated with chromosomal anomalies responsible for POF development (Beck-Peccoz & Persani, 2006). However, numerous other genes have been implicated in females with premature ovarian failure, including BMP15, FMR1, FMR2, LHR, FSHR, INHA, FOXL2, FOXO3, ERa, SF1, ERb and CYP19A1 genes (Cordts et al., 2011). Clinically, the presentation is characterized by primary amenorrhea in adolescents without secondary female characteristics, or disappearance of menses in women with normal pubertal development, palpitations, flushes, tiredness and depression. Endocrine evaluation shows high basal gonadotropins levels and low estradiol and inhibin values (Beck-Peccoz & Persani, 2006).

3.5 Endocrinopathies

The spectrum of endocrinopathies is broad and includes adrenal diseases (including 17-a-Hydroxylase deficiency, 17,20-Lyase deficiency, aromatase deficiency), thyropathies, poorly controlled diabetes and ovarian disorders (Deligeoroglou et al., 2010).

3.6 Chronic oligo- or anovulation

Chronic oligo- or anovulation refers to p*olycystic ovary syndrome,* an eterogeneous endocrinopathy characterized by a broad spectrum of clinical and biochemical features. In fact, this complex disorder requires the presence of several phenotypes, including hyperandrogenism and/or hyperandrogenemia, and normoovulation or oligoovulation with or without polycystic ovaries (Azziz et al., 2006). This phenomenon has been described in at least 6% of women during the reproductive years (Rosenfield, 2007). However, it has been recently reported that using different diagnostic criteria the prevalence of polycystic ovary syndrome was approximately 18% (March et al., 2010). The etiopathogenesis of polycystic ovary syndrome is still unclear although it seems a combination of genetic and environmental factors. In particular, two conditions have been recognized as playing a major role: insulin resistance with hyperinsulinemia and hyperandrogenism (Teede et al., 2010). In addition, hypothalamic/pituitary disorders, ovarian disorders failure and obesity are implicated in the pathogenesis of polycystic ovary syndrome (Doi et al., 2005; Legro & Strauss, 2002). This syndrome becomes symptomatic already during adolescence (Azziz et al., 2004; Franks et al., 2006) with psychological, metabolic and reproductive symptoms, including depression, anxiety (Deeks et al., 2010), hirsutism, oligoamenorrhea or amenorrhoea, infertility (Boomsma et al., 2006), metabolic syndrome, type 2 diabetes and cardiovascular diseases (Apridonidze et al., 2005; Legro et al., 1999). In particular, 70% to 80% of women with polycystic ovary syndrome show oligoamenorrhea or amenorrhoea caused by chronic oligo-ovulation/anovulation (Brassard et al., 2008; Teede et al., 2010).

4. The assessment and investigation of amenorrhea

According to the American Society for Reproductive Medicine, the investigation of amenorrheic girls should be started by 15 years of age in girls with normal secondary sexual development as well as in girls presenting thelarche before 10 years of age but without menses within 5 years, and in girls without secondary sexual development until 13 years of age (The Practice Committee of American Society for Reproductive Medicine, 2008). Diagnostic features of primary and secondary amenorrhea are reported in Table 2.

4.1 Medical history

The first step in the evaluation of amenorrheic girl should be based on the *patient and family history* (Master-Hunter & Heiman, 2006). The physician should conduct a complete patient history including growth and pubertal pattern, congenital anomalies, preceding or existing chronic or autoimmune diseases, anosmia, galactorrhea, recurring abdominal and/or pelvic pain, headache, vomiting, nausea, visual changes or double vision, preceding central nervous system radiation or chemotherapy and/or pelvic radiation, legal or illegal drug utilize, psychological distress, nutritional and exercise pattern, menarche, menstrual history, sexual life. In particular, date of menarche and records of menses should be extremely accurate. The family history should include growth and pubertal pattern, menarche and menstrual history of mothers and sisters, infertility, genetic disorders, chronic or autoimmune diseases, disorders or signs of androgen excess, hypo/hypertrichosis of pubis.

4.2 Physical examination

A complete *physical evaluation* should be carefully performed (Master-Hunter & Heiman, 2006), including anthropometric measurements [height, height standard deviation score, weight, body mass index, body mass index standard deviation score, growth velocity], staging of pubertal development according to the criteria of Marshall and Tanner (Marshall & Tanner, 1969), signs of androgen excess (acne, hirsutism, deepening of the voice), signs or

	Clinical aspects	Laboratoristic features	Instrumental procedures
Anatomic genital defects	-Frequent abdominal and pelvic pain -Hematometra/hematocolpos -Normal secondary female characteristics, except in: • mild androgen insensitivity syndrome (male external genitalia) • partial androgen insensitivity syndrome (partial masculinization of external genitalia) -Scarce or absent pubic/axillary hair, inguinal masses (complete androgen insensitivity syndrome)	-In Mayer-Rokitansky- Küster-Hauser syndrome: • normal levels of basal gonadotropins and sex steroids • no hyperandrogenism • 46,XX karyotype -In complete androgen insensitivity syndrome: • high levels of basal LH and testosterone, frequently with high levels of estradiol • 46,XY karyotype	-Pelvic ultrasonography and magnetic resonance imaging: • anatomic defects -Hysteroscopy or salpingogram: • intrauterine synechiae
Hypothalamic causes	-Low body weight (functional hypothalamic amenorrhea) -Absence of secondary sexual characteristics, hyposmia/anosmia (Kallman syndrome) -Normal olfaction with a phenotype deriving from pre- and postnatal gonadotropins and sex steroid deficiency (idiopathic hypogonadotropic hypogonadism)	-Insufficient secretion of GnRH leading to low levels of basal gonadotropins and estradiol -After stimulation with exogenous GnRH, gonadotropins secretion is in the physiological range -Low levels of leptin	Magnetic resonance imaging: • normal or altered anatomy/ development of the hypothalamus
Pituitary causes	-Galactorrhea (prolactinomas)	-High levels of prolactin -Suppression of GnRH release -Reduction of estradiol levels	Magnetic resonance imaging: • empty sella • normal or altered anatomy/ development of the pituitary gland
Ovary insufficiency	-Lack of pubertal development, webbing of the neck, misshapen ears, widely spaced nipples, cardiac malformations, renal diseases, short stature (Turner syndrome) -Female external or ambiguous genitalia with normal vagina and uterus (Swyer syndrome) -Primary amenorrhea without secondary characteristics, or secondary amenorrhea in girls with normal puberty (ovarian failure)	-High FSH and LH levels -Estrogen deficiency -Low inhibin levels -Karyotype: • 46,XX • 45,X • 46,XX/45,X mosaicism • 46,XY	Pelvic ultrasonography: • streak gonads • absent or reduced follicular activity
Chronic oligo- or anovulation	-Signs of androgen excess: acne, hirsutism, deepening of the voice -Obesity, metabolic syndrome, type 2 diabetes, cardiovascular diseases -Oligoamenorrhea or amenorrhoea	-Hyperandrogenemia -Insulin resistance -Hyperinsulinemia	Pelvic ultrasonography: • polycystic ovaries

Table 2. Diagnostic features of primary and secondary amenorrhea

symptoms of systemic diseases or endocrine disorders (goiter, central obesity, purplish skin striae, muscle weakness), and stigmata of genetic anomalies (short stature, misshapen ears, broad chest, widely spaced nipples, cubitus valgus). Systolic blood pressure and diastolic blood pressure should be measured to exclude hypertension. Therefore, the physician should perform a careful examination of the external genitalia to assess clitoris, hymen permeability and vaginal and uterine development (Adams Hillard, 2008).

4.3 Laboratory evaluation

Laboratory evaluation of amenorrheic adolescents should include the measurements of basal plasma gonadotropins, estradiol, progesterone, free and total testosterone, dehydroepiandrosterone sulphate, delta4-androstenedione, 17-OHprogesterone, thyroid function tests (free triiodothyronine, free thyroxine, thyrotropin, anti-thyroglobulin antibodies, anti-thyroid peroxidase antibodies, anti-thyrotropin receptor antibodies), prolactin, fasting insulin and glucose, insulin resistance indexes, adrenocorticotropic hormone, cortisol, markers of ovarian tumours. Because pregnancy represents the most frequent cause of secondary amenorrhea, urine or serum pregnancy test is obligatory in adolescents with irregular menses (Master-Hunter & Heiman,2006). It has been suggested to perform the "progesterone challenge test" in those females with secondary amenorrhea and androgen in the normal range in order to measure circulating estrogens values and identify an insufficient endometrial estrogenization (Deligeoroglou et al., 2010).

It can be also very important to detect peak plasma gonadotropins response to exogenous gonadotropin-releasing hormone to detect a defect of hypothalamic-pituitary axis. Karyotype should be requested in case of suspected genetic anomalies.

4.4 Instrumental evaluation

The *instrumental procedures* are crucial in the evaluation of primary and secondary amenorrhea. Pelvic transabdominal ultrasonography scanning should be performed by a trained and experienced operator to measure length, breadth, and depth of uterus and ovaries, and endometrial thickness. Furthermore, magnetic resonance imaging of the hypothalamus and pituitary gland, and magnetic resonance imaging of the pelvis are of pivotal importance. In some cases, it can be necessary to perform hysteroscopy or hysterosalpingogram to assess the presence of intrauterine synechiae (The Practice Committee of American Society for Reproductive Medicine, 2008).

5. Treatment of amenorrhea

Amenorrhea and the related disorders require appropriate treatments (Table 3).

	Therapeutic approaches
Anatomic genital defects	- Surgical correction - Gonadectomy followed by exogenous estrogens (complete androgen insensitivity syndrome)
Hypothalamic causes	- Estrogens and progestin replacement therapy - Calcium and vitamin D supplementation - Reduced physical activity, weight gain - Surgical removal of tumours
Pituitary causes	- Dopamine agonists: cabergoline or bromocriptine (prolactinomas) - Surgical removal (tumours) - Estrogens and progestin replacement therapy
Ovary insufficiency	- Estrogens replacement therapy at approximately 12 years of age at low-doses, followed by a gradual augment over 2-4 years. Progestin should be started after at least 2 years or at uterine bleeding. Calcium supplementation (Turner syndrome) - Estrogens replacement therapy after gonadectomy at approximately 11 years of age (Swyer syndrome) - Estrogens replacement therapy until the normal age of menopause; for females having a whole uterus combined estrogens and progestin hormone therapy; physical activity, diet rich in calcium and vitamin D (premature ovarian failure)
Endocrine diseases	Appropriate therapy
Chronic oligo- or anovulation	- Increased physical activity, reduced food intake - Estrogen replacement therapy at low doses combined with cyclic progestin - Insulin-sensitising drugs (metformin)

Table 3. Therapeutic approaches for primary and secondary amenorrhea

5.1 Treatment of the anatomic defects of the genital tract

Every anatomic defect of the genital tract requires appropriate surgical procedures. In particular, transverse vaginal septum require the excision, imperforate hymen necessitates the elimination of the tissue in a triangular form and intrauterine synechiae require their removal. Furthermore, cervical agenesis may require hysterectomy while cervical dysgenesis may necessitate cervical canalization (Deligeoroglou et al., 2010).

Regarding to Mayer-Rokitansky-Küster-Hauser syndrome, patients may benefit by surgical formation of a neovagina; undeveloped uterus should be removed in presence of functional endometrium as it can be responsible for uterus swelling and recurrent lower abdominal pain. Finally, in girls with diagnosis of androgen insensitivity syndrome a vaginal length adequate for intercourse could be reached through non surgical dilatation. However, in some cases surgical correction of genital tract anomalies should be performed in order to create a neovagina. Both in girls affected by Mayer-Rokitansky-Küster-Hauser syndrome and androgen insensitivity syndrome it is imperative to guarantee a constant psychological support (Deligeoroglou et al., 2010).

5.2 Treatment of hypothalamic and pituitary disorders

Hypothalamic amenorrhea should be treated according to its aetiology. In particular, treatment of functional hypothalamic amenorrhea should be finalised to the appearance or regulation of menstrual cycles by starting estrogens and progestin therapy. Furthermore, this therapy should prevent the development of osteoporosis. Respect to oral estrogens, it has been demonstrated that transdermal hormone replacement therapy has better effects on bone density than oral hormone replacement therapy due to the absence of the first-pass hepatic metabolism (Jayasinghe et al., 2008). In addition, calcium and vitamin D supplementation is highly suggested (Master-Hunter & Heiman, 2006). In particular, in athletes with the "female athlete triad" treatment targets to restore menses through reduced physical activity, weight gain, calcium supplementation and estrogen therapy (American Academy of Pediatrics Committee on Sports Medicine and Fitness, 2000).
Regarding to the Kallmann syndrome, the treatment targets to promote breast development through estrogens and progestin replacement therapy in girls and to promote virilization through testosterone replacement therapy in males. Furthermore, hormonal treatments can be offered as a valid method for restoring fertility in these patients. Both pulsatile gonadotropin-releasing hormone or gonadotropins administration have been utilized to stimulate ovulation in females and spermatogenic activity in males (Buchter et al., 1998). Also in the majority of subjects affected by idiopathic hypogonadotropic hypogonadism, long-term exogenous pulsatile gonadotropin-releasing hormone therapy has been proven to be efficient because it induces testicular growth and development of sperm in the ejaculate, favours sexual life and improves reproductive prognosis. However, a minor part of this population did not respond to gonadotropin-releasing hormone replacement, suggesting that pituitary and testicular defects in these subjects are improbable to be totally consequences of gonadotropin-releasing hormone deficiency (Sykiotis et al., 2010).
Regarding to prolactinomas, therapy should target to restore menses and guarantee fertility. Dopamine agonists are the favourite treatment of hyperprolactinemia because they are able to reduce prolactin levels, to decrease the tumor size and to restore gonadal function (Iyer & Molitch, 2011). Actually, two dopamine agonists are used to treat prolactinomas: bromocriptine and cabergoline. In particular, cabergoline has been shown to be more efficacious with less adverse effects than bromocriptine in females with microadenomas (Webster et al., 1994). Therefore, cabergoline represents the principal therapeutic approach. Also females with macroadenoma can benefit by dopamine agonists or, in some cases, they must underwent surgical removal of tumours (Master-Hunter & Heiman, 2006).
Sheehan's syndrome requires the general standard of treatment of patients presenting with hypopituitarism, aiming to replace the endocrine deficits. In particular, because these patients are at increased risk of developing partial loss of feminization, amenorrhea and osteoporosis, they should start hormone replacement therapy (Kelestimur, 2003).

5.3 Treatment of ovary insufficiency-related diseases

Turner syndrome requires growth-promoting treatments aimed to obtain a normal progression of puberty and the achievement of a normal adult height. Growth hormone represents the focus of growth-promoting therapy as this therapy is able to improve growth velocity and final height (Bondy et al., 2007). Regarding to the induction of puberty, it is opportune to dose gonadotropins levels before starting hormone replacement therapy to rule out a delayed puberty. Recent data have demonstrated that treatment with estrogens should begin at approximately 12 years of age to promote a normal pubertal development without interfering with growth hormone therapy on final height. Actually, oral estrogens as well as transdermal and injectable depot forms of estradiol are available (Ankarberg-Lindgren et al., 2001; Rosenfield et al., 2005). Estradiol therapy is generally initiated at low-doses (from 1/10 to 1/8 of the adult dose) followed by a gradual augment over 2–4 years, while progestin should be started after at least 2 years or when uterine bleeding happens to permit a regular uterine and breast development (Bondy et al., 2007). In addition, calcium supplementation has been highly suggested in Turner syndrome.

In Swyer syndrome, estrogens replacement therapy should be started after gonadectomy at approximately 11 years of age in order to allow a normal pace of puberty (Han et al., 2008).

Women with diagnosis of premature ovarian failure should undergo estrogens replacement therapy until the normal age of menopause to replace deficit of ovarian estrogens and to counter menopausal symptoms. In particular, for those females having a whole uterus it is preferable to start combined estrogens and progestin hormone therapy to avoid hyperplasia of the endometrium (Shelling, 2010). Due to estrogen deficiency, women with premature ovarian failure are also at risk of osteoporosis (Rebar, 2009); for this reason, physical activity, diet rich in calcium and vitamin D without smoking or alcohol consumption are mandatory.

5.4 Treatment of chronic oligo- or anovulation

Overweight or obese women with polycystic ovary syndrome presenting oligomenorrhoea or amenorrhoea should underwent structured lifestyle interventions, including increased physical activity and reduced food intake (Moran et al., 2009). In fact, it has been demonstrated that a weight loss of 5-10% is associated with beneficial effects on reproductive system (Huber-Buchholz et al., 1999). Regarding to pharmacological treatment, actually there is no therapy able to completely resolve hormonal disturbances in polycystic ovary syndrome. Furthermore, pharmacological treatments should not substitute the lifestyle interventions (Teede et al., 2010). Estrogen replacement therapy at low doses combined with cyclic progestin can be started leading to a reduction of hyperandrogenism. Furthermore, insulin-sensitising drugs represent a valid approach to reduce insulin resistance in polycystic ovary syndrome (Meyer et al., 2007). In particular, metformin has been proven to improve ovulation and regulate menstrual periods (Tang et al., 2009).

6. Conclusion

Future research is needed to clarify amenorrhea and the related endocrine disorders in order to make an early diagnosis and to identify the more appropriate strategies during reproductive years of life.

7. References

Adams Hillard, P.J. (2008). Menstruation in adolescents: what's normal, what's not. *Annals of the New York Academy of Sciences*,1135:29-35

Ameh, E.A., Mshelbwala, P.M. & Ameh, N. (2011). Congenital vaginal obstruction in neonates and infants: recognition and management. *Journal of Pediatric and Adolescent Gynecology*. 24(2):74-78

American Academy of Pediatrics Committee on Sports Medicine and Fitness. (2000). Medical concerns of the female athlete. *Pediatrics*,106: 610-613

American College of Obstetricians and Gynecologist Committee on Adolescent Health Care. (2006). ACOG Committee Opinion No. 355. Vaginal agenesis: diagnosis, management, and routine care. *Obstetrics and Gynecology*,108(6):1605-1609

Ankarberg-Lindgren, C., Elfving, M., Wikland, K.A. & Norjavaara, E. (2001). Nocturnal application of transdermal estradiol patches produces levels of estradiol that mimic those seen at the onset of spontaneous puberty in girls. *Journal of Clinical Endocrinology and Metabolism*,86:3039-3044

Apridonidze, T., Essah, P.A., Iuorno, M.J. & Nestler, J.E. (2005). Prevalence and characteristics of the metabolic syndrome in women with polycystic ovary syndrome. *Journal of Clinical Endocrinology and Metabolism*,90:1929-1935

Asa, S.L. & Ezzat, S. (2009). The pathogenesis of pituitary tumors. *Annual Review of Pathology*,4:97-126

Azzizz, R., Woods, K.S., Reyna, R., Key, T.J., Knochenhauer, E.S. & Yildiz, B.O. (2004). The prevalence and features of the polycystic ovary syndrome in an unselected population. *Journal of Clinical Endocrinology and Metabolism*,89(6):2745-2749

Azziz, R., Carmina, E., Dewailly, D., Diamanti-Kandarakis, E., Escobar-Morreale, H.F., Futterweit, W., Janssen, O.E., Legro, R.S., Norman, R.J., Taylor, A.E. & Witchel, S.F. (2006). Positions statement: criteria for defining polycystic ovary syndrome as a predominantly hyperandrogenic syndrome: an Androgen Excess Society guideline. *Journal of Clinical Endocrinology and Metabolism*,91(11)4237-4245

Bachmann, G. & Kemmann, E. (1982). Prevalence of oligomenorrhea and amenorrhea in a college population. *American Journal of Obstetrics and Gynecology*,144:98-102

Barbaro, M., Oscarson, M., Schoumans, J., Staaf J., Ivarsson S.A. & Wedell, A. (2007). Duplication Containing the DAX1 Gene Isolated 46,XY Gonadal Dysgenesis in Two Sisters Caused by a Xp21.2 Interstitial. *Journal of Clinical Endocrinology and Metabolism*,92:3305-3313

Bean, E.J., Mazur, T. & Robinson, A.D. (2009). Mayer-Rokitansky-Küster-Hauser syndrome: sexuality, psychological effects, and quality of life. *Journal of Pediatric and Adolescent Gynecology*,22(6):339-346

Beck-Peccoz, P. & Persani, L. (2006). Premature ovarian failure. *Orphanet Journal of Rare Diseases*,1:9 doi:10.1186/1750-1172-1-9

Becker, A.E., Grinspoon, S.K., Klibanski, A. & Herzog, D.B. (1999). Eating disorders. *New England Journal of Medicine*, 340,1092-1098

Bianco, S.D. & Kaiser, U.B. (2009). The genetic and molecular basis of idiopathic hypogonadotropic hypogonadism. *Nature Reviews Endocrinology*,5:569-576

Boechat, M.I., Westra, S.J. & Lippe, B. (1996). Normal US appearance of ovaries and uterus in four patients with Turner's syndrome and 45,X karyotype. *Pediatric Radiology*,26:37-39

Boehmer, A.L., Brinkmann, O. & Bruggenwirth, H. (2001). Genotype versus phenotype in families with androgen insensitivity syndrome. *Journal of Clinical Endocrinology and Metabolism*,86:4151

Bondy, C.A. for The Turner Syndrome Consensus Study Group. (2007). Care of Girls and Women with Turner Syndrome: A Guideline of the Turner Syndrome Study Group. *Journal of Clinical Endocrinology and Metabolism*,92:10-25

Boomsma, C.M., Eijkemans, M.J., Hughes, E.G., Visser, G.H., Fauser, B.C. & Macklon, N.S. (2006). A meta-analysis of pregnancy outcomes in women with polycystic ovary syndrome. *Human Reproduction Update*,12:673-683

Brassard, M., AinMelk, Y. & Baillargeon, J.P. (2008). Basic infertility including polycystic ovary syndrome. *The Medical Clinics of North America*,92:1163-1192

Brennan, A.M. & Mantzoros, C.S. (2006). Drug Insight: the role of leptin in human physiology and pathophysiology--emerging clinical applications. *Nature Clinical Practice Endocrinology & Metabolism*,2(6):318-327

Brenner, S.H., Lessing, J.B., Quagliarello, J. & Weiss, G. (1985). Hyperprolactinemia and associated pituitary prolactinomas. *Obstetrics and Gynecology*,65:661-664

Brinkmann, A.O., Faber, P.W., van Rooij, H.C., Kuiper, G.G., Ris, C., Klaassen, P., van der Korput, J.A., Voorhorst, M.M., van Laar, J.H., Mulder, E. (1989) The human androgen receptor: domain structure, genomic organization and regulation of expression. *Journal of Steroid Biochemistry*,34(1-6):307-310

Brioude, F., Bouligand, J., Trabado, S., Francou, B., Salenave, S., Kamenicky, P., Brailly-Tabard, S., Chanson, P., Guiochon-Mantel, A. & Young, J. (2010). Non-syndromic congenital hypogonadotropic hypogonadism: clinical presentation and genotype-phenotype relationships. *European Journal of Endocrinology*,162:835-851

Buchter, D., Behre, H.M., Kliesch, S. & Nieschlag, E. (1998). Pulsatile GnRH or human chorionic gonadotropin/human menopausal gonadotropin as effective treatment for men with hypogonadotropic hypogonadism: a review of 42 cases. *European Journal of Endocrinology*,139:298-303

Carranza-Lira, S., Forbin, K. & Martinez-Chéquer, J.C. (1999). Rokitansky syndrome and MURCS association-clinical features and basis for diagnosis. *International Journal of Fertility and Women's Medicine*,44(5):250-255

Chumlea, W.C., Schubert, C.M., Roche, A.F., Kulin, H.E., Lee, P.A., Himes, J.H. & Sun, S.S. (2003). Age at menarche and racial comparisons in US girls. *Pediatrics*,111(1):110-113.

Conway, G.S., Kaltsas, G., Patel, A., Davies, M.C. & Jacobs, H.S. (1996). Characterization of idiopathic premature ovarian failure. *Fertility and Sterility*,64:337-341

Cordts Barchi, E., Christofolini, D.M., Amaro dos Santos, A., Bianco, B. & Parente Barbosa, C. (2011). Genetic aspects of premature ovarian failure: a literature review. *Archives of Gynecology and Obstetrics*,283:635-643

Cramer, D.W., Xu, H. & Harlow, B.L. (1995). Family history as a predictor of early menopause. *Fertility and Sterility*,64:740-745

Cremers, C.W., Strübbe, E.H. & Willemsen, W.N. (1995). Stapedial ankylosis in the Mayer-Rokitansky-Kuster-Hauser syndrome. *Archives of Otolaryngology Head & Neck Surgery*,121(7):800-803

Deeks, A.A., Gibson-Helm, M.E. & Teede, H.J. (2010). Anxiety and depression in polycystic ovary syndrome: a comprehensive investigation. *Fertility and Sterility*,93:2421-2423

Deligeoroglou, E., Athanasopoulos, N., Tsimaris, P., Dimopoulos, K.D., Vrachnis, N. & Creatsas, G. (2010). Evaluation and management of adolescent amenorrhea. *Annals of the New York Academy of Sciences*,1205:23-32

Diaz, A., Laufer M.R. & Breech, L.L. (2006). Menstruation in girls and adolescents: using the menstrual cycle as a vital sign. *Pediatrics*,118:2245-2250

Dodé, C., Levilliers, J., Dupont, J.M., De Paepe, A., Le Dù, N., Soussi-Yanicostas, N., Coimbra, RS., Delmaghani, S., Compain-Nouailles, S., Baverel, F., Pecheux, C., Le Tessier, D., Cruaud, C., Delpech, M., Speleman, F., Vermeulen, S., Amalfitano, A., Bachelot, Y., Bouchard, P., Cabrol, S., Carel, J.C., Delemarre-van de Waal, H., Goulet-Salmon, B., Kottler, M.L., Richard, O., Sanchez-Franco, F., Saura, R., Young, J., Petit, C. & Hardelin, J.P. (2003). Loss-of-function mutations. in FGFR1 cause autosomal dominant Kallmann syndrome. *Nature Genetics*,33:463-465

Dodé, C., Teixeira, L., Levilliers, J., Fouveaut, C., Bouchard, P., Kottler, M.L., Lespinasse, J., Lienhardt-Roussie, A., Mathieu, M., Moerman, A., Morgan, G., Murat, A., Toublanc, J.E., Wolczynski, S., Delpech, M., Petit, C., Young, J. & Hardelin, J.P. (2006). Kallmann syndrome: mutations in the genes encoding prokineticin-2 andprokineticin receptor-2. *PLoS Genetics*,2:1648-1652

Dodé, C. & Hardelin, J.P. (2009). Kallmann syndrome. *European Journal of Human Genetics*,17:139-146

Doi, S.A., Al-Zaid, M., Towers, P.A., Scott, C.J. & Al-Shoumer, K.A. (2005). Ovarian steroids modulate neuroendocrine dysfunction in polycystic ovary syndrome. *Journal of Endocrinological Investigation*,28:882-892

European Society of Human Reproduction and Embryology Capri Workshop Group. (2006). Nutrition and reproduction in women. *Human Reproduction Update*,12(3):193-207

Falardeau, J., Chung, W.C., Beenken, A., Raivio, T., Plummer, L., Sidis, Y., Jacobson-Dickman, E.E., Eliseenkova, A.V., Ma, J., Dwyer, A., Quinton, R., Na, S., Hall, J.E., Huot, C., Alois, N., Pearce, S.H., Cole, L.W., Hughes, V., Mohammadi, M., Tsai, P. & Pitteloud, N. (2008). Decreased FGF8 signaling causes deficiency of gonadotropin-releasing hormone in humans and mice. *Journal of Clinical Investigation*,118:2822-2831

Fedele, L., Bianchi, S., Tozzi, L., Borruto, F. & Vignali, M. (1996). A new laparoscopic procedure for creation of a neovagina in Mayer-Rokitansky-Kuster-Hauser syndrome. *Fertility and Sterility*,66(5):854-857

Ferguson-Smith, M.A. (1965). Karyotype-phenotype correlations in gonadal dysgenesis and their bearing on the pathogenesis of malformations. *Journal of Medical Genetics*,2:142-155

Flug, D., Largo, R.H. & Prader, A. (1984). Menstrual patterns in adolescent Swiss girls: a longitudinal study. *Annals of Human Biology*,11:495-508

Franco, B., Guioli, S., Pragliola, A. Incerti, B., Bardoni, B., Tonlorenzi, R., Carrozzo, R., Maestrini, E., Pieretti, M, Taillon-Miller, P., Brown, C.J., Willard, H.F., Lawrence, C., Graziella Persico, M., Camerino, G. & Ballabio, A. (1991). A gene deleted in Kallmann's. syndrome shares homology with neural cell adhesion and axonal path-finding molecules. *Nature*;353:529-536

Franks, S., McCarthy, M.I. & Hardy, K. (2006). Development of polycystic ovary syndrome: involvement of genetic and environmental factors. *International Journal of Andrology*,29(1):278-285

Frisch, R.E. & McArthur, J.W. (1974). Menstrual cycles: fatness as a determinant of minimum weight for height necessary for their maintenance or onset. *Science*,949-951

Frisch, R.E. (1987). Body fat, menarche, fitness and fertility. *Human Reproduction*,2:521-533

Golden, N.H. & Carlson, J.L. (2008). The pathophysiology of amenorrhea in the adolescents. *Annals of the New York Academy of Sciences*,1135:163-178

Goswami, D. & Conway, G.S. (2007). Premature ovarian failure. *Hormon Research*,68(4):196-202

Grumbach, M.N. (2003). Disorders of sex differentiation, In: *Williams Textbook of Endocrinology,* Larsen P.R., pp. 842-1002, Saunders, Philadelphia

Han, T.S., Goswami, D., Trikudanathan, S., Creighton, S.M. & Conway, G.S. (2008). Comparison of bone mineral density and body proportions between women with complete androgen insensitivity syndrome and women with gonadal dysgenesis. *European Journal of Endocrinology*,159(2):179-185

Hardelin, J.P., Levilliers, J., del Castillo, I., Cohen-Salmon, M., Legouis, R., Blanchard, S., Compain, S., Bouloux, P., Kirk, J., Moraine, C., Chaussain, J.L., Weissenbach, J. & Petit, C. (1992). X chromosome-linked. Kallmann syndrome: stop mutations validate the candidate gene. *Proceedings of the National Academy of Sciences of the United States of America*,89: 8190-8194

Hovatta, O. (1999). Pregnancies in women with Turner syndrome. *Annals of Medicine*,31:106-110

Huber-Buchholz, M.M., Carey, D.G. & Norman, R.J. (1999). Restoration of reproductive potential by lifestyle modification in obese polycystic ovary syndrome: role of insulin sensitivity and luteinizing hormone. *Journal of Clinical Endocrinology and Metabolism*,84:1470-1474

Hughes, I.A. & Deeb, A. (2006). Androgen resistance. *Best Practice & Research Clinical Endocrinology & Metabolism*,20(4):577-598

Iyer, P. & Molitch, M.E. (2011). Positive Prolactin Response to Bromocriptine in Two Patients with Cabergoline Resistant Prolactinomas. *Endocrine Practice*,16:1-11

Jana, M. & Kumar, A. (2010). Kallmann syndrome in an adolescent boy. *Pediatric Radiology*,40(1):S164

Jayasinghe, Y., Grover, S.R. & Zacharin, M. (2008). Current concepts in bone and reproductive health in adolescents with anorexia nervosa. *BJOG*,115(3):304-315

Jorgensen, P.B., Kjartansdòttir, K.R. & Fedder, J. (2010). Care of women with XY karyotype: a clinical practice guideline. *Fertility and Sterility*,94(1):105-113

Kelestimur, F. (2003). Sheehan's Syndrome. *Pituitary*,6:181-188

Laughlin, G.A., Dominguez, C.E. & Yen, S.S. (1998). Nutritional and endocrine metabolic aberrations in women with functional hypothalamic amenorrhea. *Journal of Clinical Endocrinology and Metabolism*,83,25-32

Layman, L.C., McDonough, P.G., Cohen, D.P., Maddox, M., Tho, S.P. & Reindollar, R.H. (2001). Familial gonadotropin-releasing hormone resistance and hypogonadotropic hypogonadism in a family with multiple affected individuals. *Fertility and Sterility*,75:1148-1155

Legro, R.S. & Strauss, J.F. (2002). Molecular progress in infertility: polycystic ovary syndrome. *Fertility and Sterility*,78:569-576

Legro, R.S., Kunselman, A.R., Dodson, W.C. & Dunaif, A. (1999). Prevalence and predictors of risk for type 2 diabetes mellitus and impaired glucose tolerance in polycystic ovary syndrome: a prospective, controlled study in 254 affected women. *Journal of Clinical Endocrinology and Metabolism*,84:165-169

Manuel, M., Katayama, P.K. & Mand Jones, H.W.Jr. (1976). The age of occurrence of gonadal tumors in intersex patients with a Y chromosome. *American Journal of Obstetrics and Gynecology*,124:293-300

March, W.A., Moore, V.M., Willson, K.J., Phillips, D.I., Norman, R.J. & Davies, M.J. (2010). The prevalence of polycystic ovary syndrome in a community sample assessed under contrasting diagnostic criteria. *Human Reproduction*,25:544-551

Marshall, W.A. & Tanner, J.M. (1969). Variations in pattern of pubertal changes in girls. *Archives of Disease in Childhood*,44(235):291-303

Master-Hunter, T. & Heiman, D.L. (2006). Amenorrhea: evaluation and treatment. *American Family Physician*,73(8):1374-1382

Mendelsohn, F.A. & Warren, M.P. (2010). Anorexia, bulimia, and the female athlete triad: evaluation and management. *Endocrinology and Metabolism Clinics in North America*,39(1):155-167

Meyer, C., McGrath, B.P. & Teede, H.J. (2007). Effects of medical therapy on insulin resistance and the cardiovascular system in polycystic ovary syndrome. *Diabetes Care*,30:471-478

Miller, K.K., Grinspoon, S.K., Ciampa, J., Hier, J., Herzog, D. & Klibanski, A. (2005). Medical findings in outpatients with anorexia nervosa. *Archives of Internal Medicine*,165:561-566

Moran, L.J., Pasquali, R., Teede, H.J., Hoeger, K.M. & Norman, R.J. (2009). Treatment of obesity in polycystic ovary syndrome: a position statement of the Androgen Excess and Polycystic Ovary Syndrome Society. *Fertility and Sterility*, 92:1966-1982

Morcel, K. & Camborieux, L. (2007). Programme de Recherches sur les Aplasies Müllériennes, Guerrier, D. Mayer-Rokitansky-Kuster-Hauser (MRKH) syndrome. *Orphanet Journal of Rare Diseases*,14;2:13

Morgan, T. (2007). Turner Syndrome: Diagnosis and Management. *American Family Physician*,76:405-410

Nielsen, J. & Wohlert, M. (1991). Chromosome abnormalities found among 34.910 newborn children: results from a 13-year incidence study in Arhus, Denmark. *Human Genetics*,87:81-83

Oakes, M.B., Eyvazzadeh, A.D., Quint, E. & Smith, Y.R. (2008). Complete androgen insensitivity syndrome-a review. J *Pediatric and Adolescent Gynecology*,21(6):305-310

Pasquino, A.M., Passeri, F., Pucarelli, I., Segni, M. & Municchi, G. (1997). Spontaneous pubertal development in Turner's syndrome. *Journal of Clinical Endocrinology and Metabolism*,82:1810-1813

Patel, S.S. & Bamigboye, V. (2007). Hyperprolactinaemia. *Journal of Obstetrics and Gynaecology*,27:455-459

Pettersson, F., Fries, H. & Nillius, S.J. (1973). Epidemiology of secondary amenorrhea. I. Incidence and prevalence rates. *American Journal of Obstetrics and Gynecology*,117:80-86

Quinton, R., Duke, V.M., Robertson, A., Kirk, J.M., Matfin, G., de Zoysa PA, Azcona, C., MacColl, G.S., Jacobs, H.S., Conway, G.S., Besser, M., Stanhope, R.G. & Bouloux, P.M. (2001). Idiopathic gonadotrophin deficiency: genetic questions addressed through phenotypic characterization. *Clinical Endocrinology* (Oxf),55:163-174

Rebar, R.W. (2009). Premature ovarian failure. *Obstetrics and Gynaecology*,113:1355-1363

Rock, J.A., H.A. Zacur, A.M. Dlugi, Jones, H.W.Jr & Telinde, R.W. (1982). Pregnancy success following surgical correction of imperforate hymen and complete transverse vaginal septum. *Obstetrics and Gynecology*,59:448-451

Rosenfield, R.L., Devine, N., Hunold, J.J., Mauras, N., Moshang, T.Jr & Root, A.W. (2005). Salutary effects of combining early very low-dose systemic estradiol with growth hormone therapy in girls with Turner syndrome. *Journal of Clinical Endocrinology and Metabolism*,90:6424-6430

Rosenfield, RL. (2007). Identifying children at risk of polycystic ovary syndrome. *Journal of Clinical Endocrinology and Metabolism*,92(3):787-796

Santoro, N. (2003). Mechanisms of premature ovarian failure. *Annals of Endocrinology*,64:87-92

Sarpel, U. (2005). The incidence of complete androgen insensitivity in girls with inguinal hernias and assessment of screening by vaginal length measurement. *Journal of Pediatric Surgery*,40:133

Seminara, S.B., Hayes, F.J. & Crowley, W.F.Jr. (1998). Gonadotropin-releasing hormone deficiency in the human (idiopathic hypogonadotropic hypogonadism and Kallmann's syndrome): pathophysiological and genetic considerations. *Endocrine Reviews*,19:521-539

Shelling, A.N. (2010). Premature ovarian failure. *Reproduction*,140(5):633-641

Strübbe, E.H., Cremers, C.W., Dikkers, F.G. & Willemsen, W.N. (1994). Hearing loss and the Mayer-Rokitansky-Kuster-Hauser syndrome. *The American Journal of Otology*,15(3):431-436

Swenson, I. & Havens, B. (1987). Menarche and menstruation: a review of the literature. *Journal of Community Health Nursing*,4(4):199-210

Sykiotis, G.P., Hoang, X.H., Avbelj, M. & Hayes, F.J., Thambundit, A., Dwyer, A., Au, M., Plummer, L., Crowley, W.F.Jr. & Pitteloud, N. (2010). Congenital Idiopathic Hypogonadotropic Hypogonadism: Evidence of Defects in the Hypothalamus, Pituitary, and Testes. *Journal of Clinical Endocrinology and Metabolism*,95(6):3019-3027

Tang, T., Lord, J.M., Norman, R.J., Yasmin, E. & Balen, A.H. (2009). Insulin-sensitising drugs (metformin, rosiglitazone, pioglitazone, D-chiro-inositol) for women with polycystic ovary syndrome, oligo amenorrhoea and subfertility. *Cochrane Database of Systematic Reviews*,4:CD003053

Teede, H., Deeks, A. & Moran, L. (2010). Polycystic ovary syndrome: a complex condition with psychological, reproductive and metabolic manifestations that impacts on health across the lifespan. *BMC Medicine*,8:41

The Practice Committee of American Society for Reproductive Medicine. (2008). Current evaluation of amenorrhea. *Fertility and Sterility*,90(5 Suppl):S219-225

Thomas, F., Renaud, F., Benefice, E., de Meeüs, T., Guegan, J.F. (2001). International variability of ages at menarche and menopause: patterns and main determinants. *Human Biology*,73(2):271-290

Timmreck, L.S. & Reindollar, R.H. (2003). Contemporary issues in primary amenorrhea. *Obstetrics and Gynecology Clinics of North America*,30(2):287-302

Torgerson, D.J., Thomas, R.E. & Reid, D.M. (1997). Mothers and daughters menopausal ages: is there a link? *European Journal of Obstetrics, Gynecology and Reproductive Biology*,74:63-66

Turner, H.H. (1938). A syndrome of infantilism, congenital webbed neck, and cubitus valgus. *Endocrinology*,23:566–574

Ullrich, O. (1930). U ber typische Kombinationsbilder multipler Abartungen. *Zeitschrift fur Kinderheilkunde*,49:271-276

Van Kasteren, Y.M. & Schoemaker, J. (1999) Premature ovarian failure: a systematic review on therapeutic interventions to restore ovarian function and achieve pregnancy. *Human Reproduction Update*,5:483-492

Warren, M.P. & Goodman, L.R. (2003). Exercise-induced endocrine pathologies. *Journal of Endocrinological Investigation*,26(9):873-878

Watson, T.L. & Andersen, A.E. (2003). A critical examination of the amenorrhea and weight criteria for diagnosing anorexia nervosa. *Acta Psychiatrica Scandinavica*,108:175-182

Webster, J., Piscitelli, G., Polli, A., Ferrari, C.I., Ismail, I. & Scanlon, M.F. (1994). A comparison of cabergoline and bromocriptine in the treatment of hyperprolactinemic amenorrhea. Cabergoline Comparative Study Group. *New England Journal of Medicine*,331(14):904-909

Welt, C.K., Chan, J.L., Bullen, J., Murphy, R., Smith, P., DePaoli, A.M., Karalis, A. & Mantzoros, C.S. (2004). Recombinant human leptin in women with hypothalamic amenorrhea. *New England Journal of Medicin*e,35:987-997

World Health Organization task force on adolescent reproductive health. (1986). World Health Organization multicenter study on menstrual and ovulatory patterns in adolescent girls. II. Longitudinal study of menstrual patterns in the early postmenarcheal period, duration of bleeding episodes and menstrual cycles. *Journal of Adolescent Health Care*,7:236-244

21

The Management of Dysfunctional Uterine Bleeding

Aytul Corbacioglu
Bakirkoy Women's and Children's Teaching Hospital, Department of Obstetrics and Gynaecology Turkey

1. Introduction

Abnormal uterine bleeding is one of the most common reasons for women to seek for care. Dysfunctional uterine bleeding describes the spectrum of abnormal bleeding patterns in the abscence of a medical illness or pelvic pathology. It is responsible for about half of the women with abnormal uterine bleeding in reproductive age (Ewenstein, 1996). It mainly presents as menorrhagia, hence, the term generally refers to heavy, prolonged and frequent bleeding of uterine origin which is not due to any recognisable cause (Farrell, 2004). It is a debiliating disorder both medically and socially. In addition, it is the commonest cause of iron deficinecy in the developed world and of chronic illness in the developing world (Royal College of Obstetrics and Gynaecology [RCOG], 1998). The number of menses experienced by women in their lifetimes increased as a result of the reduction of family size leading to shorter periods of childbearing and lactational amenorrhoea. As a consequence, abnormal menstruation is especially a problem of the twentieth century (Farquhar & Brown, 2009). The prevelance of abnormal uterine bleeding in reproductive age group ranges from 9% to 30% (Coulter et al.,1991). One in 20 women aged 30-49 in the UK consult their General Practitioner each year with menorrhagia, and it accounts for 12% of all gynaecology referrals (Vessey t al., 1992).

Dysfunctional uterine bleeding is a diagnosis of exclusion. Menstrual history and physical examination are the mainstay of evaluation of cases. Laboratory tests, imaging studies and histologic examinations may be indicated, as well. Its management is complicated and variable according to the case. Although hysterectomy was the first option in the 1960s, medical treatment and less invasive surgical procedures have evolved recently. The aim of this chapter is to discuss the diagnostic steps and new treatment modalities of dysfunctional uterine bleeding based on a review of the literature.

2. Definition of normal and abnormal uterine bleeding

The usual duration of menstrual flow is 2-7 days with an interval of 21-35 days. The average volume of blood loss is between 30-80 ml. The traditional definitions of abnormal menstrual bleeding are:

- Menorrhagia: Menstrual bleeding with excessive flow or duration. Intervals are regular.
- Metrorrhagia: Irregular menstrual bleeding.

- Menometrorrhagia: Menstrual bleeding with excessive flow or duration. Intervals are irregular.
- Intermenstrual bleeding: Variable amounts of bleeding between normal regular menstrual periods.
- Polymenorrhea: Menstrual bleeding with intervals of less than 21 days.
- Oligomenorrhea: Menstrual bleeding with intervals of greater than 35 days.
- Heavy menstrual bleeding is both menorrhagia and menometrorrhagia, and refers to the menstrual blood loss of higher than 80 ml per month.

3. Measurement of menstrual blood loss

Although heavy menstrual bleeding is defined as menstrual blood loss higher than 80 mL, up to 50% of women complaining of heavy menstrual bleeding have an objective blood loss lower than this level (Gannon et al., 1996). The assessment of menstrual blood loss is a complicated issue. The duration of menses and the number of sanitary pads worn do not correspond to the woman's actual blood loss (Chimbira et al., 1980; Haynes et al., 1977), as the number of tampons worn reflects personal hygiene more than menstrual blood loss (Fraser et al., 1984). For this reason, many techniques have been investigated for a long time, however, none of the objective methods are practical enough for clinical use.

3.1 Direct measurement by using the alkaline hematin test

The alkaline hematin test is an objective way of assessing menstrual blood loss by extracting hemoglobin from used sanitary pads, and converting it to hematin which is than measured spectrophotometrically (Hallberg & Nillson, 1964; Shaw et al., 1972). In many studies it was shown to be the accurate and simple method of measuring menstrual blood loss (Cheyne & Shepherd, 1970; Van Eijkeren et al., 1986; Vasilenko et al., 1988; Jannsen et al, 1995; Pendergrass et al, 1984). However, this is an impractical method that is rarely used outside of a research setting as it demands collecting the used feminine hygiene products (O'Flynn N & Britten, 2000; Chapple et al., 2001; Wyatt et al., 2001).

3.2 Indirect measurement by using Pictorial Blood Loss Assessment Charts (PBAC)

As the alkaline hematin technique was not appropriate for routine clinical use, a pictorial blood loss assessment chart was developed (Higham et al., 1990). In this method women assess the degree of staining of their used sanitary pads or tampons, and assign a numerical score. When this score was compared with the objective menstrual blood loss measurements, a sensitivity of 86% and a specificity of 89% were achieved with a PBAC score of >100 being positive (Higham et al., 1990). Recently it has been shown that a PBAC score of >150 for diagnosing menstrual blood loss >80 ml provided best precision and accuracy (Zakherah et al, 2011). It is accepted as a simple and accurate method of assessing blood loss that can be used in clinical practice (Zakherah et al., 2011; Barr et al., 1999). However, there are some studies questioning the discriminatory power as a diagnostic test (Deeny & Davis, 1994; Reid et al., 2000). As most of the studies ignored the extraneous blood loss, that is, blood not collected on feminine hygiene products, in one study participants were instructed to mark down the loss each time they changed their napkin or tampon (Wyatt et al., 2001). The authors concluded that some women also lose a significantly large amount of extraneous blood, which cannot be assessed by the alkaline hematin method.

3.3 Self-assessment measures

The symptoms that may signify heavy menstrual bleeding include (Farrell, 2004):

- an unusual increase in blood loss
- more than 7 days of bleeding
- bleeding or flooding not contained within pads or tampons (particularly if wearing the largest size)
- clots larger than 3 cm.

As the first two methods are impractical, measuring menstrual blood loss is not recommended except for research settings. Heavy menstrual bleeding is accepted as excessive menstrual loss which interferes with the woman's physical, emotional and social quality of life. Whether menstrual blood loss is a problem, is advised to be determined not by measuring blood loss but by the women herself (National Collaborating Centre for Women's and Children's Health, 2007).

There are many studies that compare the clinical parameters with objective menstrual blood volume. While some of them were unable to show a correlation between subjective assessment of menstrual blood loss and actual blood volume (Chimbira et al., 1980), the others revealed some correlation between menstrual blood volume and duration of menses, as well as clot size, ferritin level and frequency of pad change (Snowden & Christian, 1983; Higham & Shaw, 1999; Warner et al., 2004) .

4. Pathogenesis of dysfunctional uterine bleeding

4.1 Mechanism of normal menstruation

The seat of normal menstrual bleeding is located in the upper two-thirds of the endometrial mucosa. It is characterized by tissue necrosis, disruption of microvasculature, migratory leukocytes, and platelet/fibrin thrombi in microvessels (Ferenczy, 2003). Menstruation is initiated by the enzymatic degradation of the endometrium as a result of estrogen-progesterone withdrawal. In the first half of the secretory phase of the menstrual cycle, acid phosphatase, and other potent lytic enzymes are confined to lysosomes. The release of these enzymes is inhibited by progesterone which stabilizes the lysosomal membranes. During the second half of the secretory phase, due to the withdrawal of estradiol and progesterone, the enzymes are released into the cytoplasmic substance and intercellular space. In the vascular endothelium lytic-enzyme release leads to platelet deposition, release of prostaglandins, vascular thrombosis, extravasation of red blood cells, and tissue necrosis (Ferenczy, 2003). In addition, the withdrawal of progesterone up-regulates key inflammatory mediators. Among the stimulated agents the α-chemokine CXCL8 (neutrophil chemotactic factor, IL-8) and the β-chemokine CCL-2 (monocyte chemotactic peptide-1, MCP-1), as well as the inducible enzyme, COX-2 are responsible for the synthesis of prostaglandins (Jabbour et al., 2006).

Immediately before and during menstruation, there is the induction of the expression, secretion, and activation of matrix metalloproteinases which have the capacity to degrade all of the components of extracellular matrix (Salamonsen, 2003). Progesterone inhibits endometrial metalloproteinase expression, an action mediated by transforming growth factor-β (Brunnel et al., 1995). As a result of progesterone withdrawal, metalloproteinase secretion and activation are increased, followed by dissolution of the extracellular matrix (Irwin et al., 1996). The enzymatic degradation of endometrium extends to the deepest

extent of functional layer, where the rupture of basal arterioles contribute to bleeding that caused by the dissolution of the surface membrane. A cleavage plane develops at the junction of the loose, vascular, edematous stroma with the basal layer. Desquamation begins in the fundus and gradually extends towards the isthmus (Speroff & Fritz, 2005).
Immediately after separation of the functional layer of the endometrium, endometrial regeneration and vessel growth are initiated by the influence of estradiol. TGF-α, EGF, and platelet derived growth factor (PDGF) are mitogens for epithelial cells that origin from the basal layer (Chan et al., 2004). Vascular endothelial growth factor (VEGF) together with FGF and PDGF are known to stimulate angiogenesis in the endometrium (Weston & Rogers, 2000). Early in menstruation the hemostasis is provided by platelet and fibrin plug formation. However, the cessation of menstrual bleeding depends on vasoconstriction of the denuded spiral arterioles in the basal layer and possibly of the radial arteries of superficial myometrium, an action that is promoted by endothelins and prostaglandins in the menstrual endometrium (Ferenczy, 2003).
In summary, normal menstruation is a process initiated by the release of lysosomal enzymes which leads to the shedding of the functional layer of endometrium, and terminated by the restructuring of the endometrium, and the vasoconstriction of the spiral arterioles and the radial arteries.

4.2 Mechanism of dysfunctional uterine bleeding

There are two types of dysfunctional uterine bleeding; ovulatory (10%) and anovulatory (90%). In ovulatory cycles the menstrual pattern is uniform, regular and heavy but of normal duration. On the contrary, in anovulatory cycles the pattern is variable, irregular and the duration may be longer (Speroff & Fritz, 2005). Ovulatory dysfunctional uterine bleeding is the major pattern in 30s, whereas anovulatory dysfunctional uterine bleeding is more likely to occur at the extremes of reproductive years and in women who have polycystic ovarian syndrome.
In ovulatory dysfunctional uterine bleeding, generally circulating ovarian hormone levels are normal and endometrial histology shows changes identical to women without dysfunctional uterine bleeding. Therefore, the major proposed mechanism of ovulatory dysfunctional uterine bleeding is impaired hemostatic mechanisms. A shift in the ratio of endometrial vasoconstrictor ($PGF_{2\alpha}$) to vasodilator (PGE_2), and an increase in total endometrial prostaglandins have been demonstrated in ovulatory dysfunctional uterine bleeding patients (Ferenzcy, 2003). Platelet and plug formation are poor due to prolonged vasodilation . In addition, a potent vasodilator parathyroid hormone- related protein and high proteolytic lysosomal enzyme activity are increased in women with ovulatory dysfunctional uterine bleeding (Casey & Mac Donald, 1996). As a result, in ovulatory dysfunctional uterine bleeding, treatment with prostaglandin synthetase inhibitors are more effective than hormonal treatment. However, there are rare hormonal conditions that cause abnormal uterine bleeding in ovulatory cycles. The most common one is midcycle bleeding due to abrupt fall in estrogen levels just before the ovulation which is called as 'estrogen withdrawal bleeding'. Another one is the luteal phase defect which is characterized by spotting before the menstruation because of insufficient progesterone secretion, and known as 'progesterone withdrawal bleeding'.
Anovulatory dysfunctional bleeding occurs as a result of endometrial response to abnormal levels of steroid hormones. As normal menstruation results from estrogen-progesterone withdrawal, hyperestrogenic or hyperprogestogenic states end with anovulatory bleeding.

While estrogen is the principal hormone which is effective on the endometrial glands and vasculature, progesterone mainly affects the stroma. In normal menstruation cycle, estrogen and progesterone stimulus is balanced leading to stable endometrial epithelium, stroma, and microvasculature. Random breakdown is avoided, and endometrial shedding occurs uniformly throughout the endometrial cavity. Prolonged hyperestrogenism unopposed by progesterone, leads to proliferative endometrium and hyperplasia with a poor stromal matrix (Ferenzcy, 2003). The bleeding caused by focal stromal breakdown is called 'estrogen breakthrough bleeding'. Endometrial shedding is irregular, and not universal. There is constantly changing patchwork of small repairs instead of organized and well structured remodeling. In persistent proliferative endometrium, spiral arterioles are often suppressed and venous capillaries are dilated and increased in number (Ferenczy, 2003). Also, the sensitivity of abnormal vasculature in hyperestrogenic endometrium is suspected to be greater to vasodilation by prostaglandins than to their vasoconstrictor counterparts (Smith et al., 1982). In addition, a potent vasoconstrictor, angiotensin-2 is decreased in endometrial hyperplasia (Li & Ahmed, 1996). Anovulatory dysfunctional uterine bleeding is initiated by an increase in vascular density with abnormal structural abnormalities leading to rupture or degradation of the microvascular system (Ferenzcy, 2003). As tissue loss involves the superficial endometrium only focally, vasoconstriction of basal and radial arteries does not occur and this causes abnormalities in hemostasis. This is the mechanism of bleeding in chronic anovulation. The amount and duration of bleeding can vary according to the amount and duration of unopposed estrogen exposure (Speroff & Fritz, 2005). Low level chronic estrogen stimulation typically results in intermittent spotting, whereas sustained high level estrogen exposure commonly results in acute episodes of profuse bleeding.

Anovulatory dysfunctional uterine bleeding due to hyperprogestogenism, known as 'progesterone breakthrough bleeding' manifests in continuous progestin or low-dose oral contraceptive users. Endometrial histology is chiefly influenced by progesterone and ranges from severe atrophy with or without stromal decidualization to mixed proliferative/secretory patterns according to the duration and amount of progesterone exposure (Ferenczy, 2003). As the progesterone/estrogen ratio increases, secretory-type atrophy becomes prominent with a gland-stroma ratio largely in favour of the stroma. Histologically there is a decrease in the number and turtuoisity of spiral arterioles and many of the subepithelial microvessels are dilated and lined by a very thin endothelial cell layer (Hickey et al., 2000). Since the basement membrane is poorly formed or absent, and there are gaps between endothelial cells, pools of extravasated red blood cells are often seen (Hourihan et al., 1986). These structural alterations and vascular fragility lead to breakdown and bleeding.

5. Differential diagnosis

Dysfunctional uterine bleeding is a diagnosis of exclusion. In half of women with menorrhagia there is no organic cause (Pitkin, 2007). In the first place, the aim is to exclude the structural and histological abnormalities and dysfunctional uterine bleeding is diagnosed when all of the organic causes are ruled out. Table 1 shows the list of etiologic factors leading to abnormal uterine bleeding.

Pregnancy is the most important etiologic factor that should be excluded primarily. Ectopic pregnancy, abortion, placental abnormalities and gestational trophoblastic diseases are the major causes of abnormal uterine bleeding.

Structural abnormalities of uterus such as leimyoma, polyp or endometrial hyperplasia manifest as heavy menstrual bleeding. In addition, abnormal uterine bleeding is the most frequent symptom of women with cervical and endometrial malignancies. Adenomyosis is characterized with heavy painful bleeding with dyspareunia. Furthermore, women with chronic endometritis and cervicitis can experience irregular bleeding. A woman who has multiple partners, and complains for the symptoms of heavy menstrual bleeding and dysmenorrhea should be evaluated for pelvic inflammatory disease (PID).

Endocrine abnormalities account for an important proportion of abnormal uterine bleeding. Both hypotyroidism and hypertyroidism are associated with abnormal uterine bleeding. Hyperprolactinemia and diabetes mellitus are associated with anovulation. Policytic ovary syndrome (PCOS) is the most common cause of anovulation with a prevelance of 5% to 8% (Azziz et al., 2004). The diagnostic criteria for PCOS include at least two of the following (The Rotterdam ESHRE/ASRM-sponsored PCOS consensus workshop group, 2004):

1. Menstrual irregularity due to oligo- or anovulation.
2. Signs of androgen excess, either on physical examination (eg, hirsutism, acne) or laboratory testing (eg, elevated testosterone)
3. Evidence of polycystic ovaries by ultrasound.

Conditions that should be ruled out include congenital adrenal hyperplasia (manifested by an elevated early morning 17-hydroxyprogesterone), androgen-secreting tumors (manifested by a serum testosterone >200 ng/dl or dehydroepiandrosterone sulfate >800 μg/dl), and hyperprolactinemia (Ely et al., 2006).

Coagulopathies and anticoagulant drug intake should be taken into account during the evaluation of heavy menstrual bleeding. Von Willebrand disease is a common cause of pubertal menorrhagia. Besides, a systemic review of 11 studies from Europe and the USA showed an overall prevalence of 13% in reproductive years (Shankar et al., 2004). Trombocytopenia and leukemia also may cause abnormal uterine bleeding.

6. Diagnostic evaluation

Detailed menstrual history can provide most of the information needed to differentiate anovulatory bleeding from the other causes of abnormal uterine bleeding. Intermenstrual intervals, volume and duration of bleeding, previous menstrual patterns, associated symptoms and temporal associations, such as postcoital or postpartum, should be asked. Medications, especially exogenous hormones and systemic diseases, such as renal or liver dysfunction, should be considered during the evaluation. Physical examination is necessary to determine the origin of bleeding and to exclude vaginal and cervical pathologies. Vaginal discharge, uterus size and contour, and uterine tenderness should be noted.

Imaging studies may be needed for differential diagnosis. Transvaginal ultrasound is the first-line diagnostic tool for identifying structural abnormalities in dysfunctional uterine bleeding (National Collaborating Centre for Women's and Children's Health, 2007). It is performed for the diagnosis of fibroid, endometrial polyp, intrauterine and ectopic pregnancy. Saline infusion sonography is a noninvasive imaging study which has a high sensitivity in diagnosis of endometrial polyp and submucous myom. Hysteroscopy should be used as a diagnostic tool only when ultrasound results are inconclusive, for example in order to determine the exact location of a fibroid or the exact nature of the abnormality (National Collaborating Centre for Women's and Children's Health, 2007). In addition, CT and MRI can be used for the evaluation of pelvic masses and malignancies.

Pregnancy-related bleeding	Ectopic pregnancy Abortion Gestational trophoblastic diseases Placenta previa Ablatio placenta
Anatomic causes	Fibroids Endometrial and endocervical polyps Endometrial hyperplasia Adenomyosis
Infectious causes	Endometritis Cervicitis
Neoplasia	Endometrial cancer Cervical cancer
Endocrine causes	Hypothyroidism and hyperthyroidism Hyperprolactinemia Adrenal gland dysfunction Hypothalamic and pituitary dysfunction Estrogen producing tumors Polycytic ovary syndrome Diabetes mellitus
Hematologic causes	Coagulopathies: von Willebrand disease Thrombocytopenia Leukemia
Exogenous hormones and the other iatrogenic causes	Contraceptive hormones Intrauterine devices Anticoagulants Corticosteroids Antipsychotics
Systemic illnesses	Chronic renal failure Chronic liver diseases Obesity Anorexia Depression Alcoholism
Dysfunctional uterine bleeding	Ovulatory Anovulatory

Table 1. Causes of abnormal uterine bleeding

Complete blood count should be performed in all cases to determine the level of anemia and to estimate the amount of bleeding. β-hCG is necessary in order to exclude pregnancy. Women with family history or additional bleeding symptoms, adolescents with acute bleeding, and those who have abnormal bleeding since menarche should be investigated for hematologic diseases with platelet count, prothrombin time and partial thromboplastin time. Also in chronic liver disease and alcoholism coagulation parameters should be considered. Tyroid stimulating hormone (TSH) should be screened early in the evaluation (Ely et al., 2006). Prolactin level is evaluated in the presence of galactorrhea or oligomenorrhea. Follicule stimulating hormone (FSH) and estradiol levels may be assessed in perimenopausal women. FSH, LH, testosterone, 17-OH progesterone and DHEAS are performed if polycystic ovary syndrome is suspected. Liver and renal function tests are not recommended during the first evaluation, but should be assessed according to the medical history of patient.

Pap-smear should be a part of clinical examination. Endometrial sampling is mandatory in the evaluation of women older than 35 years of age (ACOG, 2001). Also, it should be performed to the younger women with the history of chronic anovulation in order to exclude endometrial carcinoma and hyperplasia. In addition, any cervical mass should be investigated with a biopsy. Table 2 summarizes the diagnostic evaluation of abnormal uterine bleeding.

History	Intermenstrual interval Volume of bleeding (number of sanitary pads or tampons per day) Duration of bleeding Associated symptoms (dysmenorrhea, hirsutism, galactorrhea, pelvic pain) Temporal associations (postcoital, postpartum, postpill, weight change) Systemic illnesses Medications
Physical examination	Origin of bleeding Structural abnormalities Malignancies Infections
Imaging studies	Transvaginal ultrasonography Saline infusion sonography Hysteroscopy CT and MRI
Laboratory tests	Complete blood count B-hCG Tyroid function tests Prolactin FSH, LH, estradiol Testosterone, 17-OH- P, DHEAS PT, APTT Renal and liver function tests
Histologic examination	Pap-smear Endometrial sampling Cervical biopsy

Table 2. Summary of diagnostic evaluation of abnormal uterine bleeding.

7. Treatment of dysfunctional uterine bleeding

Hysterectomy was the most commonly performed treatment for menorrhagia in the past. 80% of the women treated for menorrhagia had no uterine abnormality and over a third of the women undergoing hysterectomies for heavy menstrual bleeding had a normal uterus removed (Gath et al., 1982; Clarke et al,. 1995). Today, in spite of the high patient satisfaction rate of hysterectomy, medical therapies or less invasive surgical procedures are preferred instead of hysterectomy in order to avoid its serious complications. Need for contraception, contraindications for treatment and patient choices are the factors influencing the selection of therapy. Iron supplements should be prescribed in addition to any kind of therapy. Table 3 shows a list of treatment modalities of dysfunctional uterine bleeding.

1. Medical treatment
   - I. Hormonal medications
     - a. Progestogens
     - b. Estrogen
     - c. Oral contraceptives
     - d. Danazol
     - e. GnRH analogues
   - II. Non-hormonal medications
     - a. Nonsteroidal anti-inflammatory drugs (NSAIDs)
     - b. Tranexamic acid
   - III. Levonorgestrel-releasing intrauterine system
2. Surgical treatment
   - I. Hysterectomy
   - II. Endometrial resection and ablation
     - a. First generation techniques
     - b. Second generation techniques

Table 3. Treatment of dysfunctional uterine bleeding

7.1 Medical management

Medical therapy is the first-line therapy in dysfunctional uterine bleeding. Cyclic progestogens are the most common prescribed drugs for dysfunctional uterine bleeding. Combined oral contraceptives and levonorgestrel intrauterine system provide additional contraceptive effect. Nonsteroidal anti-inflammatory drugs and tranexamic acid are medications that offer a simple therapy to be taken only during menses. Although danazol and gonadotropin-releasing hormone analogues are highly effective, they are not used frequently due to their side effects and high costs. They can be used for a short period in women waiting for surgery. Effective use of medical therapies reduces the number of surgical procedures. A combination of two or more of these agents may be required to successfully control the abnormal uterine bleeding.

7.1.1 Hormonal medications

7.1.1.1 Progestogens

Progestogens are the mainstay of the treatment of anovulatory bleeding. Progestogens account for 55% of the total prescribed drugs for menorrhagia and norethisterone is the most commonly prescribed progestogen in the UK (Coulter et al., 1995). In anovulatory women with menorrhagia, progestin treatment control the bleeding coordinating regular uterine shedding. Progestogens have an anti-mitotic effect on the endometrium, because they stimulate 17β-hydroxysteroid dehydrogenase and sulfotransferase activity, the enzymes that convert estradiol to estrone sulfate (Gurpide et al., 1976). They also inhibit estrogen's induction of its own receptor and suppress estrogen-mediated transcription of oncogens (Kirkland et al., 1992). As a consequence of these effects, continuous progestogens induce endometrial atrophy, and prevent estrogen-stimulated endometrial proliferation (Hichey et al., 2007).

Progestogens are administered in luteal phase from day 15 or 19 to day 26 in anovulatory cycles. In a comparison of 5 mg norethisteron three times daily with 10 mg medroxyprogesterone acetate three times daily for 14 days, no obvious difference was observed between these two progestogens (Fraser et al., 1990). Recently an increase in the duration and dosage has been investigated in patients with ovulatory dysfunctional uterine bleeding, and administration of oral progestogens from day 5 to day 26 of the cycle produced a significant reduction in bleeding (Lethaby et al., 2008). The studies which compared luteal progestogens with the other medical therapies have revealed that oral progestogens were less effective in reducing menstrual blood loss when compared with tranexamic acid, danazol and progesterone-releasing intrauterine system, whereas there was no significant difference when compared with nonsteroidal anti-inflammatory drugs (Lethaby et al., 2008). In addition, it is shown that progestogens were less effective than levonorgestrel-releasing intrauterine system, but had a lower incidence of intermenstrual bleeding and breast tenderness (Irvine et al., 1998).

For emergency suppression of heavy menstrual bleeding norethisteron at least 15 mg per day, or medroxyprogesterone acetate at least 30 mg per day is prescribed until bleeding ceases and a maintenance dose should be continued until the woman has 3-4 weeks free of bleeding (Farrell, 2004).

Fatigue, mood changes, weight gain, nausea, bloating, edema, headache, depression, loss of libido, irregular bleeding and atherogenic changes in the lipid profile can be associated with the prolonged use of high-dose progestogens (Lethaby et al., 2008).

7.1.1.2 Estrogen

Estrogen is mostly administered in acute and heavy bleeding when the endometrium is grossly denuded. Intravenous administration of 25 mg conjugated equine estrogens every 4 hours until bleeding subsides or for 24 hours is very effective in reducing heavy bleeding (DeVore et al, 1982). In less severe cases high dose oral estrogen (1.25 mg conjugated estrogens or 2.0 mg micronized estradiol every 4-6 hours for 24 hours) can control bleeding (Speroff & Fritz, 2005). After the bleeding lightens the dose should be tapered to once a day for another 7-10 days. If the bleeding is lighter single daily dose of 1.25 mg conjugated

estrogen or 2 mg micronized estradiol for 7-10 days is enough to control bleeding (Speroff & Fritz, 2005). After the initial estrogen therapy a progestogen should be added and continued until the 21st day of therapy in order to generate a withdrawal bleeding.
Due to chronic low level estrogen stimulation, the endometrium becomes very thin and denuded resulting in intermittent spotting and staining. In these cases, progestin therapy cannot be used because progesterone affect only the endometrium stimulated by estrogen previously. Thus, estrogen therapy is preferred in women with a thin endometrium assessed by transvaginal ultrasound. Similarly, in progesterone breakthrough bleeding owing to depot forms of progestin therapy or low dose estrogen-progestin contraceptives, 1.25 mg oral conjugated estrogen or 2 mg oral micronized estradiol is added to therapy for 7-10 days.

7.1.1.3 Oral contraceptives

Oral contraceptives reduce the amount of bleeding by 40% in dysfunctional uterine bleeding (Fraser & McCarron, 1991). When taken in a cyclical fashion it induces regular shedding of a thinner endometrium and inhibits ovulation. Good cycle control together with the provision of contraception makes it more acceptable long term therapy for menorrhagia (Farquer & Brown, 2009). It is also a good option in cases of heavy bleeding when the endometrium thickness is uniformly increased. Although it contains both estrogen and progestin, the main action is performed by the progestin (Speroff & Fritz, 2005). One common oral contraceptive regimen for severe acute bleeding is one pill four times daily for four days followed by three times daily for three days, followed by twice daily for two days, followed by once daily for three weeks. Then after a break of one week, oral contraceptive is taken on a regular basis using three weeks on and one week off, for at least three months (Ely et al., 2006).
In anovulatory cycles in order to prevent the recurrence of heavy bleeding, it should be administered daily throughout following cycles as a maintenance therapy. If there is any contraindication for oral contraceptive use, cyclic progestogens are chosen instead, however, they do not avoid pregnancy. The contraindications of oral contraceptives are; previous thromboembolic event or stroke, history of estrogen-dependent tumor, active liver disease, pregnancy, hypertriglyceridemia and smoking > 15 cigarettes per day of women older than 35 years (Ely et al., 2006). In addition, long-term use of oral contraceptives are not preferred by many women as a therapy of menorrhagia.

7.1.1.4 Danazol

Danazol is a drug chemically derived from testosterone. It reduces the menstrual blood loss because it inhibits ovulation, reduces estrogen level and causes endometrial atrophy (Beaumont et al., 2007). The standard dose is 200 mg/day, although the studies did not show any difference in effectiveness or frequency of adverse effects when compared with a lower dose of 100 mg/day (Chimbira et al., 1980) and a reducing dose regimen (Higham & Shaw, 1993). Danazol is found to be more effective than progestogens, nonsteroidal anti-inflammatory drugs and oral contraceptive pills, although it caused more severe side effects in comparison to progestogens and nonsteroidal anti-inflammatory drugs (Beaumont et al., 2007). When the treatment is discontinued, the effects of danazol persist for two to three cycles before blood loss returns to pre-treatment levels (Chimbira et al., 1979).
As it is derived from testosterone, it has androgenic effects which may result in acne, seborrhoea, hirsutism, and hoarseness. Also, it may cause weight gain, nausea, tiredness, irritability, musculoskeletal pains, hot flushes, breast atrophy and benign hepatic adenomas

in case of its prolonged administration (Beaumont et al., 2007). Moreover, an additional contraceptive is required because of its teratogenic effect .

7.1.1.5 GnRH analogues

They have a limited role in the treatment of dysfunctional uterine bleeding, but can be used as pretreatment before endometrial ablation. The success of hysteroscopic procedure depends on complete endometrial destruction. The radius of a standard electrosurgical loop used for endometrial resection is about four mm and the dept of tissue destruction with Nd:YAG laser or a roller ball electrode is four to six mm (Goldrath, 1990; Duffy, 1992). The success rate increases if surgery is undertaken in the immediate post-menstrual phase or following the administration of hormonal agents which induce endometrial thinning or atrophy (Sowter, 2002). GnRH analogues are the most common evaluated drugs in the studies. Danazol is also used for this purpose, but less frequently. The use of goserelin acetate (GnRH analogue) before hysteroscope shortens operating time, and reduces intra-operative distension medium absorption (Donnez, 1997). Also it provides an ease of surgery and a higher rate of post-operative amenorrhea after 12 months of surgery (Vilos, 1996; Sowter, 2002). However, in MISTLETOE study in over 10000 endometrial resections, the use of endometrial thinning agents was not associated with any reductions in complication rates (Overton, 1997). Also patient satisfaction is highly irrespective of the use of GnRH-analogues (Sowter, 2002).

7.1.2 Non-hormonal medications

7.1.2.1 Nonsteroidal Anti-Inflammatory Drugs (NSAIDs)

The endometrium of women with menorrhagia has been found to have higher levels of PGE_2 and F_{2a} when compared with normal menses (Willman et al., 1976). Also, the ratio of prostaglandin E_2 to F_2, and the ratio of prostaglandin I_2 to thromboxane are elevated resulting in deranged hemostasis (Smith et al., 1981; Makarainen & Ylikorkala, 1986). Nonsteroidal anti-inflammatory drugs inhibiting prostaglandin synthesis by the enzyme cyclo-oxgenase, reduce the menstrual blood loss approximately 20-40% and to a greater extent in those with excessive bleeding (Hall et al., 1987; Shaw et al, 1994).

Mefenamic acid, naproxen, ibuprofen, flurbiprofen, meclofenamic acid, diclofenac, indomethacin and asetylsalicyclic acid are used for the treatment of heavy menstrual bleeding. There are no differences in clinical efficiency between individual prostaglandin inhibitors. However, there are some women who seem to respond well to one agent but less well to another (Lethaby et al, 2007). As a group, Nonsteroidal anti-inflammatory drugs are less effective than tranexamic acid, danazol and levonorgestrel releasing intrauterine system, whereas there was no significant difference in efficacy in comparison with oral luteal progestogen, ethamsylate, and oral contraceptive pill (Lethaby et al, 2007).

The advantage of this treatment is the low incidence of side effects as the drug is used only during the bleeding period. Also, it provides relief from dysmenorrhea which is often related to heavy menstrual bleeding. Side effects of nonsteroidal anti-inflammatory drugs include headache and gastroinstestinal symptoms such as nausea, vomiting, diarrhea and dyspepsia. Contraindications are gastrointestinal disorders such as ulcers, intolerance to nonsteroidal anti-inflammatory drugs, or asthma (Farrell, 2004).

7.1.2.2 Tranexamic acid

Tranexamic acid is an anti-fibrinolytic. Plasminogen activators, the enzymes that cause fibrinolysis, are found in higher levels in the endometrium of women with heavy menstrual bleeding than those with normal menstrual bleeding (Gleeson, 1994). Thus, anti-fibrinolytic drugs are used in the treatment of menorrhagia. Tranexamic acid is more effective than either nonsteroidal anti-inflammatory drugs and oral luteal phase progestogens (Lethaby et al., 2000). Also the studies comparing tranexamic acid with oral progestogens for changes in quality of life showed that the former is more effective in improving flooding and leakage problems and sex life (Lethaby et al., 2000). It is prescribed on only the heavy days of the menses, with a dose of 1 g 3-4 times daily (Farrell, 2004). However, in a study a dose of 2 g/day is shown to be more effective than 10 mg twice-daily medroxyprogesterone acetate (Kriplani et al, 2006). Tranexamic acid may be considered as a first-line treatment for ovulatory dysfunctional uterine bleeding, especially for patients in whom hormonal treatment is either not recommended or not wanted (National Health Committee New Zealand, 1998; Wellington & Wagstaff, 2003).

Although it is known to reduce the menstrual blood loss by 50% (Higham & Shaw,1991), tranexamic acid has not been used widely because of its possible side effects. Since it is an anti-fibrinolytic drug, it is suggested to be associated with thrombogenic disease. However, the studies were unable to show increased rates of thrombogenic disease with tranexamic acid administration in comparison to placebo (Rybo, 1991). The recent studies proved that tranexamic acid is an effective and safe form of medical therapy in women with menorrhagia without any serious adverse effects (Kriplani et al., 2006; Srinil & Jaisamrarn, 2005; Lukes et al., 2010).

Eythamsylate is a drug used rarely in heavy menstrual bleeding. Even though it is not a true anti-fibrinolytic, it affects in a similar mechanism. It reduces capillary bleeding by correcting abnormal platelet function (Lethaby et al, 2000).

7.1.3 Levonorgestrel-releasing intrauterine system

Levonorgestrel-releasing intrauterine system has been developed primarily as a contraceptive device which does not suppress ovulation. It consists of a T-shaped intrauterine device sheated with a reservoir of levonorgestrel that is released at the rate of 20 μg daily. This low level of hormone minimizes the systemic progestogenic effects, and patients are more likely to continue with this therapy than with cyclical progestogen therapy (Irvine et al., 1998). It prevents the endometrial proliferation and reduces both the duration and amount of bleeding (Silverberg et al., 1986). It is accepted as an alternative to surgery with a reduction in menstrual blood loss up to 90% (Milsom, 2007; Andersson et al., 1994). It is more effective than the other medical therapies (Lethaby et al, 2005). A study comparing the efficacy of levonorgestrel-releasing intrauterine system to oral contraceptives, showed a more pronunced clinical benefit with levonorgestrel-releasing intrauterine system therapy in terms of decreasing menstrual blood loss score after 6 months of treatment (Endricat et al., 2009). This is a more acceptable treatment than norethisterone taken for 21 days of the cycle for the women, and they are more satisfied with this therapy (Irvine et al., 1998). Levonorgestrel-releasing intrauterine system treatment has been compared to either transcervical resection of the endometrium or balloon ablation (Lethaby et al., 2005). Although there was a higher rate of successful treatment in those undergoing transcervical resection or balloon ablation in four trials, rates of satisfaction and change in quality of life were similar, but women with levonorgestrel-releasing intrauterine system had a greater incidence of progestogenic side effects within a year. In two studies, 82% and 64% of women on a waiting list of hysterectomy cancelled their surgery after using levonorgestrel-releasing intrauterine system (Barrington & Bowen-Simpkins, 1997;

Lähteenmaki et al., 1998). Another study comparing levonorgestrel-releasing intrauterine system with hysterectomy, revealed that there was no significant difference in quality of life scores, but the former treatment had lower costs than the latter (Hurskainen et al., 2001).
Side effects are ectopic pregnancy, expulsion of device and progestogenic effects such as bloating, weight gain and breast tenderness (Lethaby et al., 2005). Irregular bleeding and spotting are temporary and generally seen in the first three months. However, after 12 months of therapy, there is a major reduction in blood loss up to 97%, thus, most of the women have a light bleeding and 20% of them have amenorrhea. As amenorrhea and altered bleeding patterns may be undesirable to some women (Chi, 1993), counselling before insertion is very important. Relief from dysmenorrhea and reduced incidence of pelvic inflammatory disease due to the thickening of the utero-cervical mucus are additional advantages of levonorgestrel-releasing intrauterine system (Andersson et al., 1994). An increased incidence of transient ovarian cysts has been reported with levonorgestrel-releasing intrauterine system use (Brache et al., 2002).
Due to its high efficacy in reducing menstrual blood loss without disturbing fertility, this method offers a first-line therapy for dysfunctional uterine bleeding in women of any reproductive age who wish a contraceptive method and accept hormonal drug use.

7.2 Surgical treatment

Surgical procedures are performed when medical therapy fails or there is an associated symptom such as pain. Also, some of the patients prefer surgery instead of long-term use of medications. These techniques should not be performed to women who wish to have further pregnancies. These procedures include hysterectomy, endometrial resection and ablation. Dilatation and curettage is no longer accepted as a therapeutic treatment (National Collaborating Centre for Women's and Children's Health, 2007).
All of the surgical procedures are much more successful than oral medications (Cooper et al.,1997, Kupperman et al., 2004). In addition, the rate of satisfaction and overall quality of life were higher in women who had surgery (Marjoribanks et al., 2006). Also, when conservative surgery (endometrial resection and ablation) was compared with levonoregtrel-releasing intrauterine system, conservative surgery was more effective in controlling bleeding at one year, however, patients satisfaction rates and quality of life were not different between these two groups (Marjoribanks et al., 2006).

7.2.1 Hysterectomy

Hysterectomy has been traditionally regarded as the definitive surgical treatment for menorrhagia and menstrual disorders have been the leading indication of hysterectomy (Farquhar & Steiner, 2002). There are three types of hysterectomy; laparoscopically assisted, vaginal and abdominal. The laparoscopically assisted hysterectomy by a competent and experienced operator is the most appropriate technique with less morbidity (Farrell, 2004). Hysterectomy is associated with 100% success in treating heavy menstrual bleeding and a high patient satisfaction up to 95% (Marjoribanks et al., 2006), but have complications and rarely operative mortality. For this reason, hysterectomy should not be as a fist-line treatment (National Callobarating Centre for Women's and Children's Health, 2007). It should be only considered when other treatment options have failed or there is a wish for amenorrhea, as well as when the woman has no longer wishes to retain her uterus and fertility.

7.2.2 Endometrial resection and ablation

These procedures involve the destruction of the full thickness of endometrium together with the superficial myometrium including the deep basal glands (Lethaby et al., 2009). First generation techniques utilize hysteroscope, and require general or regional anesthesia, surgical skill and hospital admission (Marjoribanks et al., 2006). By contrast, second generation techniques do not use hysteroscope, do not require surgical skill and can be done as one day or outpatient surgery with a local anaesthetic (Jack et al., 2005). Compared to hysterectomy, endometrial destruction techniques have a shorter operation time and hospital stay, quicker recovery, and fewer postoperative complications (Marjoribanks et al., 2006). On the other hand, hysterectomy is more successful in improvement in heavy menstrual bleeding and higher satisfaction rates compared to endometrial ablation (Lethaby et al., 1999). Repeat surgery due to the failure of the initial treatment, was more likely after endometrial ablation than hysterectomy (3 to 18% versus 1%) (Lethaby et al., 1999). The initial cost of endometrial destruction is significantly lower than hysterectomy, but, since re-treatment is often necesssary, the cost difference narrows over time (Lethaby et al, 1999). Although hysterectomy is much more successful than these procedures, there is now evidence that it is used less frequently in clinical practice (Reid, 2007).

Endometrial resection and ablation should be offered to the women who do not wish further childbearing. However, unlike hysterectomy, pregnancy after endometrial ablation is possible although it is not often (Kdous et al., 2008). Premenopausal women should have a post-operative contraception method, because serious complications such as spontaneous abortion, prematurity, uterine rupture, and placenta adhesion complications in the pregnancies after endometrial ablation have been reported (Laberge, 2008; Kuzel et al., 2010; Yin , 2010).

7.2.2.1 First generation techniques

The first effective ablation of the endometrium under hysteroscopic vision for the treatment of dysfunctional uterine bleeding was performed using laser photovapourisation (Goldrath et al., 1981). A few years later rollerball ablation with electrosurgical equipment (Lin et al,. 1988; Vaincaillie, 1989) and transcervical resection of the endometrium (TCRE) with resectoscope (DeCherney et al., 1983, 1987) began to be performed. These procedures have the advantage of diagnosis polyps as they directly visualize the endometrial cavity. Overall complication rate has been reported as 4.4% and ablation either by laser or rollerball were safer than endometrial resection (Overton et al., 1997). The risk of immediate hemorrhage was three times greater and the risk of uterine perforation was four times greater with resection than ablation. In a multicentre study, of the 1866 women followed up for at least one year after laser endometrial ablation, 56% developed complete amenorrhea, 38% reported continuing but satisfactorily reduced menstruation, and 7% patients failed to improve with the first treatment. Overall, 93% had a satisfactory response to laser ablation and only 1.8% required subsequent hysterectomy (Erian, 1994). It is reported that amenorrhea is best attained when complete preoperative atrophy is achieved, by either depot goserelin (GnRH analogue) or danazol, although goserelin appears to be more effective and better tolerated than danazol (Alford & Hopkins, 1996; Garry et al., 1996; Fraser et al., 1996).

7.2.2.2 Second generation techniques

Second generation procedures except hydrothermal ablation and endometrial laser intrauterine thermal therapy are performed without direct visualization through a hysteroscope (Lethaby et al., 2009). These procedures include cryoablation (Pitroff et al., 1993), hot saline solution irrigation (Baggish et al.,1995), diode laser hyperthermy (heating) (Donnez et al.,1996), microwave ablation (Sharp et al., 1995), a heated balloon system (Singer et al.,1994) and photodynamic therapy (intrauterine light delivery) (Fehr et al.,1995). A meta-analysis of 21 studies with 3395 premenopausal women showed that when these procedures were compared with first generation techniques, there were no significant difference in reducing menstrual blood loss and the rate of re-intervention and satisfaction (Lethaby et al., 2009). Second generation techniques were easier to perform with shorter surgery times using local anaesthesia. While intra and postoperative complications such as fluid overload, perforation, cervical lacerations and hematometra, were more common with first generation, other types of complications, nausea, vomiting, and uterine cramping and pain, were more common with second generation techniques (Lethaby et al, 2009). These methods are complex which have the potential of mechanical breakdown. Considerable experience in intrauterine cavity assessment and manipulation is required for safely use of these devices.

8. Conclusion

Dysfunctional uterine bleeding is a common, debiliating condition. There is no practical method of measuring the amount of bleeding, and the assessment of menstrual blood loss is based on the complains of woman. While anovulatory dysfunctional uterine bleeding is commonly seen at both ends of the reproductive years because of hypothalamic immaturity and perimenopausal changes, ovulatory type is majorly seen in the 30s and its mechanism is less well understood. Physical examination and diagnostic tests are performed with the aim of exclusion of pregnancy and organic diseases. There are many different types of therapy, and the selection is mainly depends on the wishes and conditions of the patient. The treatment of anovulatory dysfunctional uterine bleeding is simple as it is usually treated effectively by replacing the missing component, progesterone, in the luteal phase. However, the treatment of ovulatory dysfunctional uterine bleeding is more complex. Nonsteroidal anti-inflammatory drugs or tranexamic acid is the current first-line treatment for those that wish to conceive or do not accept hormonal treatment. Also, they are preferred while investigations and definite treatment are being organized. Combined oral contraceptives, progestogens from days 5 to 26 of the menstrual cycle, or levonorgestrel-releasing intrauterine system are acceptable for the other women, although the latter seems to be best option when long term use is anticipated. On the other hand, danazol and GnRH analogues are not used routinely. Surgical treatment is considered when bleeding is a severe impact on a woman's quality of life and there is no wish of further conception. Although hysterectomy was the most commonly performed procedure in the past, the recently evolved conservative surgeries are preferred today. Second generation endometrial ablation procedures are going to become more prevalent in the future. However, more studies with longer duration of follow-up are needed to clarify the long-term benefits.

9. References

ACOG practice bulletine management of anovulatory bleeding. International Journal of Gynecology & Obstetrics 2001;72:263-71.

Alford WS & Hopkins MP. Endometrial rollerball ablation. Journal of Reproductive Medicine 1996;41(4):251-4.

Andersson K, Odlind V & Rybo G. Levonorgestrel-releasing and copper-releasing (Nova T) IUDs during five years of use: a randomized comparative trial. Contraception 1994;49:56-72.

Azziz R, Woods KS, Reyna R, Key TJ, Knochenhauer ES & Yildiz BO. The prevelance and features of the polycystic ovary syndrome in an unselected population. Journal of Clinical Endocrinology and Metabolism 2004;89:2745-2749.

Baggish MS, Paraiso M, Brexnock EM & Griffey S. A computer- controlled, continuously circulating hot irrigating system for endometrial ablation. American Journal of Obstetrics and Gynecology. 1995;173:1842-8.

Barr F, Brabin L & Agbaje O. A pictorial chart for managing common menstrual disorders in Nigerian adolescents. International Journal of Gynecology and Obstetrics 1999;66(1):51-3.

Barrington JW & Bowen-Simpkins P. The levonorgestrel intrauterine system in the management of menorrhagia. British Journal of Obstetrics and Gynaecology 1997;104:614-16.

Brunel KL, Rodger WH, Gold LI, Kore M, Hargrove JT, Matrisian LM & Osteen KG. Transforming growth factor-beta mediates the progesterone suppression of an epithelial metalloproteinase by adjacent stroma in the human endometrium. Proceedings of the National Academy of Sciences 92:7362,1995.

Beaumont HH, Augood C, Duckitt K & Lethaby A. Danazol for heavy menstrual bleeding. Cochrane Database of Systemic Reviews 2007, Issue 3. Art. No.: CD001017. DOI: 10.1002/14651858.CD001017.pub2.

Brache V, Faundes A, Alvarez F & Cochon L. Nonmenstrual adverse events during use of implantable contraceptives for women: data from clinical trials. Contraception 2002;65:63-74.

Casey ML & Mac Donald PC: The endothelin-parathyroid hormone related protein vasoactive peptide system in human endometrium: modulation by transforming growth factor-beta. Human Reproduction 1996:62-82.

Chan RW, Schwab KE & Gargett CE. Cloneginicity of human endometrial epithelial and stromal cells. Biology of Reproduction 2004;70:1738-50.

Chapple A, May C & Ling M. Is objective testing for menorrhagia in general practice practical? Results from a qualitative study. European Journal of General Practice 2001;7(1):13-17.

Cheyne GA & Shepherd MM. Comparison of chemical and atomic absorption methods for estimating menstrual blood loss. Journal of Medical Laboratory Technology 1970;27(3): 350-4.

Chi IC. The TCu-380A(AG), MLCu375 and Nova T IUDs and the IUD daily releasing 20 μg levonorgestrel-four pillars of IUD contraceptive for the nineties and beyond? Contraception 1993;47:325-347.

Chimbira TH, Cope E, Anderson ABM & Bolton G. The effect of danazol on menorrhagia, coagulation mechanisms, hematological indices and body weight. British Journal of Obstetrics and Gynaaecology 1979;86:46-50.

Chimbira TH, Anderson ABM & Turnbull AC. Relation between measured blood loss and patients subjective assessment of loss, duration of bleeding, number of sanitary towels used, uterine weight and endometrial surface area. British Journal of Obstetrics and Gynaecology 1980;87(7):603-609.

Chimbira TH, Anderson ABM, Naish C, Cope E & Turnbull AC. Reduction of menstrual blood loss by Danazol in unexplained menorrhagia: Lack of effect of placebo. British Journal of Obstetrics and Gynaecology 1980;87(12):1152-58.

Clarke A, Black N, Rowe P, Mott S & Howle K. Indications for and outcome of total abdominal hysterectomy for benign disease: a prospective cohort study. British Journal of Obstetrics and Gynaecology. 1995;102:611-20.

Cooper KG, Parkin DE, Garrartt AM & Grant AM. A randomised comparison of medical and hysteroscopic management in women consulting a gynaecologist for treatment of heavy menstrual loss. British Journal of Obstetrics and Gynaecology 1997;104:1360-6.

Coulter A, Bradlow J, Agass M, Bartin-Bates C & Tulloch A. Outcomes of referrals to gynecology outpatient clinics for menstrual problems: an aussit of general practice records. British Journal of Obstetrics and Gynaaecology. 1991;98: 789-796.

Coulter A, Kelland J, Peto V & Rees MCP. Treating menorrhagia in primary care. International Journal of Technology Assessment in Health Care 1995;11(3):456-71.

Crosgiani PG, Vercellini P, Mosconi P, Oldani S, Cortesi I & De Giorgi O. Levonorgestrel-releasing intrauterine device versus hysteroscopic endometrial resection in the treatment of dysfunctional uterine bleeding. Obstetrics and Gynecology 1997;90: 257-63.

DeCherney AH & Polan ML. Hysteroscopic management of intrauterine lesions and intractable uterine bleeding. Obstetrics and Gynecology 1983;61:392-7.

DeCherney AH, Diamond MP, Lavey G & Polan ML. Endometrial ablation for intractable uterine bleeding: hysteroscopic resection. Obstetrics and Gynecology 1987;70: 668-70.

Deeny M & Davis JA. Assessment of menstrual blood loss in women referred for endometrial ablation. European Journal of Obstetrics, Gynecology, and Reproductive Biology 1994;57(3):179-80.

DeVore GR, Owens O & Kase N. Use of intravenous premarin in the treatment of dysfunctional uterine bleeding- a double-blind randomized control study. Obstetrics and Gynecology 59:285;1982.

Donnez J, Polet R, Mathieu PE, Konwitz , Nisolle M & Casans-Roux F. Endometrial laser interstitial hyperthermy: a potential modality for endometrial ablation. Obstetrics and Gynecology 1996,87:459-64.

Donnez J, Vilos G, Gannon MJ, Stampe-Sorensen S, Klinte I & Miller RM. Goserelin acetate (Zoladex) plus endometrial ablation for dysfunctional uterine bleeding: a large randomized, double-blind study. Fertility and Sterility 1997;68(1):29-36.

Duffy S, Reid P & Sharp F. In vivo studies of uterine electro surgery. British Journal of Obstetrics and Gynecology 1992;99:579-82.

Ely JW, Kennedy CM, Clark EC & Bowdler NC. Abnormal uterine bleeding: A management algorithm. The Journal of the American Board of Family Medicine 2006;19:590-602.

Endrikat J, Shapiro H, Lukkari-Lax E, Kunz M, Schmidt W & Fortier M. A Canadian, multicentre study comparing the efficacy of levonorgestrel-relasing intrauterine system to an oral contraceptive with idiopathic menorrhagia. Journal of Obstetrics and Gynaecology Canada, 2009;31(4):340-7.

Erian J. Endometrial ablation in the treatment of menorrhagia. British Journal of Obstetrics and Gynaecology 1994;101(Suppl 11):19-22.
Ewenstein BM. The pathophysiology of bleeding disorders presenting as abnormal uterine bleeding. American Journal of Obstetrics and Gynecology 1996;175:770-7.
Farquhar C & Steiner C. Hysterectomy rates in the United States 1990-1997. Obstetrics and Gynaecology 2002;99:229-34.
Farquhar C & Brown J. Oral contraceptive pill for heavy menstrual bleeding. Cochrane Database of Systemic Reviews 2009, Issue 4. Art. No.: CD000154, DOI: 10.1002/14651858.CD000154.pub2.
Farrell E. Dysfuntional uterine bleeding. Australian Family Physician 2004;33(11):906-8.
Fehr MK, Madsen SJ, Svaasand LO, Tromberg BJ, Eusebio J, Berns MW & Tadir Y. Intrauterine light delivery for photodynamic therapy of the human endometrium. Human Reproduction 1995;10:3067-72.
Fraser IS, McGarron G & Markham R. A preliminary study of factors influencing the perception of menstrual blood loss in patients complaining of menorrhagia. Obstetrics and Gynecology 1984;149:788-93.
Fraser IS. Treatment of ovulatory and anovulatory dysfunctional uterine bleeding with oral progestogens. Australian & New Zealand Journal of Obstetrics and Gynaecology 1990;30:353-6.
Fraser IS & McCarron G. Randomized trial of 2 hormonal and 2 prostaglandin-inhibiting agents in women with a complaint of menorrhagia. Australian & New Zealand Journal of Obstetrics and Gynaecology 1991;31:66.
Fraser IS, Healy DL, Torode H, Song JY, Mamers P & Wilde F. Depot goserelin and danazol pre-treatment before rollerball endometrial ablation for menorrhagia. Obstetrics and Gynecology 1996;87(4):544-50.
Ferenczy A. Pathophysiology of endometrial bleeding. Maturitas 2003;45:1-14.
Gannon MJ, Day P, Hammadieh N & Johnson N. A new method for measuring blood loss and its use in screening women before endometrial ablation. British Journal of Obstetrics and Gynaaecology 1996; 103: 1029-33.
Garry R, Khair A, Mooney P & Stuart M. A comparison of goserelin and danazol as endometrial thinning agents prior to endometrial laser ablation. British Journal of Obstetrics and Gynaecology 1996;103(4):339-44.
Gath D, Cooper P & Day A. Hysterectomy and psychiatric disorder. I: Levels of psychiatric morbidity before and after hysterectomy. British Journal of Psychiatry 1982;140:335-342.
Gleeson NC. Cyclic changes in endometrial tissue plasminogen activator and plasminogen activator inhibitor type 1 in women with normal menstruation and essential menorrhagia. American Journal of Obstetrics and Gynaecology 1994;171(1):178-83.
Goldrath MH, Fuller TA & Segal S. Laser photovaporization of endometrium for the treatment of menorrhagia. American Journal of Obstetrics and Gynecology 1981;140:14-9.
Goldrath M. Use of danazol in hysteroscopic surgery for menorrhagia. Journal of Reproductive Medicine 1990;35:91-6.
Gurpide E, Gusperg S & Tseng L. Estradiol binding and metabolism in human endometrial hyperplasia and adenocarcinoma. Journal of Steroid Biochemistry 1976;7:891.

Hall P, Maclachlan N, Thorn N, Nudd MWE, Taylor CG & Garrioch DB. Control of menorrhagia by the cyclo-oxygenase inhibitors naproxen sodium and mefenamic acid. British Journal of Obstetrics and Gynaecology 1987;94:554.

Hallberg L & Nilsson L. Determination of menstrual blood loss. Scandinavian Journal of Clinical Laboratory Investigations 1964;16:244-8.

Hallberg L, Hogdahl AM, Nilson L & Rybo G. Menstrual blood loss- a population study: Variation at different ages and attemps to define normality. Acta Obstetrica et Gynecologica Scandinavica 1966;45:320-51.

Haynes PJ, Hodgson H, Anderson ABM & Turnbull AC. Measurement of menstrual blood loss in patients complaining of menorrhagia. British Journal of Obstetrics and Gynaecology 1977; 84: 763-768.

Hickey M, Dwarte D & Fraser IS. Superficial endometrial vascular fragility in Norplant users and in women with ovulatory dysfunctional uterine bleeding. Human Reproduction 2000;15:1509-14.

Hickey M, Higham JM & Fraser I. Progestogens versus oestrogens and progestogens for irregular uterine bleeding associated with anovulation. Cochrane Database of Systematic Reviews 2007, Issue 4. Art. No.: CD001895. DOI: 10.1002/14651858. CD0018895.pub2.

Higham JM, O'Brien PM & Shaw RM. Assessment of menstrual blood loss using a pictorial chart. British Journal of Obstetrics and Gynaecology 1990;97(8):734-9.

Higham J & Shaw R. Risk-benefit assessment of drugs used for the treatment of menstrual disorders. Drug Safety 1991;6:183-91.

Higham JM & Shaw RW. A comparative study of Danazol, a regimen of decreasing doses of danazol, and norethindrone in the treatment of objectively proven unexplained menorrhagia. American Journal of Obstetrics and Gynaecology 1993;169:1134-9.

Higham JM & Shaw RW. Clinical associations with objective menstrual blood volume. European Journal of Obstetrics, Gynecology, and Reproductive Biology 1999;82(1):73-6.

Hourihan HM, Sheppard BL & Bonnar J. A morphometric study of the effects of oral norethisterone and levonorgestrel on endometrial blood vessels. Contraception 1986;34:603-12.

Hurskainen R, Teperi J, Rissanen P, Aalto AM, Grenman S, Kivelä A, Kujansuu E, Vuorma S, Yliskosi M & Paavonen J. Quality of life and cost-effectiveness of levonorgestrel-releasing intrauterine system versus hysterectomy for treatment of menorrhagia: a randomised trial. Lanset 2001;357(9252):273-7.

Irvine GA, Campbell-Brown MB, Lumsden MA, Heikkila A, Walker JJ & Cameron IT. Randomised comparative trial of the levonorgestrel intrauterine system and norethisterone for treatment of idiopathic menorrhagia. British Journal of Obstetrics and Gynaecology 1998;105(6):592-8.

Irwin JC, Kirk D, Gwatkin RBL, Navre M, Cannon P & Giudice LC. Human endometrial matrix metalloproteinase-2, a putative menstrual proteinase. Hormonal regulation in cultured stromal cells and messenger RNA expression during the menstrual cycle. Journal of Clinical Investigation 97:438,1996.

Jabbour HN, Kelly RW, Fraser HM & Critchley OD. Endocrine regulation of menstruation. Endocrine Reviews 2006:27(1):17-46.

Jack SA, Cooper KG, Seymour J, Graham W, Fitzmaurice A & Perez J. A randomised controlled trial of microwave endometrial ablation without endometrial preparation in the outpatient setting: patient acceptability, treatment outcome and costs. BJOG 2005;112:1109-16.

Jannsen CA, Scholten PC & Heintz AP. A simple visual assessment technique to discriminate between menorrhagia and normal menstrual blood loss. Obstetrics and Gynecology 1995;85(6):977-82.

Kdous M, Jacob D, Gervaise A, Risk E & Sauvanet E. Thermal balloon ablation for dysfunctional uterine bleeding: technical aspects and results. A prospective cohort study of 152 cases. Tunisie Medicale 2008;86(5):473-8.

Kirckland JL, Murthy L & Stancel GM. Progesterone inhibits the estrogen-induced expression of c-fos messenger ribonucleic acid in the uterus. Endocrinology 1992;130:3223.

Kriplani A, Kulshrestha V, Agarwal N & Diwakwar S. Role of tranexamic acid in management of dysfunctional uterine bleeding in comparison with medroxyprogesterone acetate. Journal of Obstetrics and Gynaecology, 2006;26(7): 673-8.

Kupperman M, Varner RE, Dummith RL, Learmen LA, Ireland C, Vittinghoff E, Stewart AL, Lin F, Richter HE, Showstack J, Hulley SB, Washington AE & Ms Research Group. Effects of hysterectomy vs medical treatment on health-related quality of life and sexual functioning: the medicine or surgery(Ms) randomised trial. JAMA 2004;291(12):1447-55.

Kuzel D, Bartosova L, Rezabek K, Toth D, Cindr J & Mara M. Successful pregnancy after thermal balloon endometrial ablation followed by in vitro fertilization and embryo transfer. Fertility and Sterility 2010; 93(3): 1006.

Laberge PY. Serious and deadly complications from pregnancy after endometrial ablation: two case reports and review of the literature. Journal of Gynecology, Obstetrics and Biology of Reproduction 2008;37(6):609-13.

Lähteenmaki P , Haukkamaa M, Puolakka J, Riikonen U, Sainio S, Suvisaari J & Nilsson CG, Open randomised study of use of levonorgestrel releasing intrauterine system as an alternative to hysterectomy. BMJ 1998;316:1122-1126.

Lethaby A, Sheppard S, Farquhar C & Cooke I. Endometrial resection and ablation versus hysterectomy for heavy menstrual bleeding. Cochrane Database of Systematic Reviews 1999, Issue 2. Art. No.: CD000329. DOI: 10.1002/14651858. CD000329.

Lethaby A, Farquhar & Inez Cooke. Antifibrinolytics for heavy menstrual bleeding. Cochrane Database of Systematic Reviews 2000, Issue 4. Art. No.: CD000249. DOI: 10.1002/14651858. CD000249.

Lethaby A, Cooke I & Rees MC. Progesterone or pregesteron-releasing intrauterine systems for heavy menstrual bleeding. Cochrane Database of Systematic Reviews 2005, Issue 4.Art. No.: CD002126.DOI: 10.1002/14651858.CD002126.pub2.

Lethaby A, Augood C, Duckitt K & Farquhar C. Nonsteroidal anti-inflammatory drugs for heavy menstrual bleeding. Cochrane Database of Systematic Reviews 2007, Issue 4.Art. No.: CD000400. DOI: 10.1002/14651858.CD000400.pub.2.

Lethaby A, Irviner GA & Cameron IT. Cyclic progestogens for heavy menstrual bleeding. Cochrane Database of Systematic Reviews 2008, Issue 1. Art. No.: CD001016. DOI: 10.1002/14651858.CD001016.pub2.

Lethaby A, Hickey M, Garry R & Penninx J. Endometrial resection/ablation techniques for heavy menstrual bleeding. Cochrane Database of Systematic Reviews 2009, Issue 4.Art.No.: CD001501. DOI: 10.1002/14651858.CD001501. pub3.

Li XF & Ahmed A. Expression of angiotensin II and its receptor subtypes in endometrial hyperplasia: a possible role in dysfunctional menstruation. Laboratory Investigation 1996;75:137-45.

Lin BL, Miyamoto N & Tomomatu M. The development of a new hysteroscopic resectoscope and its clinical applications on transcervical resection and endometrial ablation. Japanese Journal of Gynecological and Obstetrical Endoscopy 1988;4:6-9.

Lukes AS, Moore KA, Muse KN, Gersten JK, Hecht BR, Edlund M, Richter HE, Eder SE, Attia GR, Patrick DL, Rubin A &

Shangold GA. Tranexamic acid treatment for heavy menstrual, bleeding: a randomized controlled trial. Obstetrics and Gynecology 2010;116(4):865-75.

Makarainen L & Ylikorkala O. Primary and myoma-associated menorrhagia: role of prostaglandin and effects of ibuprofen. British Journal of Obstetrics and Gynaecology 1986;93:974-8.

Marjoribanks J, Lethaby A & Farquhar C. Surgery versus medical therapy for heavy menstrual bleeding. Cochrane Database of Systematic Reviews 2006, Issue 2. Art.No.: CD003855. DOI: 10.1002/14651858. Cd003855.pub2.

Milsom I. The levonorgestrel-releasing intrauterine system as an alternative to hysterectomy in peri-menopausal women. Contraception 2007;75(6 Suppl): S 152-4.

National Collaborating Centre for Women's and Children's Health. NICE clinical guideline 44. Heavy menstrual bleeding. London: RCOG Press, 2007.

National Health Committee. Guidelines for the management of heavy menstrual bleeding. New Zealand, 1998.

O'Flynn N & Britten N. Menorrhagia in general practice–disease or illness. Social Science and Medicine 2000;50(5):651-61.

Overton C, Hargreaves J & Maresh M. A national survey of the complications of endometrial destruction for menstrual disorders: the MISTLETOE study. British Journal of Obstetrics & Gynaecology 1997;104(12):1351-59.

Pendergrass PB, Scott JN & Ream LJ. A rapid, noninvasive method for evaluation of total menstrual loss. Gynecologic and Obstetric Investigation 1984;17(4):174-8.

Pitkin J. Dysfunctional uterine bleeding. BMJ 2007;334:1110-1

Pitroff R, Maija S & Murray A. Initial experience with transcervical cryoablation using saline as a uterine distension medium. Minimally Invasive Therapy 1993;2:69-73.

Reid PC, Coker A & Coltard R. Assessment of menstrual blood loss using a pictorial chart: a validation study. BJOG: an International Journal of Obstetrics and Gynaecology 2000;107(3):320-2.

Reid PC. Endometrial ablation in England- coming of age? An examination of hospital episode statistics 1989/1990 to 2004/2005. European Journal of Obstetrics and Gynecology 2007;135:191-4.

The Rotterdam ESHRE/ASRM-sponsored PCOS consensus workshop group. Revised 2003 consensus on diagnostic criteria and long-term health risks related to polycystic ovary syndrome (PCOS). Human Reproduction 2004; 19: 41–7

Royal College of Obstetrics and Gynaecologists. National evidence-based clinical guidelines. The initial management of menorrhagia. London: RCOG, 1998.

Rybo G. Tranexamic acid therapy effective treatment in heavy menstrual bleeding: Clinical update on safety. Therapeutic Advances 1991;4:1-8.

Salamonsen LA. Tissue injury and repair in the female human reproductive tract. Reproduction 2003;125:301-311.

Shangold GA. Tranexamic acid treatment for heavy menstrual bleeding: a randomized controlled trial. Obstetrics and Gynecology 2010;116(4):865-75.

Shankar M, Lee CA, Sabin CA., Evonomides DL & Kadir RA. Von Willebrand disease in women with menorrhagia: a systematic review. BJOG 2004;11:734-740.

Sharp NC, Cronin N, Feldberg I, Evans M, Hodgson D & Ellis S. Microwaves for menorrhagia: a new fast technique for endometrial ablation. Lancet 1995;346(8981):1003-4.

Shaw ST Jr, Aaronson DE & Moyer DL. Quantitation of menstrual blood loss-further evaluation of the alkaline hematin method. Contraception 1972;5(6):497-513.

Shaw RW. Assessment of medical treatments for menorrhagia. British Journal of Obstetrics and Gynaecology 1994;101(Suppl 11).

Silverberg SG, Haukkamaa M, Arko H, Nillson CG & Luukkainen T. Endometrial morphology during long-term use of levonorgestrel-releasing intrauterine devices. International Journal of Gynecologic Pathology 1986;5:235-41.

Singer A, Almanza R, Guiterrez A, Haber G, Bolduc L & Neuwirth R. Preliminary clinical experience with thermal balloon endometrial ablation method to treat menorrhagia. Obstetrics & Gynecology 1994;83:732-7.

Smith SK, Abel MH, Kelly RW & Baird DT. Prostaglandin synthesis in the endometrium of women with ovulatory dysfunctional uterine bleeding. British Journal of Obstetrics and Gynaecology 1981;88:434-442.

Smith SK, Abel MH, Kelly RW & Baird DT. The synthesis of prostaglandins from persistent proliferative endometrium. Journal of Clinical Endocrinology and Metabolism 1982;55:284-9.

Snowden R & Christian B. Patterns and Perceptions of Menstruation. A World Health Organization International Collaborative Study. London: Croon Helm;1983.

Sowter MC, Lethaby A & Singla AA. Pre-operative endometrial thinning agents before endometrial destruction for heavy menstrual bleeding. Cochrane Database of Systematic Reviews 2002, Issue 3. Art. No.: CD001124.DOI:10.1002/14651858.CD001124.

Speroff L & Fritz MA. (2005) Dysfunctional uterine bleeding, In: *Clinical Gynecologic Endocrinology and Infertility*, Speroff L, Fritz MA, pp. 547-573. Lippincott Williams & Wilkins, 0-7817-4795-3, Philadelphia.

Srinil S & Jaisamrarn U. Treatment of idiopathic menorrhagia with tranexamic acid. Journal of Medical Association of Thailand. 2005;88(Suppl 2):S1-6.

Vaincaillie TG. Electrocoagulation of the endometrium with the ball-ended resectoscope. Obstetrics and Gynecology 1989;74:425-7.

Van Eijkeren MA, Scholten PC, Christiaens GC, Alsbach GP & Haspels AA. The alkaline hematin method for measuring menstrual blood loss- a modification and its clinical use in menorrhagia. European Journal of Obstetrics, Gynecology, and Reproductive Biology 1986;22(5-6):345-51.

Vasilenko P, Kraicer PF, Kaplan R, deMasi A & Freed N. A new and simple method of menstrual blood loss. Journal of Reproductive Medicine 1988;33(3):293-7.

Vessey MP, Villard-Mackintosh L, McPherson K, Coulter A & Yeates D. The epidemiology of hysterectomy: findings in a large cohort study. British Journal of Obstetrics and Gynaecology 1992;99:402-7.

Vilos GA, Donnez J, Gannon MJ, Stampe-Sorensen S, Klinte I & Miller RM. Goserelin acetate as adjunctive therapy for endometrial ablation in women with dysfunctional uterine bleeding. The Journal of the American Assocation of Gynecologic Laparoscopy. 1996; 3(4, Suppl):S54-5.

Warner PE, Critchley HO, Lumsden MA, Campbell-Brown M, Douglas A & Murray GD. Menorrhagia II: Is the 80-ml blood loss criterion useful in management of complaint of menorrhagia? American Journal of Obstetrics and Gynecology 2004;190(5):1224-9.

Wellington K & Wagstaff AJ. Tranexamic acid: a review of its use in the management of menorrhagia. Drugs 2003;63(13): 1417-33.

Weston G & Rogers PA. Endometrial angiogenesis. Bailliere's Best Practice & Research: Clinical Obstetrics & Gynaecology 2000:14:919-36.

Willman EA, Collins WD & Clayton SC. Studies on the involvement of prostaglandins in uterine symptomatology and pathology. British Journal of Obstetrics and Gynaecology 1976;83:337-341.

Wyatt KM, Dimmock PW, Walker TJ & O'Brien PM. Determination of total menstrual blood loss. Fertility and Sterility 2001;76(1):125-31.

Yin CS. Pregnancy after hysteroscopic endometrial ablation without endometrial preparation: a report of five cases and a literature review. Taiwanese Journal of Obstetrics and Gynecology 2010;49(3):311-9.

Zakherah MS, Sayed GH, El-Nashar SA & Shaaban MM. Pictorial blood loss assessment chart in the evaluation of heavy menstrual bleeding: Diagnostic accuracy compared to alkaline hematin. Gynaecologic and Obstetric Investigation 2011 Jan 13 (Epub ahead of print).